Clinical Manual of Geriatric Psychopharmacology

Clinical Manual of Geriatric Psychopharmacology

Sandra A. Jacobson, M.D.

Assistant Professor, Department of Psychiatry and Human Behavior,
Brown Medical School, Providence, Rhode Island

Ronald W. Pies, M.D.

Clinical Professor of Psychiatry, Tufts University School of Medicine,
Boston, Massachusetts

Ira R. Katz, M.D.

Professor of Psychiatry and Director, Section of Geriatric Psychiatry,
University of Pennsylvania, Philadelphia, Pennsylvania

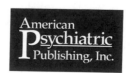

American
Psychiatric
Publishing, Inc.

Washington, DC
London, England

Note: The authors have worked to ensure that all information in this book is accurate at the time of publication and consistent with general psychiatric and medical standards, and that information concerning drug dosages, schedules, and routes of administration is accurate at the time of publication and consistent with standards set by the U.S. Food and Drug Administration and the general medical community. As medical research and practice continue to advance, however, therapeutic standards may change. Moreover, specific situations may require a specific therapeutic response not included in this book. For these reasons and because human and mechanical errors sometimes occur, we recommend that readers follow the advice of physicians directly involved in their care or the care of a member of their family.

Copyright © 2007 American Psychiatric Publishing, Inc.
ALL RIGHTS RESERVED
Manufactured in the United States of America on acid-free paper
11 10 09 08 07   5 4 3 2 1
First Edition
Typeset in Adobe's Formata and AGaramond.
American Psychiatric Publishing, Inc., 1000 Wilson Boulevard, Arlington, VA 22209-3901, www.appi.org

Library of Congress Cataloging-in-Publication Data
Jacobson, Sandra A., 1953–
    Clinical manual of geriatric psychopharmacology / by Sandra A. Jacobson, Ronald W. Pies, Ira R. Katz. — 1st ed.
        p. ; cm.
    Includes bibliographical references and index.
    ISBN 1-58562-252-4 (pbk. : alk. paper)
    1. Geriatric psychopharmacology—handbooks, manuals, etc.
    I. Pies, Ronald W., 1952– . II. Katz, Ira R. III. Title.
    [DNLM: 1. Psychotropic Drugs—pharmacokinetics. 2. Psychotropic drugs—therapeutic use. 3. Aged—psychology. 4. Aging—metabolism. 5. Mental Disorders—drug therapy. 6. Psychopharmacology— methods. QV 77.2 J17c 2007]
RC451.4.A5J334 2007
615'.78—dc22   2006025880

British Library Cataloguing in Publication Data
A CIP record is available from the British Library.

Contents

The Practice of Geriatric Psychopharmacology

Introduction

Few areas of current psychiatric practice present a challenge quite as daunting as that of geriatric psychopharmacology, which is complicated not only by the effects of normal aging but by medical disease and coadministered medications. Elderly patients often present with subclinical syndromes or symptoms that are modified by comorbid disease or partial treatment. Since the psychotropic regimen for an individual patient may be a composite of prescriptions from the hospital, clinic, and long-term-care facility, there may be duplicate medications (e.g., two antipsychotics), drug interactions may be significant, dosing may be inappropriate (e.g., inadequate dose of an antidepressant because of lack of titration), or dosing schedules for various medications may be out of synchrony. It is clearly in the interest of such patients to have an identified primary care provider—one who not only keeps the patient's medication regimen as trim as possible but oversees drug trials for specific indications and either titrates or discontinues medications as appropriate. Consultation with a clinician who has a good knowledge of geriatric psychopharmacology can be an invaluable component of care for the elderly patient.

For the psychiatric consultant, communication with the primary care physician is essential because the patient's detailed medical history has to be known and a physical examination must be documented before a psychotropic medication can be prescribed. Table 1–1 lists recommended routine screening procedures for this purpose (Thompson et al. 1983). The evaluation of cognitive function is important and should precede any effort to obtain informed consent for treatment, since substituted judgment may be required. Whenever possible, nonpharmacologic measures such as supportive/educative psychotherapy and environmental modification should be used and other somatic treatments, such as electroconvulsive therapy, should be considered so that polypharmacy is minimized.

Maximizing Therapeutic Effects

The three major determinants of effectiveness in pharmacotherapy include making a correct diagnosis, using a proven treatment, and persisting to ensure adequacy of the intervention. For all the reasons noted in the section above, the risk of misdiagnosis in geriatrics is higher than in the general population. Extra care has to be taken to obtain an accurate longitudinal history and to corroborate that history by speaking with family members or other caregivers. Furthermore, the patient's psychotropic-free baseline should be observed whenever possible and the patient should be detoxified from alcohol and other nonprescribed drugs.

Criteria such as those in DSM-IV-TR or ICD can be used to make specific diagnoses. In areas where these criteria may not be detailed enough for geriatrics (e.g., in specific etiologies of dementia), complete diagnostic criteria from original sources are included in the appropriate chapters throughout this book. For each medication trial, the first step is to identify and characterize target symptoms; whenever possible, objective ratings of pathology should be used, employing standardized scales with published normative data (Burns et al. 1999; Rush et al. 2000; Sajatovic and Ramirez 2003). For convenience, selected scales are reproduced throughout this volume. Although the practice of geriatric psychopharmacology has been limited in the past by a scant evidence base, this is now changing, and it is becoming easier to identify proven treatments for elderly patients. A survey of the Cochrane Database of Systematic Reviews (using the terms *elderly, geriatric, older, dementia,* or *Alzheimer's disease* and culling records pertinent to the discussions in the following chapters) revealed that of 21 com-

Table 1–1. Routine screening for psychotropic use in elderly patients

History

Is a medical illness causing the "psychiatric" symptoms?

Is a drug the patient is currently taking causing the psychiatric symptoms? This includes over-the-counter drugs and herbal preparations as well as prescribed medications. The patient/caregiver should be asked to bring current medication bottles to each visit.

Has the patient had these or other psychiatric symptoms in the past?

If so, what was the diagnosis and what medication, if any, was therapeutically effective? What side effects, if any, developed?

Physical examination

Is there evidence of neurologic, renal, hepatic, or other medical diseases that would further increase the elderly patient's risk for side effects?

Establish baseline function: pulse, blood pressure; orthostatic pulse and blood pressure.

Mental status

Is there a psychiatric illness of recent onset?

Is there evidence of dementia or delirium?

Laboratory studies

Is there evidence of decreased hepatic synthetic function (i.e., decreased serum albumin) or decreased renal function (i.e., decreased creatinine clearance)?

Is there evidence from a laboratory evaluation that a medical illness is causing the psychiatric symptoms?

Establish baseline labs: complete blood count with platelets, basic chemistries (glucose, blood urea nitrogen, creatinine, electrolytes including Ca^{++}), thyroid-stimulating hormone, cholesterol, triglycerides, and electrocardiogram.

Drug interactions

What adverse drug interactions might develop if the psychotropic drug were added to medications the patient is currently taking?

Source.   Adapted from Thompson TL, Moran MG, Nies AS: "Psychotropic Drug Use in the Elderly: Part 2." *New England Journal of Medicine* 308:194–199, 1983. Used with permission.

pleted reviews relevant to geriatric psychopharmacology, only 11 found sufficient data on which to base a recommendation. Six of those 11 reviews were published in 2006. Information needed to access these reviews is shown in Table 1–2.

Throughout this manual, available evidence of the efficacy of various drugs is presented to help guide treatment decisions. To best utilize this information, the reader should also be familiar with expert consensus guidelines and algorithms for sequencing and combining treatments for patients who do not respond adequately to an initial trial. In the absence of geriatric data, algorithms developed for mixed-age or nonelderly populations should be used. The specific choice of drug for an elderly patient is influenced by several factors, including comorbid medical or neurologic diagnoses, hypothesized neurotransmitter derangements, expected side-effect profile for that patient, and prior positive responses to drugs in the target class. Interactions with existing medications must also be considered.

The final determinant of effectiveness is adequacy of the drug trial. An *adequate trial* is defined as a trial in which a sufficient amount of drug is administered for a sufficient period of time. What constitutes *sufficient time* varies widely among drugs and classes: for both pharmacodynamic and pharmacokinetic reasons, sufficient time periods to observe responses in elderly patients are often much longer than those for younger patients. For a limited number of drugs in current use, *sufficient amount* can be confirmed by serum drug levels: in obtaining a drug level, optimal sampling time is the period just before a regular dose is administered (*trough level*), after the patient has achieved steady state at that dose.

The value of drug level monitoring for determining adequacy of a trial is limited when the "therapeutic range" is not established or when active metabolites are not assayed. Aside from confirming adequacy, however, drug levels are sometimes obtained to confirm suspected nonadherence (looking for a negligible detectable level) or toxicity (looking for a level that is one order of magnitude or more above the laboratory reference value). Theoretically, the level of any drug could be determined for these two purposes, with the number of drugs that could be tested being limited only by the laboratory's ingenuity in generating reference values for what constitutes a negligible amount and what constitutes a toxic level. When drug level is being considered as an explanation for clinical toxicity in a geriatric

Table 1–2. Cochrane Reviews: geriatric psychopharmacology

Evidence	Title	Authors	Year	Digital object identifier
S	Antidepressants for depressed elderly	Mottram P, Wilson K, Strobl J	2006	10.1002/14651858.CD003491.pub2
I	Antipsychotic medication for elderly people with schizophrenia	Marriott RG, Neil W, Waddingham S	2006	10.1002/14651858.CD005580
S	Cholinesterase inhibitors for Alzheimer's disease	Birks J	2006	10.1002/14651858.CD005593
S	Donepezil for dementia due to Alzheimer's disease	Birks J, Harvey RJ	2006	10.1002/14651858.CD001190.pub2
S	The effectiveness of atypical antipsychotics for the treatment of aggression and psychosis in Alzheimer's disease	Ballard C, Waite J	2006	10.1002/14651858.CD003476.pub2
S	Galantamine for Alzheimer's disease and mild cognitive impairment	Loy C, Schneider L	2006	10.1002/14651858.CD001747.pub3
S	Cholinesterase inhibitors for Parkinson's disease dementia	Maidment I, Fox C, Boustani M	2006	10.1002/14651858.CD004747.pub2
S	Memantine for dementia	McShane R, Areosa Sastre A, Minicaran N	2006	10.1002/14651858.CD003154.pub5

Table 1–2.   Cochrane Reviews: geriatric psychopharmacology *(continued)*

Evidence	Title	Authors	Year	Digital object identifier
I	Trazodone for agitation in dementia	Martinon-Torres G, Fioravanti M, Grimley Evans J	2004	10.1002/14651858.CD004990
I	Valproate preparations for agitation in dementia	Lonergan ET, Luxenberg J	2004	10.1002/14651858.CD003945.pub2
I	Cholinesterase inhibitors for dementia with Lewy bodies	Wild R, Pettit T, Burns A	2003	10.1002/14651858.CD003672
I	Antipsychotic drug treatment for elderly people with late-onset schizophrenia	Arunpongpaisal S, Ahmed I, Aqeel N, Paholpak S	2003	10.1002/14651858.CD004162
I	Electroconvulsive therapy for the depressed elderly	Van der Wurff FB, Stek ML, Hoogendijk WL, Beekman ATF	2003	10.1002/14651858.CD003593
I	Ibuprofen for Alzheimer's disease	Tabet N, Feldman H	2003	10.1002/14651858.CD004031
S	Selegiline for Alzheimer's disease	Birks J, Flicker L	2003	10.1002/14651858.CD000442
I	Folic acid with or without vitamin B_{12} for cognition and dementia	Malouf R, Grimley Evans J, Areosa Sastre A	2003	10.1002/14651858.CD004514

Table 1–2. Cochrane Reviews: geriatric psychopharmacology *(continued)*

Evidence	Title	Authors	Year	Digital object identifier
I	Antidepressants for treating depression in dementia	Bains J, Birks JS, Dening TD	2002	10.1002/14651858.CD003944
S	Haloperidol for agitation in dementia	Lonergan E, Luxenberg J, Colford J, Birks J	2002	10.1002/14651858.CD002852
S	Antidepressants versus placebo for the depressed elderly	Wilson K, Mottram P, Sivananthan A, Nightingale A	2001	10.1002/14651858.CD000561
I	Thioridazine for dementia	Kirchner V, Kelly CA, Harvey RJ	2001	10.1002/14651858.CD000464
S	Rivastigmine for Alzheimer's disease	Birks J, Grimley Evans J, Iakovidou V, Tsolaki M	2000	10.1002/14651858.CD001191

Note. I=insufficient evidence found for any recommendation to be made; S=sufficient evidence found for a recommendation to be made.
Source. The Cochrane Database of Systematic Reviews. Available at: http://www.update-software.com/publications/cochrane/. Accessed March 2006.

patient, however, it is worth remembering that in some cases, toxicity can occur even at apparently therapeutic blood levels. Serum drug levels do not always reflect the amount of the drug acting in the brain.

A basic rule in geriatric psychopharmacology is to do one thing at a time. This applies particularly to nonurgent situations; in these cases, monotherapy is used for as long as possible before changes or additions to treatment are made. In more urgent situations (i.e., the hospital admission of a delirious patient receiving multiple psychotropic medications, or treatment of depression with psychotic features), it is often true that several drugs are withheld or started simultaneously.

An initial treatment plan can provide needed ballast to help maintain the course of a treatment trial in spite of small setbacks that invariably occur. During the waiting period before a patient's response is seen, periodic determinations of partial response versus no response are made in order to decide whether the trial should be continued. For example, it would be generally unwise to maintain that a patient with major depression take sertraline for 12 weeks if no response at all were seen by 6 weeks at an adequate dose (e.g., 100–150 mg/day). If partial response were seen, the trial should be continued, since a small percentage of patients with limited early response to a selective serotonin reuptake inhibitor may still respond as late as 12 weeks into treatment.

For drugs prescribed to elderly patients on an as-needed basis (prn), clear guidelines regarding target symptoms must be provided, and administration of as-needed medications should be supervised or monitored by someone other than the patient in many cases. Prolonged daily administration of as-needed medications may signify insufficient standing doses of medication, a missed diagnosis, ineffective pharmacotherapy, or a combination of these factors. Thus, as-needed orders that have been executed daily for weeks or months should be regarded with some skepticism.

Improving Treatment Adherence

Medication nonadherence among community-dwelling adults that are 60 years of age and older is said to range from 26% to 59% (van Eijken et al. 2003). The risk of nonadherence increases with the number of prescribed medications, limitations on drug coverage under existing insurance plans (Piette et al. 2004), certain personality traits (Cohen et al. 2004), and higher levels of physical and cognitive disability (Corlett 1996; Ostrom et al. 1985). Cognitive functions influencing adherence include not only memory but also executive function and selective attention (Rosen et al. 2003).

It is not uncommon for elderly patients with chronic illnesses to self-limit prescribed medications because of cost (Tseng et al. 2004). Other factors contributing to nonadherence among elderly patients include lack of information about how to take medication, lack of understanding of the importance of medications in managing disease symptoms, irrational fears about side effects, and actual experience with side effects, particularly unexpected ones (Corlett 1996). Internet searches for answers to questions regarding medications may lead to biased information of poor quality, making it more difficult for the patient to maintain adherence. In general, consumers are poorly educated on how to find and interpret Internet-based medical information (Peterson et al. 2003). The following Internet sources can be recommended to patients for reliable and up-to-date information:

- www.healthfinder.gov
- www.mdadvice.com
- www.medicinenet.com
- www.medem.com

Patients should be advised to access one of these sites and then to search for the topic of interest. A general search (e.g., Google) for the topic of interest is more likely to bring up biased information or advertisements.

Research has shown that certain personality factors may affect adherence. In a nongeriatric sample, personality factors identified by the NEO Five-Factor Inventory—Revised that were associated with poor adherence with antidepressant medication included extraversion (especially elevation on the "activity" facet) and openness to experience (elevation on the "feelings" facet); in contrast, one personality factor identified as being associated with better adherence was agreeableness (elevation on the "modesty" facet) (Cohen et al. 2004).

Strategies identified as effective in improving treatment adherence include close collaboration between the doctor, patient, and caregiver (Morrow et al. 1996); education about prescribed drugs by the pharmacist, particularly before hospital discharge (Al-Rashed et al. 2002); simplification of the medication regimen; reduction of medication costs (Sharkey et al. 2005); certain memory aids, such as telephone reminders (van Eijken et al. 2003); medication boxes with marked compartments; and attention to medication packaging to take into account physical limitations, such as poor eyesight.

Simplification of the treatment plan has perhaps the greatest effect on adherence. For most nonactivating psychotropics, the best schedule is once-daily dosing at bedtime. For medications that have to be taken more often, actual times should be decided jointly by the patient, caregiver, and doctor and then written on the prescription. Varying schedules, such as every-other-day regimens, should be avoided as far as possible.

Available strategies to reduce out-of-pocket medication costs have been fairly limited in the past, although it is well established that cost prohibits adherence among a substantial number of elderly patients, even for the treatment of life-threatening chronic illnesses (Piette et al. 2004; Tseng et al. 2004). Most elders in the United States have no insurance covering prescription drugs. In an attempt to provide coverage for this vulnerable population, Medicare Part D was introduced, effective January 1, 2006. During the enrollment period, many elders were unsure about eligibility, bewildered at the array of plans available, and unclear about what to do with existing policies such as Medigap. It is too soon to tell with certainty whether Medicare Part D will be effective in reducing drug costs for those who elect to participate. It will be incumbent on prescribers to become familiar with the various Medicare Part D plans available and with which drugs are covered by each plan.

It will continue to be important for prescribers to be familiar with private drug plans for patients who retain their own insurance because their existing drug coverage is "creditable" (i.e., it is equal or superior to a standard Part D plan). For most private plans, copayments are required and most are higher for branded than for generic drugs. Copayments can of course be reduced by providing more doses per prescription (e.g., a 3-month rather than 1-month supply).

For patients who continue without insurance, the prescriber will need to know about the relative costs of drugs and about medication assistance and discount programs available through pharmacies and pharmaceutical companies. Drug costs vary widely among markets (e.g., United States vs. Canada), among suppliers (Internet vs. local pharmacy), and between branded and generic medications. Although it may be illegal for U.S. citizens to order prescription drugs from abroad, those who fill prescriptions for supplies of 90 days or less (i.e., for individual use) are not pursued for prosecution at present. This is a controversial issue at both the state and federal levels of government, with regulations and enforcement procedures currently under review.

Obtaining information about comparative drug costs from different sources (local pharmacies and Internet sources) is not straightforward. In general, Internet sites represent business interests and have little incentive to provide information other than for their own drugs or retail sites. The consumer is left to make price inquiries from each local and Internet pharmacy individually. It is of course still true that generic formulations cost much less than branded products, even when purchased locally. Generic formulations are generally acceptable substitutes for branded drugs, although idiosyncratic reactions or inefficacy is occasionally seen with generic drugs, even with supposedly bioequivalent formulations.

Effective communication between the doctor and the patient and the caregiver during each visit—and the fact that this communication goes both ways—cannot be overemphasized. It is usually a good idea for the patient or caregiver to repeat oral instructions to ensure that they are correctly understood. It is always a good idea for the doctor to give the patient time to voice concerns (i.e., about medication compatibility or side effects). Because questions often do arise after the visit, it is helpful to provide written information and instructions (Newell et al. 1999), remembering that visually impaired patients may require large-type instructions. Telephone reminder systems (usually computer-linked) have been identified as particularly effective in improving adherence (van Eijken et al. 2003). Other memory aids should be tailored to the individual patient's situation: pillboxes, calendar-style written medication schedules, and cuing devices such as a wristwatch or pillbox alarm to remind patients of medication times can be useful. Maintaining contact with the patient's caregiver also helps to increase adherence.

Physical incapacities are particularly important to note in elders who self-administer medications (Thwaites 1999). For those with disabling conditions such as arthritis, nonchildproof caps may be required. For those with visual deficits, large-print labels may be needed. For those who have trouble swallowing pills, liquid preparations or sprinkles can be considered.

Minimizing Adverse Effects and Drug Interactions

One tenet of prescribing for geriatric patients is that certain medications are best avoided in elderly patients. Since the early 1990s, Beers and colleagues have been cataloging medications and surveying colleagues using Delphi methods to determine the collective experience of elderly patients and their health care providers as to which medications should be avoided altogether in this population and which should be avoided in patients with particular medical conditions (Beers 1997; Beers et al. 1991; Fick et al. 2003). The Beers criteria are reproduced in Tables 1–3 and 1–4.

For pharmacokinetic and pharmacodynamic reasons noted above, effective doses of medications that are used for geriatric patients are often much lower than those for younger patients, on the order of one-third to one-half the "usual" dose. Keeping medication at the lowest effective dose is the single most important step in minimizing side effects for geriatric patients.

Another variable that can be manipulated to minimize adverse effects is that of between-dose fluctuation in drug level. A drug given at a dosage of 10 mg one time a day has a higher peak and lower trough level than the same drug given at a dosage of 5 mg two times a day, despite yielding the same average steady-state concentration. Since peak levels can be associated with symptoms of toxicity, dividing the dose often has the effect of reducing toxic effects. The trade-off in doing so is that the potential for nonadherence probably increases. Moreover, some side effects (e.g., sexual dysfunction) may not be related to peak blood levels.

As noted above, monodrug therapy is preferred to polydrug therapy to treat conditions responsive to one drug. Effective treatment for many

Table 1–3. Beers 2002 criteria for potentially inappropriate medication use in older adults: independent of diagnoses or conditions

Drug	Concern	Severity rating
Propoxyphene (Darvon) and combination products (Darvon with aspirin, Darvon-N, and Darvocet-N)	Offers few analgesic advantages over acetaminophen, yet has the adverse effects of other narcotic drugs.	Low
Indomethacin (Indocin and Indocin SR)	Of all available NSAIDs, this drug produces the most CNS adverse effects.	High
Pentazocine (Talwin)	Narcotic analgesic that causes more CNS adverse effects, including confusion and hallucinations, more commonly than other narcotic drugs. Additionally, it is a mixed agonist and antagonist.	High
Flurazepam (Dalmane)	This benzodiazepine hypnotic has an extremely long half-life in elderly patients (often days), producing prolonged sedation and increasing the incidence of falls and fractures. Short- or medium-acting benzodiazepines are preferable.	High
Doxepin (Sinequan)	Because of its strong anticholinergic and sedating properties, doxepin is rarely the antidepressant of choice for elderly patients.	High
Reserpine at doses >0.25 mg	May induce depression, impotence, sedation, and orthostatic hypotension.	Low

Table 1–3. Beers 2002 criteria for potentially inappropriate medication use in older adults: independent of diagnoses or conditions *(continued)*

Drug	Concern	Severity rating
Amitriptyline (Elavil), chlordiazepoxide-amitriptyline (Limbitrol), and perphenazine-amitriptyline (Triavil)	Because of its strong anticholinergic and sedative properties, amitriptyline is rarely the antidepressant of choice for elderly patients.	High
Muscle relaxants and antispasmodics: methocarbamol (Robaxin), carisoprodol (Soma), chlorzoxazone (Paraflex), metaxalone (Skelaxin), cyclobenzaprine (Flexeril), and oxybutynin (Ditropan). (Do not consider the extended-release Ditropan XL.)	Most muscle relaxants and antispasmodic drugs are poorly tolerated by elderly patients because they cause anticholinergic adverse effects, sedation, and weakness. Additionally, their effectiveness at doses tolerated by elderly patients is questionable.	High
Meprobamate (Miltown and Equanil)	This is a highly addictive and sedating anxiolytic. Those using meprobamate for prolonged periods may become addicted and may need to be withdrawn slowly.	High
Diphenhydramine (Benadryl)	May cause confusion and sedation. Should not be used as a hypnotic, and when used to treat emergency allergic reactions, it should be used in the smallest possible dose. Significant inhibitor of CYP2D6.	High

Table 1–3. Beers 2002 criteria for potentially inappropriate medication use in older adults: independent of diagnoses or conditions *(continued)*

Drug	Concern	Severity rating
Doses of short-acting benzodiazepines: doses >lorazepam (Ativan), 3 mg; oxazepam (Serax), 60 mg; alprazolam (Xanax), 2 mg; temazepam (Restoril), 15 mg; triazolam (Halcion), 0.25 mg	Because of increased sensitivity to benzodiazepines in elderly patients, smaller doses may be effective as well as safer. Total daily doses should not exceed the suggested maximums.	High
Long-acting benzodiazepines: chlordiazepoxide (Librium), chlordiazepoxide-amitriptyline (Limbitrol), clidinium-chlordiazepoxide (Librax), diazepam (Valium), clorazepate (Tranxene), quazepam (Doral), halazepam (Paxipam),	These drugs have a long half-life in elderly patients (often several days), producing prolonged sedation and increasing the risk of falls and fractures. Short- and intermediate-acting benzodiazepines are preferred if a benzodiazepine is required.	High
Ferrous sulfate >325 mg/day	Dosages > 325 mg/day do not dramatically increase the amount absorbed but greatly increase the incidence of constipation.	Low
Long-term use of stimulant laxatives: bisacodyl (Dulcolax), cascara sagrada except in the presence of opiate analgesic use.	May exacerbate bowel dysfunction.	High

Table 1–3. Beers 2002 criteria for potentially inappropriate medication use in older adults: independent of diagnoses or conditions *(continued)*

Drug	Concern	Severity rating
Long-term use of full-dosage, longer half-life, non-COX-selective NSAIDs: naproxen (Naprosyn, Anaprox and Aleve), oxaprozin (Daypro), and piroxicam (Feldene)	These drugs have the potential to produce GI bleeding, renal failure, high blood pressure, and heart failure.	High
Gastrointestinal antispasmodic drugs: dicyclomine (Bentyl), hyoscyamine (Levsin and Levsinex), propantheline (Pro-Banthine), belladonna alkaloids (Donnatal and others), and clidinium-chlordiazepoxide (Librax)	GI antispasmodic drugs are highly anticholinergic and have uncertain effectiveness. These drugs should be avoided (especially for long-term use).	High
Anticholinergics and antihistamines: chlorpheniramine (Chlor-Trimeton), diphenhydramine (Benadryl), hydroxyzine (Vistaril and Atarax), cyproheptadine (Periactin), promethazine (Phenergan), tripelennamine, dexchlorpheniramine (Polaramine)	All nonprescription and many prescription antihistamines may have potent anticholinergic properties. Nonanticholinergic antihistamines are preferred in elderly patients when treating allergic reactions.	High

Table 1–3. Beers 2002 criteria for potentially inappropriate medication use in older adults: independent of diagnoses or conditions (*continued*)

Drug	Concern	Severity rating
All barbiturates (except phenobarbital) except when used to control seizures	Are highly addictive and cause more adverse effects than most sedative or hypnotic drugs in elderly patients.	High
Meperidine (Demerol)	Not an effective oral analgesic in doses commonly used. May cause confusion and has many disadvantages compared with other narcotic drugs.	High
Ticlopidine (Ticlid)	Has been shown to be no better than aspirin in preventing clotting and may be considerably more toxic. Safer, more effective alternatives exist.	High
Ketorolac (Toradol)	Intermediate- and long-term use should be avoided in older persons because a significant number have asymptomatic GI pathologic conditions.	High
Amphetamines and anorectic agents	These drugs have potential for causing dependence, hypertension, angina, and myocardial infarction.	High
Daily fluoxetine (Prozac)	Long half-life of drug and risk of producing excessive CNS stimulation, sleep disturbance, and increased agitation. Safer alternatives exist.	High
Thioridazine (Mellaril)	Greater potential for CNS and extrapyramidal adverse effects. High potential for QTc prolongation on electrocardiogram.	High

Table 1–3. Beers 2002 criteria for potentially inappropriate medication use in older adults: independent of diagnoses or conditions *(continued)*

Drug	Concern	Severity rating
Mesoridazine (Serentil)	CNS and extrapyramidal adverse effects. High potential for QTc prolongation on electrocardiogram.	High
Clonidine (Catapres)	Potential for orthostatic hypotension and CNS adverse effects.	Low
Desiccated thyroid	Concerns about cardiac effects. Safer alternatives available.	High
Amphetamines (excluding methylphenidate hydrochloride and anorectics)	CNS stimulant effects.	High
Estrogens only (oral)	Evidence of the carcinogenic (breast and endometrial cancer) potential of these agents and lack of cardioprotective effect in older women.	Low

Note.   CNS=central nervous system; COX=cyclooxygenase; CYP=cytochrome P450; GI=gastrointestinal; NSAIDs=nonsteroidal anti-inflammatory drugs. Severity rating possibilities are "high" and "low."

Source.   Adapted from Fick DM, Cooper JW, Wade WE, et al: "Updating the Beers Criteria for Potentially Inappropriate Medication Use in Older Adults." *Archives of Internal Medicine* 163:2716–2724, 2003. Used with permission.

Table 1–4. Beers 2002 criteria for potentially inappropriate medication use in older adults: considering diagnoses or conditions

Disease or condition	Drug	Concern	Severity rating
Hypertension	Phenylpropanolamine hydrochloride (removed from market in 2001), pseudoephedrine, diet pills, and amphetamines	May produce elevation of blood pressure secondary to sympathomimetic activity.	High
Gastric or duodenal ulcers	NSAIDs and aspirin (>325 mg) (coxibs excluded)	May exacerbate existing ulcers or produce new/additional ulcers.	High
Seizures or epilepsy	Clozapine (Clozaril), chlorpromazine (Thorazine), thioridazine (Mellaril), and thiothixene (Navane)	May lower seizure threshold.	High
Blood clotting disorders or receiving anticoagulant therapy	Aspirin, NSAIDs, dipyridamole (Persantine), ticlopidine (Ticlid), and clopidogrel (Plavix)	May prolong clotting time and elevate INR values or inhibit platelet aggregation, resulting in an increased potential for bleeding.	High
Bladder outflow obstruction	Anticholinergics and antihistamines, gastrointestinal antispasmodics, muscle relaxants, oxybutynin (Ditropan), flavoxate (Urispas), antidepressants, decongestants, and tolterodine (Detrol)	May decrease urinary flow, leading to urinary retention.	High

Table 1–4.   Beers 2002 criteria for potentially inappropriate medication use in older adults: considering diagnoses or conditions *(continued)*

Disease or condition	Drug	Concern	Severity rating
Stress incontinence	α-Blockers (doxazosin, prazosin, and terazosin), anticholinergics, tricyclic antidepressants (imipramine, doxepin, amitriptyline), and long-acting benzodiazepines	May produce polyuria and worsening of incontinence.	High
Arrhythmias	Tricyclic antidepressants (imipramine, doxepin, and amitriptyline)	Concern due to proarrhythmic effects and ability to produce QT interval changes.	High
Insomnia	Decongestants, theophylline (Theo-Dur), methylphenidate (Ritalin), MAOIs, and amphetamines	Concern due to CNS stimulant effects.	High
Parkinson's disease	Metoclopramide (Reglan), conventional antipsychotics, and tacrine (Cognex)	Concern due to their antidopaminergic/cholinergic effects.	High
Cognitive impairment	Barbiturates, anticholinergics, antispasmodics, muscle relaxants, and CNS stimulants (dextroamphetamine, methylphenidate, methamphetamine, and pemoline)	Concern due to CNS-altering effects.	High

Table 1–4. Beers 2002 criteria for potentially inappropriate medication use in older adults: considering diagnoses or conditions *(continued)*

Disease or condition	Drug	Concern	Severity rating
Depression	Long-term benzodiazepine use. Sympatholytic agents (methyldopa [Aldomet], reserpine, and guanethidine [Ismelin])	May produce or exacerbate depression.	High
Anorexia and malnutrition	CNS stimulants (dextroamphetamine, methylphenidate, methamphetamine, pemoline, and fluoxetine)	Concern due to appetite-suppressing effects.	High
Syncope or falls	Short- to intermediate-acting benzodiazepines and tricyclic antidepressants (imipramine, doxepin, and amitriptyline)	May produce ataxia, impaired psychomotor function, syncope, and additional falls.	High
SIADH/ Hyponatremia	SSRIs (fluoxetine [Prozac], citalopram [Celexa], fluvoxamine [Luvox], paroxetine [Paxil], and sertraline [Zoloft])	May exacerbate or cause SIADH.	Low
Seizure disorder	Bupropion (Wellbutrin)	May lower seizure threshold.	High
Obesity	Olanzapine (Zyprexa)	May stimulate appetite and increase weight gain.	Low

Table 1–4.   Beers 2002 criteria for potentially inappropriate medication use in older adults: considering diagnoses or conditions *(continued)*

Disease or condition	Drug	Concern	Severity rating
Chronic obstructive pulmonary disease	Long-acting benzodiazepines (chlordiazepoxide [Librium], chlordiazepoxide-amitriptyline [Limbitrol], clidinium-chlordiazepoxide [Librax], diazepam [Valium], quazepam [Doral], halazepam [Paxipam], and clorazepate [Tranxene]), and β-blockers (propranolol)	CNS adverse effects. May induce respiratory depression. May exacerbate or cause respiratory depression.	High
Chronic constipation	Calcium channel blockers, anticholinergics, and tricyclic antidepressants (imipramine, doxepin, and amitriptyline)	May exacerbate constipation.	Low

Note.   CNS=central nervous system; INR=international normalized ratio; MAOI=monoamine oxidase inhibitor; NSAIDs=nonsteroidal anti-inflammatory drugs; SIADH=syndrome of inappropriate antidiuretic hormone; SSRI=selective serotonin reuptake inhibitor. Severity rating possibilities are "high" and "low."

Source.   Adapted from Fick DM, Cooper JW, Wade WE, et al: "Updating the Beers Criteria for Potentially Inappropriate Medication Use in Older Adults." *Archives of Internal Medicine* 163:2716–2724, 2003. Used with permission.

Table 1–5. Summary guidelines: the practice of geriatric psychopharmacology

- Clarify diagnosis.
- Obtain a psychotropic-free baseline, if possible.
- Identify target symptoms.
- Use objective ratings of effect.
- Use doses and titration schedules recommended for geriatrics.
- Make only one medication change at a time, if possible.
- Use monotherapy as far as possible.
- Consider drug cost and affordability.
- Simplify instructions to the patient.
- Give instructions in writing.
- Use pillboxes and other adherence aids.
- Monitor patient closely for changes in vital signs, bowel/bladder function, vision, and so on, or for development of abnormal limb or mouth movements.
- Ask explicitly about relevant side effects.
- At regular intervals, reassess need for drug.
- Obtain drug levels when indicated.
- Document adequacy of all drug trials.

geriatric patients, however, requires informed polypharmacy. For this reason, it is essential that the geriatric psychopharmacologist become knowledgeable about drug interactions in addition to adverse drug effects. Interacting drugs should be avoided if possible; if such drugs must be coprescribed, they should be administered as far apart in time as feasible. For medications with particularly dangerous potential interactions, such as monoamine oxidase inhibitors, it is recommended that patients wear identification bracelets and/or carry cards warning against the dangers of administering drugs such as meperidine (Demerol) or pressor amines (Jenike 1989).

It is often true that bad outcomes with medication can be minimized if developing side effects are detected early. For this reason, it is critically important that patients and their families and caregivers be fully educated about the signs of potentially serious reactions as well as expectable nuisance side effects. In addition, in this population, there should be a low threshold for obtaining tests such as electrocardiograms to monitor cardiac side effects. Table 1–5 provides a set of basic guidelines for the practice of geriatric psychopharmacology.

Chapter Summary

- Medications are administered to elderly patients in smaller initial doses, with smaller dosing increments, and on a more slowly titrating schedule than for younger patients.
- Sufficient time periods required to observe responses in elderly patients are often much longer than those for younger patients.
- When considering drug level as an explanation for clinical toxicity in a geriatric patient, it is worth remembering that in some cases, these patients can become toxic even at apparently therapeutic levels.
- Although many strategies are effective in improving adherence, simplifications of the treatment plan and minimizing drug costs have the greatest effect.

References

Beers MH: Explicit criteria for determining potentially inappropriate medication use by the elderly. Arch Intern Med 157:1531–1536, 1997

Beers MH, Ouslander JG, Rollingher I, et al: Explicit criteria for determining inappropriate medication use in nursing home residents. Arch Intern Med 151:1825–1832, 1991

Burns A, Lawlor B, Craig S: Assessment Scales in Old Age Psychiatry. London, Martin Dunitz Ltd, 1999

Cohen NL, Ross EC, Bagby RM, et al: The 5-factor model of personality and antidepressant medication compliance. Can J Psychiatry 49:106–113, 2004

Corlett AJ: Aids to compliance with medication. BMJ 313:926–929, 1996

Fick DM, Cooper JW, Wade WE, et al: Updating the Beers criteria for potentially inappropriate medication use in older adults. Arch Intern Med 163:2716–2724, 2003

Jenike MA: Geriatric Psychiatry and Psychopharmacology: A Clinical Approach. Chicago, IL, Year Book Medical Publishers, 1989

Morrow DG, Leirer VO, Andrassy JM, et al: Medication instruction design: younger and older adult schemas for taking medication. Hum Factors 38:556–573, 1996

Newell SA, Bowman JA, Cockburn JD: A critical review of interventions to increase compliance with medication-taking, obtaining medication refills, and appointment-keeping in the treatment of cardiovascular disease. Prev Med 29:535–548, 1999

Ostrom JR, Hammarlund ER, Christensen DB, et al: Medication usage in an elderly population. Med Care 23:157–164, 1985

Peterson G, Aslani P, Williams KA: How do consumers search for and appraise information on medicines on the Internet? a qualitative study using focus groups. J Med Internet Res 5:e33, 2003

Piette JD, Heisler M, Wagner TH: Cost-related medication underuse among chronically ill adults: the treatments people forgo, how often, and who is at risk. Am J Public Health 94:1782–1787, 2004

Al-Rashed SA, Wright DJ, Roebuck N, et al: The value of inpatient pharmaceutical counselling to elderly patients prior to discharge. Br J Clin Pharmacol 54:657–664, 2002

Rosen MI, Beauvais JE, Rigsby MO, et al: Neuropsychological correlates of suboptimal adherence to metformin. J Behav Med 26:349–360, 2003

Rush AJ, Pincus HA, First MB, et al: Handbook of Psychiatric Measures. Washington, DC, American Psychiatric Association, 2000

Sajatovic M, Ramirez LF: Rating Scales in Mental Health, 2nd Edition. Hudson, OH, Lexi-Comp Inc, 2003

Sharkey JR, Ory MG, Browne BA: Determinants of self-management strategies to reduce out-of-pocket prescription medication expense in homebound older people. J Am Geriatr Soc 53:666–674, 2005

Thompson TL, Moran MG, Nies AS: Psychotropic drug use in the elderly: part 2. N Engl J Med 308:194–199, 1983

Thwaites JH: Practical aspects of drug treatment in elderly patients with mobility problems. Drugs Aging 14:105–114, 1999

Tseng CW, Brook RH, Keeler E, et al: Cost-lowering strategies used by Medicare beneficiaries who exceed drug benefit caps and have a gap in drug coverage. JAMA 292:952–960, 2004

van Eijken M, Tsang S, Wensing M, et al: Interventions to improve medication compliance in older patients living in the community. Drugs Aging 20:229–240, 2003

2

Basic Psychopharmacology
and Aging

Introduction

Aging is associated with changes in the function of various organ systems and receptors. The variability of these changes among individuals contributes significantly to the observed heterogeneity in pharmacologic response in the geriatric population. Further heterogeneity is introduced by genetic determinants of drug response because genes encoding drug-metabolizing enzymes, drug transporters, and drug targets also show variability. In general, this genetic endowment remains stable into old age. Thus, genetic heterogeneity with regard to pharmacologic response is amplified by aging effects.

New research in pharmacokinetics has taken us beyond phase I processes of oxidative metabolism. More is now known about the P-glycoprotein pump, the "gatekeeper" that influences not only what gets into the general circulation from the gut but also what gains access to the brain and what is excreted. In addition, more is known about phase II processes, particularly glucuronidation. It turns out that not all glucuronidated drugs are inactive: some have pharmacologic effects, which are at times more potent than those of their parent compounds (Liston et al. 2001). Furthermore, inactive glucuronides are not always rapidly excreted and may accumulate during long-term therapy. It has been speculated that these metabolites might serve as a storage depot from which active parent drugs can be recruited through deconjugation (de Leon 2003).

27

The practice of psychopharmacology is not only more complex but also more interesting than it was a few short years ago. One thing that is becoming clear is that it is no longer possible to practice psychopharmacology without at least a basic understanding of related genetic topics. We will soon enter a more sophisticated era of prescribing, one in which it will be possible to predict drug efficacy, dosing, adverse effects, and interactions using genotyping of known and to-be-discovered polymorphisms.

Pharmacokinetics and Aging

Pharmacokinetics involves the way a drug moves through the body and includes processes of absorption, distribution, metabolism, and elimination (clearance). Figure 2–1 shows the disposition of a drug administered by various routes, from ingestion to elimination.

Absorption

A psychotropic drug taken orally passes from the stomach to the proximal small intestine, where most absorption takes place. This was once considered a passive process, but it is now known that cells lining the gut (enterocytes) express not only the drug-metabolizing enzyme cytochrome P450 (CYP) 3A4 but also P-glycoprotein (Fromm 2004). The P-glycoprotein pump ("P" for "permeability") acts as an efflux pump to get the absorbed drug back into the lumen of the gut, as shown in Figure 2–2. Because P-glycoprotein is often found in proximity to CYP3A4 enzymes, the drug has yet another chance to be metabolized after efflux rather than reabsorbed into the system. By this mechanism, P-glycoprotein as the gatekeeper at the level of the gut wall is an important determinant of how much drug gets into the system (i.e., the drug's bioavailability) (Kivisto et al. 2004). The effects of aging on P-glycoprotein activity are not yet known.

As shown in Table 2–1, P-glycoprotein acts on particular substrates, both endogenous (steroids, cytokines) and exogenous (drugs), and has identified inhibitors and inducers, just as do CYP450 isoenzymes. Also like the P450 system, P-glycoprotein inhibitors are associated with increased substrate concentrations, whereas inducers are associated with decreased

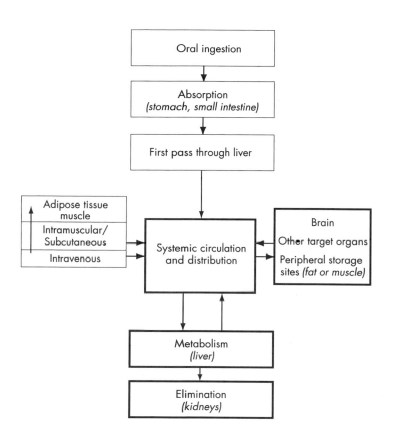

Figure 2–1.   Drug disposition: absorption, distribution, metabolism, and elimination.

Note.   Heavy-ruled boxes indicate processes most affected by aging.

substrate concentrations. Inhibitors have the effect of increasing concentrations of substrate drugs because of reduced efflux action, whereas inducers have the effect of decreasing concentrations of substrate drugs because of increased efflux action. One notable inducer is St. John's wort. This herbal preparation is actually known as a double inducer because of its capacity to induce not only P-glycoprotein but also CYP3A4. Double inhib-

Table 2–1.   Selected P-glycoprotein substrates, inhibitors, and inducers

Substrates	Inhibitors	Inducers
aldosterone	amiodarone	dexamethasone
amitriptyline	amitriptyline	doxorubicin
amoxicillin	atorvastatin	?nefazodone (chronic)
amprenavir	bromocriptine	phenobarbital
carbamazepine	chloroquine	prazosin
chloroquine	chlorpromazine	rifampin
cimetidine	clarithromycin	ritonavir (chronic)
ciprofloxacin	cyclosporine	St. John's wort
colchicine	cyproheptadine	trazodone
corticosteroids	desipramine	?venlafaxine
cyclosporine	diltiazem	
digitoxin	erythromycin	
digoxin	felodipine	
diltiazem	fentanyl	
docetaxel	fluphenazine	
L-dopa	garlic	
doxorubicin	grapefruit juice	
enoxacin	green tea (catechins)	
loperamide	midazolam	
losartan	nefazodone (acute)	
lovastatin	nelfinavir	
mibefradil	ofloxacin	
morphine	omeprazole	
nelfinavir	orange juice (Seville)	
nortriptyline	pantoprazole	
ondansetron	phenothiazines	
phenytoin	pimozide	
quetiapine	piperine	
quinidine	probenecid	
ranitidine	progesterone	
rifampin	propafenone	
ritonavir	propranolol	
saquinavir	quinidine	
tacrolimus	ritonavir (initial)	
talinolol	saquinavir	
teniposide	simvastatin	

Table 2–1.   Selected P-glycoprotein substrates, inhibitors, and inducers *(continued)*

Substrates		Inhibitors		Inducers
erythromycin	terfenadine	haloperidol	spironolactone	
estradiol	vinblastine	hydrocortisone	tamoxifen	
fexofenadine	vincristine	hydroxyzine	terfenadine	
grepafloxacin		imipramine	testosterone	
indinavir		itraconazole	trifluoperazine	
irinotecan		ketoconazole	valspodar	
lansoprazole		lansoprazole	verapamil	
		lidocaine	vinblastine	
		lovastatin	vitamin E	
		maprotiline		
		methadone		
		mibefradil		

Source.   Adapted from Cozza et al. 2003. Used with permission.

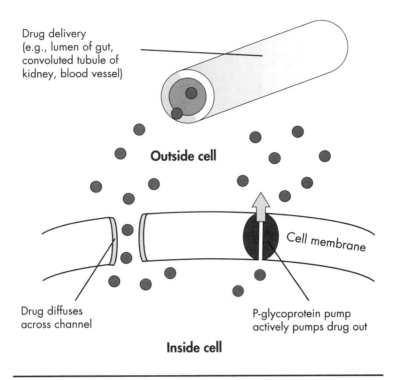

Figure 2–2. The P-glycoprotein pump.

itors include erythromycin and ketoconazole. Dietary inhibitors include black pepper, grapefruit juice, and Seville oranges (Cozza et al. 2003).

The rate of absorption partly determines how quickly an oral drug takes effect—that is, its onset of action. Among elderly individuals, the rate can be slowed by reduced gastric motility or delayed emptying, but in the absence of overt disease, the extent of absorption is relatively unaffected (Greenblatt et al. 1982b). Consumption of antacids or cathartics containing aluminum, magnesium, or calcium may delay absorption, as may fiber supplements (von Moltke et al. 2005).

Parenteral administration of drugs (intramuscular or intravenous) usually results in a faster onset of action because it circumvents gastrointestinal absorption and first-pass effects. This can be useful clinically, for example, in sedation of the dangerously agitated patient. It can also mean that side effects such as hypotension come on more quickly and so can pose a hazard to those unprepared for immediate parenteral effects.

Distribution

From the small intestine, the drug passes through the portal circulation to the liver, as shown in Figure 2–1. A portion of the drug is passed on through the liver to the systemic circulation. For some psychotropics, a much larger portion is metabolized in the liver (and gut wall) before it enters the circulation, a process known as *first-pass metabolism*. It is now understood that P-glycoprotein activity in the liver is an important determinant of the extent of this first-pass effect (Fromm 2004). Metabolites leaving the liver then enter the systemic circulation, and those that have been transformed into water-soluble compounds (*conjugated*) may be excreted directly by the kidneys.

Pharmacokinetic processes up to this point in Figure 2–1 (*systemic circulation*) are circumvented by parenteral drug administration (intramuscular or intravenous). Because first-pass metabolism is avoided, bioavailability of parenteral drugs is nearly 100%, and the intramuscular or intravenous dose required is usually smaller than the oral dose. However, it is important to note that the relatively small muscle mass of the average elderly patient makes intramuscular dosing very painful and renders absorption erratic. For these reasons, the intramuscular route of drug administration is the least desirable for geriatric patients.

Drugs in the systemic circulation are distributed to target organs (such as the brain) and then to the liver, to the kidneys, or to peripheral storage sites, such as fat or muscle. Distribution to these peripheral sites is significantly influenced by age because fat stores show a relative increase and lean body mass a relative decrease with aging. These changes in the aging individual result in an increasing volume of distribution for lipophilic (fat-soluble) drugs, including almost all psychotropics (Thompson et al. 1983a). Since drug half-life is directly related to volume of distribution, this change has important effects on drug prescribing, as detailed below in the "Drug Half-Life" section (Greenblatt et al. 1986). For lithium and other hydrophilic (water-soluble) drugs, the volume of distribution decreases with aging, so more of the drug is present in the systemic circulation and proportionately more drug reaches the brain. This is one reason that smaller doses of lithium are required as patients age (although the major reason relates to reduced renal clearance, as noted in the "Clearance" section later in this chapter).

The relatively larger volume of distribution for lipophilic drugs in the aging population has another consequence: a highly lipophilic drug, such as diazepam, entering the systemic circulation is rapidly taken up by adipose tissue, such that its concentration in plasma falls more quickly below the minimum effective threshold (von Moltke et al. 1995). The duration of effect with initial dosing is therefore brief. The drug is removed slowly from adipose stores, so that with repeated dosing, there is the potential for considerable accumulation (von Moltke et al. 1995).

Other properties determining a drug's distribution include its affinity for different tissues and the extent of its plasma protein binding (von Moltke et al. 1995). As Figure 2–1 suggests, the various sites of distribution are actually in competition with the brain for the drug. The greater the uptake in peripheral sites (such as larger adipose stores taking up more lipophilic drug), the less drug there is in the systemic circulation and the less drug there is available to brain receptors. In fact, only a small proportion of most administered drugs ever reaches these target receptors (von Moltke et al. 1995).

At the blood-brain barrier, drugs may gain entry to the central nervous system by passive diffusion or other means. Drugs that are substrates for the P-glycoprotein pump, located in capillary endothelial cells, may be returned to the general circulation by the efflux action of the pump (Fromm 2004). Psychotropic medications listed as substrates for the P-glycoprotein pump (Table 2–1) include carbamazepine, amitriptyline, nortriptyline, and quetiapine. The extent to which the pump's action can be inhibited by drugs listed as inhibitors (Table 2–1) is an area of current research. When the pump is inhibited, however, not only substrate drugs but also neurotoxins can be present in the brain at higher-than-usual concentrations (Fromm 2004).

Metabolism

Drug metabolism involves two phases: phase I (oxidation) and phase II (most importantly, glucuronidation). However, drugs undergoing metabolism do not necessarily proceed through both phases or proceed through them in order. That is, although some drugs are in fact oxidized and then glucuronidated, others are glucuronidated and then oxidized. Still others are either oxidized or glucuronidated, or undergo both processes simultaneously. The principal drug-metabolizing enzymes include cytochrome P450, also known as CYP (phase I), and uridine 5'-diphosphate glucuronosyltransferase, also known as UGT (phase II). These enzymes exist as gene superfamilies, with individual proteins (isoenzymes) differing in substrate and inhibitor specificities (Miners et al. 2003). Both CYP and UGT enzymes are found in tissues throughout the body, but their most important actions occur in the liver.

Phase I oxidation reactions of several CYP450 enzymes involved in the metabolism of psychotropic drugs are significantly affected by aging (Greenblatt et al. 1986). In contrast, phase II processes of conjugation (also known as glucuronidation), acetylation, and methylation are unaffected by normal aging (Greenblatt et al. 1986; Hammerlein et al. 1998), although they may be affected by other factors as noted below. Medications metabolized primarily through conjugation may thus be preferred in the elderly population.

Aging is associated with decreased hepatic blood flow and reduced hepatic metabolism of many medications (Thompson et al. 1983b). For example, demethylation reactions converting tertiary amines to secondary amines, such as amitriptyline to nortriptyline, are less efficient in elderly patients, which may be associated with accumulation of more active tertiary compounds.

Phase I Metabolism: Oxidation via the Cytochrome P450 System

Three CYP450 families are of particular interest in human psychopharmacology: CYP1, CYP2, and CYP3 (Nemeroff et al. 1996). As shown in Table 2–2, each CYP enzyme has specific substrate drugs, enzyme inhibitors, and enzyme inducers (Cozza et al. 2003; Richelson 1997). Some drugs (e.g., carbamazepine) appear on more than one list, as substrates for or inhibitors or inducers of one or more enzymes. For most drugs, substrates are oxidatively metabolized by CYP enzymes to inactive or less active metabolites. In the presence of enzyme inducers, the oxidation reaction is facilitated, and the active parent compound is metabolized more rapidly. In the presence of enzyme inhibitors, the proportion of active parent compound stays high relative to that of inactive metabolite. The degree of enzyme inhibition may be additive when more than one inhibitor is administered.

Genetic differences (polymorphisms) expressed as the presence or activity of certain CYP enzymes account for much of the observed variability among individuals in serum levels of certain psychotropic drugs seen with the same administered dose. *Poor metabolizers* (also called *slow metabolizers*), having low or no activity of an enzyme, could be expected to have difficulty metabolizing and excreting substrates for that enzyme, resulting in high levels of active drug. For example, poor metabolizers of risperidone were noted to have a high incidence of adverse drug reactions and drug discontinuation (de Leon et al. 2005). *Average metabolizers* are considered normal (although in the older literature, they may have been called *extensive* or *rapid metabolizers*) (Cozza et al. 2003). An average metabolizer could be converted to a poor metabolizer by sufficient P450 inhibition. *Ultraextensive metabolizers* (formerly called *ultrarapid metabolizers*) may need more administered drug than usual because of the speed at and extent to which they metabolize. When a prodrug such as codeine is given to an ultraextensive metabolizer, toxicity can result, even from a small dose (Gasche et al. 2004). The ultraextensive metabolizer polymorphism is uncommon; it is seen in an estimated 1%–3% of the population (Cozza et al. 2003). Ethnic differences in prevalence of the poor metabolizer phenotype have also been seen (Nemeroff et al. 1996; Richelson 1997). As of this writing, laboratory methods exist to identify poor metabolizers at CYP2D6 and CYP2C19 by genotyping. It is expected that these tests soon will become available for clinical use.

CYP1A2. This isoenzyme is of interest to psychiatrists because it is induced by smoking and modafinil, inhibited by fluvoxamine, and includes caffeine, clozapine, and cyclobenzaprine among its substrates (see Table 2–2.) Approximately 12% of Caucasians, African Americans, and Asians are poor metabolizers at CYP1A2 (Richelson 1997). CYP1A2 activity declines with aging and is significantly inhibited by commonly used medications such as fluvoxamine and ciprofloxacin (Cozza et al. 2003; Ereshefsky et al. 1996). Starting or stopping smoking may be par-

Table 2–2. Drugs metabolized by known CYP450 isoenzymes

Substrates

1A2	2B6	2C8	2C19	2C9	2D6	2E1	3A4,5,7
amitriptyline	bupropion	paclitaxel	amitriptyline	amitriptyline	alprenolol	acetaminophen	alfentanil
caffeine	cyclophos-phamide	torsemide	carisoprodol	celecoxib	amitriptyline	aniline	alprazolam
clomipramine	efavirenz	amodiaquine	citalopram	diclofenac	amphetamine	benzene	amlodipine
clozapine	ifosfamide	cerivastatin	clomipramine	fluoxetine	aripiprazole	chlorzoxazone	aripiprazole
cyclobenzaprine	methadone	repaglinide	cyclophosphamide	fluvastatin	atomoxetine	enflurane	atorvastatin
estradiol			diazepam	glimepiride	bufuralol	ethanol	buspirone
fluvoxamine			hexobarbital	glipizide	carvedilol	formamide	Cafergot
haloperidol			imipramine	glyburide	chlorpheniramine	(N,N-dimethyl)	caffeine
imipramine			indomethacin	ibuprofen	chlorpromazine	halothane	cerivastatin
mexiletine			lansoprazole	irbesartan	clomipramine	isoflurane	chlorphenir-amine
naproxen			mephenytoin (S)	losartan	codeine	methoxyflurane	cilostazol
olanzapine			mephobarbital (R)	meloxicam (S)	debrisoquine	sevoflurane	clarithromycin
ondansetron			moclobemide	naproxen	desipramine	theophylline	cocaine
phenacetin			nelfinavir	nateglinide	dextromethor-phan		codeine
propranolol			nilutamide	phenytoin	duloxetine		cyclosporine
riluzole			omeprazole	piroxicam	encainide		dapsone
ramelteon			pantoprazole	rosiglitazone			

Table 2–2.   Drugs metabolized by known CYP450 isoenzymes *(continued)*

Substrates *(continued)*

1A2	2B6	2C8	2C19	2C9	2D6	2E1	3A4,5,7
ropivacaine			phenobarbitone	sulfamethoxazole	flecainide		dextromethorphan
tacrine			phenytoin	suprofen	fluoxetine		diazepam
theophylline			primidone	tamoxifen	fluvoxamine		diltiazem
tizanidine			progesterone	tolbutamide	haloperidol		docetaxel
verapamil			proguanil	torsemide	imipramine		domperidone
warfarin (R)			propranolol	warfarin (S)	lidocaine		eplerenone
zileuton			rabeprazole		metoclopramide		erythromycin
zolmitriptan			teniposide		metoprolol (S)		estradiol
			warfarin (R)		mexiletine		eszopiclone
					minaprine		felodipine
					nebivolol		fentanyl
					nortriptyline		finasteride
					ondansetron		haloperidol
					paroxetine		hydrocortisone
					perhexiline		imatinib mesylate
							indinavir

Table 2–2. Drugs metabolized by known CYP450 isoenzymes *(continued)*

Substrates *(continued)*

1A2	2B6	2C8	2C19	2C9	2D6	2E1	3A4,5,7
					perphenazine		irinotecan
					phenacetin		LAAM
					phenformin		lercanidipine
					propafenone		lidocaine
					propranolol		lovastatin
					risperidone		methadone
					sparteine		midazolam
					tamoxifen		nateglinide
					thioridazine		nelfinavir
					timolol		nifedipine
					tramadol		nisoldipine
					venlafaxine		nitrendipine
							ondansetron
							paclitaxel
							pimozide
							progesterone
							propranolol
							quinidine

Table 2–2. Drugs metabolized by known CYP450 isoenzymes *(continued)*

Substrates *(continued)*

1A2	2B6	2C8	2C19	2C9	2D6	2E1	3A4,5,7
							quinine
							ritonavir
							salmeterol
							saquinavir
							sildenafil
							simvastatin
							sirolimus
							tacrolimus
							tamoxifen
							telithromycin
							terfenadine
							testosterone
							trazodone
							triazolam
							verapamil
							vincristine
							zaleplon
							zolpidem

Table 2–2. Drugs metabolized by known CYP450 isoenzymes (*continued*)

Inhibitors

1A2	2B6	2C8	2C19	2C9	2D6	2E1	3A4,5,7
amiodarone	thiopeta	gemfibrozil	chloramphenicol	amiodarone	amiodarone	diethyldithio-carbamate	amiodarone
cimetidine	ticlopidine	glitazones	cimetidine	fluconazole	bupropion	disulfiram	aprepitant
fluoroquinolones		montelukast	felbamate	fluvastatin	celecoxib		chloram-phenicol
fluvoxamine		quercetin	fluoxetine	fluvoxamine	chlorpheniramine		cimetidine
furafylline		trimethoprim	fluvoxamine	isoniazid	chlorpromazine		ciprofloxacin
interferon			indomethacin	lovastatin	cimetidine		clarithromycin
methoxsalen			ketoconazole	phenylbuta-zone	citalopram		delavirdine
mibefradil			lansoprazole	probenecid	clemastine		diethyldithio-carbamate
ticlopidine			modafinil	ritonavir	clomipramine		diltiazem
			omeprazole	sertraline	cocaine		efavirenz
			oxcarbazepine	sulfamethox-azole	diphenhydramine		erythromycin
			probenecid	sulfaphenazole	doxepin		fluconazole
			ticlopidine	teniposide	doxorubicin		fluvoxamine
			topiramate	trimethoprim	duloxetine		gestodene
				zafirlukast	escitalopram		grapefruit juice
					fluoxetine		
					halofantrine		

Table 2–2. Drugs metabolized by known CYP450 isoenzymes *(continued)*

Inhibitors *(continued)*

1A2	2B6	2C8	2C19	2C9	2D6	2E1	3A4,5,7
					haloperidol (red)		indinavir
					H$_1$ receptor antagonists		itraconazole
					hydroxyzine		ketoconazole
					levomepromazine		mibefradil
					methadone		mifepristone
					metoclopramide		nefazodone
					mibefradil		nelfinavir
					moclobemide		norfloxacin
					paroxetine		norfluoxetine
					perphenazine		ritonavir
					quinidine		star fruit
					ranitidine		telithromycin
					ritonavir		troleandomycin
					sertraline		verapamil
					terbinafine		
					ticlopidine		
					tripelennamine		

Table 2–2. Drugs metabolized by known CYP450 isoenzymes *(continued)*

Inducers

1A2	2B6	2C8	2C19	2C9	2D6	2E1	3A4,5,7
broccoli	pheno-barbital	rifampin	carbamazepine	rifampin	dexamethasone	ethanol	barbiturates
brussels sprouts	phenytoin		norethindrone	secobarbital	rifampin	isoniazid	carbamazepine
char-grilled meat	rifampin		prednisone				efavirenz
insulin			rifampin				glucocorticoids
methyl-cholanthrene							modafinil
modafinil							nevirapine
nafcillin							oxcarbazepine
β-naphthoflavone							phenobarbital
omeprazole							phenytoin
tobacco							pioglitazone
							rifabutin
							rifampin
							St. John's wort
							troglitazone

Note. LAAM=levo-α acetylmethadol. A comprehensive review of drug interactions involving CYP450 isoenzymes, UGTs, and P-glycoproteins in Cozza et al. 2003 is the source of several tables included in this book. Another source of information about drugs metabolized by CYP450 isoenzymes is the Web site prepared by Dr. David Flockhart at Indiana University (http://medicine.iupui.edu/flockhart/table.htm), which site is regularly updated.
Source. Adapted from Cozza et al. 2003; Flockhart 2006.

ticularly problematic because the effect on 1A2 activity takes several weeks to manifest, at which point the patient might be in a different setting (e.g., discharged from the hospital). A patient who quit smoking could potentially experience toxicity while taking a medication like clozapine or theophylline. The interaction of clozapine with fluvoxamine also may be significant, since fluvoxamine is known to inhibit every one of clozapine's CYP450 metabolic pathways.

CYP1A2 is a low-affinity, high-capacity enzyme when compared with 2D6, 2C9, and 2C19. This means that when a drug metabolized by either 2D6 or 1A2 is given, it will be metabolized first by 2D6 (a high- affinity, low-capacity enzyme). Then, when 2D6 becomes overwhelmed (being low capacity), 1A2 will take over, creating a significant problem if 1A2 is inhibited in an individual who is a poor metabolizer at 2D6 (Cozza et al. 2003).

CYP2C9. This enzyme is of particular interest in geriatrics because S-warfarin (the active form) is a substrate, and drugs that significantly inhibit this enzyme could result in high warfarin levels and bleeding. Major inhibitors include ritonavir, fluconazole, and fluvoxamine. It is not clear whether fluoxetine, paroxetine, and sertraline are potent enough inhibitors to be problematic when administered with warfarin. It does appear, however, that fluoxetine's inhibitory potential is sufficient to increase levels of phenytoin when these drugs are given together. Other substrates important to geriatrics are oral hypoglycemics of the sulfonylurea class, including tolbutamide, glipizide, and glyburide. Inhibition of CYP2C9 in the presence of one of these drugs could produce increased drug levels, resulting in hypoglycemia.

CYP2C19. This isoenzyme is found in several tissues but has its primary drug-metabolizing actions in the liver. As with CYP2D6 (described in the next section), genetic variants of CYP2C19 can be associated with a poor metabolizer phenotype (Cozza et al. 2003). Approximately 10%–20% of Africans, 15%–20% of Asians, 3%–5% of Caucasians, and 38%–79% of Pacific Islanders have been found to be poor metabolizers (Flockhart 1995). Fluvoxamine is the most potent inhibitor of CYP2C19, and ticlopidine is also fairly potent. Rifampin is the strongest inducer.

CYP2D6. The CYP2D6 isoenzyme is one of the workhorses of human drug metabolism and is important to psychiatrists because its substrates and inhibitors include numerous commonly used psychotropics, as shown in Table 2–2. CYP2D6 works mainly in the liver but is found in tissues such as heart, prostate, bone marrow, and brain (Cozza et al. 2003). In the brain, CYP2D6 is found in proximity to areas where the dopamine transporter functions, and it is thought that it might have a role as a neuroprotectant (de Leon 2003).

For most drugs, oxidative metabolism by CYP2D6 yields less active metabolites; the exceptions include analgesics such as codeine and tramadol, which are administered as prodrugs and must be metabolized in order to have the desired pharmacodynamic effects (Poulsen et al. 1996). CYP2D6 is a low-capacity, high-affinity enzyme, so it may preferentially metabolize substrates but may become saturated at higher substrate concentrations (Cozza et al. 2003). Available data suggest that CYP2D6 activity does not decline with normal aging (Ereshefsky et al. 1996).

Significant inhibitors of CYP2D6 include fluoxetine, paroxetine, sertraline at dosages of 100 mg/day or more, bupropion, cimetidine, quinidine, ritonavir, and terbinafine. Among the selective serotonin reuptake inhibitor (SSRI) antidepressants, the relative strength of inhibition is as follows: paroxetine > fluoxetine > sertraline > fluvoxamine > citalopram, escitalopram. According to Flockhart 2006, inducers of CYP2D6 include only dexamethasone and rifampin.

Polymorphisms at CYP2D6 give rise to a poor metabolizer phenotype in 3%–10% of Caucasians and 0%–2% of African Americans and Asian Americans (Cozza et al. 2003; Richelson 1997). When a poor metabolizer at CYP2D6 ingests a drug usually metabolized by this enzyme, the drug may accumulate or be metabolized by a secondary enzyme such as CYP3A4, a process that can be less efficient (Cozza et al. 2003). Alternatively, drugs such as codeine or tramadol that must be metabolized to active forms may be ineffective in a poor metabolizer. Interestingly, mutations giving rise to the poor metabolizer phenotype have been associated with Parkinson's disease and dementia with Lewy bodies as well as acute and tardive movement disorders in patients treated with antipsychotics (Cozza et al. 2003).

CYP2E1.   This isoenzyme is of interest because of its role in the metabolism of ethanol and general anesthetics and its ability to generate free radicals and promote carcinogenesis (Cozza et al. 2003). Increased activity of

CYP2E1 has been linked to esophageal, stomach, and liver cancers. Activity of CYP2E1 is induced by chronic alcohol consumption, poorly controlled diabetes, and obesity. CYP2E1 is also the enzyme partly responsible for the higher risk of liver damage in alcoholic persons who ingest acetaminophen.

CYP3A.   Members of the CYP3A subfamily are the most abundant of the CYP enzymes and are important in the metabolism of a large and diverse group of drugs, both psychotropic and nonpsychotropic. These enzymes are expressed in both the intestinal wall and the liver. In the intestine, CYP3A works in tandem with the P-glycoprotein pump in the pre-hepatic phase of first-pass metabolism. Drugs known to inhibit both CYP3A and P-glycoprotein include ketoconazole, quinidine, verapamil, propranolol, and ritonavir (von Moltke and Greenblatt 2000).

Psychotropic substrates of CYP3A include antidepressants, antipsychotics, and sedative-hypnotics. Significant inhibitors include antifungals, certain antibiotics, and grapefruit juice. Among psychotropics, inhibitors include nefazodone and the SSRIs. Certain of the antihistamine substrates for this enzyme (including terfenadine and astemizole) and the gastric motility drug cisapride are highly cardiotoxic at high serum levels, causing *torsades de pointes* tachycardia when their metabolism by CYP3A4 is inhibited; all three drugs have now been withdrawn from the U.S. market. Inducers of CYP3A4 include carbamazepine, rifampin, phenytoin, St. John's wort, phenobarbital, steroids such as dexamethasone, chronic ethanol consumption, and hydrocarbons inhaled in cigarette smoke. Clearance of drugs metabolized primarily by CYP3A does appear to decrease with aging (Pollock 1998).

Phase II Metabolism: Glucuronidation via the UGT System

Through the mechanism of glucuronidation, the family of UGT enzymes provides an important function in the detoxification and clearance of drugs, dietary chemicals, environmental pollutants, and endogenous compounds (Miners et al. 2003). Endogenous compounds include bilirubin, thyroid hormones, serotonin, and gonadal hormones (de Leon 2003). Glucuronidation is a low-affinity, high-capacity process (see above discussion) that takes place primarily in the liver, although UGTs are also found in the gastrointestinal (GI) tract, kidneys, steroid target tissues, and brain. UGTs in the GI tract and liver are poised to participate with CYP3A and P-glycoprotein in first-pass metabolism. UGT enzymes also have polymorphic expression, further adding to variations between individuals in drug bioavailability (Fisher et al. 2001).

To date, two subfamilies of UGTs are recognized in human psychopharmacology: UGT1A and UGT2B. Note that these enzymes are named in a manner analogous to CYP enzymes. Table 2–3 lists currently identified UGT substrates. Carbamazepine, the "great inducer" of P450 isoenzymes, also is an inducer of UGTs (de Leon 2003). Little other information is available about inhibitors or inducers, except what is noted below in the discussion of UGT1A.

UGT1A. Substrates for UGT1A1 include buprenorphine and naltrexone. UGT1A1 metabolizes endogenous bilirubin. It can be induced by phenobarbital, which has been used as a treatment for congenital hyperbilirubinemias (Fisher et al. 2001). Lorazepam and buprenorphine can inhibit this enzyme and thus be associated with jaundice (Fisher et al. 2001). UGT1A3 and UGT1A4 include a number of psychotropics as substrates, as noted in Table 2–3. Lamotrigine is primarily metabolized by UGT1A4 (de Leon 2003).

UGT2B. Valproate is a substrate of UGT2B7 and to a lesser extent of UGT1A3, 1A6, and 1A9 (de Leon 2003). Glucuronidation is thought to be the most important metabolic pathway for valproate, accounting for up to 60% of its metabolism (de Leon 2003). Other substrates of 2B7 include lorazepam, oxazepam, temazepam, codeine, and morphine.

Age has a relatively insignificant effect on glucuronidation, but sex, body habitus, smoking, and certain disease states do affect these processes. Glucuronidation is increased in males, in those who are overweight, and in those who smoke; and decreased in females, those who are underweight, and those with cirrhosis, fulminant hepatitis, hypothyroidism, or HIV/AIDS (Liston et al. 2001).

Protein Binding

Most psychotropic drugs are moderately to highly protein bound, meaning that they travel in tandem with plasma proteins such as albumin and α_1-acid

Table 2–3.   UGT substrates

UGT1A1	UGT1A3	UGT1A4	UGT1A6	UGT1A9	UGT2B7	UGT2B15
acetaminophen	amitriptyline	amitriptyline	acetaminophen	acetaminophen	androsterone	dienestrol
atorvastatin	atorvastatin	androsterone	entacapone	clofibrate	bile acid	entacapone
bilirubin	buprenorphine	chlorpromazine	flutamide metabolite	dapsone	chloramphenicol	estrogens (catechol)
buprenorphine	cerivastatin	clozapine/desmethyl metabolite	ketoprofen	diclofenac	clofibrate	2-OH-estrone
cerivastatin	chlorpromazine	cyproheptadine	nafazone	diflunisal	codeine	oxazepam (S)
ciprofibrate	clozapine	diphenhydramine	serotonin	2-OH-estradiol	cyclosporine	phenytoin metabolites
clofibrate	cyproheptadine	doxepin	SN-38	ethinyl estradiol	diclofenac	testosterone
estriol	diclofenac	imipramine		estrone	entacapone	tolcapone
ethinyl estradiol	diflunisal	lamotrigine		flavonoids	epirubicin	
flutamide metabolite	diphenhydramine	loxapine		furosemide	fenoprofen	
gemfibrozil	doxepin	meperidine		ibuprofen	hydromorphone	
nalorphine	estrones	olanzapine		ketoprofen	ibuprofen	
naltrexone	fenoprofen	progestins		labetalol	ketoprofen	
simvastatin	gemfibrozil	promethazine		mefenamic acid	lorazepam	
SN-38	ibuprofen	retigabine		naproxen	losartan	
telmisartan	imipramine	4-OH-tamoxifen		oxazepam (R)	morphine	
troglitazone	losartan			propofol	nalorphine	
	loxapine			propranolol	naloxone	

Table 2–3. UGT substrates *(continued)*

UGT1A1	UGT1A3	UGT1A4	UGT1A6	UGT1A9	UGT2B7	UGT2B15
	morphine			retinoic acid	naltrexone	
	nalorphine			*SN-38*	naproxen	
	naloxone			thyroxine	norcodeine	
	naltrexone			tolcapone	oxazepam (*R*)	
	naproxen			*valproate*	oxycodone	
	naringenin				tacrolimus	
	norbuprenorphine				temazepam	
	promethazine				*tolcapone*	
	simvastatin				valproate	
	SN-38				zidovudine	
	4-OH-tamoxifen				zomepirac	
	tripelennamine					
	valproate					

Note. Italic type indicates that UGT is a minor pathway for the substrate. UGT = uridine 5'-diphosphate glucuronosyltransferase.
Source. Adapted from Cozza KL, Armstrong SC, Oesterheld JR: *Concise Guide to Drug Interaction Principles for Medical Practice*, 2nd Edition. Washington, DC, American Psychiatric Publishing, 2003. Used with permission.

glycoprotein. In general, albumin levels decrease with aging. Because it is unbound drug that diffuses out of the systemic circulation to sites of action, such as the brain, concern has been raised about the effect of changes in protein levels on drug action. Even among elderly patients, reduced protein levels and protein binding of drugs turn out to have little clinical effect (von Moltke et al. 2005). It has also been thought that one drug could displace another protein-bound drug by competing for the protein binding site and that the displaced drug could have increased clinical effect by virtue of being unbound. Although displacement would be associated with a transient increase in unbound drug, that drug would be available not only for distribution to the target organ but for metabolism and excretion. Important drug interactions due to displacement from proteins are in fact very rare (von Moltke et al. 2005).

Change in protein binding does, however, affect interpretation of total drug concentrations. In general, when the unbound percentage of a drug is high because of lowered albumin levels, the measured concentration of the drug will underestimate the amount of drug acting on the target organ. This is because the laboratory measurement is of total drug concentration rather than free drug concentration, unless the latter is specifically reported as such (Greenblatt et al. 1982a). In other words, when albumin levels are low, it is of potential concern that the patient could develop toxic symptoms at apparently therapeutic drug levels. Aside from this, altered protein binding is not generally an overriding clinical concern in the elderly population.

Clearance

Clearance is the rate at which a drug is removed from the systemic circulation by hepatic metabolism and renal excretion, measured in units of cubic centimeters per minute. Clearance is the most significant physiologic determinant of steady-state plasma concentration and is inversely related to that quantity as follows: concentration at steady state = dosing rate/clearance.

P-glycoprotein resident in the canalicular membrane of hepatocytes and the luminal membrane of proximal tubule cells promotes clearance from the liver and kidneys through its action as an efflux pump (Fromm 2004). As has been noted, the effects of aging on the function of this pump are not yet known. What is clear is that aging is associated with reduced clearance of many drugs because of declines in glomerular filtration rate (GFR) and hepatic blood flow (Greenblatt et al. 1982b). Reduced clearance results in increased steady-state concentration, with enhanced therapeutic effects as well as toxicity. Reduced clearance can be offset by a decrease in dosing rate, using smaller doses and/or longer intervals such that the total dose per unit of time is lower (Greenblatt et al. 1982b). Reduced clearance is a major physiologic reason for the "start low and go slow" maxim in geriatric psychopharmacology.

For drugs cleared partly or entirely by renal excretion of intact drug, clearance declines with age in proportion to the decline in GFR (Greenblatt et al. 1982b). This applies to lithium as well as hydroxylated metabolites of various drugs, some of which are pharmacologically active, such as hydroxy-nortriptyline, hydroxy-bupropion, hydroxy-venlafaxine, and hydroxy-risperidone (Pollock 1998). Starting at 20–30 years of age, there is a decline in GFR each year of about 1 mL/minute per 1.73 m^2 of body surface area (BSA), which is the average BSA for an adult; the mean GFR at 70 years of age for males is 70 mL/minute (Skorecki et al. 2005). This rate of reduction of renal function is not universal, however; as many as one-third of individuals show no decline in GFR with aging (Rowe et al. 1976). Because of this heterogeneity, dosing adjustments for reduced GFR are based on the individual patient's creatinine clearance. Ideally, this is measured by a timed urine collection. When this is not feasible, creatinine clearance (CC) can be roughly calculated using the Cockcroft-Gault equation, as follows:

$$CC \text{ (mL/minute)} = \frac{(140 - \text{age}) \times \text{weight (kg)}}{72 \times \text{serum creatinine (mg/dL)}}$$

For females, the resulting value of creatinine clearance is multiplied by a correction factor of 0.85. It should be noted that the use of this equation for individuals with reduced muscle mass secondary to age, disease, or undernutrition has been justifiably questioned. More accurate means of determining GFR using inulin clearance or ethylenediaminetetraacetic acid (EDTA) are available (Denker and Brenner 2005).

Although oxidative metabolism may be significantly impaired in old age because of changes in liver microsomal enzyme systems, decreased hepatic blood flow with aging is an even more significant factor in reduced hepatic clearance (Greenblatt et al. 1982b). Compared with young adults, elderly individuals may have an estimated 40%–45% reduction in total blood flow to the liver (Greenblatt et al. 1982b). This is one of the main reasons that dosage adjustments are made for hepatically metabolized drugs in elderly patients. Unfortunately, there is no predictable relationship between reduced blood flow and reduced hepatic clearance. Moreover, liver function tests as used and reported clinically do not correlate well with drug-metabolizing ability (Greenblatt et al. 1982b).

Drug Half-Life

Drug half-life ($t_{1/2}$) is related to clearance as follows:

$$t_{1/2} = 0.693 \times \text{volume of distribution/clearance}$$

Note that half-life is dependent on *both* volume of distribution and clearance, either one of which could be significantly affected by aging (von Moltke et al. 2005). In recognition of the two processes by which a drug is removed from the circulation, the concepts of $t_{1/2}$ alpha (distribution half-life) and $t_{1/2}$ beta (elimination half-life) have been introduced. Where alpha or beta is not specified, the elimination (beta) half-life is usually implied. The elimination half-life has clinical utility in calculating the time to steady state and the time to washout of a drug. Steady state is reached in four to five times the half-life for a given drug. During titration, time to steady state determines how soon to increase or decrease the dose. When a drug with a narrow therapeutic index, such as lithium, is prescribed to an elderly patient, waiting for steady state during dose titration will reduce the risk of overshooting and causing toxicity. On discontinuation of a drug, washout takes four to five times the half-life. Because clearance time is reduced in the elderly, the half-life of many psychotropic drugs is increased. For lipophilic drugs used in elderly patients, the distribution half-life may be decreased while the elimination half-life is further increased because of relatively larger fat stores.

As noted in the drug summary data appearing throughout this manual, half-lives vary considerably among drugs. Drugs with very short half-lives can generally be associated with between-dose rebound or withdrawal symptoms and can be problematic if doses are missed. Conversely, and much more importantly for elderly patients, drugs or drug metabolites with long half-lives can accumulate over time and lead to toxic effects. This could occur, for example, with amitriptyline or with flurazepam and its metabolite desalkylflurazepam.

Pharmacodynamics and Aging

The pharmacodynamic changes of aging—the effects of aging on the body's response to drugs—have been little studied. Increased pharmacodynamic sensitivity to drugs with aging has been postulated but not conclusively demonstrated. In general, pharmacodynamic response is a function of neuronal receptor number and affinity, signal transduction, cellular response, and homeostatic regulation (Tumer et al. 1992). Reduced density of muscarinic, μ opioid, and dopaminergic D_2 receptors has been noted as a concomitant of aging (Hammerlein et al. 1998; Pollock 1998). The ability to up-regulate or down-regulate postsynaptic receptors also may decrease with aging. The activities of a number of enzymes are reduced with aging, except for monoamine oxidase B activity, which is increased. The functional results of these changes are likely to be significant but are at this time poorly characterized.

Chapter Summary

- Genetic heterogeneity with regard to pharmacologic response is amplified by aging effects.
- As an individual ages, fat stores increase and lean body mass decreases, resulting in a relative increase in volume of distribution for lipophilic (fat-soluble) drugs, including almost all psychotropics.
- Aging is associated with reduced clearance of many drugs because of declines in glomerular filtration rate and hepatic blood flow.
- Reduced clearance can be offset by a decrease in dosing rate, using smaller doses and/or longer intervals such that the total dose per unit time is lower; this is the basis for the "start low and go slow" maxim in geriatric psychopharmacology.
- Of the two most important CYP450 isoenzymes, CYP3A activity does appear to decrease with aging, while CYP2D6 activity does not.
- The phase II process of glucuronidation is little affected by aging but may be affected by body habitus, smoking, and certain disease states.
- The effect of aging on function of P-glycoprotein is not known.
- In elderly patients, drugs or drug metabolites with long half-lives can accumulate over time and lead to toxic effects.

References

Cozza KL, Armstrong SC, Oesterheld JR: Concise Guide to Drug Interaction Principles for Medical Practice, 2nd Edition. Washington, DC, American Psychiatric Publishing, 2003

de Leon J: Glucuronidation enzymes, genes and psychiatry. Int J Neuropsychopharmacol 6:57–72, 2003

de Leon J, Susce MT, Pan RM, et al: The CYP2D6 poor metabolizer phenotype may be associated with risperidone adverse drug reactions and discontinuation. J Clin Psychiatry 66:15–27, 2005

Denker BM, Brenner BM: Azotemia and urinary abnormalities, in Harrison's Principles of Internal Medicine. Edited by Kasper DL, Braunwald E, Fauci AS, et al. New York, McGraw-Hill, 2005, pp 246–252

Ereshefsky L, Riesenman C, Lam YW: Serotonin selective reuptake inhibitor drug interactions and the cytochrome P450 system. J Clin Psychiatry 57 (suppl 8):17–25, 1996

Fisher MB, Paine MF, Strelevitz TJ, et al: The role of hepatic and extrahepatic UDP-glucuronosyltransferases in human drug metabolism. Drug Metab Rev 33:273–297, 2001

Flockhart DA: Drug interactions and the cytochrome P450 system: a role of cytochrome P450 2C19. Clin Pharmacokinet 29 (suppl 1):45–52, 1995

Flockhart D: Drugs Metabolized by Cytochrome P450 Isoforms. August 29, 2006. Available at: http://medicine.iupui.edu/flockhart/table.htm. Accessed September 2, 2006.

Fromm MF: Importance of P-glycoprotein at blood-tissue barriers. Trends Pharmacol Sci 25:423–429, 2004

Gasche Y, Daali Y, Fathi M, et al: Codeine intoxication associated with ultrarapid CYP2D6 metabolism. N Engl J Med 351:2827–2831, 2004

Greenblatt DJ, Sellers EM, Koch-Weser J: Importance of protein binding for the interpretation of serum or plasma drug concentrations. J Clin Pharmacol 22:259–263, 1982a

Greenblatt DJ, Sellers EM, Shader RI: Drug disposition in old age. N Engl J Med 306:1081–1088, 1982b

Greenblatt DJ, Abernethy DR, Shader RI: Pharmacokinetic aspects of drug therapy in the elderly. Ther Drug Monit 8:249–255, 1986

Hammerlein A, Derendorf H, Lowenthal DT: Pharmacokinetic and pharmacodynamic changes in the elderly. Clin Pharmacokinet 35:49–64, 1998

Kivisto KT, Niemi M, Fromm MF: Functional interaction of intestinal CYP3A4 and P-glycoprotein. Fundam Clin Pharmacol 18:621–626, 2004

Liston HL, Markowitz JS, DeVane CL: Drug glucuronidation in clinical psychopharmacology. J Clin Psychopharmacol 21:500–515, 2001

Miners JO, Smith PA, Sorich MJ, et al: Predicting human drug glucuronidation parameters: application of in vitro and in silico modeling approaches. Annu Rev Pharmacol Toxicol 44:1–25, 2003

Nemeroff CB, DeVane CL, Pollock BG: Newer antidepressants and the cytochrome P450 system. Am J Psychiatry 153:311–320, 1996

Pollock BG: Psychotropic drugs and the aging patient. Geriatrics 53 (suppl 1):S20–S24, 1998

Poulsen L, Arendt-Nielsen L, Brosen K, et al: The hypoalgesic effect of tramadol in relation to CYP2D6. Clin Pharmacol Ther 60:636–644, 1996

Richelson E: Pharmacokinetic drug interactions of new antidepressants: a review of the effects on the metabolism of other drugs. Mayo Clin Proc 72:835–847, 1997

Rowe JW, Andres R, Tobin JD: Age-adjusted standards for creatinine clearance. Ann Intern Med 84:567–569, 1976

Skorecki K, Green J, Brenner BM: Chronic renal failure, in Harrison's Principles of Internal Medicine. Edited by Kasper DL, Braunwald E, Fauci AS, et al. New York, McGraw-Hill, 2005, pp 1653–1663

Thompson TL, Moran MG, Nies AS: Psychotropic drug use in the elderly: part 1. N Engl J Med 308:134–138, 1983a

Thompson TL, Moran MG, Nies AS: Psychotropic drug use in the elderly: part 2. N Engl J Med 308:194–199, 1983b

Tumer N, Scarpace PJ, Lowenthal DT: Geriatric pharmacology: basic and clinical considerations. Annu Rev Pharmacol Toxicol 32:271–302, 1992

von Moltke LL, Greenblatt DJ: Drug transporters in psychopharmacology—are they important? J Clin Psychopharmacol 20:291–294, 2000

von Moltke LL, Greenblatt DJ, Harmatz JS, et al: Psychotropic drug metabolism in old age: principles and problems of assessment, in Psychopharmacology: The Fourth Generation of Progress. Edited by Bloom FE, Kupfer DJ. New York, Raven Press, 1995, pp 1461–1469

von Moltke LL, Abernethy DR, Greenblatt DJ: Kinetics and dynamics of psychotropic drugs in the elderly, in Clinical Geriatric Psychopharmacology, 4th Edition. Edited by Salzman C. Philadelphia, PA, Lippincott Williams & Wilkins, 2005, pp 87–114

3

Antipsychotics

Introduction

With the introduction of the atypical antipsychotics, the 1990s were a time of significant resurgence in antipsychotic drug prescribing for elderly patients (Briesacher et al. 2005). These drugs were heavily promoted for a wide variety of indications, and the comfort level in prescribing them was high, even among nonpsychiatrists. More recently, serious concerns have been raised about the safety of this class of medications, particularly with respect to their relation to stroke risk and metabolic syndrome, and their use has been associated with an increased risk of death among elderly patients with dementia (Schneider et al. 2005).

Initial reports about atypical antipsychotics in the treatment of schizophrenia suggested that these agents would be particularly useful in elderly patients, with demonstrated superiority to reference "typical" agents, efficacy in both positive and negative symptoms, mood-stabilizing and antidepressant effects, lower relapse rates when used chronically, lower incidence of associated extrapyramidal side effects (EPS) and tardive dyskinesia, and improvement in cognitive function (Pickar 1995). Although some of that initial promise was borne out by subsequent clinical experience, recent studies also have questioned the efficacy of these drugs.

The results from the Clinical Antipsychotic Trials in Intervention Effectiveness (CATIE) schizophrenia study are pertinent here, even though the study population was nonelderly: aside from olanzapine, the atypical agents were no more efficacious than the conventional drug perphenazine

(Lieberman et al. 2005). A preliminary report from Phase 1 of the CATIE Alzheimer's disease (CATIE-AD) study was presented at the 2005 annual meeting of the American Psychiatric Association. This study was designed to investigate the effectiveness of three atypical antipsychotic drugs versus placebo in the treatment of psychosis, agitation, and aggression in community-dwelling patients with Alzheimer's disease. Findings included overall rates of termination comparable for all three drugs (olanzapine, quetiapine, and risperidone), rates of termination due to lack of efficacy lower for active treatments versus placebo, and rates of termination due to adverse effects greater for active treatments versus placebo (Tariot 2005).

Even more important is that significant concerns have been raised about the safety of atypical antipsychotics for elderly patients, particularly those with dementia. In April 2005, the U.S. Food and Drug Administration (FDA) issued a warning regarding the nearly doubled risk of death in this population for those treated with atypical agents versus placebo. Preliminary findings from the CATIE-AD study raised similar concerns, suggesting that the benefits of these drugs may not outweigh the risks. Moreover, the risks may not be limited to the atypical drugs; a retrospective cohort study suggested that conventional antipsychotics are at least as likely to increase the risk of death in elderly patients as the atypical drugs (Wang et al. 2005).

Expert Consensus Guidelines (Alexopoulos et al. 2004) for the use of antipsychotic agents in older patients suggest not only indications for antipsychotic use but conditions for which antipsychotic agents are not generally indicated. Antipsychotic agents are not recommended for treatment of generalized anxiety disorder, panic disorder, hypochondriasis, nonpsychotic major depression, insomnia or other sleep disturbance, primary irritability or hostility, motion sickness, neuropathic pain, or nausea and vomiting due to chemotherapy. However, contrary to the recommendations, it is not uncommon to encounter an elderly patient who has been prescribed an atypical agent for the treatment of conditions such as insomnia, frequent anxiety, or irritability. Whether this prescribing practice is more common among nonpsychiatrists is not clear.

Pharmacokinetics

In general, antipsychotics are well absorbed in the gastrointestinal (GI) tract. Rate of absorption may be affected by antacids or by anticholinergic drugs through decreased gut motility (von Moltke et al. 2005). Bioavailability of most low-potency antipsychotics (chlorpromazine, thioridazine, mesoridazine, clozapine, and quetiapine) is variable so that dosing ranges are wide and no single "correct" dose is associated with optimal response. Dose ranges for higher-potency agents (haloperidol, risperidone, and olanzapine) are narrower, and titration is therefore more routine. For agents with few active metabolites (e.g., clozapine), serum levels could theoretically be used to determine dose range for an individual patient, but therapeutic blood levels are not established for most drugs, particularly for use by the elderly population.

Antipsychotics are highly lipid soluble. In the average elderly patient, these drugs have a large volume of distribution and slow elimination and achieve high concentrations in the brain relative to plasma. As discussed in Chapter 2, "Basic Psychopharmacology and Aging," the large volume of distribution also limits the duration of action of a single dose of antipsychotic. Antipsychotics are highly protein bound—mainly to albumin but also to α_1-acid glycoprotein (AGP). As noted in Chapter 2, albumin concentration declines with aging, disease, and malnutrition. AGP is an acute-phase reactant that increases in acute disease and may be chronically elevated in rheumatologic or other inflammatory conditions. Changes in serum protein concentrations are of concern because they can affect interpretation of laboratory tests measuring serum drug levels.

Antipsychotics are metabolized primarily in the liver, first undergoing oxidation by enzymes of the cytochrome P450 (CYP) system and then undergoing glucuronidation before being excreted in the urine. Some drugs (e.g., clozapine) undergo demethylation, a type of oxidation reaction that becomes less efficient with aging, resulting in longer times to steady state and to elimination. As noted in Chapter 2, the activity of certain CYP enzymes such as CYP1A2 declines with aging, and clearance of substrates such as clozapine and olanzapine is thus decreased (Ereshefsky 1996). In contrast, activity of CYP2D6 is unaffected by aging alone (Pollock and Mulsant 1995) but may be affected to a minor degree by smoking and more significantly by CYP2D6 genotype (Pan et al. 1999). The CYP2D6 poor metabolizer phenotype, for example, has been associated with adverse drug reactions to risperidone (de Leon et al. 2005). Table 3–1 lists metabolic pathways for atypical and conventional antipsychotics.

Clearance of a particular antipsychotic medication depends in part on the age of the patient and the class of drug (Ereshefsky 1996). The effects of aging on hepatic and renal clearance are described in Chapter 2. Reduced clearance of antipsychotic medication in the elderly patient dictates careful application of the "start low and go slow" rule. Although atypical antipsychotics are generally associated with smaller clearance decrements with aging than are typical agents (Ereshefsky 1996), reduced clearance in elders has been found for risperidone (Snoeck et al. 1995), quetiapine (DeVane and Nemeroff 2001), and ziprasidone (Wilner et al. 2000). A gender difference may prove to be clinically important; the atypical agents have been found experimentally to be cleared more rapidly in men than women (Ereshefsky 1996). Smoking status may substantially affect metabolism of agents cleared primarily via CYP1A2 (Cozza et al. 2003).

Antipsychotic medications are released slowly from lipid storage sites, so when toxic effects develop, they can last for weeks. Moreover, measurable antipsychotic drug metabolites can persist in urine for as long as 3 months after discontinuation (Ereshefsky 1996).

Pharmacodynamics and Mechanism of Action

For conventional antipsychotics, the proportion of occupied dopamine D_2 receptors is a major determinant of antipsychotic effect as well as EPS. Data from positron emission tomography studies have suggested that usual doses of conventional drugs result in a range of basal ganglia D_2 occupancy values among treated patients, and that those patients with EPS tend to have values at the upper end of this range (Farde et al. 1992). Moreover, it appears that D_2 occupancy values in the same range can occur with conventional agents at smaller-than-usual dosages, such as haloperidol at 2 mg/day (Kapur et al. 1996). These studies have provided some of the rationale for the substantially lower doses used to treat elderly patients.

In contrast to conventional agents, clinically effective doses of most atypical antipsychotics are associated with a much greater serotonin 5-HT_2

Table 3–1. Antipsychotics: known metabolic pathways

Drug	Metabolic pathways	Enzyme(s) inhibited
Atypical antipsychotics		
Aripiprazole	CYP2D6, 3A4	None
Clozapine	CYP1A2, 3A4, 2D6, 2C19; UGT1A4, UGT1A3	2D6 (mild)
Olanzapine	CYP1A2, 2D6; UGT1A4	None
Quetiapine	CYP3A4, sulfation	None
Risperidone	CYP2D6, 3A4	2D6 (moderate)
Ziprasidone	Aldehyde oxidase, CYP3A4, 1A2	None
Conventional antipsychotics		
Chlorpromazine	**CYP2D6,** 1A2, 3A4; UGT1A4, UGT1A3	**2D6**
Fluphenazine	**CYP2D6,** 1A2	**2D6,** 1A2
Haloperidol	**CYP2D6, 3A4,** 1A2	**2D6**
Loxapine	UGT1A4, UGT1A3	None
Mesoridazine	CYP2D6, 1A2	None
Perphenazine	**CYP2D6, 3A4,** 1A2, 2C19	**2D6,** 1A2
Pimozide	CYP3A4, 1A2	**2D6, 3A4**
Thioridazine	**CYP2D6,** 1A2, 2C19, FMO$_3$	**2D6**

Note. Bold type indicates major pathway or potent inhibition.
Source. Adapted from Cozza KL, Armstrong SC, Oesterheld JR (eds): "Psychiatry," in *Concise Guide to Drug Interaction Principles for Medical Practice,* 2nd Edition. Washington, DC, American Psychiatric Publishing, 2003, pp. 360, 368. Used with permission.

receptor occupancy rate than dopamine D_2 occupancy rate (Nordstrom et al. 1995). In fact, one of the mechanisms originally proposed to underlie atypicality was potent $5\text{-}HT_2$ antagonism coupled with relatively weak D_2 antagonism, leading to good efficacy and low potential for EPS (Pickar 1995). It was noted, however, that this $5\text{-}HT_2 > D_2$ antagonism does not distinguish all atypical from conventional antipsychotics; the atypical antipsychotic amisulpride (not available in the United States) is not a serotonin receptor antagonist (Davis et al. 2003), and the conventional antipsychotic loxapine does block $5\text{-}HT_2 > D_2$ (Gardner et al. 2005). D_2 antagonism itself may be the mechanism underlying most antipsychotic action, particularly against positive symptoms, although this is not necessarily the only mechanism (Gardner et al. 2005).

Aripiprazole is unique among atypical agents, being a partial agonist at the D_2 receptor (both pre- and postsynaptic) as well as a partial agonist at $5\text{-}HT_{1A}$ and antagonist at $5\text{-}HT_{2A}$ receptors (Harrison and Perry 2004). A partial dopamine agonist has either agonist or antagonist activity, depending on the intensity of dopamine receptor stimulation and the level of endogenous ligand (Harrison and Perry 2004). In low-dopamine states, aripiprazole acts as a D_2 agonist, and in high-dopamine states, it acts as a D_2 antagonist.

Adverse motor effects of antipsychotics are related to binding at dopamine D_2 receptors in the basal ganglia. Other adverse effects are related to binding at other receptors: sedation and weight gain to histamine (H_1) receptor blockade, hypotension to peripheral adrenergic (α_1) receptor blockade, and anticholinergic effects such as constipation and confusion to muscarinic (M_1) receptor blockade. Side-effect profiles of individual agents differ because relative affinities for each of these receptor populations differ. Table 3–2 shows details of receptor binding for atypical antipsychotics and a representative conventional antipsychotic. In the treatment of elderly patients, agents with affinity for H_1, α_1, and M_1 receptors are best avoided because of problems with weight gain, hypotension, and anticholinergic side effects, as discussed later in this chapter.

Age-related pharmacodynamic changes render the dopaminergic system increasingly sensitive to pharmacologic manipulation. It has been demonstrated with some antipsychotics that therapeutic effects are achieved and toxic effects are seen at lower serum drug levels in older pa-

Table 3–2. Antipsychotic receptor binding

Drug	Adrenergic		Dopaminergic				H$_1$	M$_1$	NRI	SRI	Serotonergic 5-HT						
	α$_1$	α$_2$	D$_1$	D$_2$	D$_3$	D$_4$					1A	1D	2A	2C	3	6	7
Conventional antipsychotic	X			X			X	X									
Haloperidol	X		X														
Aripiprazole	X		X	X	X	X	X			X	X		X	X			X
Clozapine	X	X	X	X	X	X	X	X			X		X	X	X	X	X
Olanzapine	X		X	X	X	X	X	X					X	X	X	X	
Quetiapine	X	X	X	X			X						X			X	X
Risperidone	X	X		X								X	X			X	X
Ziprasidone	X			X	X				X	X	X	X	X	X			X

Note. H$_1$ = histaminergic receptor; M$_1$ = muscarinic type 1 receptor; NRI = norepinephrine reuptake inhibitor; SRI = serotonin reuptake inhibitor.

tients compared with younger patients—particularly in older patients with dementia. This finding presumably reflects age-related changes in neuronal sensitivity. With haloperidol, for example, serum levels associated with therapeutic improvement in older patients with schizophrenia (0–10.4 ng/mL) and older patients with dementia (0.32–1.44 ng/mL) (Lacro et al. 1996) were significantly lower than serum levels associated with therapeutic improvement in younger patients (2–15 ng/mL) (Van Putten et al. 1992).

Drug Interactions

Significant drug interactions involving antipsychotics are shown in Table 3–3. In general, atypical antipsychotic agents appear to have little potential to interfere with the metabolism of other drugs as CYP450 inhibitors or inducers. As shown in Table 2–2 in Chapter 2, however, several of the conventional antipsychotics are CYP2D6 inhibitors. All antipsychotics are themselves substrates for CYP isoenzymes, mostly CYP2D6 and/or CYP3A4, and some are also uridine 5'-diphosphate glucuronosyltransferase (UGT) substrates, so *their* metabolism may be significantly affected by *other* drugs.

A potentially serious interaction of clozapine and benzodiazepines involves cardiovascular and respiratory depression and has been associated with sudden death (Grohmann et al. 1989). Benzodiazepines are best discontinued before clozapine is initiated in elderly patients, and if needed, they should be added to an existing clozapine regimen only after clozapine titration is complete. Another potentially serious interaction could occur if ziprasidone were coadministered with another QTc-prolonging drug or with a CYP3A4 inhibitor, because a serious ventricular dysrhythmia could result, including *torsades de pointes*. For this reason, the patient's current medication regimen should be scrutinized carefully before ziprasidone is added. In addition, other risk factors for QTc prolongation, such as hypokalemia, should be addressed.

Indications

Antipsychotic medications can be appropriately used in the management of various disorders associated with psychotic symptoms, including schizo-

Table 3–3. Antipsychotic drug interactions

Antipsychotic drug	Interacting drug	Potential interaction
All antipsychotics	Antacids (e.g., Maalox)	Delayed absorption
	Antihypertensives	Complex effects depend on specific agents; hypotension or hypertension
	β-Blockers	Increased levels of both
	Ethanol; other CNS depressants	Additive CNS depression
	Tricyclic antidepressants	Increased levels of both
All antipsychotics except clozapine and quetiapine	Levodopa	Decreased antiparkinsonian effect
Low-potency typical antipsychotics, olanzapine, clozapine	Anticholinergics	Additive anticholinergic effects
Typical antipsychotics	Lithium	Neurotoxicity; increased EPS
Fluphenazine and haloperidol	Alprazolam	Increased antipsychotic level
Clozapine	Benzodiazepines	Respiratory depression/arrest
	Carbamazepine	Decreased clozapine level; increased risk of bone marrow suppression
	CYP1A2 inhibitors: fluoroquinolone antibiotics, fluvoxamine, mexiletine, etc.	Increased clozapine level

Table 3–3. Antipsychotic drug interactions (*continued*)

Antipsychotic drug	Interacting drug	Potential interaction
Clozapine (*continued*)	CYP1A2 inducers: caffeine, carbamazepine, omeprazole, ritonavir, certain foods (broccoli, cabbage), smoking	Decreased clozapine level
Pimozide, quetiapine, risperidone, and ziprasidone	CYP3A4 inhibitors: norfluoxetine, nefazodone, certain antibiotics/antifungals, certain antiretrovirals, grapefruit juice, etc.	Increased antipsychotic level
	CYP3A4 inducers: carbamazepine, phenobarbital, phenytoin, rifampin, St. John's wort, etc.	Decreased antipsychotic level
Olanzapine	CYP1A2 inhibitors: fluoroquinolone antibiotics, fluvoxamine, mexiletine, etc.	Increased olanzapine level
	CYP1A2 inducers: caffeine, carbamazepine, omeprazole, ritonavir, certain foods, smoking, etc.	Decreased olanzapine level
Risperidone, haloperidol, and aripiprazole	CYP2D6 inhibitors: bupropion, diphenhydramine, duloxetine, fluoxetine, paroxetine, cimetidine, metoclopramide, ritonavir, etc.	Increased antipsychotic level
Ziprasidone	Any QTc-prolonging drug	Additive effects, with potential for ventricular dysrhythmia

Note. CNS=central nervous system; CYP=cytochrome P450; EPS=extrapyramidal side effects.
Source. Adapted from Pies RW: "Antipsychotics," in *Handbook of Essential Psychopharmacology*, 2nd Edition. Washington, DC, American Psychiatric Publishing, 2005, pp. 175–177.

phrenia, mania with psychotic symptoms, dementia with delusions and agitation/aggression, major depression with psychotic features, delusional disorder, delirium, and psychotic disorders secondary to medical conditions. The use of antipsychotic medications to treat some of these conditions (e.g., delirium) is of necessity off-label. DSM-IV-TR codes for psychotic disorders affecting the elderly are shown in Table 3–4.

The use of antipsychotic medications to treat nonpsychotic behavioral disturbances in the context of dementia in elderly patients has been controversial. Specific behavioral problems for which antipsychotics have been prescribed include "agitation," wandering, irritability, repetitive vocalization, belligerence, insomnia, and aggression. Conventional antipsychotics have been widely used for these indications for a number of years with moderate success but with growing concern about adverse effects (particularly tardive dyskinesia). Although it has generally been believed that atypical antipsychotics are more efficacious in treating behavioral disturbances in dementia, there is no good evidence that this is the case. Moreover, both atypical and conventional antipsychotic drugs are under close scrutiny now with regard to safety in the elderly population. It is likely that nonantipsychotic medications will be increasingly used to treat or prevent behavioral disturbances in dementia. These alternatives are discussed further in Chapter 9 of this volume, "Medications to Treat Dementia and Other Cognitive Disorders."

Efficacy

Clozapine, as the prototype atypical antipsychotic, set a new standard of efficacy in the treatment of schizophrenia, ameliorating not only positive symptoms but negative symptoms, abnormal movements, and certain cognitive impairments (Jann 1991; Jibson and Tandon 1998; Pickar 1995). Clozapine has been shown to be superior to chlorpromazine in long-term treatment and in cases of treatment resistance. No other atypical drug has been proven to be equivalent to clozapine. In fact, in the CATIE study, only olanzapine among the atypical antipsychotics studied (quetiapine, risperidone, ziprasidone) proved to be more efficacious than the conventional antipsychotic perphenazine (Lieberman et al. 2005).

Table 3–4.   DSM-IV-TR psychotic disorders affecting the elderly

293.0	Delirium due to a general medical condition
780.09	Delirium not otherwise specified
290.3	Dementia of the Alzheimer's type, late onset, with delirium
290.20	Dementia of the Alzheimer's type, late onset, with delusions
296.34	Major depressive disorder, recurrent, severe, with psychotic features
296.24	Major depressive disorder, single episode, severe with psychotic features
296.xx	Bipolar I disorder—depressed/manic/mixed, severe with psychotic features
298.8	Brief psychotic disorder
295.70	Schizoaffective disorder
295.xx	Schizophrenia
295.40	Schizophreniform disorder
297.1	Delusional disorder
291.x	Alcohol-induced psychotic disorder
291.0	Alcohol intoxication delirium
291.0	Alcohol withdrawal delirium
293.xx	Psychotic disorder due to a general medical condition

Clinical Use

Choice of Antipsychotic

Antipsychotic preparations are shown in Table 3–5. In recent years, alternative formulations of several atypical antipsychotics have become available, expanding the treatment options for patients unable or unwilling to swallow pills and for patients requiring emergent sedation or long-term treatment.

The choice of a specific drug depends not only on demonstrated efficacy and safety in the elderly population but on the particular condition being treated, comorbid medical conditions that might limit the use of cer-

Table 3–5. Antipsychotic preparations

Generic name	Trade name	Relative potency	Tablets (mg)	Capsules (mg)	SR forms (mg)	Liquid concentrate	Liquid suspension or elixir	Injectable form
Conventional antipsychotics								
chlorpromazine	Thorazine	100	10, 25, 50, 100, 200		30, 75, 150, 30 mg/mL 200, 300 100 mg/mL			10 mg/mL 25 mg/mL
fluphenazine	Prolixin	2	1, 2.5, 5, 10			5 mg/mL	0.5 mg/mL 2.5 mg/5 mL	2.5 mg/mL
fluphenazine decanoate	Prolixin D							25 mg/mL
haloperidol	Haldol	2	0.2, 1, 2, 5, 10, 20			2 mg/mL		5 mg/mL
haloperidol decanoate	Haldol D							50 mg/mL 100 mg/mL
loxapine	Loxitane	10		5, 10, 25, 50		25 mg/mL		50 mg/mL
mesoridazine	Serentil	50	10, 25, 50, 100			25 mg/mL		25 mg/mL
molindone	Moban	10	5, 10, 25, 50, 100			20 mg/mL		

Table 3–5.   Antipsychotic preparations *(continued)*

Generic name	Trade name	Relative potency	Tablets (mg)	Capsules (mg)	SR forms	Liquid concentrate	Liquid suspension or elixir	Injectable form
Conventional antipsychotics (continued)								
perphenazine	Trilafon	8	2, 4, 8, 16			16 mg/5 mL		5 mg/mL
pimozide	Orap	1	2					
thioridazine	Mellaril	95	10, 15, 25, 50, 100, 150, 200			30 mg/mL 100 mg/mL	25 mg/5 mL 100 mg/5 mL	
thiothixene	Navane	5		1, 2, 5, 10, 20		5 mg/mL		2 mg/mL 5 mg/mL
trifluoperazine	Stelazine	5	1, 2, 5, 10			10 mg/mL		2 mg/mL
Atypical antipsychotics								
aripiprazole	Abilify	5	5, 10, 15, 20, 30				1 mg/mL	
clozapine	Clozaril	100	12.5, 25, 100 Branded: 25, 100 FazaClo: 25, 100					
	FazaClo[a]							

Table 3–5. Antipsychotic preparations (*continued*)

Generic name	Trade name	Relative potency	Tablets (mg)	Capsules (mg)	SR forms (mg)	Liquid concentrate	Liquid suspension or elixir	Injectable form
Atypical antipsychotics (*continued*)								
olanzapine	Zyprexa	5	2.5, 5, 7.5, 10, 15, 20					
	Zyprexa Zydis		5, 10, 15, 20					
	Zyprexa IM							10-mg vial
quetiapine	Seroquel	100	25, 50, 100, 200, 300, 400					
risperidone	Risperdal	1–2	0.25, 0.5, 1, 2, 3, 4				1 mg/mL	
	Risperdal M-Tabs[a]		0.5, 1, 2					
risperidone (long-acting injectable)	Risperdal Consta							25-, 37.5-, 50-mg dose packs
ziprasidone	Geodon	40	20, 40, 60, 80					20 mg

Note. IM=intramuscular; SR=sustained-release. [a]Orally disintegrating.

tain drugs, prior response to treatment, and the potential for noncompliance (for which long-acting, injectable formulations may be used).

Delirium is the only indication in geriatrics for which a conventional antipsychotic (haloperidol) continues to be used routinely in many settings. For conditions other than delirium, atypical antipsychotics are widely considered the drugs of choice for elderly patients. Nevertheless, atypical agents have to be used with caution in the geriatric population, not only because of newly recognized stroke and mortality risks but because of associated orthostatic hypotension, sedation, anticholinergic effects, weight gain, glucose dysregulation, and hyperlipidemia. As discussed below, these agents are not all equal with regard to risk for introducing these adverse effects. With clozapine in particular, the risk of agranulocytosis overshadows most other concerns. Agranulocytosis can occur even with scrupulous white blood cell (WBC) monitoring and can be fatal in rare cases. For this reason, in spite of its proven superiority, clozapine is still reserved for patients with schizophrenia who do not respond to or do not tolerate other antipsychotic medications. It is also used for the specific purpose of treating psychosis with comorbid tardive dyskinesia or psychosis in Parkinson's disease (PD; Small et al. 1987). Specific recommendations for antipsychotic use in selected patient populations are shown in Table 3–6.

Alternative Formulations

As shown in Table 3–5, most typical antipsychotics and several atypical antipsychotics are available in different formulations. In terms of the speed with which a medication enters the systemic circulation, intravenous formulations are the fastest, followed by short-acting intramuscular, oral liquid, oral capsule, oral tablet, and long-acting (depot) intramuscular. The time to onset of action for oral liquids is approximately the same as that for intramuscularly administered drugs (Ereshefsky 1996). Some side effects (e.g., hypotension) may occur because of too-rapid onset of action, making this another factor to consider in selecting a formulation for a particular patient.

Although there has been no consensus regarding the use of decanoate antipsychotics in the elderly population, advocates have reported good success with the use of these agents, and no greater incidence of adverse

Table 3–6. Antipsychotic agents: specific recommendations for selected patient groups

Medical condition	Recommended treatment
Diabetes	Avoid clozapine and olanzapine. Consider aripiprazole.
Glaucoma (narrow- or closed-angle)	Avoid thioridazine and clozapine. Consider aripiprazole, risperidone, and quetiapine.
Hepatic insufficiency	Reduce antipsychotic dose.
Hyperlipidemia	Avoid clozapine and olanzapine. Consider aripiprazole.
Hypotension	Avoid low-potency agents, clozapine, and risperidone. Consider aripiprazole.
Obesity	Avoid clozapine and olanzapine. Consider aripiprazole and molindone.
Orthostasis	Avoid low-potency agents, clozapine, and quetiapine. Consider aripiprazole.
Parkinson's disease or parkinsonism	Avoid haloperidol and risperidone. Consider low-dose clozapine and quetiapine.
Prostatic hypertrophy	Avoid thioridazine, clozapine, and olanzapine. Consider aripiprazole, risperidone, and quetiapine.
QTc prolongation	Avoid thioridazine and ziprasidone. Consider olanzapine.
Renal insufficiency	Antipsychotic dose adjustment generally not required.
Seizures	Avoid clozapine. Consider haloperidol and molindone.
Tardive dyskinesia	Avoid conventional antipsychotics. Consider clozapine, olanzapine, quetiapine, and aripiprazole.
Xerophthalmia (dry eyes) or xerostomia (dry mouth)	Avoid thioridazine and clozapine. Consider aripiprazole, risperidone, and quetiapine.

effects than with oral formulations. Masand and Gupta (2003) have published guidelines for the use of decanoate and long-acting, injectable medications in elders. Long-acting formulations are convenient and ensure compliance in patients for whom this is an otherwise insurmountable problem, and at least haloperidol decanoate may be associated with a low incidence of acute EPS because of slow release. On the other hand, injections are painful, injected drugs may be erratically absorbed in patients with small muscle mass, and in general these drugs have been understudied in the elderly population. In addition, with fluphenazine decanoate, a significant fraction of the injected dose is released within hours, introducing a greater risk of EPS. Despite their drawbacks, decanoate medications have a place in the treatment of a subset of elderly patients with chronic psychosis and persistent compliance problems and may be both effective and well tolerated in this population.

The equivalent geriatric decanoate dose of a stable oral dose of haloperidol can be estimated by multiplying the daily oral dose (in milligrams) by a factor of 10 and administering this dose intramuscularly every 4 weeks. A daily oral dose of 2 mg, for example, could be substituted by 20 mg of haloperidol decanoate given every 4 weeks. Fluphenazine decanoate is usually initiated in geriatric patients at a dose of 6.25 mg (0.25 cc), which is added to the patient's oral regimen. If tolerated, a second dose of 6.25 mg can then be given after 2–4 weeks, after which the oral medication should be tapered slowly and discontinued. The effective dose and dosing interval for fluphenazine decanoate are then determined empirically; intervals range from 2 weeks to 2 months.

The long-acting, injectable form of risperidone (Risperdal Consta) differs from the decanoate drugs in the mechanics and speed of its release; whereas the decanoate drugs are released over hours to days via hydrolysis, risperidone is contained in microspheres within muscle tissue (usually gluteal) and active drug is released only after 3–4 weeks. When the release process begins, therapeutic drug levels are then maintained for about 2 weeks. When treatment with long-acting, injectable risperidone is initiated, oral antipsychotic must be administered in tandem for the first 3 weeks. As with younger patients, injections are administered every 2 weeks. A dose of 25 mg every 2 weeks would be equivalent to 2–4 mg/day given orally.

Controlled trials of the use of long-acting, injectable risperidone in elderly patients have not yet been published, leaving it unclear whether this medication should be recommended for use in geriatrics. One group reported good results in a 1-year, open-label maintenance study of stable schizophrenic and schizoaffective elders, but the numbers were small and not all outcomes were reported (Lasser et al. 2005). Theoretically, the long-acting formulation could confer an advantage over the oral formulation in that the mean peak concentration at steady state would be lower and there would be less fluctuation in active drug levels over time (Eerdekens et al. 2004). It is not yet clear, however, whether long-acting, injectable risperidone is as effective as oral risperidone (Chue et al. 2005; Taylor et al. 2004). Furthermore, the drug is much more expensive than oral medication.

Pretreatment Evaluation

Prior to initiating treatment with an antipsychotic medication, the elderly patient should be assessed for involuntary movements, have orthostatic blood pressure and pulse checked, and have the following baseline laboratory studies: fasting blood sugar, lipid panel (including total cholesterol, low-density lipoprotein [LDL] cholesterol, and triglycerides), WBC count with differential, liver function panel (aspartate transaminase, alanine transaminase, alkaline phosphatase, and bilirubin), and electrocardiogram (ECG; with QTc read or calculated). This is in addition to the basic diagnostic evaluation described in Chapter 1 of this volume, "The Practice of Geriatric Psychopharmacology."

Dose and Dose Titration

Suggested initial doses, titration rates, and dose ranges for individual antipsychotic drugs are shown in the Specific Drug summaries at the end of this chapter. For all elderly patients, therapy is initiated at the lowest feasible dose, and some patients never require more than this minimum. Others will require upward dose titration, depending on factors such as age ("young-old" versus "old-old"), creatinine clearance, hepatic function, and diagnosis. In general, elders with schizophrenia require higher doses and those with dementia-related psychotic symptoms require lower doses of antipsychotics (Lacro et al. 1996).

Antipsychotic medications are titrated as rapidly as tolerated to target doses presumed to be therapeutic, as detailed in the Specific Drug summary. In practice, initial titration usually proceeds at a rate of one to two dose increases per week. For frail elders or those who are medically compromised, titration can be even slower. For medications with a wide dosing range (e.g., quetiapine), increases above the initial target dose are made after steady state is attained in order to avoid overshooting the minimal therapeutic dose for the individual patient.

During the initial stages of antipsychotic dose titration, it may be advisable to split doses (two to three times a day) to minimize problems from side effects such as orthostatic hypotension. For clozapine, quetiapine, ziprasidone, and low-potency typical agents, continued divided dosing (usually two times a day) is recommended (Ereshefsky 1996). For olanzapine, risperidone, aripiprazole, and high-potency typical antipsychotics, single bedtime doses may be used (Ereshefsky 1996).

PRN Use of Antipsychotics

When antipsychotic medications are used to control psychosis, standing rather than prn doses should be used, based on the hypothesis that consistent levels of drug at the receptor site are required for antipsychotic effect. Drugs other than clozapine can be used prn in situations such as the following: the prn dose is being used to supplement a small standing dose, with the intention of "adding" the total amount ingested to adjust the dose upward; the prn dose is used to minimize the amount of drug given, where the intention is to lower the dose; or the prn dose is used to control unexpected behaviors that cannot be managed using environmental or behavioral interventions. In the latter case, limits as to how many prn doses can be given apply to patients in long-term-care facilities. When antipsychotic medications are used prn, the effect of an individual dose is probably more related to general sedation than to specific antipsychotic effects.

Monitoring Treatment

Consensus Guidelines (Alexopoulos et al. 2004) suggest a schedule for follow-up appointments with geriatric patients who are prescribed antipsychotic medications:

- After an antipsychotic is started, the patient should be seen within 1–2 weeks.
- After a dose change, the patient should be seen in 10 days to 1 month.
- For monitoring, once the patient has been stable while taking the same dose of medication for 1 month, the patient should be seen every 2–3 months.
- During the maintenance phase, once the patient has been stable while taking the same antipsychotic for 6 months, the patient should be seen every 3–6 months.

In addition to scales used to measure improvement in targeted symptoms, other parameters are monitored to ensure patient safety. A suggested monitoring schedule is shown in Table 3–7. Vital signs, including temperature as well as orthostatic blood pressure and pulse, should be taken at least daily during dose titration for inpatients, and orthostatic vital signs (blood pressure and pulse) should be taken at each visit during dose titration for outpatients. During maintenance treatment, it is a reasonable practice to complete a scale for the assessment of abnormal movements such as the Abnormal Involuntary Movement Scale (AIMS) every 3–6 months. Weight should be checked monthly for 3 months during the initial stage of treatment, and then quarterly thereafter. Measurement of height at baseline will allow the use of a nomogram to calculate body mass index (BMI). (See discussion in "Metabolic Syndrome.") Waist circumference should be measured at least annually. Clozapine treatment requires more intensive hematologic surveillance; see discussion in "Hematologic Adverse Effects."

Serum Levels

For any antipsychotic, extreme values reported on serum level measurement may be helpful: a zero level could confirm suspected noncompliance or possibly suggest that a patient might be an ultraextensive metabolizer; conversely, a very high level could confirm suspected toxicity. Most commercial laboratories will perform these measurements. For purposes of therapeutic-level monitoring, only drugs with few active metabolites are usefully assayed, and not all of these drugs have been adequately studied.

Table 3–7. Suggested schedule for monitoring adverse effects of antipsychotic treatment

	Baseline	4 weeks	8 weeks	12 weeks	Quarterly	Every 6 months	Annually	Every 5 years
Abnormal Involuntary Movement Scale	X	X	X			X		
Blood pressure and pulse (orthostatics)	X	X	X	X			X	
Electrocardiogram	X							
Fasting plasma glucose	X			X			X	
Fasting lipid profile	X			X				X
Liver function tests	X					X		
White blood cell count with differential	X	X				X		
Waist circumference	X						X	
Weight and height (body mass index calculation)	X	X	X	X	X			

Among antipsychotics, only clozapine, haloperidol, fluphenazine, thiothixene, and perphenazine have anything resembling established therapeutic ranges, and these are usually inapplicable to the geriatric population.

Managing Treatment Resistance

Initial management of apparent treatment resistance follows a logical sequence of confirming the diagnosis, ruling out comorbid substance abuse or other confounding conditions, ascertaining compliance, and adjusting the medication dose. Dose adjustments are usually made on the basis of clinically observed therapeutic effects and adverse effects, but drug levels can be checked to determine extreme values (zero or orders of magnitude above therapeutic range). The patient functioning poorly on an antipsychotic in the presence of EPS or akathisia may benefit more from a dose decrease than a dose increase, since the adverse effect may be overwhelming the therapeutic benefit.

True treatment resistance is defined by nonresponse to two adequate antipsychotic trials. In general, patients with schizophrenia that is truly treatment resistant should first be switched to a third atypical agent other than clozapine and maintained on an adequate dose of that agent for 6–12 weeks (Marder 1996). If there is a partial response, the trial should be maintained up to 16 weeks. If there is still an inadequate response, a trial of clozapine should be considered. This trial should be continued, if possible, for a period of 6–12 months. Adjunctive therapies such as mood stabilizers could be used to augment a partial response (Marder 1996).

Switching Antipsychotics

When switching from one antipsychotic to another, it is generally safer to taper and discontinue one agent before starting the second. When this is not feasible because of severity of psychotic symptoms, the second drug can be added to the first, which can then be tapered and discontinued. This strategy is termed *cross-tapering*. During the course of antipsychotic cross-tapering, careful attention should be paid to cardiac conduction and other potential adverse effects such as orthostasis and EPS. One-step switching, in which the first antipsychotic is stopped and the second started (often at a therapeutic or near-therapeutic dose), has not been demonstrated to be safe in elderly patients. It has been reported to be done safely in nonelderly patients with aripiprazole (Casey et al. 2003). It cannot be done with clozapine.

In the course of cross-tapering to switch from a conventional antipsychotic to an atypical agent, a therapeutic response is sometimes seen that is followed by clinical worsening as the cross-taper proceeds. In this situation, it is difficult to know whether the problem is the decreasing level of conventional drug, the increasing level of atypical drug, or some interaction. If clinically reasonable, it may be best to complete the cross-taper to give the second medication an adequate trial as monotherapy. This is consistent with current guidelines advocating antipsychotic monotherapy as the gold standard of treatment. Although the combination of a conventional and an atypical antipsychotic is not recommended in the treatment of elderly patients, it is sometimes used in practice.

In switching a patient from an oral agent to a decanoate formulation, it is necessary to determine first that the patient tolerates the particular medication (haloperidol or fluphenazine) by giving several doses of the oral drug. When the injection is then given, the oral agent is continued for a minimum of 3–5 days while the deposited drug undergoes hydrolysis, a prerequisite to absorption.

To switch a patient from oral risperidone to long-acting, injectable risperidone, the manufacturer recommends continuing oral risperidone for a minimum of 3 weeks. In practice, some clinicians have found it necessary to continue the oral drug for as long as 4–6 weeks to maintain symptom stability (Masand and Gupta 2003).

Duration of Treatment

Consensus Guidelines include suggestions as to the usual duration of antipsychotic medication treatment for various indications, which are shown in Table 3–8.

Discontinuation

Elders with schizophrenia are best maintained long-term with a stable, low dose of antipsychotic—preferably an atypical agent. For those without

Table 3–8. Suggested durations of antipsychotic treatment

Disorder	Duration of treatment	
	Before changing dose or switching if response is inadequate	After response, before trying to discontinue
Delirium	1 day	1 week
Dementia with agitation and delusions	5 days	3 months
Dementia with agitation without delusions	7 days	3 months
Schizophrenia	2 weeks	Indefinitely
Delusional disorder	2 weeks	6 months–indefinitely
Nonpsychotic major depression with agitation	1 week	2 months
Psychotic major depression	1 week	6 months
Nonpsychotic major depression with severe anxiety	2 weeks	2 months
Mania with psychosis	5 days	3 months
Mania without psychosis	1 week	2 months

Source. Adapted from Alexopoulos GS, Streim JE, Carpenter D, et al: "Using Antipsychotic Agents in Older Patients." *Journal of Clinical Psychiatry* 65 (suppl 2):5–104, 2004. Used with permission.

schizophrenia, periodic attempts to reduce the dose of the antipsychotic medication are recommended and even mandated for patients in long-term-care facilities. Unless adverse effects necessitate abrupt discontinuation, dose reduction should proceed slowly to minimize withdrawal symptoms. Conventional antipsychotics given at the recommended geriatric (low) doses should be tapered over 2 weeks, at a minimum. Clozapine withdrawal is complicated by the drug's anticholinergic and antiadrenergic activity as well as by the potential for rebound psychosis, such that the taper is best performed over a minimum of 4 weeks in elderly patients. An only slightly less protracted withdrawal period may apply to thioridazine because of its anticholinergic properties.

Overdose in Elderly Patients

Recommendations regarding overdose of atypical antipsychotics are specific to individual drugs, and are discussed in the Specific Drug summaries at the end of this chapter. Conventional antipsychotics are usually nonlethal when taken alone in overdose. Exceptions include highly anticholinergic drugs and drugs associated with significant prolongation of the QTc interval at high doses (haloperidol, thioridazine, mesoridazine, and fluphenazine). Signs of overdose with a conventional agent include tachycardia, hypotension, sedation, restlessness, delirium, and severe EPS. The syndrome can progress to cardiorespiratory arrest, coma, and death. Management includes gastric lavage and/or emesis while the patient is still conscious; activated charcoal if given within 1 hour of ingestion; control of hypotension, seizures, and EPS; and general supportive measures (including airway protection by intubation if needed and intravenous fluids). Antipsychotic drugs are not removed by dialysis. In monitored settings, anticholinergic (M_1 receptor) effects can be reversed with physostigmine 1–2 mg intravenously or intramuscularly (Schneider 1993), although this carries the risk of inducing bradycardia.

Adverse Effects

It has long been recognized that conventional antipsychotics place elderly patients at particular risk of EPS and tardive dyskinesia, and this has been a driving force for the increase in atypical antipsychotic use in geriatrics. In recent years, however, evidence has mounted that atypical antipsychotics carry their own host of nontrivial adverse effects, including an approximate 1.6- to 1.7-fold increased risk of death in elderly patients with dementia, even with short-term use (Schneider et al. 2005). Although investigation and debate continue regarding these issues, the FDA now requires boxed warnings for atypical antipsychotics regarding increased risk of mortality in geriatric patients with dementia. In addition, warnings are now required regarding the increased risk of stroke with risperidone, olanzapine, and aripiprazole. With longer-term use of atypical drugs (e.g., in elders with schizophrenia or bipolar disorder), other major issues will relate to weight gain, glucose dysregulation, and dyslipidemia, the constellation of signs making up the metabolic syndrome, as discussed later in this chapter.

Tables 3–9 and 3–10 show the relative severity of selected adverse effects for various conventional and atypical antipsychotics. Metabolic effects of atypical agents are included in a separate table and discussed in a later section of this chapter.

Adverse effects that are particularly problematic for elderly patients include QTc prolongation, orthostasis or hypotension, sedation, anticholinergic effects, and metabolic effects such as weight gain, glucose dysregulation, and dyslipidemia over the longer term. In addition, for certain patient populations, hyperprolactinemia can be problematic. These adverse effects and their management are discussed later in this chapter. The incidence of hypotensive and sedative effects may be influenced by the rate of titration; hence the recommendation to start low and go slow in older patients. Other factors include the rate of absorption and the frequency of dosing. Because of the potential for adverse antipsychotic effects in the elderly population, it is advisable to give small doses, divide doses (at least initially), titrate slowly, and use caution with oral liquid and short-acting parenteral preparations.

Clozapine use is fraught with its own set of risks not specific to the geriatric population, including agranulocytosis (discussed below), myocarditis, cardiomyopathy, and venous thromboembolism (Hagg et al. 2000). Sialorrhea, whether due to impaired swallowing (Pearlman 1994; Rabinowitz et al. 1996) or to increased salivary flow (Wirshing 2001),

Table 3–9.   Adverse effects of conventional antipsychotics: relative severity

Drug		Adverse effects			
Generic name	Trade name	Sedation (H₁ receptor)	Extrapyramidal (dopamine receptor)	Anticholinergic (M₁ receptor)	Orthostasis (α₁ adrenergic receptor)
chlorpromazine	Thorazine	+++	+	+++	+++
fluphenazine	Prolixin	+	+++	+	+
haloperidol	Haldol	+	+++	+	+
loxapine	Loxitane	++	++	+	++
mesoridazine	Serentil	+++	+	++	++
molindone	Moban	+	++	+	+
perphenazine	Trilafon	+	++	+	++
pimozide	Orap	+	+++	+	+
thioridazine	Mellaril	+++	+	+++	+++
thiothixene	Navane	+	+++	+	+
trifluoperazine	Stelazine	+	+++	+	+

Note.   + = mild severity; ++ = moderate severity; +++ = substantial severity; H_1 = histamine; M_1 = muscarinic.
Source.   Adapted from Pies RW: "Antipsychotics," in *Handbook of Essential Psychopharmacology*, 2nd Edition. Washington, DC, American Psychiatric Publishing, 2005, p. 162. Used with permission.

Table 3–10. Adverse effects of atypical antipsychotics: relative severity

Generic name	Trade name	Adverse effects					
		Sedation	EPS	Anticholinergic	Orthostasis	Increased QTc	Increased prolactin
aripiprazole	Abilify	0	+	+/−	0/+	0	0
clozapine	Clozaril	+++	0	+++	+++	+	0
olanzapine	Zyprexa	++	0/+	++	+/++	0/+	0/+
quetiapine	Seroquel	++	0	+	++	++	0/+
risperidone	Risperdal	+	+/++	+	++	+/++	++/+++
ziprasidone	Geodon	+	+	+	+	+++	0/+

Note. This table does not include metabolic adverse effects, which are shown in Table 3–13. 0=none or almost none; +/−=equivocal or minor; +=mild; ++=moderate; +++=substantial; EPS=extrapyramidal side effects.
Source. Adapted from Pies 2005.

places the elderly patient at risk of aspiration, especially at night. Adverse effects of clozapine that do inordinately affect elderly patients include hypotension and sedation, and because these effects are so common, they likely represent significant risks with clozapine use in elders.

Anticholinergic Effects

Peripheral effects of cholinergic receptor blockade include dry mouth, blurred vision, exacerbation of glaucoma, constipation, urinary retention, and tachycardia, any of which could be serious in the elderly patient. Central effects of muscarinic receptor blockade include drowsiness, irritability, disorientation, impaired memory and other cognitive dysfunction, assaultiveness, and delirium. Patients with dementia characterized by cholinergic hypofunction (e.g., Alzheimer's disease, dementia with Lewy bodies [DLB]) are likely to be particularly affected. When these symptoms are mistaken for escalating psychosis, the dose of antipsychotic may be increased, resulting in worsening dysfunction. Among conventional antipsychotics, chlorpromazine, thioridazine, and mesoridazine are the most anticholinergic, and among atypical antipsychotics, clozapine and olanzapine are the most anticholinergic. Although in younger patients the anticholinergic effects of olanzapine are considered negligible at usual therapeutic doses, this may not be the case in the geriatric population, particularly among those with dementia (Mulsant et al. 2004).

Cardiovascular and Related Effects

Hypotension/Orthostasis

Significant hypotension is defined as a systolic blood pressure less than 90 mmHg, and significant orthostatic hypotension is defined as a drop in systolic blood pressure of more than 15–20 mmHg, when the patient sits up from lying or stands. These effects are related to α_1 adrenoceptor antagonism. Relative severity of orthostatic effects of conventional and atypical antipsychotics is shown in Tables 3–9 and 3–10. Orthostasis is more common in elderly patients, in those with reduced cardiac output, and in those taking other α_1-blocking medications. The importance of this problem in older patients cannot be overstated. Both hypotension and orthostatic hypotension are associated with falls, myocardial infarction, and cerebral ischemia, including stroke. In most cases, these effects develop early in the course of antipsychotic treatment. Because they are highly dependent on speed of absorption and peak plasma level of drug with α_1 effects, it is likely that they occur more frequently with parenterally administered or oral liquid preparations. For patients with baseline orthostasis, an antipsychotic medication with low affinity for the α_1 receptor such as aripiprazole is preferred. Standard management of orthostasis is discussed in Chapter 4 of this volume, "Antidepressants," in the section on antidepressant adverse effects.

QTc Prolongation

As shown in Figure 3–1, the QT interval spans the time from the start of ventricular depolarization (the Q wave of the QRS complex) to the end of ventricular repolarization (the T wave). The QT shortens as the heart rate increases and is corrected for heart rate (QTc) by one of several algorithms. The Bazett correction formula is shown in Figure 3–1. QTc prolongation is defined as a QTc value > 450 ms for men or > 470 ms for women (Taylor 2003). The use of a percentage increase over baseline is problematic because determination of the baseline value is complicated; the quantity normally varies even over the course of a day. In one study of subjects with normal heart rates, the difference between daytime and nighttime QT values ranged from 35–108 ms, with nighttime values being higher (Morganroth et al. 1991).

Usually, QTc prolongation results from delayed or prolonged repolarization, which may enable early after-depolarizations to occur and set the stage for extrasystoles and eventual *torsades de pointes*. This condition may result in dizziness or syncope or may progress to ventricular fibrillation and sudden death (Taylor 2003). QTc intervals > 500 ms are particularly worrisome, since they are associated with a significant risk of ventricular dysrhythmia and sudden death.

Antipsychotic medications are known to affect the QTc in a dose- and level-dependent manner (Taylor 2003). In one large epidemiologic study, patients taking antipsychotics in dose-equivalents of more than 100 mg thioridazine had a 2.4-fold increase in rate of sudden death (Ray et al. 2001). A comparative study of antipsychotics in a nongeriatric sample examined serial ECGs and found that although none of the QTc in-

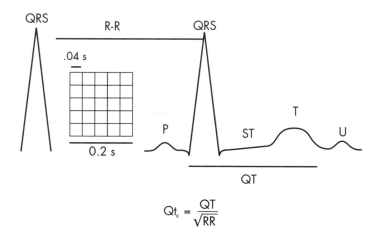

Figure 3–1. The QTc interval on the electrocardiogram.

Source. Adapted from Adler J: "QTc Calculator," July 31, 2003. Available at: http://www.pocket-doc.com/QTc.htm. Accessed October 30, 2005. Used with permission.

tervals of treated patients was over 500 ms, the antipsychotics affected the QTc differentially (Harrigan et al. 2004). The rank order of antipsychotics from most to least effect on QTc was as follows: thioridazine (30.1 ms), ziprasidone (15.9 ms), haloperidol (7.1 ms), quetiapine (5.7 ms), risperidone (3.9 ms), olanzapine (1.7 ms) (Harrigan et al. 2004). Aripiprazole and clozapine were not included in the study.

The risk of using antipsychotics is amplified in the presence of other risk factors for QTc prolongation. These include preexisting cardiovascular disease (including congenital and other occult cardiac lesions), electrolyte abnormalities (particularly hypokalemia or hypomagnesemia), thyroid disease, and structural brain disease (stroke, trauma) (Vieweg 2002). Significant liver disease may also increase risk, possibly only if acute (Tei et al. 2004).

If a prolonged QTc is encountered clinically, the following actions have been recommended (Vieweg 2002):

1. Repeat the ECG.
2. Check potassium, magnesium, and calcium levels, as well as thyroid-stimulating hormone level or thyroid panel.
3. Reassess cardiac history, including family history of syncope or sudden death. (These factors can modify risk and influence decisions regarding future treatment.)
4. In cases of confirmed QTc prolongation (especially if QTc > 500 ms), syncope, presyncope, or palpitations, urgent consultation with a cardiologist is recommended.

Urgent treatment of prolonged QTc includes discontinuing all offending medications; suppressing early after-depolarizations by administration of intravenous magnesium, potassium, and lidocaine; and increasing the heart rate to shorten the QT interval by pacing or administration of isoproterenol. The patient may require sedation during the treatment period.

Stroke

The FDA has issued a warning regarding the risk of stroke among elderly patients with dementia and psychosis or other behavioral disturbances who are treated with risperidone, olanzapine, or aripiprazole. It is not yet clear whether other atypical or conventional antipsychotics should be included in this warning.

Possible mechanisms by which atypical antipsychotics could cause stroke include thromboembolic effects (e.g., on coagulation or platelet function), orthostasis, cardiac dysrhythmias, or oversedation leading to hemoconcentration or dehydration; as yet there is no evidence favoring one particular mechanism. In fact, two large, population-based, retrospective cohort studies comparing atypical to conventional antipsychotics showed no increased stroke risk for atypical agents (Gill et al. 2005; Herrmann et al. 2004), and a review of data from 11 randomized controlled trials also failed to show evidence of increased risk (Herrmann and Lanctot 2005). Because these comparisons were made against conventional antipsychotics that might themselves confer increased risk, it is difficult to come to a reasonable conclusion without more definitive information. In the interim, because of the potential risk of stroke and sudden death, the recommended course of action is to raise the threshold for prescribing antipsychotic drugs to elderly patients (particularly those with dementia), to do a thoughtful risk-benefit analysis before deciding to use one of these agents, and to obtain fully informed consent from the patient or substitute decision-maker before proceeding with treatment (Katz 2004). It should be noted that this would represent a change from current practice for many clinicians.

Hematologic Effects

A decline in WBC counts can be seen with typical antipsychotics, particularly low-potency phenothiazines. Agranulocytosis (absolute neutrophil count $< 500/mm^3$) is a potentially life-threatening condition associated with clozapine therapy and much more rarely with other phenothiazines (chlorpromazine, fluphenazine, perphenazine, thioridazine, and trifluoperazine). Case reports have appeared in the literature of agranulocytosis associated with olanzapine and quetiapine use, but a clear cause-effect relationship has not been established for these drugs. The risk of agranulocytosis with clozapine and other medications is highest in the first few months of treatment, but it can occur at any time and is not a dose-dependent development. The overall risk is less than 1% but may be higher in the geriatric population.

Because of the risk of agranulocytosis, weekly WBC checks are required for at least the first 6 months of clozapine treatment and for a minimum of 4 weeks after clozapine discontinuation. If cell counts remain acceptable during the first 6 months of treatment (WBC count at least $3,000/mm^3$ and absolute neutrophil count at least $1,500/mm^3$), WBC checks can be done every other week thereafter for the next 6 months. If cell counts remain acceptable during the second 6 months of treatment, WBC checks can thereafter be done monthly. Other drugs with the potential for bone marrow suppression, including amoxicillin, carbamazepine, captopril, sulfonamides, and propylthiouracil, should be avoided in combination with clozapine (McEvoy et al. 2006). Specific recommendations for management of leukopenia and agranulocytosis with clozapine treatment are shown in Table 3–11.

Table 3–11. Hematologic monitoring with clozapine

Situation	Hematologic values for monitoring	Frequency of WBC and ANC monitoring
Initiation of therapy[a]	WBC $\geq$3,500/mm^3 ANC $\geq$2,000/mm^3	Weekly for 6 months
6–12 months of therapy	All results for WBC $\geq$3,500/mm^3 and ANC $\geq$2,000/mm^3	Every 2 weeks for 6 months
12 months of therapy	All results for WBC $\geq$3,500/mm^3 and ANC $\geq$2,000/mm^3	Every 4 weeks ad infinitum
Immature forms present	N/A	Repeat WBC and ANC
Discontinuation of therapy	N/A	Weekly for at least 4 weeks from day of discontinuation or until WBC >3,500/mm^3 and ANC >2,000/mm^3
Substantial drop in WBC or ANC	Single drop or cumulative drop within 3 weeks of WBC $\geq$3,000/mm^3 or ANC $\geq$1,500/mm^3	1. Repeat WBC and ANC. 2. If repeat values are 3,000/mm^3 $\leq$ WBC $\leq$3,500/mm^3 and ANC <2,000/mm^3, then monitor twice weekly.
Mild leukopenia/ Mild granulocytopenia	3,500/mm^3 > WBC$\geq$ 3,000/mm^3 and/or 2,000/mm^3 >ANC$\geq$ 1,500/mm^3	Twice weekly until WBC >3,500/mm^3 and ANC> 2,000/mm^3, then return to previous monitoring frequency

Table 3–11. Hematologic monitoring with clozapine (*continued*)

Situation	Hematologic values for monitoring	Frequency of WBC and ANC monitoring
Moderate leukopenia/ Moderate granulocytopenia	$3,000/mm^3 > WBC \geq 2,000/mm^3$ and/or $1,500/mm^3 > ANC \geq 1,000/mm^3$	1. Interrupt therapy 2. Daily until $WBC > 3,000/mm^3$ and $ANC > 1,500/mm^3$ 3. Twice weekly until $WBC > 3,500/mm^3$ and $ANC > 2,000/mm^3$ 4. May rechallenge when $WBC > 3,500/mm^3$ and $ANC > 2,000/mm^3$ 5. If rechallenged, monitor weekly for 1 year before returning to the usual monitoring schedule of every 2 weeks for 6 months and then every 4 weeks ad infinitum.
Severe leukopenia/ Severe granulocytopenia	$WBC < 2,000/mm^3$ and/or $ANC < 1,000/mm^3$	1. Discontinue treatment and do not rechallenge patient 2. Monitor until normal and for at least 4 weeks from day of discontinuation as follows: Daily until $WBC > 3,000/mm^3$ and $ANC > 1,500/mm^3$ Twice weekly until $WBC > 3500/mm^3$ and $ANC > 2,000/mm^3$ Weekly after $WBC > 3,500/mm^3$

Table 3–11. Hematologic monitoring with clozapine *(continued)*

Situation	Hematologic values for monitoring	Frequency of WBC and ANC monitoring
Agranulocytosis	ANC ≤500/mm^3	1. Discontinue treatment and do not rechallenge patient. 2. Monitor until normal and for at least 4 weeks from day of discontinuation as follows: Daily until WBC >3,000/mm^3 and ANC >1,500/mm^3 Twice weekly until WBC >3,500/mm^3 and ANC >2,000/mm^3 Weekly after WBC >3,500/mm^3

Note. ANC=absolute neutrophil count; WBC=white blood cell count.
[a]Do not initiate clozapine in patients with a history of myeloproliferative disorder or in those with clozapine-induced agranulocytosis or granulocytopenia.

Source. Adapted from *Physicians' Desk Reference,* 60th Edition. Oradell, NJ, Medical Economics, 2006, p. 2176.

Metabolic Syndrome

Metabolic syndrome is defined by abnormal values in the following variables: waist circumference, fasting blood glucose, blood pressure, triglycerides, and high-density lipoproteins (HDL) cholesterol. As shown in Table 3–12, metabolic syndrome is diagnosed when three or more of five criteria are met. The metabolic syndrome parameters represent an important target of risk-reduction therapy for coronary heart disease, approaching elevated LDL cholesterol in significance (National Cholesterol Education Program 2001). Prothrombotic and proinflammatory states are factors in the development of the metabolic syndrome that have not been included in the defining criteria (National Cholesterol Education Program 2001). Thakore (2005) and others have raised the question as to whether chronic stress with associated hypercortisolemia might also be implicated in the development of the syndrome.

Although randomized, head-to-head, prospective studies are lacking, it appears that individual atypical antipsychotics differ in the degree of associated risk for the development of the metabolic syndrome. In general, clozapine and olanzapine may confer the greatest risk and aripiprazole and ziprasidone the least risk. Data for quetiapine and risperidone are conflicting and difficult to interpret, particularly with regard to glucose dysregulation and dyslipidemia. Table 3–13 displays a risk data summary with regard to individual atypical drugs (American Diabetes Association et al. 2004).

The link between psychotropic medications and risk factors for coronary heart disease has clear implications for the practice of geriatric psychopharmacology. It is no longer tenable to partition patient care into "psychiatric" versus "medical" domains; all prescribers need to be aware of the risks, know how they are measured or assayed, work closely with primary care providers, and be ready to refer patients to specialists (cardiologists or endocrinologists) when appropriate.

When treatment with an atypical antipsychotic is being considered for an elderly patient, the clinician should first determine whether the patient is overweight or obese, has pre-diabetes or diabetes, is hypertensive, or has preexisting dyslipidemia. To establish whether a patient is overweight, the clinician determines the patient's BMI using currently measured weight and height. These measurements are used with a nomogram

Table 3–12. National Cholesterol Education Program Adult Treatment Panel III: definition of metabolic syndrome

Three or more of the following:

Waist circumference	Males: >40 inches (>102 cm)
	Females: >35 inches (>88 cm)
Fasting glucose	≥100 mg/dL
Blood pressure	≥130/85
Triglycerides	≥150 mg/dL
HDL cholesterol	Males: <40 mg/dL
	Females: <50 mg/dL

Source. Reprinted from Expert Panel on Detection, Evaluation, and Treatment of High Blood Cholesterol in Adults: "Executive Summary of the Third Report of the National Cholesterol Education Program (NCEP) (Adult Treatment Panel III)." *Journal of the American Medical Association* 285:2486–2497, 2001. Used with permission.

Table 3–13. Adverse metabolic effects of atypical antipsychotics: relative severity

Drug	Weight gain	Diabetes risk[a]	Dyslipidemia
Clozapine	+++	+	+
Olanzapine	+++	+	+
Risperidone	++	C	C
Quetiapine	++	C	C
Aripiprazole	+/–	–	–
Ziprasidone	+/–	–	–

Note. +=increased effect; –=no significant effect; C=conflicting data.
[a]The U.S. Food and Drug Administration has now issued a blanket, class-effect warning regarding glycemic dyscontrol for all atypical antipsychotics. Long-term data are more limited with the newer drugs aripiprazole and ziprasidone.
Source. Reprinted from American Diabetes Association, American Psychiatric Association, American Association of Clinical Endocrinologists, et al: "Consensus development conference on antipsychotic drugs and obesity and diabetes." *Diabetes Care* 27:596–601, 2004. Copyright 2004, American Diabetes Association. Used with permission.

like that shown in Figure 3–2 to determine BMI. As noted, a patient with a BMI of 25–29.9 would be classified as overweight, while a patient with a BMI of ≥30 would be classified as obese. Fasting blood glucose levels of ≥100–125 mg/dL would be consistent with pre-diabetes, while levels of ≥126 mg/dL would be consistent with diabetes. Blood pressure >140/90 is considered high, but note that the metabolic syndrome guidelines place the cutoff at >130/85. Lipid levels are stratified and high levels posited as follows (American Diabetes Association et al. 2004):

- LDL cholesterol: <100, optimal; 100–129, near or above optimal; 130–159, borderline high; 160–189, high; ≥190, very high
- Total cholesterol: <200, desirable; 200–239, borderline high; ≥240 high
- HDL cholesterol: <40, low; ≥60, high

For patients with LDL or total cholesterol falling into the high or borderline high ranges or HDL cholesterol falling in the low range, the clinician should not hesitate to refer back to the primary care physician or to an appropriate specialist.

During the course of treatment with an antipsychotic, metabolic syndrome parameters must be monitored. The prescribing clinician may work in tandem with the patient's primary care physician, but he or she should not assume that these labs will be checked routinely. A very specific set of recommendations has been set forth by the Consensus Development Conference on Antipsychotic Drugs and Obesity and Diabetes regarding scheduled monitoring, as shown in Table 3–14 (American Diabetes Association et al. 2004).

For elderly patients with schizophrenia who develop metabolic syndrome or one of its components on an atypical antipsychotic, the clinician should consider a switch to another agent such as aripiprazole or ziprasidone. If this is not feasible or if the trial of the new agent fails, the patient could still be treated with the offending antipsychotic, but he or she should be maintained at the lowest effective dose and should be monitored in close accordance with the American Diabetes Association (ADA) guidelines (Melkersson and Dahl 2004). It is not yet clear which of the metabolic syndrome parameters is reliably related to antipsychotic dose.

	Body mass index (kg/m²)												
	19	20	21	22	23	24	25	26	27	28	29	30	35	40
	Normal						Overweight					Obese		
Height (inches)	Weight (lb)												
58	91	96	100	105	110	115	119	124	129	134	138	143	167	191
59	94	99	104	109	114	119	124	128	133	138	143	148	173	198
60	97	102	107	112	118	123	128	133	138	143	148	153	179	204
61	100	106	111	116	122	127	132	137	143	148	153	158	185	211
62	104	109	115	120	126	131	136	142	147	153	158	164	191	218
63	107	113	118	124	130	135	141	146	152	158	163	169	197	225
64	110	116	122	128	134	140	145	151	157	163	169	174	204	232
65	114	120	126	132	138	144	150	156	162	168	174	180	210	240
66	118	124	130	136	142	148	155	161	167	173	179	186	216	247
67	121	127	134	140	146	153	159	166	172	178	185	191	223	255
68	125	131	138	144	151	158	164	171	177	184	190	197	230	262
69	128	135	142	149	155	162	169	176	182	189	196	203	236	270
70	132	139	146	153	160	167	174	181	188	195	202	207	243	278
71	136	143	150	157	165	172	179	186	193	200	208	215	250	286
72	140	147	154	162	169	177	184	191	199	206	213	221	258	294
73	144	151	159	166	174	182	189	197	204	212	219	227	265	302
74	148	155	163	171	179	186	194	202	210	218	225	233	272	311
75	152	160	168	176	184	192	200	208	216	224	232	240	279	319
76	156	164	172	180	189	197	205	213	221	230	238	246	287	328

Figure 3–2. Determination of body mass index.

Note. Parameters for normal based on National Institutes of Health: "Clinical Guidelines on the Identification, Evaluation, and Treatment of Overweight and Obesity in Adults— The Evidence Report." *Obesity Research* 6 (suppl 2): 51S–201S, 1998.

Weight Gain

Significant weight gain may occur with atypical antipsychotic use, often within the first 6–12 weeks of treatment (Wetterling 2001). Patients with lower BMI at baseline may be at higher risk for weight gain. Once weight has been gained, it is very difficult to lose; only small reductions are seen with either pharmacologic or behavioral programs (Faulkner et al. 2003). Note that the ADA guidelines (Table 3–14) suggest weight checks monthly for the first 3 months and then only quarterly. Patients should be encouraged to check weight at home weekly between visits and

Table 3–14.   Schedule for monitoring: metabolic syndrome parameters

	Baseline	4 weeks	8 weeks	12 weeks	Quarterly	Annually	Every 5 years
Personal/Family history	X					X	
Weight (body mass index)	X	X	X	X	X		
Waist circumference	X					X	
Blood pressure	X			X		X	
Fasting plasma glucose	X			X		X	
Fasting lipid profile	X			X			X

Source.   Reprinted from American Diabetes Association, American Psychiatric Association, American Association of Clinical Endrocrinologists, et al: "Consensus Development Conference on Antipsychotic Drugs and Obesity and Diabetes." *Diabetes Care* 27:596–601, 2004. Copyright 2004, American Diabetes Association. Used with permission.

to schedule an earlier appointment if a significant weight gain (> 2 kg in 2 weeks) occurs at any time (Wetterling 2001). For a cumulative gain of ≥5% of initial weight, a switch to another antipsychotic should be considered and a weight management plan implemented.

The mechanism by which antipsychotics induce weight gain is not understood completely. It may relate to histamine H_1 or specific serotonin receptor ($5\text{-}HT_{2C}$) binding. Research focused on leptins has shown that serum leptin levels increase with weight gain and are correlated with the amount of weight gain, but apparently weight gain itself precedes leptin level increases (McIntyre et al. 2003a). More recently, it has been found that among olanzapine-treated patients, serum ghrelin levels also increased as leptin levels and body fat increased (Murashita et al. 2005), and that patients with high BMI treated with other atypical antipsychotics had high ghrelin levels (Palik et al. 2005). Normally, ghrelin levels are *inversely* proportional to leptin levels and body fat, and ghrelin has a role in appetite stimulation, so this finding may provide an important clue as to mechanism.

Summarizing the literature with regard to risk of weight gain with individual drugs among patients of unselected age, the rank order of atypical antipsychotics, from most to least weight gain, is as follows: clozapine > olanzapine >> risperidone, quetiapine >> ziprasidone, aripiprazole (Allison et al. 1999). The results of the CATIE trial support this general ranking; in that trial, olanzapine was associated with the greatest weight gain and ziprasidone the least (Lieberman et al. 2005). The risk of weight gain with quetiapine is actually controversial: some studies have found an association with weight gain, and it has been speculated that this relates to the dibenzodiazepine structure that quetiapine has in common with olanzapine and clozapine (McIntyre et al. 2003b). Among conventional antipsychotics, the higher-potency agents such as fluphenazine and haloperidol are at the lower end of the weight-gain continuum, while the lower potency agents chlorpromazine and thioridazine/mesoridazine are at the higher end (more weight gain) (Allison et al. 1999). Molindone also has little potential to induce weight gain (Richelson 1996).

Diabetes Mellitus

The mechanism by which atypical antipsychotics induce glucose dysregulation and overt diabetes mellitus is not fully understood. It is not completely explained by weight gain (Howes et al. 2004). Diabetes appears to be reversible on discontinuation of antipsychotic or dose lowering in only some patients (Koller et al. 2001). Rechallenge results in recurrence of diabetes in the majority of patients and in some patients within days of restarting the medication (Koller et al. 2001). A similar rank-ordering of atypical antipsychotics may apply to the potential for glucose dysregulation as to other elements of the metabolic syndrome; from most to least glucose dysregulation: clozapine, olanzapine >> quetiapine > risperidone > ziprasidone, aripiprazole (Koller et al. 2004; Lindenmayer et al. 2003). In the CATIE study, quetiapine and risperidone were equally implicated in glucose dysregulation (Lieberman et al. 2005).

Glucose dysregulation can occur in any patient who is treated with an atypical agent but is most problematic for patients with preexisting insulin-dependent diabetes. These patients can develop diabetic ketoacidosis, a serious condition that is sometimes fatal. The signs of diabetic ketoacidosis include rapid onset of polyuria and/or polydipsia, weight loss, nausea, vomiting, dehydration, rapid respiration, and clouding of sensorium (American Diabetes Association et al. 2004).

Hyperlipidemia

As with other elements of the metabolic syndrome, the risk for hyperlipidemia is not distributed equally among the atypical antipsychotic agents. The rank order of medications from most to least lipid-elevating effect is as follows: clozapine, olanzapine >> quetiapine > risperidone >> ziprasidone, aripiprazole (Casey 2004; Lieberman et al. 2005). Less commonly, extremely high elevations of cholesterol and triglycerides are seen and have been reported with olanzapine as well as quetiapine (Meyer 2001).

Treatment options for a developing hyperlipidemia include switching to aripiprazole or ziprasidone (Kingsbury et al. 2001) and adding a lipid-lowering drug. Among the statins, pravastatin and fluvastatin are recommended for patients with psychotic illness. Other lipid-lowering drugs have significant potential for drug interactions or cause abdominal discomfort (Baptista et al. 2004).

Musculoskeletal System Effects

Treatment with atypical antipsychotics and haloperidol has been associated with a variable elevation in serum creatine kinase (CK) level (MM form) in the absence of obvious musculoskeletal pathology in about 10% of patients (Meltzer et al. 1996). In a minority of these, the elevation is extreme, in the range seen with rhabdomyolysis, although no evidence has been found of consequent impairment of renal function. It has been hypothesized that the increased CK activity might reflect changes in cell membrane permeability particularly affecting skeletal muscle in susceptible individuals (Meltzer et al. 1996). In the workup of elevated CK in the individual patient, this asymptomatic elevation serves as a diagnosis of exclusion, after conditions such as acute myocardial infarction or neuroleptic malignant syndrome (NMS) have been ruled out.

Neuropsychiatric Effects

Extrapyramidal Side Effects

A substantial amount of literature supports the belief that atypical antipsychotic agents are associated with rates of EPS significantly lower than those of typical agents. The results of the CATIE study, which compared perphenazine with atypicals in a nonelderly cohort of patients with schizophrenia, call this belief into question. In that study, no significant difference was found in the rate of EPS with perphenazine compared with olanzapine, quetiapine, risperidone, or ziprasidone over a course of 18 months (Lieberman et al. 2005). In fact, looking at actual percentages, perphenazine had a lower rate of associated EPS than either olanzapine or risperidone. These findings are confounded by the fact that patients with preexisting tardive dyskinesia were excluded from the perphenazine group and by the possibility that the dose of perphenazine used in the study may not have been equivalent to the atypical doses (Lieberman et al. 2005). Moreover, any attempt to interpret findings for application to the geriatric population is hindered by the fact that the doses of medications used were higher than the ceiling doses recommended for elders, as listed in the Specific Drug summaries at the end of this chapter.

Neither clozapine nor aripiprazole was included in the CATIE study. Clozapine is not associated with parkinsonian symptoms at any dose and has a low prevalence of associated akathisia (Chengappa et al. 1994). Among the other atypical agents, quetiapine is most like clozapine in its profile of EPS. In past studies, actual improvement of EPS has been noted with added clozapine, olanzapine (Sajatovic et al. 1998), and aripiprazole (Madhusoodanan et al. 2004). (Case reports of EPS and akathisia with aripiprazole have been confounded by coadministered drugs.) Risperidone is poised between the typical and atypical agents in its extrapyramidal profile; at doses above 4 mg in elders, it may have effects as pronounced as those of the conventional agents, whereas at low doses (1 mg/day or less), it has little extrapyramidal effect, except perhaps akathisia. Patients who are CYP2D6 poor metabolizers are at risk for EPS with certain drugs (e.g., fluphenazine, risperidone) (Schillevoort et al. 2002). For these patients, doses should be lowered or a drug not metabolized by CYP2D6 should be used. With the conventional agent haloperidol, parenteral as opposed to oral administration is associated with a greatly reduced incidence of parkinsonian symptoms but probably not of akathisia.

The pattern of EPS affecting elderly patients differs in some important ways from that found in younger populations. The risk of akathisia decreases with age, with a rate of 3% found in those over 65 years of age (Wirshing 2001). Likewise, the risk of dystonia decreases with age, with a rate of 15% found in those over 65 years of age (Wirshing 2001). Drug-induced parkinsonism, on the other hand, is more common among antipsychotic-treated elders. This syndrome resembles idiopathic parkinsonism, with symptoms of bradykinesia, rigidity, impaired righting reflex, dysphagia, sialorrhea, autonomic instability, and even seborrhea (Wirshing 2001). Symptoms do not usually manifest immediately, but after 1–2 weeks of treatment (Wirshing 2001).

Parkinsonian symptoms are the hallmark of diseases associated with α-synuclein accumulation, including PD, Parkinson's disease with dementia (PDD), and DLB (Aarsland et al. 2005). A particularly worrisome syndrome found most commonly in those with DLB (but also in PDD) is neuroleptic sensitivity reaction. This can occur in response to any antipsychotic, including atypical agents. It is characterized by the sudden onset of sedation, increased confusion, rigidity, and immobility (Aarsland et al. 2005).

Parkinsonian symptoms greatly influence the quality of life for the treated elder by affecting functional ability, including walking and eating, and increasing the incidence of events such as falls. In spite of this, routine prophylaxis with antiparkinsonian drugs is not recommended for elders, even in the initial phases of treatment, since almost all such drugs have anticholinergic effects that are seriously problematic in most older people. When antipsychotic-treated elders develop EPS, attempts are made to discontinue or lower the dose of medication or to add or switch to an atypical agent. If the offending antipsychotic is discontinued, EPS should resolve within several weeks, but in some cases signs and symptoms persist for a year or more (Eimer 1992). If additional treatment of parkinsonism is required, amantadine can be used; this is a dopamine reuptake blocker and D_2 receptor agonist well tolerated at low dosages (e.g., 12.5–50 mg two times a day).

Neuroleptic Malignant Syndrome

The central features of NMS include high fever, muscle rigidity, change in level of consciousness (often fluctuating), and autonomic instability. Different diagnostic criteria exist, and not all require the *simultaneous* presence of fever and rigidity. Laboratory abnormalities frequently include elevations in CK, WBC count, and liver transaminases (AST and ALT). Three serious medical events may ensue: rhabdomyolysis, renal failure, and disseminated intravascular coagulation. The development of renal failure is an ominous sign that may herald a fatal outcome. More rarely, liver failure is seen. The syndrome occurs most often with antipsychotic treatment but also can occur with dopamine agonist withdrawal (e.g., with levodopa or pramipexole) and other prescribed and abused drugs (Fink and Taylor 2003).

In practice, NMS is seen more commonly in younger adults than in the elderly, but its incidence may be increased by neurologic disease (particularly PD and related α-synucleinopathies) or debilitation, or by a rapid rate of initial antipsychotic titration. Although NMS is usually associated with conventional antipsychotics, similar symptoms have been reported in connection with every atypical antipsychotic currently on the market. Mortality rates appear to be lower with atypical agents, but this could be attributed to increasing vigilance and earlier detection of the syndrome in recent years (Ananth et al. 2004). Use of serum CK to guide diagnosis is sometimes confounded by the association of CK elevation with atypical antipsychotic treatment or with psychosis itself in the absence of other signs or symptoms of NMS, as discussed earlier under "Musculoskeletal System Effects."

NMS represents a medical emergency that should be managed in a monitored setting, with aggressive hydration and treatment of comorbid medical illnesses. The offending antipsychotic (or other drug) should be discontinued. It remains controversial whether benzodiazepines treat NMS per se (as a form of catatonia) or only serve to alleviate anxiety. When CK levels are very high or still increasing, or when there is persistent rigidity or fever, dantrolene and/or bromocriptine may be useful. Electroconvulsive therapy (ECT) has been reported to be effective in facilitating a rapid resolution of the syndrome (Fink and Taylor 2003). NMS is discussed more fully in Chapter 8 of this volume, "Treatment of Movement Disorders."

Sedation

Histamine (H_1) receptor binding underlies sedation and at least contributes to weight gain, both commonly seen in antipsychotic-treated patients. Tables 3–9 and 3–10 show relative sedative effects of various typical and atypical agents. Sedation in elderly patients is associated with decreased oral intake, increased risk of falls, and increased risk of aspiration. Tolerance to sedative effects from antipsychotic medication often develops within a few days to several weeks. For certain patients, particularly those on a combination of medications, sedation persists. When these patients require treatment over an extended period, high-potency (less sedating) antipsychotic drugs are preferred.

Seizures

Low-potency typical antipsychotic agents and clozapine are associated with an increased risk of seizures (McEvoy et al. 2006). For any antipsychotic, there is an increased incidence of seizures wherever there is a history of past seizure or structural brain disease. The correlation of clozapine and seizures is dose dependent; in patients of mixed age, the rate is 1% at doses <300 mg/day (Casey 1997), but approaches 4%–6% at doses >600 mg/day (Meltzer 1995). Tonic-clonic seizures may be preceded by myoclonus or drop attacks. In addition, epileptiform activity on electroencephalograms may predict the later development of seizures. Patients with any of these risk factors or who develop clinical seizures should be treated with dose reduction and more gradual titration or with addition of an anticonvulsant in consultation with a neurologist.

Tardive Dyskinesia

Tardive dyskinesia is a syndrome of abnormal involuntary movements associated with antipsychotic medication treatment. The syndrome occurs more frequently among elderly patients, women, patients with diabetes (Caligiuri and Jeste 2004), and patients without schizophrenia (Wirshing 2001). In general, the cumulative incidence is related to duration of antipsychotic use. The prevalence of tardive dyskinesia among elderly patients after 3 years of treatment with conventional antipsychotics is 60% (Jeste et al. 1995), and the incidence within the first few months of treatment is not trivial (Jeste et al. 1999). A variety of candidate genes have been studied as possible contributors to tardive dyskinesia susceptibility among neuroleptic-treated patients, with positive results for a *DRD3* Ser9Gly polymorphism (Lerer et al. 2002), certain CYP2D6 mutations (Nikoloff et al. 2002), and the C/C genotype of 5-HT_{2A} (Lattuada et al. 2004).

All conventional and all atypical antipsychotics have been reported in association with tardive dyskinesia, but the risk introduced by atypical antipsychotics appears to be lower than the risk with conventional agents. Although the CATIE study found no difference between perphenazine and the atypical agents in tardive dyskinesia measures, the study might have been too short to detect differences. Moreover, as noted above, patients with preexisting tardive dyskinesia were excluded from the perphenazine group but not the other groups (Lieberman et al. 2005). Further discussion of the clinical characteristics and treatment of tardive dyskinesia is found in Chapter 8.

Ocular Effects

Three types of ocular effects of antipsychotic treatment may be seen: abnormal pigmentation, pigmentary retinopathy, and lens opacification (cataracts). Pigmentation of the conjunctiva, cornea, lens, or retina is a usually benign side effect of low-potency phenothiazine antipsychotics. Pigmentary retinopathy is a serious condition that can result in irreversible visual impairment associated with use of thioridazine at high doses (greater than 800 mg in patients of mixed age) and perhaps mesoridazine. Elderly patients who are treated with thioridazine should have regular ophthalmologic examinations. Lens opacification (cataracts) can occur with phenothiazines and was formerly a concern with quetiapine. Earlier recommendations for twice-yearly ophthalmologic examinations with a slit lamp for quetiapine-treated patients have been replaced by the recommendation for routine eye examinations according to usual guidelines of the American Academy of Ophthalmology (Fraunfelder 2004).

Prolactin Elevation

Among atypical antipsychotics, risperidone is more likely than other agents to be associated with significant prolactin elevation (Montgomery et al. 2004). Aripiprazole and ziprasidone are considered prolactin-sparing drugs (Haddad and Wieck 2004; Lieberman et al. 2005). In young patients, prolactin elevations can be of concern because they may lead to hypogonadism. In elderly patients, the clinical sequelae are less clear. It has been observed that chronic use of dopamine antagonists confers a small but significant increased risk of breast cancer (Wang et al. 2002), but in fact it is unknown whether this is related to hyperprolactinemia (Haddad and Wieck 2004). On the other hand, prolactin elevation would likely be problematic for patients with existing prolactin-dependent metastatic breast carcinoma. Osteoporosis may be another concern in women with high prolactin levels (Becker et al. 2003), as may gynecomastia and galactorrhea in men.

Syndrome of Inappropriate Antidiuretic Hormone

A syndrome of inappropriate antidiuretic hormone (SIADH) secretion can occur with typical as well as atypical antipsychotic medications, especially in debilitated patients. The resulting hyponatremia may be associated with delirium, disorientation, or memory impairment and may progress to seizures, coma, and death, in severe cases. SIADH is distinguished from polydipsia (excessive water intake) by urine osmolality: relatively high urine osmolality is found with SIADH, and very low osmolality is found with polydipsia and water intoxication. As discussed in Chapter 4 of this volume, "Antidepressants," SIADH is also associated with a number of medical and neurologic diseases, and it is associated more commonly with antidepressants than antipsychotics.

Transaminase Elevation

Increases in serum transaminase levels (AST and ALT) of 1.5–2 times normal are common in the first few weeks of treatment in patients given typical or atypical antipsychotics (Casey 1997; Fuller et al. 1996). The usual clinical course is a return to normal values (Casey 1997). Higher increases in transaminase levels (three times normal or greater), elevation of alkaline phosphatase, or elevation of bilirubin should be cause for holding antipsychotic treatment. In addition, the patient should be monitored clinically for jaundice, malaise, or anorexia, all of which may precede alterations in liver function tests. Patients with a history of obstructive jaundice or preexisting liver disease should not be treated with phenothiazine antipsychotics.

Antipsychotic Treatment of Selected Syndromes and Disorders

Delirium

Delirium is a syndrome defined by a disturbed level of conscious awareness coupled with either a change in cognitive function or the development of a perceptual disturbance. Symptoms develop acutely and fluctuate over a 24-hour period. By definition, symptoms are secondary to medical illness or medications. A list of medical etiologies of delirium in elderly patients is shown in Table 3–15. It is very common among elderly patients for more than one cause to contribute to a delirium episode and for delirium to be superimposed on preexisting dementia.

Definitive treatment of the cause of delirium (e.g., correction of hyponatremia or treatment of urinary tract infection) always takes precedence over symptomatic treatment. Moreover, when environmental interventions are implemented early and consistently (Inouye et al. 1999), psychosis and agitation may be controlled without medication. Antipsychotic medications can be used to treat psychosis (hallucinations, delusions, or thought disorganization) or severe and persistent agitation in the delirious patient when these symptoms cause suffering, pose a danger, or interfere with needed care. There is currently no consensus among experts as to which antipsychotic agent is preferred; the three drugs used most commonly are haloperidol, quetiapine, and risperidone.

Table 3–15.   Selected causes of delirium in elderly patients

- Medications (especially anticholinergics, opioids, sedative-hypnotics, nonsteroidal anti-inflammatory drugs, chemotherapy drugs, certain antibiotics, digoxin)

- Infection (urinary tract infection, pneumonia, sepsis, encephalitis)

- Fluid/Electrolyte derangement (hypokalemia, hyponatremia, dehydration, constipation)

- Metabolic derangement (hypoxia, hypoglycemia, uremia, vitamin deficiency states, endocrine diseases)

- Inflammatory disease (temporal arteritis, vasculitis)

- Postoperative states (especially coronary artery bypass graft and hip fracture repair)

- Alcohol withdrawal

- Sedative withdrawal (benzodiazepines, barbiturates)

- Cardiovascular disease (severe hypertension, congestive heart failure, myocardial infarction, arrhythmia)

- Stroke or transient ischemic event

- Subdural hematoma

- Intracranial pathology (tumor, abscess, aneurysm)

- Fall with head injury

- Nonconvulsive status epilepticus

The advantages of haloperidol in the medically ill population are several: no significant hemodynamic effects at usual therapeutic doses, little or no respiratory depression, little effect on glucose regulation, and availability in intravenous form (so that ultralow doses can be used with good effect and little adverse effect). A recent report cited an association of haloperidol use with lower hospital mortality in mechanically ventilated patients (Milbrandt et al. 2005). Haloperidol is also a great deal less expensive than comparator drugs. The disadvantage of haloperidol is that high doses can prolong the QTc interval. In addition, this drug has well-documented EPS and can cause NMS and tardive dyskinesia when used long-term. These risks have been thought to be lower for the atypical agents.

The advantage of quetiapine is that it is highly sedating, and thus can quell agitation in delirium, but this medication can be overly sedating in the frail elderly patient. In addition, quetiapine can cause hypotension and glucose dysregulation, even with short-term use. Risperidone can be effective in reducing psychosis and agitation in delirium when dosed appropriately. Unfortunately, this medication is too often dosed and titrated as it is for the younger population, resulting in akathisia in the delirious elder. Risperidone also can cause hypotension.

Regardless of which agent is selected for the treatment of delirium, the course of treatment should be brief; the medication should be used until symptoms abate and then should be tapered off over 3–5 days. By limiting the duration of treatment, usual concerns about the development of tardive dyskinesia (with haloperidol) or metabolic syndrome (with quetiapine and risperidone) are not prohibitive.

Suggested dosing of antipsychotic medication for the elderly patient with delirium is as follows: haloperidol, 0.25–0.5 mg intravenously every 8 hours standing and 0.25–0.5 mg intravenously every 6 hours prn for agitation; quetiapine, 12.5–25 mg orally two to three times a day standing and 12.5–25 mg orally every 6 hours prn for agitation; risperidone, 0.25–1 mg orally two times a day standing and 0.25–1 mg orally every 6 hours prn for agitation.

For critically ill patients whose movements pose a medical hazard, such as those on ventilators or intra-aortic balloon pumps, and for terminally ill cancer patients, more aggressive treatment of agitation may be needed. Adams (1984) proposed a regimen involving a combination of intravenous haloperidol, lorazepam, and hydromorphone that is still often used in intensive care unit (ICU) settings. Although a great deal of anecdotal experience supports the use of this regimen in elderly patients, it has not been systematically studied in this population. Sedation in the ICU patient is discussed further in Chapter 6 of this volume, "Anxiolytic and Sedative-Hypnotic Medications."

Delusional Disorder

The same principles apply to delusional disorder as to schizophrenia (see "Schizophrenia and Schizoaffective Disorder" later in this chapter), except that delusional disorders may be less treatment-responsive and there is generally less need to control acute agitation. Chronic therapy may be indicated, and for this purpose the lowest effective dose of antipsychotic should be used. Atypical antipsychotics have been recommended as preferred agents. Consensus Guidelines suggest the following dosage ranges (Alexopoulos et al. 2004): risperidone, 0.75–2.5 mg/day; olanzapine, 5–10 mg/day; quetiapine, 50–200 mg/day.

Dementia With Psychotic Symptoms

Alzheimer's disease, vascular dementia, DLB, and other dementias are frequently associated with psychotic symptoms at some stage of the illness (Tariot 1996). Half of Alzheimer's disease patients develop psychotic symptoms within 3 years of initial diagnosis, and these symptoms persist at 18-month follow-up in the majority of patients (Finkel 2004). In DLB, psychotic symptoms in the form of visual hallucinations are in fact a central feature of the psychopathology. This can be a particularly vexing problem because these patients may have a neuroleptic sensitivity reaction to antipsychotic treatment, as mentioned in an earlier section.

In view of the potentially serious consequences of administering antipsychotics to patients with DLB, the differential diagnosis of dementia in elderly patients is critical (Ballard et al. 1998; McKeith et al. 1995). Furthermore, for patients with DLB, the only antipsychotics that can be used to treat psychosis without worsening motor function are clozapine and quetiapine (Baskys 2004). Both risperidone and olanzapine are associated with worsening of motor symptoms (Baskys 2004; McKeith et al. 1995). Ziprasidone and aripiprazole have been inadequately studied for this indication.

For patients with non–Lewy body dementia, typical or atypical agents can be used. These medications are best prescribed at very low doses on a standing rather than prn basis. As discussed in Chapter 9, antipsychotic medications have been used to treat aggression and dangerous agitation as well as psychosis in patients with dementia. For sundowning, the antipsychotic can be given 1–2 hours before the time of usual behavioral disturbance to take advantage of sedative effects. A randomized controlled trial of haloperidol for psychosis and disruptive behavior in Alzheimer's disease demonstrated that dosages of 2–3 mg/day provided the best balance of efficacy and side effects, with dosages below 1 mg/day being no more effective than placebo (Devanand et al. 1998). A randomized controlled trial of risperidone in a large cohort of elderly patients with dementia (Alzheimer's disease, vascular dementia, or mixed) demonstrated that an optimal dosage of risperidone of 1 mg/day was effective in reducing behavioral pathology (Katz et al. 1999; Kumar and Brecher 1999). Quetiapine (McManus et al. 1999) and aripiprazole also may also be effective for this indication; ziprasidone has not been studied.

Based in part on expert consensus guidelines, the following dosage ranges for treatment of patients with dementia and psychosis are suggested: risperidone, 0.5–2 mg/day; quetiapine, 50–200 mg/day (divided two times a day); olanzapine, 5–10 mg/day (Alexopoulos et al. 2004).

Depression With Psychotic Symptoms

The treatment of choice for elderly patients with major depression with psychotic features is ECT, which induces rapid remission. When a course of ECT is completed, the antidepressant effect must be maintained, either with antidepressant medication or with maintenance ECT treatment. Alternatively, an atypical antipsychotic such as aripiprazole or risperidone can be used in combination with an antidepressant such as venlafaxine or citalopram. Medications generally have a longer lag time to effect than ECT.

For elderly patients with psychotic depression, the Consensus Guidelines suggest that an antidepressant medication be given with an antipsychotic medication in the following dosage ranges: risperidone, 0.75–2.25 mg/day; olanzapine, 5–10 mg/day; quetiapine, 50–200 mg/day (Alexopoulos et al. 2004).

Mania

The use of atypical antipsychotic medications for the treatment of geriatric mania is increasing in spite of the absence of controlled trials exclusive to the elderly population. A recent randomized controlled trial of quetiapine versus lithium in a mixed-age sample showed that quetiapine was safe and effective at dosages of 400–800 mg/day (Bowden et al. 2005). These dosages exceed those recommended in the geriatric population. It is unclear at this writing whether growing concerns about weight gain, hyperlipidemia, glucose dysregulation, and increased mortality with the atypical agents will alter the trend favoring these drugs.

The Consensus Guidelines suggest the following atypical antipsychotic dose ranges for elderly patients with psychotic mania or severe nonpsychotic mania: risperidone, 1.25–3 mg/day; olanzapine, 5–15 mg/day; quetiapine, 50–250 mg/day (Alexopoulos et al. 2004).

Although it is not included in the consensus guideline recommendations, aripiprazole also may be useful for this indication; ziprasidone has not been studied in elderly patients. Although clozapine is effective in acute mania, it is not a drug of choice for elders because these patients are at greater risk than younger patients for developing agranulocytosis. Treatment of mania is discussed more fully in Chapter 5 of this volume, "Mood Stabilizers."

Parkinson's Disease With Psychosis

Among patients with PD, 20%–30% experience psychotic symptoms, mostly due to antiparkinsonian medications. The most common symptoms are visual hallucinations (with or without delirium), confusion, and paranoid delusions (Katz 2004). Clozapine is the most effective drug for the treatment of PD with psychosis and is the reference drug for this indication. At a dosage of 50 mg/day or less (modal dose of 25 mg), clozapine is associated with significant improvement in psychosis without exacerbation of parkinsonism (Parkinson Study Group 1999). Clozapine may also improve levodopa-induced dyskinesias (Durif et al. 2004). PD patients with psychosis who are treated with clozapine have a better prognosis over the longer term than untreated patients in terms of lowered mortality and reduced risk of nursing home placement (Fernandez et al. 2004). For patients with PD, clozapine should be initiated at a very low dosage (e.g., 6.25 mg/day) and titrated slowly. The dosage range for PD with psychosis is 6.25 mg–150 mg.

Quetiapine also shows promise in treating psychosis in patients with PD and appears to be neutral with regard to motor symptoms (Katz 2004). Because of its safer adverse-effect profile, quetiapine is rapidly becoming a drug of choice in the treatment of PD with psychosis. The dosage is usually in the range of 12.5–150 mg/day, with most patients treated effectively with ≤50 mg/day.

Olanzapine not only is ineffective for psychosis in PD but also is associated with worsening of motor deficits as well as gait and general functioning (Katz 2004). Several trials of aripiprazole have found this drug unhelpful for PD with psychosis, but initial doses were high and titration was more rapid than usual for elderly patients (Fernandez et al. 2004; Schonfeldt-Lecuona and Connemann 2004). Anecdotal evidence suggests that single doses of ziprasidone at 10 or 20 mg intramuscularly may be effective in calming agitated PD patients with psychosis without affecting motor symptoms (Oeschsner and Korchounov 2005), but there are as yet no data from controlled studies to recommend this treatment.

Anecdotal evidence also suggests that psychosis in PD may require indefinite treatment: in five out of six patients withdrawn after long-term stabilization on clozapine or quetiapine, psychosis recurred, with more severe symptoms in three patients (Fernandez et al. 2005). Finally, although the logistics of coadministration of levodopa and antipsychotic drugs are not completely clear, it makes sense to separate their administration in time (e.g., by giving the atypical antipsychotic at bedtime and the last dose of levodopa at dinnertime).

Schizophrenia and Schizoaffective Disorder

The population of elderly patients with schizophrenia is a heterogeneous one, consisting of some individuals with early-onset disease grown old, some with late-onset disease (after 40 years of age), and some with very late-onset schizophrenia-like psychosis, with onset after 60 years of age. Among patients with onset earlier in life, negative symptoms may be prominent, including affective blunting, poverty of speech and thought, apathy, anhedonia, reduced social drive, loss of motivation, lack of social interest, and inattention to social or cognitive input (Finkel 2004). In the current cohort of elders with early-onset disease, tardive dyskinesia also is commonly seen. Among patients with very late-onset schizophrenia-like psychosis, it is particularly common to note sensory deficits, especially hearing impairment, and poor insight (Rodriguez-Ferrera et al. 2004). Negative symptoms and formal thought disorder are rare in this group (Howard et al. 2000). The annual incidence of very late-onset disease is reported to increase by 11% with each 5-year increase in age (Howard et al. 2000).

In the treatment of acute psychosis in elderly patients with schizophrenia, there is no evidence favoring the "rapid neuroleptization" protocols formerly used to treat schizophrenic exacerbations. Large daily doses of any antipsychotic, conventional or atypical, greatly increase the risk of adverse effects in the geriatric population. For psychotic patients with aggression or other excessive motor behavior, quetiapine can be used for its sedative as well as its antipsychotic effects, or a second medication such as a benzodiazepine, trazodone, or gabapentin can be used for sedation.

During maintenance treatment, periodic attempts should be made to reduce the dose of antipsychotic so that the patient can be maintained at the lowest effective dose. Interruptions of treatment are not recommended because of increased risk of psychotic relapse and withdrawal-related dyskinesias.

The Consensus Guidelines suggest the following daily dose ranges for the treatment of schizophrenia in the elderly population: risperidone, 1.25–3.5 mg/day; quetiapine, 100–300 mg/day; olanzapine, 7.5–15 mg/day; aripiprazole, 15–30 mg/day (Alexopoulos et al. 2004).

Long-acting, injectable risperidone can be used in elders, but these patients are more likely to experience adverse effects such as insomnia, constipation, and (more rarely) exacerbation of psychosis (Masand and Gupta 2003).

The same principles apply to the treatment of schizoaffective disorder as to the treatment of schizophrenia in the elderly population. Some patients may have symptoms controlled with an atypical antipsychotic as monotherapy. Others may require combined therapy with a mood stabilizer or antidepressant, or ECT.

The need for lifelong treatment of schizophrenia and schizoaffective disorder places these patients at high risk for weight gain and development of the metabolic syndrome (with atypical antipsychotic use). Routine psychiatric care for this population of necessity involves regular weight and waist circumference measurements, laboratory testing as outlined above, and educational efforts directed toward increasing exercise and improving diet.

Secondary Psychotic Syndromes

Symptoms of delusions, hallucinations, or thought disorganization can occur as secondary symptoms in the context of various medical disorders, including cerebrovascular disease and endocrine dysfunction. Psychotic symptoms can occur with or without changes in level of consciousness and sensorium characteristic of delirium. Treatment first involves optimization of therapy directed at the underlying medical condition. An atypical antipsychotic may be started concurrently at a low dosage (e.g., risperidone, 0.25 mg two times a day) and titrated to effect. The antipsychotic should be tapered and withdrawn, if possible, when the medical condition has been stabilized.

Chapter Summary

- Indications for antipsychotic medications in the elderly population include schizophrenia, mania with psychotic symptoms, dementia with delusions and agitation/aggression, major depression with psychotic features, delusional disorder, delirium, and psychotic disorders secondary to medical conditions.
- When antipsychotic medications are used to control psychosis, standing rather than prn doses should be used.
- All antipsychotics are substrates for CYP isoenzymes, mostly CYP2D6 and/or CYP3A4; in addition, several of the conventional antipsychotics are potent CYP2D6 inhibitors.
- Initial titration of an antipsychotic should usually proceed at a rate of one to two dose increases per week; less for frail or medically compromised elders.
- In the treatment of acute psychosis in elderly patients with schizophrenia, there is no evidence favoring the "rapid neuroleptization" protocols formerly used to treat schizophrenic exacerbations.
- Adverse effects that are particularly problematic for elderly patients include QTc prolongation, orthostasis/hypotension, sedation, anticholinergic effects, and metabolic effects (weight gain, glucose dysregulation, and dyslipidemia) over the longer term.
- The apparently increased risk of stroke and sudden death associated with atypical antipsychotics necessitates an increased threshold for their use in elderly patients, particularly those with dementia. The same caution should be used for conventional antipsychotics in the elderly.
- Individual atypical antipsychotics differ substantially in the degree of associated risk for the development of the metabolic syndrome. In general, clozapine and olanzapine may confer the greatest risk and aripiprazole the least.
- The prevalence of tardive dyskinesia among elderly patients after 3 years of treatment with conventional antipsychotics is 60%.

References

Aarsland D, Perry R, Larsen JP, et al: Neuroleptic sensitivity in Parkinson's disease and parkinsonian dementias. J Clin Psychiatry 66:633–637, 2005

Adams F: Neuropsychiatric evaluation and treatment of delirium in the critically ill cancer patient. Cancer Bull 36:156–160, 1984

Alexopoulos GS, Streim JE, Carpenter D, et al: Using antipsychotic agents in older patients. J Clin Psychiatry 65 (suppl 2):5–104, 2004

Allison DB, Mentore JL, Moonseong H, et al: Antipsychotic-induced weight gain: a comprehensive research synthesis. Am J Psychiatry 156:1686–1696, 1999

American Diabetes Association, American Psychiatric Association, American Association of Clinical Endocrinologists, et al: Consensus development conference on antipsychotic drugs and obesity and diabetes. Diabetes Care 27:596–601, 2004

Ananth J, Parameswaran S, Gunatilake S, et al: Neuroleptic malignant syndrome and atypical antipsychotic drugs. J Clin Psychiatry 65:464–470, 2004

Ballard C, Grace J, McKeith I, et al: Neuroleptic sensitivity in dementia with Lewy bodies and Alzheimer's disease. Lancet 351:1032–1033, 1998

Baptista T, Kin NY, Beaulieu S: Treatment of the metabolic disturbances caused by antipsychotic drugs. Clin Pharmacokinet 43:1–15, 2004

Baskys A: Lewy body dementia: the litmus test for neuroleptic sensitivity and extrapyramidal symptoms. J Clin Psychiatry 65 (suppl 11):16–22, 2004

Becker D, Liver O, Mester R, et al: Risperidone, but not olanzapine, decreases bone mineral density in female premenopausal schizophrenia patients. J Clin Psychiatry 64:761–766, 2003

Bowden CL, Grunze H, Mullen J, et al: A randomized, double-blind, placebo-controlled efficacy and safety study of quetiapine or lithium as monotherapy for mania in bipolar disorder. J Clin Psychiatry 66:111–121, 2005

Briesacher BA, Limcangco MR, Simoni-Wastila L, et al: The quality of antipsychotic drug prescribing in nursing homes. Arch Intern Med 165:1280–1285, 2005

Caligiuri MP, Jeste DV: Association of diabetes with dyskinesia in older psychosis patients. Psychopharmacology (Berl) 176:281–286, 2004

Casey DE: The relationship of pharmacology to side effects. J Clin Psychiatry 58 (suppl 10):55–62, 1997

Casey DE: Dyslipidemia and atypical antipsychotic drugs. J Clin Psychiatry 65 (suppl 18):27–35, 2004

Casey DE, Carson WH, Saha AR, et al: Switching patients to aripiprazole from other antipsychotic agents: a multicenter randomized study. Psychopharmacology (Berl) 166:391–399, 2003

Chengappa KNR, Shelton MD, Baker RW, et al: The prevalence of akathisia in patients receiving stable doses of clozapine. J Clin Psychiatry 55:142–145, 1994

Chue P, Eerdekens M, Augustyns I, et al: Comparative efficacy and safety of long-acting risperidone and risperidone oral tablets. Eur Neuropsychopharmacol 15:111–117, 2005

Cozza KL, Armstrong SC, Oesterheld JR (eds): Concise Guide to Drug Interaction Principles for Medical Practice, 2nd Edition. Washington, DC, American Psychiatric Publishing, 2003

Davis JM, Chen N, Glick ID: A meta-analysis of the efficacy of second-generation antipsychotics. Arch Gen Psychiatry 60:553–564, 2003

de Leon J, Susce MT, Pan RM, et al: The CYP2D6 poor metabolizer phenotype may be associated with risperidone adverse drug reactions and discontinuation. J Clin Psychiatry 66:15–27, 2005

Devanand DP, Marder K, Michaels KS, et al: A randomized, placebo-controlled dose-comparison trial of haloperidol for psychosis and disruptive behaviors in Alzheimer's disease. Am J Psychiatry 155:1512–1520, 1998

DeVane CL, Nemeroff CB: Clinical pharmacokinetics of quetiapine: an atypical antipsychotic. Clin Pharmacokinet 40:509–522, 2001

Durif F, Debilly B, Galitzky M, et al: Clozapine improves dyskinesias in Parkinson disease. Neurology 62:381–388, 2004

Eerdekens M, Van Hove I, Remmerie B, et al: Pharmacokinetics and tolerability of long-acting risperidone in schizophrenia. Schizophr Res 70:91–100, 2004

Eimer M: Considerations in the pharmacologic management of dementia-related behavioral symptoms. Consult Pharm 7:921–933, 1992

Ereshefsky L: Pharmacokinetics and drug interactions: update for new antipsychotics. J Clin Psychiatry 57 (suppl 11):12–25, 1996

Farde L, Nordstrom AL, Wiesel FA, et al: Positron emission tomographic analysis of central D$_1$ and D$_2$ dopamine receptor occupancy in patients treated with classical neuroleptics and clozapine. Relation to extrapyramidal side effects. Arch Gen Psychiatry 49:538–544, 1992

Faulkner G, Soundy AA, Lloyd K: Schizophrenia and weight management: a systematic review of interventions to control weight. Acta Psychiatr Scand 108:324–332, 2003

Fernandez HH, Donnelly EM, Friedman JH: Long-term outcome of clozapine use for psychosis in parkinsonian patients. Mov Disord 19:831–833, 2004

Fernandez HH, Trieschmann ME, Okun MS: Rebound psychosis: effect of discontinuation of antipsychotics in Parkinson's disease. Mov Disord 20:104–115, 2005

Fink M, Taylor MA: Catatonia: A Clinician's Guide to Diagnosis and Treatment. New York, Cambridge University Press, 2003

Finkel S: Pharmacology of antipsychotics in the elderly: a focus on atypicals. J Am Geriatric Soc 52:S258–S265, 2004

Fraunfelder FW: Twice-yearly exams unnecessary for patients taking quetiapine. Am J Ophthalmol 138:870–871, 2004

Fuller MA, Simon MR, Freedman L: Risperidone-associated hepatotoxicity. J Clin Psychopharmacol 16:84–85, 1996

Gardner DM, Baldessarini RJ, Waraich P: Modern antipsychotic drugs: a critical review. CMAJ 172:1703–1711, 2005

Gill SS, Rochon PA, Herrmann N, et al: Atypical antipsychotic drugs and risk of ischaemic stroke: population based retrospective cohort study. BMJ 330:445, 2005

Grohmann R, Ruther E, Sassim M, et al: Adverse effects of clozapine. Psychopharmacology (Berl) 99(suppl):S101–S104, 1989

Haddad PM, Wieck A: Antipsychotic-induced hyperprolactinemia: mechanisms, clinical features and management. Drugs 64:2291–2314, 2004

Hagg S, Spigset O, Soderstrom TG: Association of venous thromboembolism and clozapine. Lancet 355:1155–1156, 2000

Harrigan EP, Miceli JJ, Anziano R, et al: A randomized evaluation of the effects of six antipsychotic agents on QTc, in the absence and presence of metabolic inhibition. J Clin Psychopharmacol 24:62–69, 2004

Harrison TS, Perry CM: Aripiprazole: a review of its use in schizophrenia and schizoaffective disorder. Drugs 64:1715–1736, 2004

Herrmann N, Lanctot KL: Do atypical antipsychotics cause stroke? CNS Drugs 19:91–103, 2005

Herrmann N, Mamdani M, Lanctot KL: Atypical antipsychotics and risk of cerebrovascular accidents. Am J Psychiatry 161:1113–1115, 2004

Howard R, Rabins PV, Seeman MV, et al: Late-onset schizophrenia and very-late-onset schizophrenia-like psychosis: an international consensus. Am J Psychiatry 157:172–178, 2000

Howes OD, Bhatnagar A, Gaughran FP, et al: A prospective study of impairment in glucose control caused by clozapine without changes in insulin resistance. Am J Psychiatry 161:361–363, 2004

Inouye SK, Bogardus ST, Charpentier PA, et al: A multicomponent intervention to prevent delirium in hospitalized older patients. N Engl J Med 340:669–676, 1999

Jann MW: Clozapine. Pharmacotherapy 11:179–195, 1991

Jeste DV, Caligiuri MP, Paulsen JS, et al: Risk of tardive dyskinesia in older patients: a prospective longitudinal study of 266 outpatients. Arch Gen Psychiatry 52:756–765, 1995

Jeste DV, Lacro JP, Palmer B, et al: Incidence of tardive dyskinesia in early stages of low-dose treatment with typical neuroleptics in older patients. Am J Psychiatry 156:309–311, 1999

Jibson MD, Tandon R: New atypical antipsychotic medications. J Psychiatr Res 32:215–228, 1998

Kapur S, Remington G, Jones C, et al: High levels of dopamine D_2 receptor occupancy with low dose haloperidol treatment: a PET study. Am J Psychiatry 153:948–950, 1996

Katz IR: Optimizing atypical antipsychotic treatment strategies in the elderly. J Am Geriatr Soc 52:S272–S277, 2004

Katz IR, Jeste DV, Mintzer JE, et al: Comparison of risperidone and placebo for psychosis and behavioral disturbances associated with dementia: a randomized, double-blind trial. J Clin Psychiatry 60:107–115, 1999

Kingsbury SJ, Fayek M, Trufasiu D, et al: The apparent effects of ziprasidone on plasma lipids and glucose. J Clin Psychiatry 62:347–349, 2001

Koller E, Schneier B, Bennett K, et al: Clozapine-associated diabetes. Am J Med 111:716–723, 2001

Koller EA, Weber J, Doraiswamy PM, et al: A survey of reports of quetiapine-associated hyperglycemia and diabetes mellitus. J Clin Psychiatry 65:857–863, 2004

Kumar V, Brecher M: Psychopharmacology of atypical antipsychotics and clinical outcomes in elderly patients. J Clin Psychiatry 60 (suppl 13):5–9, 1999

Lacro JP, Kuczenski R, Roznoski M, et al: Serum haloperidol levels in older psychotic patients. Am J Geriatr Psychiatry 4:229–236, 1996

Lasser RA, Bossie CA, Gharabawi GM, et al: Remission in schizophrenia: results from a 1-year study of long-acting risperidone injection. Schizophr Res 77:215–227, 2005

Lattuada E, Cavallaro R, Serretti A, et al: Tardive dyskinesia and DRD2, DRD3, DRD4, 5-HT2A variants in schizophrenia: an association study with repeated assessment. Int J Neuropsychopharmacol 7:489–493, 2004

Lerer B, Segman RH, Fangerau H, et al: Pharmacogenetics of tardive dyskinesia: combined analysis of 780 patients supports association with dopamine D_3 receptor gene Ser9Gly polymorphism. Neuropsychopharmacology 27:105–119, 2002

Lieberman JA, Stroup TS, McEvoy JP, et al: Effectiveness of antipsychotic drugs in patients with chronic schizophrenia. N Engl J Med 353:1209–1223, 2005

Lindenmayer J-P, Volavka J, Citrome L, et al: Changes in glucose and cholesterol levels in patients with schizophrenia treated with typical or atypical antipsychotics. Am J Psychiatry 160:290–296, 2003

Madhusoodanan S, Brenner R, Gupta S, et al: Clinical experience with aripiprazole treatment in ten elderly patients with schizophrenia or schizoaffective disorder: retrospective case studies. CNS Spectr 9:862–867, 2004

Marder SR: Management of treatment-resistant patients with schizophrenia. J Clin Psychiatry 57 (suppl 11):26–30, 1996

Masand PS, Gupta S: Long-acting injectable antipsychotics in the elderly. Drugs Aging 20:1099–1110, 2003

McEvoy GK, Snow EK, Kester L, et al: AHFS Drug Information. Bethesda, MD, American Society of Health-System Pharmacists, 2006, p 2364

McIntyre RS, Mancini DA, Basile V, et al: Antipsychotic-induced weight gain: bipolar disorder and leptin. J Clin Psychopharmacol 23:323–327, 2003a

McIntyre RS, Trakas K, Lin D, et al: Risk of weight gain associated with antipsychotic treatment: results from the Canadian National Outcomes Measurement Study in Schizophrenia. Can J Psychiatry 48:689–694, 2003b

McKeith IG, Ballard CG, Harrison RW: Neuroleptic sensitivity to risperidone in Lewy body dementia (letter). Lancet 346:699, 1995

McManus DQ, Arvanitis LA, Kowalcyk BB: Quetiapine, a novel antipsychotic: experience in elderly patients with psychotic disorders. J Clin Psychiatry 60:292–298, 1999

Melkersson K, Dahl M-L: Adverse metabolic effects associated with atypical antipsychotics. Drugs 64:701–723, 2004

Meltzer HY: Atypical antipsychotic drugs, in Psychopharmacology: The Fourth Generation of Progress. Edited by Bloom FE, Kupfer DJ. New York, Raven Press, 1995, pp 1277–1286

Meltzer HY, Cola PA, Parsa M: Marked elevations of serum creatine kinase activity associated with antipsychotic drug treatment. Neuropsychopharmacology 15:395–405, 1996

Meyer JM: Novel antipsychotics and severe hyperlipidemia. J Clin Psychopharmacol 21:369–374, 2001

Milbrandt EB, Kersten A, Kong L, et al: Haloperidol use is associated with lower hospital mortality in mechanically ventilated patients. Crit Care Med 33:226–229, 2005

Montgomery J, Winterbottom E, Jessani M, et al: Prevalence of hyperprolactinemia in schizophrenia: association with typical and atypical antipsychotic treatment. J Clin Psychiatry 65:1491–1498, 2004

Morganroth J, Brozovich FV, McDonald JT, et al: Variability of the QT measurement in healthy men, with implications for selection of an abnormal QT value to predict drug toxicity and proarrhythmia. Am J Cardiol 67:774–776, 1991

Mulsant BH, Gharabawi GM, Bossie CA, et al: Correlates of anticholinergic activity in patients with dementia and psychosis treated with risperidone or olanzapine. J Clin Psychiatry 65:1708–1714, 2004

Murashita M, Kusumi I, Inoue T, et al: Olanzapine increases plasma ghrelin level in patients with schizophrenia. Psychoneuroendocrinology 30:106–110, 2005

National Cholesterol Education Program: Executive Summary of the Third Report of the National Cholesterol Education Program (NCEP) Expert Panel on Detection, Evaluation, and Treatment of High Blood Cholesterol in Adults (Adult Treatment Panel III). JAMA 285:2486–2497, 2001

Nikoloff D, Shim J-C, Fairchild M, et al: Association between CYP2D6 genotype and tardive dyskinesia in Korean schizophrenics. Pharmacogenomics J 2:400–407, 2002

Nordstrom AL, Farde L, Nyberg S, et al: D_1, D_2, and 5-HT_2 receptor occupancy in relation to clozapine serum concentration: a PET study of schizophrenic patients. Am J Psychiatry 152:1444–1449, 1995

Oeschsner M, Korchounov A: Parenteral ziprasidone: a new atypical neuroleptic for emergency treatment of psychosis in Parkinson's disease? Hum Psychopharmacol 20:203–205, 2005

Palik E, Birkas KD, Faludi G, et al: Correlation of serum ghrelin levels with body mass index and carbohydrate metabolism in patients treated with atypical antipsychotics. Diabetes Res Clin Pract 68:S60–S64, 2005

Pan L, Vander Stichele R, Rosseel MT, et al: Effects of smoking, CYP2D6 genotype, and concomitant drug intake on the steady state plasma concentrations of haloperidol and reduced haloperidol in schizophrenic inpatients. Ther Drug Monit 21:489–497, 1999

Parkinson Study Group: Low-dose clozapine for the treatment of drug-induced psychosis in Parkinson's disease. N Engl J Med 340:757–763, 1999

Pearlman C: Clozapine, nocturnal sialorrhea, and choking (letter). J Clin Psychopharmacol 14:283, 1994

Pickar D: Prospects for pharmacotherapy of schizophrenia. Lancet 345:557–562, 1995

Pies RW: Antipsychotics, in Handbook of Essential Psychopharmacology, 2nd Edition. Washington, DC, American Psychiatric Publishing, 2005, pp 139–252

Pollock BG, Mulsant BH: Antipsychotics in older patients. A safety perspective. Drugs Aging 6:312–323, 1995

Rabinowitz T, Frankenburg FR, Centorrino F, et al: The effect of clozapine on saliva flow rate: a pilot study. Biol Psychiatry 40:1132–1134, 1996

Ray WA, Meredith S, Thapa PB, et al: Antipsychotics and the risk of sudden cardiac death. Arch Gen Psychiatry 58:1161–1167, 2001

Richelson E: Preclinical pharmacology of neuroleptics: focus on new generation compounds. J Clin Psychiatry 57 (suppl 11):4–11, 1996

Rodriguez-Ferrera S, Vassilas CA, Haque S: Older people with schizophrenia: a community study in a rural catchment area. Int J Geriatr Psychiatry 19:1181–1187, 2004

Sajatovic M, Perez D, Brescan D, et al: Olanzapine therapy in elderly patients with schizophrenia. Psychopharmacol Bull 34:819–823, 1998

Schillevoort I, de Boer A, van der Weide J, et al: Antipsychotic-induced extrapyramidal syndromes and cytochrome P450 2D6 genotype: a case-control study. Pharmacogenetics 12:235–240, 2002

Schneider LS: Efficacy of treatment for geropsychiatric patients with severe mental illness. Psychopharmacol Bull 29:501–524, 1993

Schneider LS, Dagerman KS, Insel P: Risk of death with atypical antipsychotic drug treatment for dementia. JAMA 294:1934–1943, 2005

Schonfeldt-Lecuona C, Connemann BJ: Aripiprazole and Parkinson's disease psychosis. Am J Psychiatry 161:373–374, 2004

Small JG, Milstein V, Marhenke JD, et al: Treatment outcome with clozapine in tardive dyskinesia, neuroleptic sensitivity, and treatment-resistant psychosis. J Clin Psychiatry 48:263–267, 1987

Snoeck E, Van Peer A, Sack M, et al: Influence of age, renal and liver impairment on the pharmacokinetics of risperidone in man. Psychopharmacology (Berl) 122:223–229, 1995

Tariot PN: Treatment strategies for agitation and psychosis in dementia. J Clin Psychiatry 57 (suppl 14):21–29, 1996

Tariot PN: An overview of main outcomes in CATIE-AD (Summary no 57A), in Syllabus and Proceedings Summary, American Psychiatric Association Annual Meeting, Atlanta, GA, May 21–26, 2005. American Psychiatric Association, 2005, p 172

Taylor DM: Antipsychotics and QT prolongation. Acta Psychiatr Scand 107:85–95, 2003

Taylor DM, Young CL, Mace S, et al: Early clinical experience with risperidone long-acting injection: a prospective, 6-month follow-up of 100 patients. J Clin Psychiatry 65:1076–1083, 2004

Tei Y, Morita T, Inoue S, et al: Torsades de pointes caused by a small dose of risperidone in a terminally ill cancer patient. Psychosomatics 45:450–451, 2004

Thakore JH: Metabolic syndrome and schizophrenia. Br J Psychiatry 186:455–456, 2005

Van Putten T, Marder SR, Mintz J, et al: Haloperidol plasma levels and clinical response: a therapeutic window relationship. Am J Psychiatry 149:500–505, 1992

Vieweg WVR: Mechanisms and risks of electrocardiographic QT interval prolongation when using antipsychotic drugs. J Clin Psychiatry 63:18–24, 2002

von Moltke LL, Abernethy DR, Greenblatt DJ: Kinetics and dynamics of psychotropic drugs in the elderly, in Clinical Geriatric Psychopharmacology, 4th Edition. Edited by Salzman C. Philadelphia, PA, Lippincott Williams & Wilkins, 2005, pp 87–114

Wang PS, Walker AM, Tsuang MT, et al: Dopamine antagonists and the development of breast cancer. Arch Gen Psychiatry 59:1147–1154, 2002

Wang PS, Schneeweiss S, Avorn J, et al: Risk of death in elderly users of conventional vs. atypical antipsychotic medications. N Engl J Med 353:2335–2341, 2005

Wetterling T: Bodyweight gain with atypical antipsychotics: a comparative review. Drug Saf 24:59–73, 2001

Wilner KD, Tensfeldt TG, Baris B, et al: Single- and multiple-dose pharmacokinetics of ziprasidone in healthy young and elderly volunteers. Br J Clin Pharmacol 49 (suppl 1):15S–20S, 2000

Wirshing WC: Movement disorders associated with neuroleptic treatment. J Clin Psychiatry 62 (suppl 21):15–18, 2001

Generic name	aripiprazole
Trade name	Abilify
Class	Quinolone derivative
Half-life	75 hours; 94 hours for dehydro-aripiprazole
Mechanism of action	D_2 partial agonist; 5-HT$_{1A}$ partial agonist; 5-HT$_{2A}$ antagonist
Available preparations	Tablets: 5, 10, 15, 20, 30 mg Oral solution: 1 mg/mL (150 mL)
Starting dose	5 mg/day
Titration	Increase by 5 mg after 2 weeks
Typical daily dose	10 mg/day
Dose range	2.5–15 mg/day
Therapeutic serum level	Not established

Comments: A recommended drug in elderly patients because of a favorable adverse-effect profile. As a dopamine D_2 partial agonist at pre- and post-synaptic receptors, aripiprazole has pro-dopaminergic effects at low dopamine levels and dopamine-blocking effects at high dopamine levels. It is well absorbed orally, taken with or without food. Peak level in plasma in 3–5 hours (delayed by a high-fat meal). Bioavailability 87%. More than 99% protein bound. It is metabolized primarily via CYP2D6 and 3A4. The active metabolite dehydro-aripiprazole has D_2 affinity similar to the parent compound. It has a very long half-life, with steady state reached in 14 days. *Drug interactions:* Aripiprazole interacts with CYP2D6 inhibitors and CYP3A4 inhibitors and inducers (see Tables 2–2 and 3–3). Like other atypical antipsychotics, confers a low risk of EPS and tardive dyskinesia. Compared with other atypicals, aripiprazole has a relatively lower risk of prolactin elevation, QTc prolongation, dyslipidemia, glucose dysregulation, and weight gain. *Common adverse effects:* Headache, agitation, anxiety, insomnia, somnolence, akathisia, light-headedness, weight gain, nausea, dyspepsia, constipation, and vomiting.

Generic name	clozapine
Trade name	Clozaril
Class	Dibenzodiazepine
Half-life	12 hours (range 4–66 hours)
Mechanism	Blockade of dopaminergic and serotonergic receptors
Available preparations	Tablets: 12.5, 25, 100 mg (scored) Orally disintegrating tablets: 25, 100 mg
Starting dose	6.25–12.5 mg/day
Titration	Increase by 6.25–12.5 mg every 7 days (may be added to a high-potency typical antipsychotic, which is tapered when clozapine dose is at target or at 100 mg/day)
Typical daily dose	Schizophrenia: 100 mg bid for acute treatment; lower dose for maintenance Psychosis in Parkinson's disease: 6.25–50 mg
Dose range	6.25–400 mg/day (divided doses)
Therapeutic serum level	350–450 ng/mL (clozapine plus norclozapine) for adult patients with schizophrenia; no clear relationship between level and response

Comments: Highly effective for schizophrenia and psychosis in Parkinson's disease and related disorders, but use is limited in elderly patients because of adverse effects. Boxed warnings regarding agranulocytosis, seizures, myocarditis, orthostasis, cardiorespiratory collapse with coadministration of benzodiazepines, and increased mortality in elders with dementia-related psychosis. Used for patients with schizophrenia who are resistant to other treatments, have severe movement disorders (e.g., tardive dykinesia), or have recurrent suicidal behaviors unresponsive to other interventions. Well absorbed orally, with no effect of food on bioavailability. 97% protein bound. Extensively metabolized in the liver to inactive metabolites. Peak level in 2.5 hours. Lowest doses (e.g., 6.25 mg) used for very elderly patients and patients with dementia. Divided doses are recommended. Not used prn. Latency to response may be seen; 6 weeks' to several months' latency is not uncommon in elderly patients. Response may not plateau for 12 months, especially for negative symptoms. *Drug interactions:* Potential interaction with benzodiazepines associated with sudden death; add benzodiazepines only after clozapine titration is complete. Other drug interactions mediated by CYP1A2, 2D6, and 3A4 (see Tables 2–2 and 3–2). *Adverse effects:* Agranulocytosis, NMS, deep venous thrombosis and pulmonary embolism, glucose dysregulation, weight gain, increased serum CK, increased serum lipids (including triglycerides), seizures (plasma levels > 1,000 ng/mL), tachycardia, confusion, sedation, dizziness, and salivary pooling. See Table 3–11 for guidelines on management of leukopenia. Routine WBC monitoring weekly for 6 months, then every other week if WBC and ANC values have been normal, then monthly if all counts normal for a second 6 months. To discontinue (for reasons other than leukopenia), decrease dose gradually over 4–6 weeks, and continue WBC monitoring for 4 weeks after discontinuation. For missed doses or if patient discontinues more than 48 hours, need to re-titrate, starting with lowest dose.

Generic name	fluphenazine
Trade name	Prolixin
Class	Piperazine phenothiazine
Half-life	Oral form (HCl): 33 hours Decanoate form: approximately 7–10 days
Mechanism	D_1 and D_2 receptor blockade
Available preparations	Tablets: 1, 2.5, 5, 10 mg Decanoate (im): 25 mg/mL
Starting dose	Oral: 0.25–0.5 mg qd to bid Decanoate: 10 mg (dementia 2.5 mg)
Titration	Oral: increase by 0.25–0.5 mg as tolerated (at 4- to 7-day intervals)
Typical dose	Oral: 1 mg bid Decanoate: 12.5–25 mg every 2–4 weeks (dementia 2.5–5 mg every 2–4 weeks)
Dose range	Oral: 0.25–4 mg/day (divided) Decanoate: 5–100 mg/month
Therapeutic serum level	0.2–2 ng/mL (unselected ages)

Comments: High-potency conventional antipsychotic, a phenothiazine derivative. Effect profile similar to that of haloperidol. Liquid form not compatible with liquids containing caffeine, tannin (tea), or pectins (apple juice). With oral preparation, onset of sedative action within 1 hour and biologic effect persists 24 hours; once-daily dosing is feasible after initial titration. Decanoate peaks in 8–36 hours, with second peak in 1–2 weeks. Decanoate can be given in small doses every 2–3 weeks. Steady state may take longer than the 3–4 months observed in younger populations. Extensively metabolized in the liver to numerous active metabolites; substrate and inhibitor of CYP2D6. *Adverse effects:* Cardiovascular effects (e.g., orthostasis, dysrhythmias), extrapyramidal effects, tardive dyskinesia, NMS, seizures, anticholinergic effects (e.g., dry mouth, constipation, urinary retention, blurred vision), sexual dysfunction, weight gain, agranulocytosis, and other hematologic abnormalities.

Generic name	haloperidol
Trade name	Haldol, Haldol Decanoate
Class	Butyrophenone
Half-life	20 hours
Mechanism	Blockade of postsynaptic dopaminergic D_1 and D_2 receptors
Available preparations	Tablets: 0.5, 1, 2, 5, 10, 20 mg Oral concentrate: 2 mg/mL Injectable: 5 mg/mL Decanoate (im): 50 mg/mL, 100 mg/mL
Starting dose	0.25–0.5 mg/day to tid
Titration	Increase by 0.25–0.5 mg as tolerated (4- to 7-day intervals)
Typical dose	Short-acting oral: 1 mg bid Short-acting intravenous: 0.5 mg bid Decanoate: 25 mg/month
Dose range	0.25–4 mg/day Decanoate: 25–100 mg/month
Therapeutic serum level	0.32–10.4 ng/mL (for elderly patients; lower end of range for patients with dementia, higher end for patients with schizophrenia)

Comments: Used to treat delirium in medically compromised elders and for rapid control of psychotic agitation in emergency settings. Onset of effect with intramuscular administration in 30–60 minutes, with substantial improvement in 2–3 hours. Faster onset with intravenous administration. Bioavailability 60% with oral administration because of first-pass metabolism. Biologic effect persists 24 hours; once-daily dosing is feasible after initial titration. Decanoate time to peak is 3–9 days, half-life is 3 weeks, dosing interval 1 month. Metabolized in liver; substrate mainly of CYP2D6 and 3A4; also moderate inhibitor of both isoenzymes. Minimal hypotensive, respiratory depressive, and anticholinergic effects. *Adverse effects:* EPS, tardive dyskinesia, and NMS.

Generic name	molindone
Trade name	Moban
Class	Dihydroindolone
Half-life	20–40 hours
Mechanism	Blockade of postsynaptic dopaminergic receptors
Available preparations	Tablets: 5, 10, 25, 50 mg
Starting dose	5 mg bid
Titration	Increase by 5–10 mg/day at 4- to 7-day intervals
Typical daily dose	20 mg
Dose range	10–100 mg
Therapeutic serum level	Not established

Comments: One of the few antipsychotics not associated with weight gain. Rapidly absorbed; peak levels in 90 minutes. Duration of action is 36 hours or more. Metabolized in the liver to active metabolites that are excreted in urine. *Drug interactions:* Metabolism inhibited by selective serotonin reuptake inhibitors and quinidine. Additive effect with other central nervous system depressants, may block effect of guanethidine, and may cause neurotoxicity with lithium. *Adverse effects:* Tardive dyskinesia, EPS, anticholinergic effects, orthostasis, sedation, and cardiac toxicity.

Generic name	olanzapine
Trade name	Zyprexa, Zyprexa Zydis, Zyprexa IntraMuscular
Class	Thienobenzodiazepine
Half-life	30 hours (range 21–54 hours)
Mechanism of action	Blockade of dopaminergic and serotonergic receptors
Available preparations	Tablets: 2.5, 5, 7.5, 10, 15, 20 mg Orally disintegrating (OD) tablets: 5, 10, 15, 20 mg Injectable: 10-mg vial
Starting dose	2.5 mg/day (hs) orally Injection: 2.5 mg
Titration	Increase by 2.5 mg after 3–4 days
Typical daily dose	2.5–10 mg (qhs)
Dose range	2.5–15 mg/day
Therapeutic serum level	>9 ng/mL (not well established)

Comments: An effective antipsychotic with a poor profile of adverse effects. Well absorbed orally without regard to food. Tablets and OD tablets are bioequivalent. OD (Zydis) preparation dissolves rapidly in saliva and can be swallowed with or without liquid. *Do not break OD tablet.* Rapidly absorbed intramuscularly. Peak concentrations in 6 hours with oral use, 15–45 minutes with intramuscular use; only intramuscular administration is rapid enough for prn dosing. Maximum plasma concentrations with intramuscular use are five times higher than with oral use. Allow at least 2–4 hours between intramuscular doses. Primarily metabolized via glucuronidation, secondarily via CYP1A2. Clearance reduced in elderly and in women; increased in smokers. See Table 3–3 for drug interactions. *Adverse effects:* Orthostatic hypotension, sedation, weight gain, glycemic dyscontrol, elevation of serum lipids (triglycerides), anticholinergic effects (e.g., constipation), nausea, dizziness (not orthostatic), tremor, insomnia, overactivation, akathisia, NMS, and tardive dyskinesia. Boxed warning regarding increased mortality in elderly patients with dementia-related psychosis and warning regarding increased stroke risk in the same population.

Generic name	perphenazine
Trade name	Trilafon
Class	Piperazine phenothiazine
Half-life	20–40 hours
Mechanism	Blockade of postsynaptic dopaminergic receptors
Available preparations	Tablets: 2, 4, 8, 16 mg
Starting dose	2–4 mg/day to bid
Titration	Increase by 2–4 mg at 4- to 7-day intervals
Typical daily dose	8 mg
Dose range	2–32 mg
Therapeutic serum level	0.8–2.4 ng/mL (unselected ages)

Comments: This was the comparator conventional antipsychotic used in the CATIE schizophrenia study. Well absorbed orally, although absorption may be affected by anticholinergic effects on GI tract. Highly lipophilic. 90% protein bound. Peak serum levels in 4–8 hours; effects persist for 24 hours. Extensive first-pass metabolism. Extensive metabolism in liver; substrate and inhibitor of CYP2D6. See Tables 2–2 and 3–3 for drug interactions. Excreted in urine and bile. *Adverse effects:* Tardive dykinesia, orthostasis, sedation, anticholinergic effects, EPS, ECG changes, hypotension (especially orthostatic), tachycardia, dysrhythmias, restlessness, anxiety, NMS, seizures, skin discoloration, rash, dry mouth, constipation, urinary retention, blurred vision, weight gain, sexual dysfunction, agranulocytosis, leukopenia, cholestatic jaundice, retinal pigmentation, and decreased visual acuity.

Generic name	quetiapine
Trade name	Seroquel
Class	Dibenzothiazepine
Half-life	6 hours
Mechanism of action	Blockade of dopaminergic and serotonergic receptors
Available preparations	Tablets: 25, 50, 100, 200, 300, 400 mg (tablets contain lactose)
Starting dose	25 mg/day (qhs)
Titration	Increase every 2–4 days by 25 mg, as tolerated
Typical daily dose	50–100 mg bid
Dose range	50–400 mg (divided bid to tid)
Therapeutic serum level	Not established

Comments: Chemical analog of clozapine and olanzapine. Rapidly absorbed orally; should be given consistently in relation to meals. Peak plasma concentration in 1–2 hours. 83% protein bound. Steady state achieved within 2 days. Metabolized in liver (possibly via CYP3A4) to inactive metabolites. Level significantly increased by inhibitors such as ketoconazole. *Adverse effects:* Sedation, orthostatic hypotension, dizziness, agitation, insomnia, headache, and NMS. Suspected association with cataracts not confirmed with further postmarketing surveillance; twice-yearly slit-lamp ophthalmologic exams no longer required. Boxed warning regarding increased mortality risk in patients with dementia-related psychosis. See text for a discussion of relative risk of weight gain, glucose dysregulation, dyslipidemia, and QTc prolongation.

Generic name	risperidone
Trade name	Risperdal, Risperdal Consta, Risperdal M-Tab
Class	Benzisoxazole
Half-life	24 hours (risperidone + 9-hydroxy metabolite)
Mechanism of action	Blockade of serotonergic and dopaminergic receptors
Available preparations	Tablets: 0.25, 0.5, 1, 2, 3, 4 mg Tablets, orally disintegrating (M-Tabs): 0.5, 1, 2 g Oral solution: 1 mg/mL (30 mL) Extended-release injectable (Consta): 25-, 37.5-, 50-mg dose packs
Starting dose	0.25–0.5 mg/day (qhs) Consta: 25 mg intramuscularly (Continue oral antipsychotic for 3 weeks after injections begin)
Titration	If tolerated, titrate to bid after 2–3 days. Then, increase slowly by 0.25–0.5 mg at 7-day intervals, as tolerated
Typical daily dose	0.5 mg bid Consta: 25 mg im every 2 weeks
Dose range	0.25–3 mg Consta: 25–50 mg im every 2 weeks
Therapeutic serum level	Not established (some evidence for a therapeutic window in the range of 15–38 ng/mL in nonelderly; poorer response above ~50 ng/mL)

Comments: Effective but questionably safe drug in elders, particularly those with dementia. Risperdal Consta inadequately studied in the geriatric population. Well absorbed orally without regard to food. Tablets 66% bioavailable, solution 70% bioavailable. Orally disintegrating tablets bioequivalent to tablets. For long-acting injectable (Consta), initial absorption only about 1%, main release at about 3 weeks; therapeutic levels maintained for about 2 weeks. For oral medication, peak plasma concentrations in 1 hour for parent compound. Metabolized extensively via CYP2D6 isoenzyme system, mainly to hydroxy-risperidone, also active. Decreased clearance in renal and hepatic disease. *Adverse effects:* Hypotension (especially orthostasis), tachycardia, dysrhythmias, ECG changes, syncope, sedation, headache, dizziness, restlessness, akathisia, anxiety, extrapyramidal effects, tardive dyskinesia, and NMS. See text for a discussion of relative risk of weight gain, glucose dysregulation, dyslipidemia, and QTc prolongation. Boxed warning regarding increased mortality in elderly patients with dementia-related psychosis and warning regarding increased stroke risk in the same population.

Generic name	ziprasidone
Trade name	Geodon
Class	Benzisothiazolylpiperazine
Half-life	Oral: 7 hours Intramuscular: 2–5 hours
Mechanism of action	Effects on serotonergic and dopaminergic receptors
Available preparations	Capsule: 20, 40, 60, 80 mg Injectable (powder for reconstitution): 20 mg
Starting dose	20 mg bid with food
Titration	Increase dose by 20 mg bid every 4–7 days
Typical daily dose	40–60 mg bid
Dose range	20–80 mg bid
Therapeutic serum level	Not established

Comments: Well absorbed with oral administration. 99% protein bound. Extensively metabolized in liver, mostly by aldehyde oxidase; less than one-third metabolized via P450 enzymes, mostly CYP3A3/4. Bioavailability 60% with food. Food increases serum levels twofold; grapefruit juice also increases levels. Time to peak 6–8 hours. Excreted mostly in feces, partly in urine, mostly as metabolites. No effect of mild to moderate hepatic or renal function on pharmacokinetics. This drug has minimal effects on lipid profile and glucose regulation and is weight-neutral for many patients. QTc prolongation may be problematic if patient is also treated with other QTc-prolonging drugs or has potassium or magnesium depletion. For other drug interactions, see Tables 2–2 and 3–3. *Adverse effects:* EPS, somnolence, headache, dizziness, nausea, and akathisia. See text for discussion regarding relative severity of other adverse effects. Boxed warning regarding increased mortality in elderly patients with dementia-related psychosis and warning regarding QTc prolongation.

4

Antidepressants

Introduction

Depression is a relatively common affliction in the geriatric population. Among community-dwelling elders, major depression has a point prevalence of 4.4% in women and 2.7% in men (Steffens et al. 2000); among medical patients, those with dementia, and individuals living in nursing homes, the prevalence is considerably higher. Even today, depression is often dismissed in these populations as an understandable reaction to adversity. This argument is hardly tenable, since adversity is neither necessary nor sufficient to induce major depression, nor does it predict the need for or a response to treatment (Alexopoulos et al. 2001).

In the elderly population, depression is associated with excess disability, medical morbidity (including myocardial infarction [MI] and stroke), mortality from medical causes, suicide, and increased health care use. Suicide is a particular risk among men over 80 years of age and among elders with severe or psychotic depression, comorbid alcoholism, recent loss or bereavement, a new disability, or sedative-hypnotic abuse (Alexopoulos et al. 2001). Treatment of depression has been shown to reduce the risk of suicide in at-risk elders (Barak et al. 2005; Bruce et al. 2004).

In spite of widening recognition of these facts, depression is still undertreated in some subgroups of the elderly population. In the Cache County study, only 35.7% of elderly depressed patients were treated with an antidepressant (most with a selective serotonin reuptake inhibitor [SSRI]), while 27.4% were treated with a sedative-hypnotic (Steffens et al. 2000). Most elderly depressed patients who receive care are diagnosed and treated by their primary care physicians, and substantial numbers are treated with suboptimal medication regimens (Wang et al. 2005). Among the patients older than 75 years of age, moreover, medication alone may not be enough to treat depression; psychosocial support also may be needed, and even together, the treatment may not be effective (Roose et al. 2004).

In current practice, medications labeled as antidepressants are used for a variety of indications beyond major depression, as listed in Table 4–1. The class of so-called SSRIs—several of which affect other neurotransmitters— has expanded the utility of antidepressants to include treatment of various anxiety disorders in elderly as in younger patients. SSRIs are still viewed by many clinicians as first-choice agents for treatment of geriatric depression. The dual-acting agents (serotonergic and noradrenergic) in turn may expand the indications for antidepressants to include pain syndromes with and without depression. Tricyclic antidepressants (TCAs) have assumed a more limited role at this time despite demonstrated efficacy, mainly because of cardiovascular side effects. St. John's wort has a wider acceptance than its efficacy and safety probably merit, but it may be useful for a selected group of depressed elders. Monoamine oxidase inhibitors (MAOIs) available in the United States are used as third-line agents, mainly in treatment-refractory cases.

Recent developments in antidepressant therapy have included the introduction of duloxetine, a serotonin-norepinephrine reuptake inhibitor (SNRI); nonapproval of reboxetine in the United States; U.S. Food and Drug Administration (FDA) approval of the selegiline patch; new recognition of adverse effects associated with SSRIs (e.g., bleeding); and greater appreciation of drug interactions mediated by cytochrome P450 (CYP) isoenzymes as well as P-glycoproteins. In addition, new discoveries related to genetic variations may explain some aspects of medication intolerance, including the CYP2D6 slow metabolizer genotype, the 102 T/C single nucleotide polymorphism in the 5-HT$_{2A}$ locus, and the *HTR2A* C/C genotype associated with intolerance of paroxetine (Murphy et al. 2003b).

Cost of antidepressant medications is an issue of increasing significance. Throughout the 1990s in North America, the overall use of antidepressant medications increased, the use of SSRIs increased while the

Table 4–1. DSM-IV-TR codes for conditions treated with antidepressants

294.11	Dementia of the Alzheimer's type, with behavioral disturbance
290.43	Vascular dementia with depression
296.xx	Major depressive disorder
300.4	Dysthymic disorder
311	Depressive disorder not otherwise specified
296.5x	Bipolar I disorder—most recent episode depressed
296.89	Bipolar II disorder—depressed
293.83	Mood disorder due to (indicate general medical condition)
xxx.xx	Substance-induced mood disorder
296.90	Mood disorder not otherwise specified
300.xx	Panic disorder with/without agoraphobia
300.23	Social phobia
300.3	Obsessive-compulsive disorder
309.81	Posttraumatic stress disorder
308.3	Acute stress disorder
300.02	Generalized anxiety disorder
293.84	Anxiety disorder due to (indicate general medical condition)
xxx.xx	Substance-induced anxiety disorder
300.00	Anxiety disorder not otherwise specified
307.xx	Pain disorder
300.7	Hypochondriasis
300.82	Somatoform disorder not otherwise specified
307.42	Primary insomnia
780.xx	Sleep disorder due to (indicate general medical condition)
V62.82	Bereavement (complicated)

Other conditions not coded by DSM-IV-TR

Chronic fatigue syndrome and fibromyalgia

Failure to thrive

Irritable bowel syndrome

Primary pain syndromes (e.g., neuropathic pain, atypical chest pain)

Stress urinary incontinence

use of TCAs decreased, and the overall cost of antidepressant therapy increased (Mamdani et al. 2000). The increasing cost of medications indirectly affects compliance: studies have shown that antidepressants make up one class of medications whose use is disrupted by the introduction of cost-sharing arrangements by health plans (Goldman et al. 2004).

Electroconvulsive therapy (ECT) is still widely used for the treatment of depressed elderly patients, and most experienced clinicians believe strongly in its safety and efficacy in this population. However, there remains a lack of controlled studies to support these views. A recent Cochrane Review of ECT for elders was unable to be completed because of unsatisfactory evidence (Van der Wurff et al. 2003). Sufficient evidence was available to complete a meta-analysis of the short-term efficacy of ECT in patients of unselected age, however, and that analysis concluded that ECT is not only effective but probably more so than pharmacotherapy (UK ECT Review Group 2003).

Preliminary studies of repetitive transcranial magnetic stimulation (rTMS), using a protocol involving high-frequency stimulation (3–20 Hz) to the left prefrontal cortex or low-frequency stimulation (< 1 Hz) to the right prefrontal cortex, show promise for the successful treatment of depression (Gershon et al. 2003). One confounding variable in the elderly population has been cerebral atrophy, which affects the distance between the magnetic stimulus and the target area of cortex. Varying degrees of atrophy require some modification to existing rTMS protocols. Even so, in a randomized controlled trial of patients with Parkinson's disease and depression involving a mixed-age sample with a mean age > 65 years, rTMS was found to be as effective as fluoxetine at 20 mg/day (Fregni et al. 2004). In that study, rTMS was administered for 10 days over a 2-week period, and the antidepressant effect was noted to last a minimum of 8 weeks (Fregni et al. 2004). Antidepressant medication may have a role in continuation and maintenance treatment of depression for patients in whom rTMS induces remission, analogous to its role in relation to ECT.

Pharmacokinetics

Antidepressant preparations are listed in Table 4–2. With the exception of fluoxetine, paroxetine, and nefazodone, antidepressants have linear kinetics over the usual therapeutic dose range, meaning that, in normal metabolizers, each dose increase yields a proportionate serum level increase. Antidepressants in general are rapidly and completely absorbed in the small intestine. Food can significantly delay absorption of many antidepressants, but this probably has little clinical relevance.

Most antidepressants are highly lipophilic. As noted in Chapter 2 of this volume, "Basic Psychopharmacology and Aging," increased fat stores in elderly patients are associated with an increased volume of distribution for lipophilic drugs, with consequent lengthening of elimination half-lives. Most antidepressants are also highly tissue and protein bound, with venlafaxine being one exception. Antidepressants undergo different degrees of first-pass metabolism, yielding a range of bioavailability values.

CYP450 isoenzymes in the intestinal mucosa and liver catalyze oxidation reactions (demethylation and hydroxylation) involved in the primary metabolic pathways for antidepressants. Known metabolic pathways for antidepressants are shown in Table 4–3. Antidepressants in general are extensively metabolized, most by CYP2D6, CYP3A4, and CYP2C9/19 isoenzymes; for fluvoxamine and TCAs, CYP1A2 is also an important pathway.

Whether the ratio of dose to concentration changes with normal aging depends largely on age-related changes in clearance for a particular drug. As noted in Chapter 2, CYP3A and CYP1A2 isoenzyme activities decline with aging, whereas CYP2D6 activity does not. As for specific drugs, clearance of tertiary TCAs (e.g., imipramine and amitriptyline) is reduced, such that lower doses of these medications are indicated in elders. Clearance of desipramine is not reduced, and full antidepressant doses of desipramine are required to treat depression in elderly patients (Nelson et al. 1995). Clearance of bupropion, nefazodone, and trazodone is decreased with aging, although variably.

Decreased renal function significantly affects clearance of water-soluble antidepressant metabolites. For drugs such as TCAs, metabolite accumulation is clinically significant. For example, the concentration of a metabolite of nortriptyline (10-hydroxy-nortriptyline) increases with a decreased glomerular filtration rate, while the clearance of the parent compound is unaffected (Young et al. 1987). The metabolite is associated with prolonged cardiac conduction, is negatively correlated with clinical

Table 4–2.   Selected antidepressant preparations

Generic name	Trade name	Tablets (mg)	Capsules (mg)	SR/CR forms (mg)	Oral liquid[a]
TCAs					
desipramine	Norpramin (generic)	10, 25, 50, 75, 100, 150			
nortriptyline	Pamelor (generic)		10, 25, 50, 75		10 mg/5 mL
SSRIs					
citalopram	Celexa (generic)	10, 20, 40			10 mg/5 mL
escitalopram	Lexapro	5, 10, 20			1 mg/mL
fluoxetine	Prozac, Sarafem (generic)		10, 20, 40		20 mg/5 mL
	Prozac Weekly (delayed-release)			90	
paroxetine	Paxil, Pexeva (generic)	10, 20, 30, 40			10 mg/5 mL
	Paxil CR			12.5, 25, 37.5	
sertraline	Zoloft	25, 50, 100			20 mg/mL
Psychostimulants					
dextroamphetamine	Dexedrine, DextroStat (generic)	5, 10		5, 10, 15	

Table 4–2.   Selected antidepressant preparations *(continued)*

Generic name	Trade name	Available preparations			
		Tablets (mg)	**Capsules (mg)**	**SR/CR forms (mg)**	**Oral liquid[a]**
methylphenidate	Ritalin, Metadate, Methylin (generic)	5, 10, 20		10, 20, 30, 40	5 mg/5 mL 10 mg/5 mL
Novel antidepressants					
bupropion	Wellbutrin (generic)	75, 100			
	Wellbutrin SR (generic)			SR: 100, 150, 200	
	Wellbutrin XL			XL: 150, 300	
duloxetine	Cymbalta		20, 30, 60		
mirtazapine	Remeron (generic)	7.5, 15, 30, 45			
	Remeron SolTab (generic)	7.5, 15, 30, 45			
nefazodone	generic only	50, 100, 150, 200, 250			
trazodone	Desyrel (generic)	50, 100, 150, 300			
venlafaxine	Effexor	25, 37.5, 50, 75, 100			
	Effexor XR			37.5, 75, 150	

Note.   CR=controlled-release; SR=sustained-release; SSRI=selective serotonin reuptake inhibitor; TCA=tricyclic antidepressant.
[a]In concentrate, suspension, or elixir form.

Table 4–3.   Antidepressants: known metabolic pathways

Drug	Metabolic pathways	Enzyme(s) inhibited
Selective serotonin reuptake inhibitors		
Citalopram	2C19, 2D6, 3A4	2D6
Escitalopram	2C19, 2D6, 3A4	2D6
Fluoxetine	2C9, 2C19, 2D6, 3A4	1A2, 2B6, 2C9, **2C19, 2D6**, 3A4
Fluvoxamine	1A2, 2D6	**1A2, 2B6**, 2C9, **2C19**, 2D6, 3A4
Paroxetine	2D6	1A2, **2B6**, 2C9, 2C19, **2D6**, 3A4
Sertraline	2B6, 2C9, 2C19, 2D6, 3A4	1A2, **2B6**, 2D6, 3A4, glucuronidation
Other antidepressants		
Bupropion	2B6	**2D6**
Duloxetine	1A2, 2D6	2D6
Mirtazapine	1A2, 2D6, 3A4	None known
Nefazodone	3A4, 2D6	**3A4**
Venlafaxine	2D6	2D6

Table 4–3. Antidepressants: known metabolic pathways *(continued)*

Drug	Metabolic pathways	Enzyme(s) inhibited
Tricyclic antidepressants		
Amitriptyline	CYP2C19, 2D6, 3A4, UGT1A4	2C19, 2D6
Clomipramine	CYP2C19, 2D6, 3A4	2D6
Desipramine	CYP2D6	2D6
Doxepin	CYP1A2, 2D6, 3A4, UGT1A4, UGT1A3	2C19, 2D6
Imipramine	CYP1A2, 2C19, 2D6, 3A4, UGT1A4, UGT1A3	2C29, 2D6
Nortriptyline	CYP2D6	2D6
Protriptyline	CYP?2D6	?
Trimipramine	CYP2C19, 2D6, 3A4	?

Note. Bold type indicates major pathway or potent inhibition; ? = unknown; CYP = cytochrome P450; UGT = uridine 5′-diphosphate glucuronosyltransferase.

Source. Adapted from Cozza KL, Armstrong SC, Oesterheld JR: "Psychiatry," in *Concise Guide to Drug Interaction Principles for Medical Practice,* 2nd Edition. Washington, DC, American Psychiatric Publishing, 2003, pp. 347, 351, 354. Copyright 2003, American Psychiatric Publishing. Used with permission.

improvement, and is half as potent as the parent compound in noradrenergic uptake effects (Pollock et al. 1992; Schneider et al. 1990). An
analogous situation applies to desipramine (Kitanaka et al. 1982), and
probably to other TCAs. Serum drug levels do not routinely take metabolite levels into account, although metabolite levels can be assayed if specifically ordered. Although desmethylvenlafaxine also is renally excreted,
evidence to date suggests that the clinical significance of accumulation of
this metabolite for normally aging patients is probably minimal (McEvoy
et al. 2006). For duloxetine, clearance does decline and half-life is prolonged with aging.

Pharmacodynamics and Mechanism of Action

Antidepressants act to optimize the concentration of neurotransmitters at
the receptor interface as well as the sensitivity of both pre- and postsynaptic receptors for that neurotransmitter. In addition, antidepressants are
known to affect neuroendocrine function, neuroimmune function, and
rapid eye movement (REM) sleep. The question of what further effects
these drugs may have via second messenger systems in the postsynaptic
neuron is the focus of intensive ongoing research; for example, gene products such as brain-derived neurotrophic factor probably play some role in
antidepressant effects (Skolnick 2002). Antidepressant classes differ from
one another not only in specific neurotransmitters affected but also in the
site of action in the cycle of synthesis, release, binding, and reuptake of
neurotransmitters into the presynaptic neuron, as shown in Figure 4–1.
MAOIs block the enzyme responsible for the breakdown of dopamine,
norepinephrine, and serotonin within the presynaptic neuron. TCAs have
broad-ranging receptor binding and reuptake inhibitory effects, including
the following: serotonin, norepinephrine, and (to a lesser extent) dopamine reuptake inhibition; and muscarinic, histaminergic, α_1 adrenergic
receptor binding (McEvoy et al. 2006). Table 4–4 shows the receptor
binding profiles of various antidepressants.

SSRI antidepressants act primarily to inhibit the serotonin transporter (5-HTT), which is responsible for taking serotonin from the synaptic cleft back into the presynaptic neuron (as shown in Figure 4–1). In
this way, SSRIs increase the amount of serotonin available for binding to

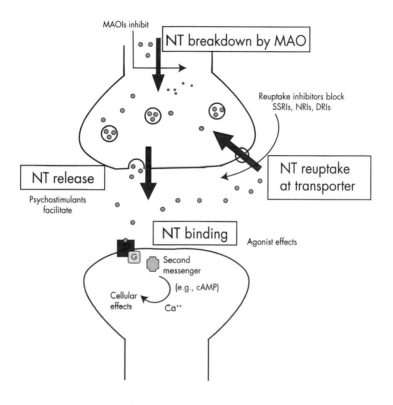

Figure 4–1. Various antidepressant mechanisms.

Note. cAMP=cyclic adenosine monophosphate; DRI=dopamine reuptake inhibitor; MAO=monoamine oxidase; MAOI=monoamine oxidase inhibitor; NRI=norepinephrine reuptake inhibitor; NT=neurotransmitter; SSRI=selective serotonin reuptake inhibitor.

target receptors. The relative potencies of SSRIs in inhibiting 5-HTT are as follows: paroxetine > citalopram > sertraline > fluvoxamine > fluoxetine. At higher doses (e.g., >60 mg fluoxetine), some SSRIs also have limited reuptake effects on norepinephrine and dopamine (Tulloch and Johnson 1992), with sertraline having the greatest dopamine reuptake blocking effects. Paroxetine also has some affinity for muscarinic recep-

Table 4–4. Antidepressants: receptor binding profiles

	Transporters			Receptors		
	Norepinephrine	Serotonin	Dopamine	H$_1$	M$_1$	α$_1$ Adrenergic
Amitriptyline	+++	++++	–	+++++	+++	+++
Clomipramine	+++	++++++	–	+++	+++	+++
Desipramine	+++++	+++	–	++	++	++
Doxepin	+++	++	0	++++++	++	+++
Imipramine	+++	+++++	–	++++	++	++
Nortriptyline	++++	+++	–	++	++	++
Citalopram	–	+++++	0	+	–	+
Escitalopram	–	+++++	0	+	–	+
Fluoxetine	++	+++++	–	–	–	–
Fluvoxamine	+	+++++	–	0	0	–
Paroxetine	+++	++++++	+	0	++	–
Sertraline	+	++++++	+++	0	+	++
Bupropion	+	–	+	–	0	–
Duloxetine	++++	++++++	+	–	–	–
Mirtazapine[a]	–	0	0	++++++	+	+
Nefazodone	++	++	++	+++	–	+++
Venlafaxine	+	++++	–	0	0	0

Note.   H$_1$=histamine type 1; M$_1$=muscarinic type 1. [a]Mirtazapine also has α$_2$ adrenergic effects.
Source.   Adapted from Richelson 2003; Pies 2005.

tors and sertraline for α_1 adrenergic receptors; otherwise, the SSRIs have negligible receptor binding effects (Richelson 2003).

Atypical antidepressants, which include the newer dual-acting medications, have various receptor binding and inhibitory effects:

- Bupropion is a noradrenergic drug with no serotonergic effects, and dopaminergic effects only at doses higher than are used clinically (McEvoy et al. 2006).
- Mirtazapine is a so-called noradrenergic and specific serotonergic antidepressant (NaSSA), with pre- and postsynaptic α_2-receptor–blocking effects, postsynaptic 5-HT$_2$ antagonist effects, 5-HT$_3$ antagonist effects, 5-HT$_1$ agonist effects, and substantial histaminergic (H$_1$) affinity (Fawcett and Barkin 1998). The antidepressant effect of mirtazapine is thought to be due primarily to enhanced release of serotonin and norepinephrine through α_2 antagonism (Pies 2005).
- Nefazodone is a potent 5-HT$_2$ antagonist with the long-term effect of decreasing the number of cortical 5-HT$_2$ receptor binding sites; it is also a weak 5-HT$_2$ and norepinephrine reuptake inhibitor (McEvoy et al. 2006). m-Chlorophenylpiperazine (mCPP), a minor metabolite of nefazodone, is an agonist at 5-HT$_{1A}$ and 5-HT$_{1C}$ sites and an antagonist at 5-HT$_2$ and 5-HT$_3$. It is speculated that 5-HT$_2$ antagonism might limit anxiogenic effects that may be associated with serotonin reuptake inhibition, so that nefazodone is possibly more anxiolytic than SSRIs.
- Trazodone is a weak serotonin reuptake inhibitor, and has differential serotonin agonist/antagonist effects, depending on dose (McEvoy et al. 2006).
- Venlafaxine is an SNRI; at doses below 150 mg/day, serotonergic effects predominate, and at doses above 150 mg, increasing noradrenergic effects are seen.
- Duloxetine is like venlafaxine (an SNRI), except that relative serotonin and norepinephrine reuptake effects are not dose dependent.
- Reboxetine is a selective norepinephrine reuptake inhibitor (NRI) used outside the United States.
- Atomoxetine is a selective NRI that is not labeled for depression but could be expected to have effects similar to reboxetine.

- For the herbal preparation St. John's wort, the antidepressant mechanism is not entirely clear but may involve serotonin reuptake inhibition and monoamine oxidase (MAO) inhibition (LaFrance et al. 2000).

Drug Interactions

Potential drug interactions with antidepressants are numerous and include both pharmacokinetic and pharmacodynamic mechanisms. Pharmacokinetic interactions primarily involve metabolic pathways such as oxidation through CYP450 isoenzymes. Pharmacodynamic interactions are often more complicated and may become apparent in the treated population only after a drug has been on the market for a time. The following tables list potential drug interactions with SSRIs and related antidepressants (Table 4–5), TCAs (Table 4–6), and MAOIs (Table 4–7). Significant interactions involving individual drugs are listed in the Specific Drug summaries at the end of this chapter.

Significant CYP450 interactions are found with fluoxetine, fluvoxamine, paroxetine, bupropion, and nefazodone. In general, these drugs act as CYP enzyme inhibitors and are associated with elevated serum levels of various substrates listed in Table 2–2 in Chapter 2; TCAs are themselves substrates but do not act as potent inhibitors. Bupropion, paroxetine, and fluoxetine are fairly potent inhibitors of the CYP2D6 isoenzyme, while sertraline and citalopram are weaker inhibitors. Sertraline may become a more potent inhibitor at dosages higher than 200 mg/day, although it is unclear whether this particular threshold applies to elders. Fluvoxamine is a very strong inhibitor of CYP1A2, with substrates including propranolol and theophylline. It also strongly inhibits CYP2C19 and moderately inhibits CYP3A4 and CYP2C9. Drug interaction through enzyme inhibition is a major reason that fluvoxamine is not a first-line drug in the treatment of elderly patients. Certain TCAs, SSRIs, and atypical antidepressants are substrates for CYP3A4, of which nefazodone is a potent inhibitor. Paroxetine is unique in being the only SSRI that is itself metabolized by only one metabolic pathway, CYP2D6, such that inhibition of that isoenzyme could be expected to have significant effects on its metabolism.

Sertraline inhibits several CYP450 isoenzymes as well as glucuronidation, but it is not a potent inhibitor of any one. Citalopram and escitalopram are nonpotent inhibitors of CYP2D6 and are themselves metabolized by several pathways.

In general, a listed P450 interaction between a substrate and inhibitor does not necessarily prohibit the coadministration of those medications. An interaction simply means that when a substrate is administered in the presence of an inhibitor, the level of that substrate could become elevated. Accordingly, caution is used when substrates with narrow therapeutic indices are prescribed, and P450 inhibition should be considered whenever adverse events occur during pharmacotherapy.

In contrast, P450 enzyme induction can be highly problematic. For example, St. John's wort is a CYP3A4 inducer and, when administered to cyclosporine-treated heart transplant patients, may be associated with subtherapeutic cyclosporine levels and transplant rejection (Ruschitzka et al. 2000). For patients receiving antiretrovirals such as indinavir, coadministration of St. John's wort also has been associated with subtherapeutic drug levels that could lead to loss of efficacy (Piscitelli et al. 2000).

Pharmacodynamic interactions often have complicated mechanisms that may be poorly understood. Examples include the significant association of upper gastrointestinal bleeding with SSRI medications given in combination with nonsteroidal anti-inflammatory drugs (NSAIDs), and serotonin syndrome with SSRI medications and nonpsychotropics such as linezolid. In general, TCAs have numerous dynamic interactions because they bind to multiple receptor types. Nonselective MAOIs interact with many foods and drugs by virtue of their mechanism of action, as discussed above.

Efficacy

The majority of depressed elderly patients will eventually respond to aggressive treatment for depression (Flint and Rifat 1996), although some elders may be slower to respond compared with younger patients. Predictors of slowed response or reduced response rate include severe depression, presence of a comorbid personality disorder or chronic physical illness, adverse life events, prior treatment failure, "near-delusional" sta-

Table 4–5. Some drugs used in clinical practice that may interact with selective serotonin reuptake inhibitors and related antidepressants

Drug class/Agent	Possible interaction effect	Possible mechanism of interaction
Antiarrhythmics (flecainide, propafenone, mexiletine)	Increased blood level of antiarrhythmic	Inhibition of CYP2D6 (which metabolizes antiarrhythmics) by SSRIs (especially paroxetine, fluoxetine)
Antibiotics (clarithromycin, erythromycin, ciprofloxacin)	Increased levels of some antidepressants (sertraline, nefazodone, citalopram)	Inhibition of CYP3A4 by antibiotics
Anticoagulant (warfarin)	Increased S-warfarin levels in presence of fluvoxamine and perhaps other SSRIs	Inhibition of CYP2C9 (which metabolizes S-enantiomer of warfarin) by fluvoxamine
Antidepressants (e.g., TCAs)[a]	Potentially both pharmacodynamic and pharmacokinetic interactions (e.g., serotonin syndrome, increased blood levels of TCAs in presence of some SSRIs) Possibly fatal serotonin syndrome when MAOIs combined with SSRIs	Combined serotonergic effects at the level of the CNS and gut; inhibition of TCA or other antidepressant metabolism by SSRI (e.g., paroxetine and fluoxetine may increase levels of desipramine)
Antifungals (ketoconazole, itraconazole)	Increased blood level of some SSRIs and other newer agents (e.g., citalopram, sertraline, nefazodone)	Inhibition of metabolism of SSRIs and nefazodone via CYP3A4

Table 4–5. Some drugs used in clinical practice that may interact with selective serotonin reuptake inhibitors and related antidepressants (*continued*)

Drug class/Agent	Possible interaction effect	Possible mechanism of interaction
Anticonvulsants (carbamazepine, oxcarbazepine, divalproex)	Variable and complex interactions (e.g., carbamazepine may decrease some SSRI levels, whereas oxcarbazepine may increase them; SSRIs may increase carbamazepine levels; concomitant use of valproate and fluoxetine may increase levels of both)	Pan-inducer such as carbamazepine enhances drug metabolism and decreases SSRI blood levels (oxcarbazepine may inhibit CYP2C19 and thus increase levels of some SSRIs) Nefazodone and some SSRIs may inhibit CYP3A4 and increase carbamazepine or oxcarbazepine levels Divalproex may inhibit CYP2D6 and other CYP enzymes involved in SSRI metabolism; fluoxetine may inhibit CYP2C9/19, which is partly involved in divalproex metabolism
Calcium channel blockers (nifedipine, verapamil, diltiazem)	Increased blood levels and cardiac effects of calcium channel blockers with some SSRIs and with nefazodone	Inhibition of calcium channel blocker metabolism by SSRIs and nefazodone via CYP3A4
Benzodiazepines	Increased benzodiazepine blood levels and CNS effects	Variable inhibition of CYP2C and 3A4, which metabolize several benzodiazepines (e.g., diazepam and alprazolam), by fluoxetine, fluvoxamine, and sertraline

Table 4–5. Some drugs used in clinical practice that may interact with selective serotonin reuptake inhibitors and related antidepressants (*continued*)

Drug class/Agent	Possible interaction effect	Possible mechanism of interaction
Antipsychotics	Increased blood levels of some antipsychotics (e.g., fluoxetine/haloperidol, fluvoxamine/olanzapine)	Inhibition of CYP2D6 (fluoxetine, paroxetine) and 1A2 (fluvoxamine) by some SSRIs, leading to increased blood levels of haloperidol and risperidone (both 2D6 substrates) and olanzapine (1A2 substrate)
	Possible increase of EPS with coprescription of an SSRI	Increased EPS may be a result of decreased dopamine function due to SSRI
Herbal or over-the-counter agents (St. John's wort, ginkgo, grapefruit juice)	Increased bleeding risk with SSRI plus ginkgo	Impairment of platelet function by SSRIs and ginkgo
	Possible serotonin syndrome with St. John's wort and potential for decreased SSRI level	St. John's wort has serotonergic effects, but also induces CYP3A4
	Possible increased SSRI blood levels with grapefruit juice	Inhibition of CYP3A4 in gut by grapefruit juice
Protease inhibitors (indinavir, ritonavir, saquinavir) and NNRTIs (efavirenz, delavirdine)	Possible serotonin syndrome with SSRI use	Initial inhibition of CYP2D6 and 3A4 by ritonavir, but after days or weeks, possible induction of 3A4 by this agent
	Increased SSRI levels with protease inhibitors and NNRTIs	Potent inhibition of CYP3A4 by NNRTIs and indinavir
	In theory, decreased SSRI levels after longer exposure to ritonavir	

Table 4–5. Some drugs used in clinical practice that may interact with selective serotonin reuptake inhibitors and related antidepressants *(continued)*

Drug class/Agent	Possible interaction effect	Possible mechanism of interaction
Narcotic analgesics (codeine, pentazocine, tramadol, methadone)	Possible decreased codeine effect with paroxetine, fluoxetine[b]	Possible reduction in conversion of codeine to active morphine by SSRI inhibition of CYP2D6[b]
	Possible increased methadone levels with fluvoxamine	Possible decreased metabolism of methadone by fluvoxamine via CYP3A4
	Possible serotonin syndrome with tramadol and SSRIs	Possible increased serotonergic effects of tramadol and/or inhibition of its metabolism by SSRIs via 2D6

Note. CNS = central nervous system; CYP = cytochrome P450; EPS = extrapyramidal side effects; MAOI = monoamine oxidase inhibitor; NNRTI = non-nucleoside reverse transcriptase inhibitor; SSRI = selective serotonin reuptake inhibitor; TCA = tricyclic antidepressant.
[a]Some antidepressant combinations may have therapeutic benefits (e.g., combination of mirtazapine and SSRI may mitigate some sexual and other SSRI side effects and augment antidepressant effect).
[b]The importance of this interaction has recently been questioned in several studies.
Source. Adapted from Pies RW: "Antidepressants," in *Handbook of Essential Psychopharmacology,* 2nd Edition. Washington, DC, American Psychiatric Publishing, 2005, pp. 61–64. Used with permission.

Table 4–6.   Tricyclic antidepressant drug interactions

Added drug	Interaction
Anticholinergic agents	Urinary retention, constipation, dry mouth, dry eyes, blurry vision
Cimetidine, neuroleptics, SSRIs, isoniazid, acetaminophen, chloramphenicol, verapamil, quinidine, epinephrine, disulfiram, methlyphenidate, methadone	Increased TCA blood levels, potential toxicity
Concomitant sympathomimetic use	Hypertension
Coumarin anticoagulants (warfarin)	Prolonged bleeding
Guanethidine, clonidine	Reduced antihypertensive effect
L-Dopa	Decreased plasma level of antidepressants
Monoamine oxidase inhibitors	CNS toxicity, hyperpyrexia, serotonin syndrome (greatest risk is with MAOI plus clomipramine, imipramine, and perhaps desipramine)
Phenytoin, barbiturates, carbamazepine, phenylbutazone, rifampin, doxycycline	Decreased level/effect of antidepressants
Quinidine, procainamide	Prolonged cardiac conduction
Sedatives, tranquilizers (including benzodiazepines)	CNS depression

Note.   CNS=central nervous system; MAOI=monoamine oxidase inhibitor; SSRI = selective serotonin reuptake inhibitor; TCA=tricyclic antidepressant.
Source.   Reprinted from Pies RW: "Antidepressants," in *Handbook of Essential Psychopharmacology,* 2nd Edition. Washington, DC, American Psychiatric Publishing, 2005, p. 60. Copyright 2005, American Psychiatric Publishing. Used with permission.

tus, and older age (Nelson et al. 1994). Elderly patients are at chronic risk of undertreatment because of low expectations regarding recovery and fears about aggressive pharmacotherapy and ECT (Heeren et al. 1997). It is very common to encounter older individuals who have been treated with the same subtherapeutic dose of antidepressant medication for years. Partial recovery is too often accepted as the end point of treatment, resulting in a high prevalence of persistent (and apparently treatment-refractory) depression in this population.

Relative efficacy of antidepressants in elderly patients is a more complicated issue. Although SSRIs have been considered first-line agents for depression treatment in this population for more than a decade, the rationale is related to a better profile of adverse effects rather than to superior efficacy. In fact, randomized controlled trials generally do not support superior efficacy of either SSRIs or older drugs (Anderson 2000). Nevertheless, TCAs and MAOIs are still considered by many clinicians to be more efficacious than SSRIs in the treatment of severe or melancholic depression. Although one recent meta-analysis did not demonstrate a clear class advantage, the study did suggest some advantage for TCAs in depressed patients who were hospitalized (Anderson 2000).

Whether newer dual-acting agents (duloxetine, mirtazapine, venlafaxine) have superior efficacy to SSRIs in elders has not yet been evaluated in any well-designed controlled trial. Those trials that have been published have been of short duration and the comparator doses of SSRIs have been unacceptably low (Goldstein et al. 2004). One controlled trial of venlafaxine versus sertraline in frail nursing home residents found that venlafaxine was no more efficacious and was less well tolerated than sertraline over 9 months (Oslin et al. 2003), but the form of venlafaxine used was immediate-release, and it was dosed one time a day. That study suggested the need for further research on the safety of venlafaxine in the old-old.

Clinical Use

The range of indications for antidepressant medications has broadened over the years, in part due to the introduction of SSRIs and other novel antidepressants with demonstrated efficacy in treating anxiety. A list of current indications for antidepressants is shown in Table 4–1. Specific treatment for most listed indications is covered in a later section.

One of the challenges of treating elderly patients is the determination of which symptoms are due to medical illness or coadministered medications and which might be attributable to depression. The inclusive ap-

Table 4–7.   Monoamine oxidase inhibitor drug
interactions

Added drug	Interaction
Atropine compounds	Increased anticholinergic effects
Fenfluramine	Confusional state (?hyperserotonergic effect)
Guanethidine, reserpine, and clonidine	Reversal of antihypertensive effect; reserpine plus MAOI may lead to hypomania
Insulin	Dangerous hypoglycemia
L-Dopa	Hypertension when used with nonselective or MAO-A-selective MAOI; appears to be safe with selective MAO-B inhibitor (selegiline 10 mg/day)
Linezolid	Additive MAOI effects; hypertensive crisis
Meperidine, fentanyl	Toxic brain syndrome/serotonin syndrome, ANS collapse, death; codeine safer but not risk free
Methadone	Minimal interaction, but needs careful monitoring
Methyldopa	CNS excitation, hypertension
Morphine	Hypotension
Other antihypertensive agents	Hypotension
Other MAOIs, sympathomimetic agents,[a] and tyramine	Hypertensive crisis when used concomitantly
Phentermine	Hypertensive reaction
Succinylcholine + phenelzine	Phenelzine may reduce cholinesterase levels, leading to increased levels of succinylcholine and prolonged apnea during ECT; tranylcypromine does not seem to have this effect

Table 4–7. Monoamine oxidase inhibitor drug interactions *(continued)*

Added drug	Interaction
Sumatriptan	Increased sumatriptan effects
Thiazide diuretic	Increased risk of hypotension
TCAs (especially imipramine, clomipramine), SSRIs, buspirone, other serotonergic agents, and dextromethorphan	Hyperserotonergic syndrome, severe confusional states, coma possible

Note. ANS=autonomic nervous system; CNS = central nervous system; EC = electroconvulsive therapy; MAO=monoamine oxidase; MAOI=monoamine oxidase inhibitor; SSRI=selective serotonin reuptake inhibitor; TCA=tricyclic antidepressant.
[a]Including ephedrine, phenylephrine, phenylpropanolamine, dopamine, amphetamines.
Source. Adapted from Pies RW: "Antidepressants," in *Handbook of Essential Psychopharmacology,* 2nd Edition. Washington, DC, American Psychiatric Publishing, 2005, p. 65. Copyright 2005, American Psychiatric Publishing. Used with permission.

proach, in which all symptoms (including anorexia and fatigue) are counted toward a diagnosis of depression, results in increased sensitivity but decreased specificity in diagnosis. The presence of "psychological" symptoms can assist the diagnostic effort, since helplessness, hopelessness, loss of self-esteem, feelings of worthlessness, excessive guilt, and the wish to die are not normal concomitants of medical illness or of normal aging (Harnett 2001).

Choice of Antidepressant

The initial decision in the treatment of depression in the geriatric patient involves a risk-benefit assessment of pharmacotherapy versus other treatments, including ECT, various psychotherapies, bright light therapy (BLT), and exercise therapy. The severity of the depression determines whether pharmacotherapy or ECT should be used in preference to other modalities. ECT remains the treatment of choice for the depressed elderly patient with psychotic symptoms. ECT appears to be more effective than pharmacotherapy in treating severe depression and induces remission rapidly, but its reputed superior safety compared with antidepressants has yet to be demonstrated by controlled study. In addition, it may be more costly than pharmacotherapy, in part because hospitalization is required in most cases (Manly et al. 2000). As an alternative to ECT, repetitive TMS would theoretically be preferred because general anesthesia is not required. As of this writing, however, rTMS remains a research tool with unknown efficacy in geriatric depression and limited availability for clinical use.

The 2001 Consensus Guidelines for the treatment of depression in elderly patients listed preferred psychotherapies as follows: cognitive-behavioral therapy (CBT), problem-solving psychotherapy, interpersonal therapy, and supportive psychotherapy (Alexopoulos et al. 2001). Behavioral therapy is often used in institutional settings, whether formally or informally, and is usually applied in tandem with other modalities. BLT can be helpful for mild seasonal depression and also can be used as an adjunct to pharmacotherapy for more severe depression. Limited data suggest that regular aerobic exercise can supplement or even supplant antidepressant medication in the treatment of mild to moderate geriatric depression; however, aerobic exercise has a slower onset of effect and requires a high level of motivation and reasonably good physical condition (Blumenthal et al. 1999).

The specific choice of antidepressant medication for the elderly patient depends not only on demonstrated efficacy of a drug (discussed earlier in this chapter) but also on its safety in the geriatric population, the medical comorbidities of the patient, any coprescribed medications, and the cost of the medication. For reasons enumerated in the section "Adverse Effects," neither TCAs nor MAOIs are first-line drugs for elderly patients. TCAs may be particularly problematic for patients with coronary heart disease (CHD), and MAOIs may be particularly problematic for patients unable to maintain compliance with dietary and over-the-counter medication limitations. A summary of specific recommendations for use of antidepressants in particular patient populations is shown in Table 4–8.

Other factors sometimes considered in choosing an antidepressant include the specific profile of symptoms (e.g., fluoxetine, venlafaxine, or bupropion for retarded depression versus mirtazapine for agitated depression), prior history of specific antidepressant response, and family history of response. There is little controlled evidence to show that symptom matching—pairing an agitated patient with a sedating antidepressant, for example—results in better long-term outcome in major depression. On the other hand, clinical experience suggests that patients may feel better during the initial days or weeks of treatment when bothersome symptoms like agitation or insomnia are adequately treated. Clinical experience also suggests that when a patient or family member is a known responder to a given antidepressant, that agent has a greater likelihood of being effective than alternative drugs, all other factors being equal. Again, there is little evidence from controlled studies to support this observation. Finally, patient preference in terms of expected "nuisance" side effects (e.g., dry mouth or blurred vision versus impotence or weight gain) should be taken into account.

Certain antidepressants are preferred for geriatric patients. In general, these drugs lack significant anticholinergic effects, are less likely than other drugs to cause orthostatic hypotension, are not associated with daytime oversedation, and (with the exception of nortriptyline) are rarely associated with cardiac dysrhythmia. Antidepressants generally preferred for elders include the SSRIs citalopram, escitalopram, and sertraline. Second-line agents include fluoxetine, paroxetine, and venlafaxine. Lack of evidence from controlled studies in the geriatric population excludes bupropion from the list, although considerable clinical experience supports the safety and efficacy of bupropion in the sustained-release formulation as well as mirtazapine in elderly patients.

Numerous randomized controlled trials have demonstrated unequivocally that TCAs are efficacious in the treatment of geriatric depression. When a TCA is used, nortriptyline is the agent most often selected, followed by desipramine; tertiary amines are avoided in this population because of sedative and anticholinergic effects (see Tables 1–3 and 1–4 in Chapter 1, "The Practice of Geriatric Psychopharmacology," detailing Beers criteria). Nortriptyline has for some time been considered the gold standard of tricyclic treatment for elderly patients because of its efficacy, linear kinetics, plasma level guidelines, relatively low potential for inducing orthostasis, and limited anticholinergic effects.

The problem in using TCAs is that these medications present a serious risk for patients with ischemic heart disease, preexisting bundle branch block, or intraventricular conduction defect (with QRS widened

Table 4–8.   Antidepressant recommendations for special populations

Clinical problem	Recommendation	Rationale
Alzheimer's disease	Avoid TCAs.	Anticholinergic effects worsen cognition.
Cardiac conduction abnormality (bundle branch block or intraventricular conduction delay)	Avoid TCAs. Use SSRI, bupropion, venlafaxine, or nefazodone.	Any TCA could worsen conduction disturbance. These medications do not prolong cardiac conduction; rarely associated with arrhythmias.
Congestive heart failure	Avoid TCAs.	May cause severe orthostatic blood pressure changes.
Diabetes	Avoid TCAs. Use SSRI, bupropion, or venlafaxine.	SSRIs have hypoglycemic effects, whereas TCAs often have hyperglycemic effects. Bupropion and venlafaxine have little effect on glucose levels.
Epilepsy	Avoid bupropion.	Increases seizure risk (dose-related).
Glaucoma	Use SSRIs, bupropion, nefazodone, or trazodone. Avoid TCAs.	These medications lack anticholinergic effects, which can precipitate angle closure. Trazodone lowers intraocular pressure in open-angle glaucoma.
Ischemic heart disease	Avoid TCAs.	TCAs create a risk of arrhythmia during ischemic episode.

Table 4–8. Antidepressant recommendations for special populations *(continued)*

Clinical problem	Recommendation	Rationale
Hepatic disease	Use short-half-life SSRIs, venlafaxine, or bupropion (if no history of seizure). Avoid TCAs (especially tertiary amines).	These medications have a wide therapeutic index; use lower start-dose. TCAs have a narrow therapeutic index.
Obesity	Use bupropion, psychostimulant, or ?nefazodone. Avoid SSRIs, TCAs, MAOIs.	These medications have a lower association with weight gain. Chronic use of TCAs may result in significant weight gain; about one-third of patients have significant weight gain with chronic use of SSRIs.
Polypharmacy (patient on multiple medications)	Use citalopram, escitalopram, sertraline, or venlafaxine.	Fewer drug interactions
Postmyocardial infarction	Avoid TCAs.	Increased mortality
Pulmonary disease: apnea, chronic obstructive pulmonary disease	Use SSRIs or trazodone.	SSRIs improve respiratory function in some cases. Trazodone does not cause respiratory depression.
Renal disease	Use SSRIs.	Metabolite clearance is less of an issue than with TCAs or bupropion.

Note. MAOI=monoamine oxidase inhibitor; SSRI=selective serotonin reuptake inhibitor; TCA=tricyclic antidepressant.

Source. Adapted from Pies RW: "Antidepressants," in *Handbook of Essential Psychopharmacology,* 2nd Edition. Washington, DC, American Psychiatric Publishing, 2005, pp. 75–77. Used with permission.

to more than 0.11 second) (Glassman and Preud'homme 1993; Roose and Dalack 1992). From the standpoint of conduction delay, no individual tricyclic is safer than any other tricyclic, including nortriptyline, desipramine, and doxepin (Glassman and Preud'homme 1993). TCAs are Type 1A antiarrhythmics and, like other drugs of this type, may increase the risk of mortality because of an interaction of the drug with ischemic myocardium, which results in an increased risk of ventricular fibrillation (Roose 2003). Nortriptyline treatment also was noted to be associated with increased triglyceride and very low-density lipoprotein levels, increased heart rate, modest changes in cardiac conduction, and significant reduction in creatinine clearance in geriatric patients after 7 months of treatment (Pollock et al. 1994). Increased heart rate and anticholinergic effects could have significant long-term impact on quality of life for the treated elder (Roose and Suthers 1998).

Despite methodological problems, studies of SSRIs have demonstrated efficacy in mild to moderate depression in outpatients, in secondary depression, and in the range of anxiety disorders listed in Table 4–1. For pharmacokinetic reasons noted above, first-line SSRIs in elderly patients include citalopram, escitalopram, and sertraline. The long half-life of fluoxetine may confer some advantage in poorly compliant patients because missed doses are not so problematic, but this advantage is almost certainly outweighed by the disadvantage that it takes many weeks to clear this drug and its active metabolite norfluoxetine if adverse effects, such as bleeding or hyponatremia, develop.

Nonselective, irreversible MAOIs are not considered first-line agents in treating elderly patients because of serious and persistent side effects (such as orthostasis) and the need for dietary and medication restrictions. Irreversible MAOIs selective for MAO-B, such as selegiline, could theoretically obviate the need for such restrictions, but in practice the doses that are effective against depression for many patients are high enough that selectivity is lost. A transdermal preparation of selegiline recently approved by the FDA may mitigate food interactions at the lowest dose of 6 mg (by bypassing the gastrointestinal tract), but all doses necessitate certain medication restrictions. In general, MAOIs are used as third-line agents in patients with atypical depression, bipolar depression, panic disorder, or depression refractory to treatment with other medications. A class of agents not available in the United States is that of the reversible MAO inhibitors (RIMAs), agents lacking many of the disadvantages noted above. Moclobemide is a RIMA selective for MAO-A that appears to have particular utility in patients with depression in the context of dementia.

Although randomized controlled trials are lacking, psychostimulants have found a treatment niche in the population of medically ill patients with depression and prominent psychomotor retardation (Pereira and Bruera 2001). Anecdotal experience is that response to either methylphenidate or dextroamphetamine is often rapid, with positive effects seen within hours or days. Energy, alertness, attention, and motivation improve; such changes likely represent nonspecific activation rather than a true antidepressant response. These medications are considered by some to be safer than TCAs in patients with medical illness. However, they can prove to be problematic in patients with significant anxiety, because restlessness can be a side effect. As a rule, tolerance to stimulant effects is not observed (Fernandez et al. 1987). The potential exists for acute worsening of depression on discontinuation of a stimulant.

Randomized controlled trials have not been conducted of newer atypical antidepressants in geriatric patients. Like the SSRIs, newer antidepressants confer the significant advantage of having little or no anticholinergic effect and, with the exception of mirtazapine and nefazodone, little α_1 adrenergic effect. Nefazodone has been associated with rare cases of hepatotoxicity, which has limited its general use. This drug is still available in the United States in generic form and is preferred by some patients because of its potent anxiolytic and hypnotic effects. Nefazodone's association with orthostasis is particularly worrisome for elderly patients. Venlafaxine in its extended-release (XR) formulation has been widely used in the elderly population, and anecdotal evidence suggests that it is effective and well tolerated, although hypertension is sometimes seen.

ECT has good short-term efficacy in the treatment of major depression among elderly patients but has a high relapse rate; to maintain the antidepressant response, antidepressant medication or maintenance ECT is required (Abrams 2001; Sackeim et al. 2001; UK ECT Review Group 2003). In the anticipation of ECT, nonessential psychotropic medications (particularly benzodiazepines and mood stabilizers) should be discontinued, although this is by no means a universal practice. ECT protocols used for geriatric patients generally involve treatments two to three times weekly; otherwise, protocols differ among centers. Some use nondominant, unilateral electrode placement, and switch to bilateral placement only for nonresponders; others start with bilateral placement (either bitemporal or bifrontal). With pulse widths now in use, bilateral placement is more effective than unilateral but may be associated with more severe cognitive impairment. A useful rule of thumb is that the patient recovering from an ECT session should have orientation to time and place return within about 10 minutes. Periods of disorientation of 45 minutes or more may predict more persistent memory impairment.

Alternative Formulations of Antidepressant Medications

The lack of available alternative formulations for antidepressants makes dosing quite inflexible. This can be a serious problem, particularly for severely depressed patients who do not have the capacity to decide about medications and refuse to take them. At present, there are no antidepressants available for parenteral use in the United States. Oral solutions of nortriptyline, fluoxetine, paroxetine, citalopram, escitalopram, sertraline, and methylphenidate are available, and sometimes these are accepted by a patient refusing to take pills. Mirtazapine is available in an orally disintegrating form, but the lowest dose is 15 mg and the tablet cannot be cut. As previously noted, a transdermal preparation of selegiline was recently approved by the FDA.

Baseline Laboratory Studies and Clinical Evaluation

Before antidepressant treatment is initiated, a careful history should be obtained and corroborated regarding alcohol and illicit drug use. Chronic alcohol overuse is common in the current elderly cohort and can be associated with significant depressive signs and symptoms. Elderly patients who are overusing alcohol should be detoxified for a minimum of 2 weeks and then reassessed for persistent depression. In many cases, depression remits with simple abstinence. If antidepressants are used after reassessment, it is important that abstinence be maintained for the duration of treatment because the combination of medication and alcohol can be hepatotoxic.

Other pertinent areas of the medical history may reveal factors that may help guide the choice of antidepressant, including the occurrence of cardiac disease, hypertension, prostatic enlargement, glaucoma, seizures, orthostasis or falls, sexual dysfunction, or drug allergies. (Side effects and warnings for specific medications and classes are described in later sections.) For patients with anxiety spectrum illness, consumption of caffeine and nicotine should be quantified. For all patients, nonpsychiatric prescription medications and over-the-counter medications should be noted. The importance of getting an accurate history regarding herbal preparations cannot be overemphasized to the patient and family, who may be reticent about revealing herbal use.

Recent stressors may be identified in the process of obtaining the history. It is a common mistake to assume that depression is a natural reaction to the stresses of aging and that antidepressant treatment is not therefore indicated. This argument becomes untenable in view of the facts that the large majority of elders endure stressors without ever becoming depressed, that even milder depressions may remit with appropriate treatment, and that the presence of a precipitating stressor predicts neither course of depression nor response to treatment. The presence of recent stressors in the life of the seriously depressed patient is a strong indication for cotreatment with medication and psychotherapy.

Physical examination includes, at minimum, orthostatic vital signs, basic cardiac and pulmonary examinations, and a neurologic examination. Neurologic examination should be directed toward uncovering focal signs suggestive of stroke, cerebellar signs suggestive of alcohol overuse, sensory abnormalities consistent with vitamin B_{12} deficiency, or abnormalities in deep tendon reflexes consistent with thyroid dysfunction. Mental status examination focuses on immediate assessment of suicide risk, presence of psychotic features (delusions or hallucinations), presence of mixed mood features (mania or hypomania and depression), and cognition. The latter is usefully assessed using the Mini-Mental State Examination (Folstein et al. 1975), possibly in combination with a clock-drawing test and other brief tests of frontal or subcortical function. Depression and anxiety rating scales are also useful, particularly in fully delineating signs and symptoms such as somatic complaints that might later be attributed to medication. Recommended depression rating scales are reproduced in a later section of this chapter.

Laboratory studies should be performed either to uncover a physical condition that may be associated with depression or anxiety symptoms (e.g., anemia, hypothyroidism, low B_{12} level), to identify factors that could complicate medication treatment (e.g., bundle branch block, chronic renal insufficiency), or to uncover factors that might interfere with treatment response such as low folate level (Fava et al. 1997). Routine studies include the following: electrocardiogram (ECG), complete blood count, serum electrolytes (including K^+, Ca^{++}, Na^+, and Mg^{++}), creatinine, liver function tests (including aspartate transaminase [AST], alanine transaminase [ALT], and lactate dehydrogenase [LDH]), B_{12} level, red blood cell (RBC) folate level, and ultrasensitive thyroid function tests (thyroid stimulating hormone [TSH]). RBC folate should be used in preference to serum folate because testing is less expensive and more closely correlated with tissue folate levels.

Antidepressant use may be associated with weight gain and the development of lipid abnormalities in some patients (Nicholas et al. 2003; Sussman and Ginsberg 1998). When significant weight gain occurs, the patient should be monitored for the development of the metabolic syndrome, as discussed in Chapter 3 of this volume, "Antipsychotics."

A number of studies have reported variable success in using other laboratory tests to confirm and monitor depression, including the dexamethasone suppression test, the thyrotropin-releasing hormone test, platelet MAO activity, platelet imipramine binding, and α_2 binding. In general, these tests are too nonspecific to be recommended for routine use.

Dose and Dose Titration

Details of initiating and titrating antidepressants are included in the Specific Drug summaries at the end of this chapter. In general, for treatment of depressive spectrum disorders, the same dose of antidepressant that induced remission is used for continuation and maintenance phase treatment.

When TCAs are used, careful attention must be paid to changes in blood pressure, orthostatic blood pressure and pulse, and reports of dizziness. For inpatients, dose increments should be made approximately every 3 days, as tolerated; for outpatients, dose increments should be made every 5–7 days. For nortriptyline, the target dose can be determined by administering a 25-mg test dose, obtaining a plasma level at 24 hours, and using a dosing nomogram (Schneider et al. 1987). Although this technique is seldom used in current practice, it can obviate the need for frequent level checks during dose titration and can help avoid overshooting the target dose in a given patient.

For SSRIs, doses should be initiated in the elderly at one-half the usual dose, and increased to the minimal effective dosage after 1–2 weeks, as tolerated. In our experience, the minimal effective dosage in elders for fluoxetine, paroxetine, and citalopram is usually 20 mg/day; the minimal effective dosage for sertraline is 50–100 mg/day; and the minimal effective dosage for escitalopram is usually 10 mg/day. The patient should be maintained at this dosage for a period of 3–4 weeks before any further increments are made, since there is evidence that increasing the dose sooner may be associated with more severe side effects but not with more rapid response (Flint 1994, 1997). All these dosing parameters assume "normal" drug metabolism (e.g., at CYP450 isoenzymes), and might not apply to patients who are poor metabolizers or ultraextensive metabolizers.

For treatment of anxiety spectrum disorders as well as other conditions such as insomnia and aggression in dementia, little information is available from systematic study to inform target dosing. In general, treatment is initiated at the lowest feasible dose and titrated slowly. Anecdotal experience suggests that elderly patients with conditions such as panic disorder may initially tolerate only doses so small as to be achievable solely with liquid formulations (e.g., citalopram, 2 mg/day). To achieve full remission of panic symptoms, however, these same patients require usual "antidepressant" doses. Furthermore, some elderly patients with panic or obsessive-compulsive disorder (OCD) may require up to 60 mg/day of fluoxetine or its equivalent for symptom control.

Course of Antidepressant Response

Although there is a great deal of between-individual variability in time to effect, in general, a minimum of 6 weeks of antidepressant treatment at a therapeutic dose should be undertaken in an elderly patient before a declaration of "no response" is made for that trial. Patients who have had no response at 6 weeks are unlikely to show remission at 12 weeks. Time to effect may be even longer for fluoxetine (Quitkin et al. 2003), presumably because of the longer interval required to reach steady state.

Early antidepressant responses (within days) may represent placebo responses that may not be sustained over time. Clinically meaningful responses usually involve a lag time of at least several weeks. Rapid dose escalation as well as use of particular agents may be associated with true early responses in some patients, as measured by statistically significant differences from placebo, but the question remains as to whether these differences translate into clinically meaningful differences among antidepressant drugs. With mirtazapine, *APOE* ε4 carriers were shown to have a more rapid response than noncarriers, and it has been speculated that this might be attributable to effects on the hypothalamic-pituitary-adrenal axis, involving lowered cortisol levels (Murphy et al. 2003a).

Little is known about the course of response of elderly patients to antidepressant medication in anxiety spectrum disorders such as panic disorder and OCD. Considering that latencies to response in younger patients are longer for these disorders than for depressive disorders, it might be reasonable to expect that latencies in elders would be especially prolonged. Some clinicians advocate continuing antidepressant treatment for OCD for 12 weeks before a declaration of "no response" is considered for that trial.

Monitoring Antidepressant Therapy

Initiation of tricyclic and MAOI antidepressant therapy in the elderly patient is often best accomplished in the inpatient setting so that important parameters such as blood pressure, orthostatic blood pressure and pulse, and ECG can be optimally monitored. Frequency of follow-up visits during the initial stages of outpatient treatment is determined by the individual situation but typically should be weekly. During continuation treatment, the patient should be seen monthly for 1 year; during maintenance treatment, the patient who is doing well on a stable dose of antidepressant medication should be seen every 3 months (Alexopoulos et al. 2001).

During the acute phase of treatment, patients taking TCAs should have a regular check of orthostatic blood pressure and pulse. At steady state, the TCA blood level and a follow-up ECG should be obtained. Patients taking duloxetine, mirtazapine, or venlafaxine should have regular determination of blood pressure, both upright and supine. Patients taking SSRIs should have pulse checks for bradycardia and serum sodium checks for hyponatremia, which is more commonly seen within the first 2 weeks of treatment. In addition, those taking SSRIs should be asked about unusual bleeding or changes in stool pattern, sexual dysfunction, and feelings of restlessness (suggesting akathisia) and should be examined for extrapyramidal symptoms (increased tone, bradykinesia, or tremor). For all patients, suicidal ideation should be monitored, in view of the particular risk for this problem in the elderly population; this is especially important during the first few weeks of drug administration. In addition, weight loss in the acute phase of treatment with fluoxetine should be followed.

During continuation and maintenance therapy, the following is suggested as a reasonable plan of monitoring for each antidepressant type:

- TCA: ECG, orthostatic blood pressure and pulse, electrolytes, serum creatinine, and liver function tests every 6 months. The TCA level should be rechecked after any dose change or after a new medication with potential CYP450 interaction has been added.
- Serotonin reuptake inhibitor: pulse checks (and ECG, if there is any indication of bradycardia), electrolytes, and liver function tests every 6 months. Periodic weight checks.
- MAOI: orthostatic blood pressure and pulse. For phenelzine, periodic liver function tests, at least during the first 6 months of therapy.

Given the association of (rare) hepatotoxicity with nefazodone, periodic checks of liver function (e.g., every 3–4 months) are suggested, even though the patient's report of malaise, anorexia, or flu-like symptoms may be a better indicator of impending hepatic failure (Konig et al. 1998).

As discussed in Chapter 1, a serum level of any antidepressant can be obtained to determine noncompliance or toxicity. With regard to therapeutic level monitoring, data are available for nortriptyline, desipramine, and imipramine. In elderly patients, nortriptyline has a therapeutic window in the range of 50–150 ng/mL. In a randomized trial of two fixed levels of nortriptyline (40–60 ng/mL vs. 80–120 ng/mL) in an elderly cohort, the lower level was associated with more residual depressive symptoms and the higher with more constipation, but there was no difference between groups in the frequency of relapse to major depression over a 3-year period (Reynolds et al. 1999). In patients with dementia and depression, therapeutic levels of nortriptyline are not established, but lower doses are used, in part because of greater sensitivity to anticholinergic effects. In addition, as noted above, nortriptyline's active hydroxy-metabolite is renally excreted, and in patients with reduced creatinine clearance, it can be elevated even when the parent drug level is in the normal range (Schneider et al. 1990). Although this metabolite can be assayed in many laboratories by special order, it is more important to follow the ECG to determine whether changes in cardiac conduction are seen.

The therapeutic threshold for desipramine in elderly patients is 105 ng/mL (Alexopoulos 1996; Nelson et al. 1995). Imipramine is not recommended for use in elderly patients. Therapeutic ranges for SSRI antidepressants have not been established, and in fact, there is a very large between-individual variation in level for a given dose because of large differences in absorption and metabolism.

One criterion used to gauge response to therapy in major depression is a 50% or greater reduction in score on a scale such as the Hamilton Rating Scale for Depression (Ham-D). This may be adequate for mildly depressed patients, but for those with higher initial scores (e.g., Ham-D = 36), the 50% score (Ham-D = 18) could still be in the significantly depressed range. For these cases, a remission criterion, defined as a Ham-D score of 7 (for the 17-item version) or 8 (for the 21-item version), is more appropriate. It is worth noting that some clinicians have suggested a slightly higher cutoff score for remission in elderly patients (10 for the 17-item version) because of substantial overlap of depressive symptoms with those of medical illness in this population. Regardless of the details, however, the idea is to return the patient to his or her predepression baseline function. In fact, failure to treat to remission results in substantially higher relapse and recurrence rates for depressive illness (McIntyre and O'Donovan 2004).

Duration of Treatment

During the acute phase of treatment for major depression, remission is induced (as discussed earlier in the chapter). Typically, this phase lasts 6–12 weeks. During the continuation phase, remission is preserved. The length of this phase depends on the number of previous episodes of depression. Consensus Guidelines offer the following suggestions for duration of antidepressant treatment (acute plus continuation phases) (Alexopoulos et al. 2001): first episode of major depression, 1 year; second episode of major depression, 2 years or more; third episode or later of major depression, >3 years.

After completing a course of antidepressant therapy, the patient is said to have recovered. At that point, maintenance phase therapy is considered for susceptible patients (i.e., those with recurrent episodes), and this therapy is continued indefinitely.

Candidates for maintenance therapy include the following: patients with a history of three or more episodes of major depression; those with two or more rapidly recurrent episodes, preexisting dysthymia, prolonged or severe individual episodes, or poor response to acute treatment; and those with coexisting anxiety disorders or substance abuse (Hirschfeld and Schatzberg 1994). For continuation as well as maintenance therapy, full acute doses of antidepressant medication are recommended, as is continuation of any adjunctive treatment, such as lithium (Flint and Rifat 2000).

Little is known about duration of treatment for anxiety disorders in elderly patients. At least a subset of patients with severe forms of panic disorder or OCD require indefinite treatment with antidepressant medication. Others may respond to CBT alone or may be able to taper off antidepressants after a course of CBT.

Managing Treatment Resistance

The treatment-resistant patient is one who has not responded to an adequate amount of medication administered for a sufficient length of time. What is an adequate amount has been reliably determined only for those medications with known therapeutic blood levels: nortriptyline, desipramine, and imipramine. In determining adequacy for all other antidepressants, it is important to note that the ratio of dose to concentration varies widely among individuals. For this reason, a significant proportion of patients with depression labeled as treatment resistant may respond to a simple increase in dose (Fava et al. 2002). For example, a patient treated with an SSRI such as citalopram at 20 mg/day who shows a partial response at 8 weeks may experience remission of symptoms with an increase in dosage to 30–40 mg/day. Furthermore, given that time to remission varies a great deal among elderly individuals, other patients may respond simply to a continuation of medication; a partial responder at 4 weeks may experience remission of symptoms at 8 weeks on the same dose. Patients with treatment-refractory dysthymia may require 16 weeks for a full response (Albert and Ebert 1996).

A substantial minority of elderly patients will not respond to an adequate initial trial of an antidepressant. For these patients, pharmacologic options include antidepressant combination treatment, augmentation with nonantidepressants, and switching. Combination and augmentation therapies are used when the response to the initial trial is partial, and switching is used when there is no response to the initial trial. All three strategies were used in a trial involving 53 elderly patients with treatment-resistant major depression who had responded inadequately to a trial of paroxetine and interpersonal therapy (Whyte et al. 2004). The patients underwent serial trials of combination therapy with bupropion and nortriptyline and augmentation therapy with lithium, and a subset were switched to extended-release venlafaxine. Overall, 60% of the patients responded to combination or augmentation treatment, and 42% responded to venlafaxine, which was better tolerated than other strategies (Whyte et al. 2004).

Effective drug combinations usually target more than one neurotransmitter system. For example, the noradrenergic antidepressant bupropion could be added to an SSRI. This practice is supported by anecdotal experience and one prospective, open-label study of 28 patients over 6 weeks (DeBattista et al. 2003). Because bupropion is stimulating, it can be associated with improvement in SSRI-associated asthenia or apathy as well as sexual dysfunction.

When fluoxetine or paroxetine is the SSRI used, however, both the dose of bupropion and the dose of SSRI should be reduced because of additive CYP2D6 inhibitory effects.

Combination therapy involving SSRIs and TCAs also can be effective. Caution is again advised, however, since serum TCA concentrations can be significantly elevated because of SSRI inhibition of CYP450 isoenzymes. As noted in Table 4–3, inhibition of CYP450 isoenzymes is especially problematic with fluoxetine, fluvoxamine, and paroxetine because of potent isoenzyme inhibition. This may be hazardous for patients with ischemic heart disease, orthostatic hypotension, or preexisting cardiac conduction abnormalities. In general, when these combinations are used, half of the usual dose of TCA is prescribed, along with a minimal effective dose of SSRI. Serum concentrations of TCA should be monitored, and the ECG should be checked periodically. Although some clinicians recommend discontinuing one agent at the time that remission is achieved (continuation monotherapy), this strategy carries the risk of relapse.

Augmentation therapy could be considered for partial responders. The advantage of augmentation therapy over switching is that it does not require tapering and discontinuation of any medication, so the response can be more rapid, theoretically. The disadvantage is that this introduces yet another medication, with the potential for drug interactions and additive adverse effects. In general, the agents that have been well studied in nonelderly populations—lithium and thyroid hormones—have not been systematically studied in the elderly, and little is known about either efficacy or safety in this population. Preliminary studies and anecdotal reports of other potential augmentation agents such as modafinil, dopamine agonists, omega-3 fatty acids, estrogen, and raloxifene have together included only a few geriatric patients, so virtually no information is available about these agents.

Lithium could be used to augment the effect of any antidepressant but may be more effective in combination with TCAs than SSRIs (Thase 2004). Lithium augmentation can be effective in elderly patients, but this drug is not necessarily benign; adverse effects may include renal dysfunction and neurotoxicity, as discussed in Chapter 5 of this volume, "Mood Stabilizers." Augmentation is usually started after a partial response is observed in a minimum 6-week trial with an adequate dose of the antidepressant. (If no initial response is seen, a switch is made instead.) Lithium should be initiated at a low dose and titrated as tolerated to maintain a serum level of about 0.4 mmol/L, although some patients may require higher levels (Nelson 1998; Rouillon and Gorwood 1998). Some patients respond within a few days of augmentation, most respond within the first 3 weeks, and some (23%) respond with a delay of 3–4 weeks (Stein and Bernadt 1993).

In the experience of the authors, both triiodothyronine (T_3) and thyroxine (T_4) appear to be effective and safe in augmenting an SSRI in individual "young-old" patients (age < 75 years) without preexisting thyroid disease. These agents cannot be recommended, however, in the absence of evidence from controlled studies. Thyroid hormone augmentation should be used with caution in patients with coronary artery disease, cardiac dysrhythmia, or heart failure, and may be problematic in other conditions that particularly affect the elderly population.

In one uncontrolled study of modafinil at 100–400 mg/day as augmentation therapy in a mixed-age sample of patients with treatment resistance, significant improvement was seen over 4 weeks in fatigue and cognition (DeBattista et al. 2004). The only randomized controlled study of modafinil in patients with treatment resistance was performed on a nongeriatric sample in which modafinil was added to SSRI monotherapy. It was concluded that modafinil is potentially effective as an adjunct for SSRI partial responders with symptoms of fatigue and sleepiness (Fava et al. 2005). In the experience of the authors, modafinil may be effective in augmenting an SSRI and safely used in individual young-old patients when started at 50 mg/day and titrated as tolerated to 100–200 mg/day (A.M. dosing). Modafinil should be used with caution in patients with angina, cardiac ischemia, left ventricular hypertrophy, mitral valve prolapse, or history of recent MI (Fuller and Sajatovic 2005).

In patients showing no response to an initial trial of antidepressant, or for those who do not respond to combination therapy or augmentation, switching is indicated. In general, switches are made to a medication with a broader spectrum of action (i.e., venlafaxine, mirtazapine, or duloxetine) or to a medication in another class.

To switch antidepressants in an elderly patient, the first drug is withdrawn gradually (over 1–2 weeks) as the second drug is titrated. Too-rapid withdrawal of venlafaxine or of short-half-life SSRIs can be associated with a withdrawal syndrome, as discussed below. It is important to monitor the patient for adverse effects and drug interactions during the switch period. For a switch from an irreversible MAOI, it is necessary to stop the MAOI and wait at least 2 weeks before starting any other antidepressant (including another MAOI), and even this washout may not be long enough for some patients. For a switch from fluoxetine to an irreversible MAOI, the waiting period is 5–6 weeks in nongeriatric patients (possibly longer in geriatric patients) because of fluoxetine's long half-life and extended time to washout.

Discontinuation of Antidepressants

Except in cases where toxicity is suspected, antidepressant medications should be tapered rather than abruptly discontinued. For most agents, tapering involves a gradual dosage reduction over a period of 2–4 weeks. For fluoxetine, the decline of serum level of drug occurs so slowly that the medication can be stopped when a dose of 10–20 mg of fluoxetine is reached. A withdrawal syndrome can be seen in the 24–48 hours after a patient treated for as little as 3–4 weeks with paroxetine, sertraline, or fluvoxamine has the dosage abruptly discontinued or decreased; this syndrome is more likely with paroxetine than with sertraline. A similar syndrome can occur with TCAs. Symptoms of this withdrawal syndrome include nausea, vomiting, fatigue, myalgia, vertigo, headache, and insomnia (Rosenbaum et al. 1998). A withdrawal syndrome with marked anxiety and agitation also may be seen with too-rapid tapering of duloxetine or venlafaxine.

Management of Antidepressant Overdose

Overdose with TCAs is serious and can be fatal. For elderly patients, even a few days' supply of TCA taken together can be fatal. The degree of QRS widening (>100 ms) is a more reliable indicator of TCA toxicity than a drug level, and is correlated with central nervous system (CNS) as well as cardiovascular compromise (Frommer et al. 1987). At a QRS duration of 150 ms, the ventricles become refractory to the next electrical impulse, and the heart begins to miss beats. The ECG would then show a 2:1 or 3:1 rhythm, which can progress to complete heart block. In addition, delayed conduction can be associated with reentry arrhythmias, and either of these developments can result in death (Glassman and Preud'homme 1993). Although TCA overdose affects many organ systems, the cause of death is usually cardiovascular. Other complications of TCA overdose include coma, seizures, hypertension, and hypotension (Frommer et al. 1987).

In general, SSRI overdose is less serious, although serotonin syndrome is a common complication, and seizures and coma can occur. Among the SSRIs, both citalopram and sertraline in overdose have been associated with significant QTc prolongation (de Boer et al. 2005; Isbister et al. 2004). Few data are available regarding newer, dual-acting antidepressants. Venlafaxine in overdose is associated with tachycardia, tremor, and seizures and is more likely than mirtazapine or nefazodone to cause serotonin syndrome (Kelly et al. 2004). Mirtazapine and nefazodone appear to be relatively safe in overdose. Little is known about the newer agent duloxetine in overdose.

Adverse Effects

Relative severities of major adverse effects of antidepressant medications are shown in Table 4–9. Effects that are particularly important in elderly patients include the following: orthostatic hypotension, cardiac conduction disturbance, bleeding, constipation, urinary retention, blurred vision, sedation, dizziness, delirium, cognitive impairment, hyponatremia or syndrome of inappropriate antidiuretic hormone (SIADH) secretion, sexual dysfunction, and weight changes. These problems may be more likely to be experienced by patients who are medically ill.

Most adverse effects occur early, usually within the first week of treatment. For most adverse effects, tolerance does not develop; no matter how low the initiating dose and how slow the titration, the problem will persist. Tolerance often does develop to sedation, dizziness, and gastrointestinal distress. Importantly, tolerance does not develop to orthostasis (Glassman and Preud'homme 1993), cardiac rhythm disturbances, or delirium; as a rule, these problems will not resolve over time.

Tricyclic Antidepressants

TCAs are noted for three important types of adverse effects: cardiac or autonomic, anticholinergic, and neuropsychiatric. Cardiac or autonomic effects include conduction delays and orthostasis. All TCAs affect cardiac conduction and are relatively contraindicated in patients with ischemic heart disease, preexisting bundle branch block, or intraventricular conduction delay (Roose and Glassman 1994). Even nortriptyline and desipramine and their hydroxy-metabolites affect cardiac conduction in vulnerable individuals (Dietch and Fine 1990). Cardiac conduction delay is manifested by prolonged QTc and widened QRS intervals. Orthostasis, which places the elderly patient at risk for stroke and falls, is secondary to α_1 antagonism of TCAs.

All TCAs also have significant peripheral and central anticholinergic effects. These effects are particularly marked for tertiary amines, which include amitriptyline, imipramine, doxepin, trimipramine, and clomipramine. Effects include constipation, urinary retention, dry mouth, and confusion. Whereas these symptoms are bothersome in younger patients, in elders they can be more serious because of their elaboration (e.g., obstipation, acute urinary retention, inability to swallow).

Neuropsychiatric effects of TCAs include dizziness (α_1 antagonism), sedation (H$_1$ [histaminergic type 1] antagonism), and cognitive impairment (M$_1$ [muscarinic type 1] antagonism). Other effects may include exacerbation of psychosis, induction of mania, excessive motor activity, myoclonus, tremors, and extrapyramidal symptoms.

Selective Serotonin Reuptake Inhibitors

With more extensive experience with SSRIs in geriatrics, the clinical view regarding adverse effects has evolved. Expected problems with nausea, diarrhea, anorexia, and overactivation have often proved transient and dose related. On the other hand, sleep disturbances and daytime somnolence have been more persistent with SSRI use, and sexual dysfunction has turned out to be more common and problematic than predicted by premarketing studies (Sussman and Ginsberg 1998). The issue of weight gain is not yet fully understood; although many patients do gain weight over time on SSRIs, for many, this could represent only a return to predepression baseline weight. More recently, hyponatremia/SIADH and upper gastrointestinal bleeding have been recognized as SSRI effects requiring vigilance and monitoring, as discussed later in this chapter. SSRIs are not associated with significant orthostasis or ventricular conduction defects (Roose and Suthers 1998), but bradycardia with fluoxetine has been reported in patients with preexisting sinus node dysfunction (Hussein and Kaufman 1994).

Table 4–9.   Relative severity of adverse effects of selected antidepressant drugs

Drug	Anticholinergic effects	Sedation or drowsiness	Insomnia or agitation	Orthostasis	Cardiac conduction effects	GI distress	Weight gain
Tricyclic/Heterocyclic antidepressants							
Amitriptyline	4	4	0.5	4	3	0.5	4
Clomipramine	3	3	0.5	3	3	0.5	3
Desipramine	1	1	1	2	3	0.5	1
Doxepin	3	4	0.5	3	2	0.5	3
Imipramine	3	3	1	4	3	1	3
Nortriptyline	1	2	0.5	1	2	0.5	2
Selective serotonin reuptake inhibitors							
Citalopram	0.5	0.5	0.5	0	0	1.5	0
Escitalopram	0.5	0.5	0.5	0	0	1	0
Fluoxetine	0	0.5	2	0	0.5	3	0
Paroxetine	2	0.5	1	0	0.5	3	0–0.5
Sertraline	0	0.5	1	0	0.5	3	0

Table 4–9. Relative severity of adverse effects of selected antidepressant drugs *(continued)*

Drug	Anticholinergic effects	Sedation or drowsiness	Insomnia or agitation	Orthostasis	Cardiac conduction effects	GI distress	Weight gain
Atypical/Novel agents							
Bupropion	0	0.5	2	0	0.5	1	0
Mirtazapine	0.5–1	4	0.5	0.5	0	0	4
Nefazodone	0.5	0.5	0	2	0.5	2	0.5
Venlafaxine	0.5	0.5	2	0	0.5	3	0

Note. 0=virtually none; 0.5=minimal; 1=modest; 1.5=moderate; 2=significant; 3=moderately high; 4=high; GI=gastrointestinal.
Source. Adapted from Pies RW: "Antidepressants," in *Handbook of Essential Psychopharmacology,* 2nd Edition. Washington, DC, American Psychiatric Publishing, 2005, pp. 49–50. Used with permission.

The possible association of SSRIs with suicide risk has been a highly controversial issue and remains a subject of intensive clinical and epidemiologic study. The FDA has now required that all antidepressants carry a boxed warning regarding suicide risk for children and adolescents. However, studies to date have shown reduced, rather than increased, suicide risk with SSRI and other antidepressant use in adults (Isacsson et al. 2005; Leon et al. 1999). When elevated suicide risk is seen, it has been shown to correlate with severity of psychopathology (Leon et al. 1999).

Atypical/Heterocyclic Antidepressants

At present, the medications included in the class of atypical or heterocyclic antidepressants include bupropion, venlafaxine, mirtazapine, nefazodone, trazodone, and duloxetine. This is a heterogeneous group in terms of mechanism and receptor effects, as shown in Table 4–4. All except bupropion have serotonergic effects. Common adverse effects for this group of drugs include headache, insomnia, dizziness, dry mouth, constipation, nausea (except with mirtazapine), and sedation (except with bupropion). Mirtazapine also is associated with increased appetite and weight gain and, in some patients, with increased cholesterol levels (Nicholas et al. 2003). Mirtazapine may be associated with neutropenia and, in rare cases, with agranulocytosis. Nefazodone now bears a boxed warning for hepatic failure and other hepatic effects.

Monoamine Oxidase Inhibitors

Use of MAOIs in the elderly is generally limited by orthostasis as well as dietary restrictions and drug interactions. Ingestion of tyramine-containing foods can precipitate a hypertensive crisis. Serious drug interactions can occur with commonly used over-the-counter medications, narcotics (especially meperidine), and SSRIs. Significant orthostasis can appear after a delay as long as 6 weeks. Pyridoxine deficiency is a potential side effect of MAOI use that can be prevented by coadministration of pyridoxine (vitamin B_6).

St. John's Wort

St. John's wort is an over-the-counter herbal supplement that has been associated with mania (Stevinson and Ernst 2004), bleeding (subarachnoid hemorrhage and subdural hematoma), photosensitivity, gastrointestinal symptoms, allergic reactions, fatigue, dizziness, and xerostomia (LaFrance et al. 2000). It is also a significant inducer of the CYP3A4 isoenzyme and can be associated with greatly reduced levels of cyclosporine, protease inhibitors, and other coadministered drugs. Patients who take St. John's wort may not divulge this fact to physicians when they are admitted to the hospital, even when given an opportunity to do so (Martin-Facklam et al. 2004).

Electroconvulsive Therapy

ECT is often cited as being safer to administer to geriatric patients than antidepressant medications. In fact, evidence to support this claim is lacking; there has yet to be a comparative study of first-line pharmacotherapy with ECT in this population. There are significant cardiovascular risks associated with ECT in elderly patients, which in some cases are minimized by pretreatment with β-blockers or calcium channel blockers. In general, however, ECT is well tolerated in the elderly—even in patients with dementia (Van der Wurff et al. 2003). ECT may be associated with transient posttreatment confusion and memory impairment. Those at increased risk for these side effects include the very old, those on psychotropic medications at the time of ECT, and those with major medical illness or prior cognitive impairment (Manly et al. 2000; Van der Wurff et al. 2003).

System-Specific Adverse Effects

Anticholinergic Effects

Anticholinergic effects can be central (delirium and memory and other cognitive impairments) or peripheral (constipation, urinary retention, visual problems, and dry mouth). These effects are amplified by excessive initial doses and too-rapid titration of medications. They can occur, however, with low starting doses and slow titration, and may be persistent. Since tolerance does not develop over time to these effects, discontinuation and a switch to another agent should be considered early. Constipation prophylaxis can be provided by regular use of a bulk laxative (Metamucil) or docusate sodium (Colace). Cathartics such as milk of magnesia should be used only intermittently. Prophylaxis and treatment of constipation are discussed more fully in Chapter 10 of this volume, "Analgesic Medications."

Urinary anticholinergic symptoms include urinary hesitancy, dribbling, reduced flow, atonic bladder, urinary retention, and in severe cases, even renal failure (Pollack and Rosenbaum 1987). Before treatment of urinary retention is initiated, it is important to establish that outflow is not obstructed (e.g., by an enlarged prostate). If not, bethanechol at 10–30 mg administered orally three times a day may be useful (Cole and Bodkin 1990); if this medication is used, however, the patient has to be monitored for signs of cholinergic excess, including diarrhea, intestinal cramping, and rhinorrhea. With urinary retention of even moderate severity, the anticholinergic medication should ordinarily be discontinued and urologic consultation obtained.

Visual blurring can be treated with 1% pilocarpine eyedrops or bethanechol at 10–30 mg administered orally three times a day (Pollack and Rosenbaum 1987), with the same monitoring recommendations noted above. For patients with narrow-angle glaucoma, tricyclics and other medications with anticholinergic effects are contraindicated. For patients with open-angle glaucoma, these medications can be used, but close follow-up is indicated.

In the patient without swallowing difficulty, dry mouth can be treated with sugarless gum or candy to stimulate salivary flow, or with artificial saliva preparations available over the counter (Pollack and Rosenbaum 1987). Oral or sublingual bethanechol also can be helpful.

Cardiac Effects

Dysrhythmias

Ventricular tachycardia, associated with TCA use, is by far the most serious of the cardiac rhythm disturbances, since it can progress to ventricular fibrillation and death. Because TCAs have been found to be proarrhythmic under conditions of ischemia such as angina or MI, they are relatively contraindicated in elderly patients with ischemic heart disease (Glassman et al. 1993), coronary artery disease, evidence of ischemia on ECG or other testing, history of angina, or history of MI. Other risk factors for TCA-induced rhythm abnormalities (including *torsades de pointes*) include a family history of long QT, older age, female gender, metabolic or cardiovascular disease, coadministration of drugs that inhibit TCA metabolism, hypokalemia, overdose of TCA, and coadministration of drugs that also prolong QT (Vieweg and Wood 2004). Among TCAs, amitriptyline and maprotiline may be most likely to induce ventricular tachycardia and *torsades de pointes* (Vieweg and Wood 2004).

TCAs and their hydroxy-metabolites also are associated with slowing of intraventricular conduction. Patients with preexisting bundle branch block (QRS duration more than 100 ms) or intraventricular conduction delay are at significant risk of progressing to a higher-degree block (Glassman and Roose 1994). Patients with first-degree atrioventricular block (PR interval greater than 200 ms) have been understudied but probably have a risk somewhat less than those with bundle branch block (Glassman and Roose 1994). Earlier claims that doxepin was safer than other tricyclics with regard to conduction delay were based on studies using subtherapeutic doses of that medication. In fact, no TCA is safe in elderly patients at risk on the basis of preexisting cardiac conduction delays.

Compared with TCAs, SSRIs have a more benign cardiac-effect profile. In fact, the risk of sudden death in SSRI-treated patients appears to be the same as for nonantidepressant users (Ray et al. 2004). Although published reports exist linking SSRIs to various supraventricular dysrhythmias, including sinus bradycardia, atrial fibrillation, atrial flutter, heart block, and supraventricular tachycardia, the overall incidence of these dysrhythmias is low (Glassman and Preud'homme 1993; Sheline et al. 1997; Spier and Frontera 1991). Patients likely to be at higher risk for the development of these problems include those with preexisting sinus node dysfunction or significant left ventricular impairment. On the other hand, some SSRIs do have significant CYP450 drug interactions with other medications used to treat dysrhythmias and related conditions (e.g., encainide and β-blockers). For this reason, caution is advised in using SSRIs in elderly patients with these cardiac problems who require cotreatment with other medications.

Trazodone may be associated with increased frequency of premature ventricular contractions (PVCs) in patients with preexisting ventricular "irritability." Although no clear guidelines exist as to when this medication is contraindicated, caution should be used in administering trazodone to patients with frequent PVCs on baseline ECGs. Venlafaxine and bupropion have minimal, if any, effect on cardiac conduction, and nefazodone has only benign effects on the ECG, such as asymptomatic slowing of heart rate (Stoudemire 1996). Preliminary evidence suggests that mirtazapine's effects on cardiac rhythm are infrequent and consist mainly of bradycardia and PVCs. Duloxetine is associated with atrial fibrillation and bundle branch block in < 1% of cases (Semla et al. 2006).

In general, cardiac dysrhythmias with antidepressants should be managed prospectively; patients considered at risk should not be treated with medications known to be associated with particular dysrhythmias. Furthermore, when cardiac rhythm disturbances develop in the course of treatment with an antidepressant, discontinuation of the antidepressant is recommended.

Myocardial Depression

TCAs were shown in an in vitro study of harvested human atrial tissue to have direct depressive effects on heart contractility, independent of conduction effects. In that study, amitriptyline effects were noted to be worse than the effects of desipramine in myocardial depression (Heard et al. 2001).

Hypertension

Medications with noradrenergic effects (TCAs, bupropion, duloxetine, mirtazapine, and venlafaxine) may be associated with blood pressure elevation. In some cases, this elevation may only be manifested in the recumbent position. It may be only diastolic or both systolic and diastolic, and the degree of elevation may be significant. In the case of venlafaxine, the risk of hypertension appears to be dose related, seen in approximately 3% of adults taking venlafaxine at dosages under 100 mg/day (Semla et al. 2006).

Orthostatic Hypotension

Orthostatic hypotension is a significant drop in systolic blood pressure (> 15–20 mmHg) with sitting and/or standing. It is problematic because of its association with falls and ischemic events such as stroke. Known risk factors for the development of orthostasis with antidepressant treatment include pretreatment orthostasis and evidence of conduction abnormality on ECGs (Halper and Mann 1988). A possible genetic predisposition was suggested by a study of nortriptyline implicating a polymorphism in the gene coding for P-glycoprotein (Roberts et al. 2002).

Trazodone-associated orthostasis peaks with the blood level 1 hour after oral administration and then lessens over several hours (Glassman and Preud'homme 1993). It is more likely to occur when the drug is taken on an empty stomach. Administration of trazodone at bedtime makes this problem moot for some patients, but such administration has to be reconsidered for patients who are up to the bathroom soon after retiring for the night.

Orthostatic hypotension usually does not resolve on its own with continuation of the antidepressant (Glassman and Preud'homme 1993). In some cases, it can be treated by lowering or dividing the dose of medication. "Ambulatory hygiene" practices may be helpful; these include rising slowly from lying or sitting, dorsiflexing the feet before standing, and crossing the legs while sitting upright (Beers and Berkow 2000). Strength training also may result in better hemodynamic response to orthostatic challenge in geriatric patients. Some patients benefit from the use of elastic stockings, abdominal binders, or footboards (Cole and Bodkin 1990).

Pharmacologic interventions used for symptomatic treatment of orthostasis are not benign, particularly in patients with conditions such as congestive heart failure, edema, sodium retention, renal insufficiency, or cirrhosis. Medications that have been used for this problem include sodium chloride tablets, fludrocortisone, midodrine, methylphenidate, ephedrine, caffeine, T_3, and T_4 (Pollack and Rosenbaum 1987; Tan and Bransgrove 1998). These medications are not necessarily recommended for use in the elderly patient with antidepressant-related orthostasis. For this problem, the best course of action may be a switch to an antidepressant in another class (e.g., an SSRI).

Endocrine Effects

Both hyponatremia and SIADH have been associated with SSRI use in elderly patients. Available data suggest that the incidence of SIADH in SSRI-treated elders is about 12% and does not appear to be dose dependent (Fabian et al. 2004). Under normal circumstances, antidiuretic hormone (ADH) secretion is stimulated when plasma osmolarity and sodium are high. When osmolarity is low, secretion of ADH is "inappropriate" and indicates the presence of a nonosmotic stimulus such as malignancy, pulmonary disorder, CNS disorder (e.g., stroke), infection, trauma, or use of a thiazide diuretic, antipsychotic, or NSAID (Fabian et al. 2004). It is speculated that serotonin itself may be a nonosmotic stimulus for ADH secretion (Fabian et al. 2004). Most cases of SIADH occur within the first 2 weeks of SSRI treatment but may occur at any time (Fabian et al. 2004). Risk factors for SIADH in elders include low body mass index and lower baseline sodium (<138 mEq/L) (Fabian et al. 2004). SIADH/hyponatremia may first manifest in elders as an unexplained change in mental status.

SIADH is diagnosed by the following laboratory values:

- Serum sodium low (usually<130 mEq/L)
- Plasma osmolarity low (<275 mOsm/kg H_2O)
- Urine sodium high (usually>20 mEq/L)
- Urine osmolarity high (>100 mOsm/kg H_2O)

When SIADH is diagnosed, the treatment involves stopping the offending agent and restricting fluid intake to 1,000 cc/day or less until the serum sodium normalizes to≥135 mEq/L. The time to normalization of sodium varies from days to weeks. Failure to detect and manage even mild hyponatremia may result in progression, with the possible development of seizures or coma; the syndrome may be fatal (Fabian et al. 2004). It has been recommended that serum sodium be checked before treatment, and at weeks 1 and 2 after treatment is commenced with an SSRI (Fabian et al. 2004).

Gastrointestinal Effects

The most commonly noted adverse effects of SSRIs are gastrointestinal: nausea, loose stools, diarrhea, and in some cases, vomiting. These effects can be reduced by slow dose titration, and tolerance may develop over time. Nausea and constipation also are seen with the heterocyclic/atypical agents. Nausea is a particular problem with venlafaxine when the dose is titrated too quickly, as well as with duloxetine (20%–22% incidence) (Semla et al. 2006). The problem of GI bleeding with SSRIs is discussed below in the section "Hematologic Effects."

Genitourinary Effects

Urinary retention may be a consequence of anticholinergic effects (discussed earlier) or other mechanisms. Among heterocyclic antidepressants, both venlafaxine and duloxetine have been associated with this effect. In rare cases, males treated with trazodone develop a persistent nonsexual penile tumescence known as priapism. In any trazodone-treated male, when erection persists long enough to be worrisome, the patient should be brought to the acute care clinic or emergency room for treatment.

Hematologic Effects

Medications that inhibit the 5-HTT carrier protein (i.e., SSRIs) also inhibit the uptake of serotonin into platelets. This serotonin store is responsible for platelet aggregation and adhesion, the processes of hemostasis. Platelets deficient in serotonin provide a possible explanation for the association of SSRI use and abnormal bleeding (Ramasubbu 2004). Theoretically, this bleeding could affect any organ system, but it is more likely to occur in areas of susceptibility, such as the upper GI tract and operative sites for certain kinds of surgeries (e.g., orthopedic surgery).

The risk of upper GI bleeding with SSRIs is about the same as that with ibuprofen (de Abajo et al. 1999) and is greatest among patients with a history of GI bleeding (van Walraven et al. 2001). A large population-based cohort study showed that the relative risk of admission to the hospital with upper GI bleeding for SSRI-treated patients is 3.6 compared with nontreated patients; with addition of an NSAID, the risk increases to 12.2; with the addition of low-dose aspirin, the risk is 5.2 (Dalton et al. 2003). The relative risk of upper GI bleeding with a combination of an SSRI with warfarin is not known, but it is expected to be high. This risk could be further increased if warfarin were given with an SSRI known to inhibit the metabolism of the active (S) form of warfarin such as fluvoxamine. For antidepressants with both serotonergic and noradrenergic actions (e.g., venlafaxine and duloxetine), the relative risk of upper GI bleeding is less compared with SSRIs, around 2.3% (Dalton et al. 2003). The association of SSRIs with bleeding is apparently dose dependent and is greatest for SSRIs with high 5-HTT affinity such as fluoxetine, paroxetine, and sertraline (Ramasubbu 2004). In some cases, mild bruising can be treated with daily vitamin C supplementation, but anything more severe, or bleeding that is recurrent, should prompt discontinuation of the offending drug.

Neuropsychiatric Effects

Anxiety

Anxiety is a potential side effect of SSRI therapy. It is more problematic in the early stages of treatment and possibly more with fluoxetine or fluvoxamine than other SSRIs (Pies 2005). This problem is best managed by slow initial titration of the drug and forewarning the patient, but short-term use of a benzodiazepine such as lorazepam is sometimes needed.

Cognitive Impairment

Antidepressant effects on cognition are probably mediated by cholinergic and histaminergic receptor blockade. In general, tertiary-amine TCAs are believed to be more problematic from a cognitive standpoint than SSRIs and newer atypical antidepressants. However, paroxetine was found in one study to correlate negatively with delayed verbal recall and paired associate learning scores in healthy elderly subjects (Furlan et al. 2001). On the other hand, venlafaxine at a dosage of 37.5 mg administered two times a day was found to be free from cognitive and psychomotor effects in a 26-week randomized controlled trial of elderly patients with moderate depression (Trick et al. 2004).

Delirium

Delirium can develop in elderly patients with the use of any antidepressant, but strongly anticholinergic drugs (e.g., TCAs such as amitriptyline) are particularly implicated, even at therapeutic doses. Often heralding the onset of anticholinergic delirium is a prodrome characterized by restlessness and nightmares. When delirium is fully developed, a central anticholinergic syndrome may be seen, marked by myoclonus, and choreoathetoid movements. Dilated pupils and flushed, dry skin also may be noted. The syndrome is usually diagnosed presumptively, although administration of physostigmine confirms the diagnosis when the patient shows transient resolution of symptoms. Physostigmine must be used with extreme caution in elderly patients because of the risk of inducing cardiac dysrhythmias.

Falls

Any medication that causes orthostasis can be associated with falls, so it is not surprising that both TCAs and MAOIs are known for this problem. What is unexpected is that elderly, SSRI-treated patients were observed in epidemiologic studies to have approximately the same risk of falling (rate ratio=1.8) as elderly, TCA-treated patients (rate ratio=2.0), while trazodone-treated patients have a slightly lower risk (rate ratio=1.2) (Thapa et al. 1998). The increased risk of falls with SSRIs and TCAs appears to be dose dependent (Thapa et al. 1998). For falls resulting in hip fracture, elderly SSRI-treated women appear to have the same risk as elderly TCA-treated women (1.7-fold increase compared to nonantidepressant users) over almost 5 years of follow-up (Ensrud et al. 2003). The equivalent risk in SSRI- and TCA-treated patients suggests that the factors contributing to falls in antidepressant-treated elderly patients likely involve more than just orthostasis.

Insomnia

Antidepressants have significant effects on sleep, particularly the amount and latency of REM sleep, but also sleep initiation and maintenance (Wilson and Argyropoulos 2005). Over time, as depression remits, both subjective and objective measures of sleep improve. In the interim before remission, and with initiation of treatment, certain medications are more likely to disturb sleep than others. Among depressed individuals, medications associated with reduced sleep continuity with initiation of treatment (first 1–2 nights) include all SSRIs, venlafaxine, reboxetine, imipramine, and clomipramine (Wilson and Argyropoulos 2005). Medications associated with improved sleep continuity with initiation of treatment include trimipramine, mianserin, mirtazapine, nefazodone, and trazodone (Wilson and Argyropoulos 2005). After 21 nights of treatment, medications still associated with reduced sleep continuity include only fluoxetine and clomipramine (Wilson and Argyropoulos 2005). (Note that no data are available here for bupropion or duloxetine.)

For some depressed patients, insomnia is so debilitating that it appears impossible to wait weeks for antidepressant effects on sleep. In these cases, a medication such as mirtazapine could be selected for treatment. Alternatively, a low dose of mirtazapine (3.75–7.5 mg at bedtime) or trazodone (12.5–50 mg at bedtime) could be used temporarily in conjunction with the selected antidepressant.

Mania

All antidepressants, including BLT and ECT, can induce mania in the predisposed patient. Antidepressants also can be associated with the induction of rapid cycling in bipolar patients, including those patients with highly recurrent unipolar depression. In general, these conditions should be treated by the taper and discontinuation of the offending drug and initiation or optimization of the dose of a mood stabilizer. ECT also can be effective treatment, followed by continuation therapy with a mood stabilizer. Antidepressants recommended by some experts as less likely to induce mania or rapid cycling include SSRIs, bupropion, and venlafaxine (Suppes et al. 2005).

Motor Dysfunction

Case reports have brought attention to the potential of SSRIs to cause extrapyramidal syndromes (i.e., parkinsonism), particularly in elderly or medically ill patients (Pies 1997b). In patients treated concurrently with SSRIs and antipsychotics, significant parkinsonism can occur. SSRI and TCA use also may be associated with a fine, distal resting tremor that may be exacerbated by caffeine, nicotine, or anxiety (Pollack and Rosenbaum 1987). Although evidence from controlled trials is lacking for this indication, an anecdotal report suggests that this tremor can be treated with 10–20 mg of propranolol administered orally three to four times a day (Pollack and Rosenbaum 1987). In the experience of the authors, akathisia developing in the course of antidepressant therapy also can be treated with 10–20 mg of propranolol three times a day, but a switch to another agent should be considered if the problem persists.

Seizures

All antidepressants are associated with lowering of the seizure threshold. In SSRI- and bupropion-treated patients who have been screened to rule out predisposition to seizures, the rate of seizure while receiving therapy is on the order of 0.1% at recommended doses (McEvoy et al. 2006).

Sedation

Sedation is a side effect of a number of antidepressants, including TCAs, nefazodone, mirtazapine, paroxetine, and to a lesser extent, other SSRIs (see Table 4–9). TCA-associated sedation is attributed to H_1 receptor binding. This problem is dose-related and can be minimized by starting at a low dose and titrating slowly. Tolerance does develop to sedative effects of antidepressant drugs over time but may be too slow to make these drugs acceptable, particularly to outpatients. Trazodone also is highly sedating and is widely used specifically as a sedative in elderly patients, whether or not depression is present.

Stroke

Serotonin is a vasoactive amine that induces constriction in larger arteries and dilatation in smaller vessels (Ramasubbu 2004). Case reports have appeared of cerebrovascular events believed to be secondary to reversible and multifocal arterial spasm in patients given serotonergic drugs (Singhal et al. 2002). Some of these patients meet criteria for Call-Fleming syndrome, characterized by sudden-onset severe headache, focal neurologic deficits, and seizures (Singhal et al. 2002). This syndrome is most common in nonelderly women. For the geriatric population, the reports raise the question of whether serotonergic antidepressants might place patients at risk of vasoconstrictive stroke (Ramasubbu 2004). Based on the wide clinical experience with SSRIs in geriatrics, it would appear that such events—if they occur—are infrequent. This is apparently also the case with intracranial or intracerebral bleeding and SSRI use; a recent review found no association between the two events (Ramasubbu 2004).

Sexual Dysfunction

The incidence of antidepressant-associated sexual dysfunction depends in part on the specific antidepressant. A prospective study involving a mixed-age sample of 1,022 patients treated in Spain found rates of sexual dysfunction as follows: >65% with paroxetine, citalopram, and venlafaxine; 58% with fluoxetine; 24% with mirtazapine; and 8% with nefazodone (Montejo et al. 2001). In the geriatric population as in younger populations, it is helpful to sort out preexisting issues affecting sexual function from treatment-related issues; baseline assessment makes it less likely that sexual dysfunction will be misattributed to antidepressant therapy. Pretreatment screening for erectile dysfunction, anorgasmia, or vaginal dryness may reveal conditions that represent an indication for urologic or gynecologic consultation.

Antidepressant-induced sexual dysfunction can relate to decreased libido, delayed orgasm or ejaculation, anorgasmia or absence of ejaculation, or erectile dysfunction or reduced vaginal lubrication (Montejo et al. 2001). Several therapeutic options exist: the offending medication can be replaced by bupropion or mirtazapine, agents less associated with adverse sexual side effects; the dose of antidepressant can be reduced (especially effective with SSRIs used at higher doses); or a low dose of bupropion or mirtazapine can be added to an established antidepressant regimen (Delgado et al. 1999). The use of drug holidays planned for a time that sexual activity is anticipated (for example, stopping sertraline or paroxetine from Thursday to Sunday) is not recommended, as it carries the risk of inducing withdrawal symptoms and probably contributes to noncompliance. Putative antidotes such as yohimbine, cyproheptadine and *ginkgo biloba* could theoretically be used, but are best avoided in elders because of adverse effects and potential drug interactions. Sildenafil was shown to be effective in treating antidepressant-induced erectile dysfunction in nongeriatric males at a dose of 50–100 mg before intercourse. The only common adverse effect was headache in that population (Nurnberg et al. 2003). The safety of various sildenafil-antidepressant combinations in older men has yet to be established, as has their efficacy for other sexual dysfunctions, such as anorgasmia in elderly women.

Toxic Effects

Serotonin Syndrome

Serotonin syndrome is a toxic syndrome defined by the triad of mental status changes, neuromuscular signs, and autonomic hyperactivity that is thought to be caused by overstimulation of postsynaptic serotonin receptors (Boyer and Shannon 2005). The syndrome has a rapid onset, with most patients presenting within 6 hours of initiation of a new serotonergic medication, a change in dose, or overdose (Boyer and Shannon 2005). It is diagnosed clinically when a serotonergic drug has been administered (within the past 5 weeks) and mental status changes occur in the presence of any of the following signs (Boyer and Shannon 2005):

- Tremor and hyperreflexia (leg>arm)
- Spontaneous clonus (leg>arm)
- Inducible clonus and either agitation or diaphoresis
- Rigidity, temperature>38°C, and either ocular clonus or inducible clonus
- Ocular clonus and either agitation or diaphoresis

Other signs and symptoms can include shivering, tachycardia, hypertension, akathisia, mydriasis, hyperactive bowel sounds, diarrhea, hypervigilance, pressured speech, agitation, easy startle, repetitive rotation of head with neck in extension, and increased muscle tone (greater in lower extremities) (Boyer and Shannon 2005; Lejoyeux et al. 1995). A hypomanic syndrome can be seen (Lejoyeux et al. 1995). Laboratory abnormalities can include metabolic acidosis, elevated creatinine, and elevated liver transaminases (AST and ALT). Serotnin syndrome can have a rapid progression; delirium, seizures, shock, rhabdomyolysis, renal failure, and disseminated intravascular coagulation may ensue. The syndrome can be fatal.

Implicated drugs include SSRIs, TCAs, MAOIs, atypical/heterocyclic antidepressants, and over-the-counter and herbal preparations such as St. John's wort. Table 4–10 is a more complete list of medications that may be implicated. CYP450 drug interactions are likely to contribute to toxic effectsm, since drugs that inhibit CYP2D6 or CYP3A4 in the presence of an SSRI could result in high SSRI concentrations. In addition, patients who are poor metabolizers of CYP2D6 may be at particular risk when given paroxetine or fluvoxamine.

The differential diagnosis of serotonin syndrome includes neuroleptic malignant syndrome (NMS) and anticholinergic syndrome. Specific medication history may be of help in making the diagnosis. In addition, compared with NMS, serotonin syndrome has a more rapid onset and progression, and symptoms are hyperkinetic rather than hypokinetic (akinesia or bradykinesia with NMS) (Boyer and Shannon 2005). Compared with the anticholinergic syndrome, serotonin syndrome has neuromuscu-

Table 4–10. Drugs and drug interactions associated with serotonin syndrome

Drugs associated with serotonin syndrome

Selective serotonin reuptake inhibitors: sertraline, fluoxetine, fluvoxamine, paroxetine, and citalopram

Antidepressant drugs: trazodone, nefazodone, buspirone, clomipramine, and venlafaxine

Monoamine oxidase inhibitors: phenelzine, moclobemide, clorgyline, and isocarboxazid

Anticonvulsants: valproate

Analgesics: meperidine, fentanyl, tramadol, and pentazocine

Antiemetic agents: ondansetron, granisetron, and metoclopramide

Antimigraine drugs: sumatriptan

Bariatric medications: sibutramine

Antibiotics: linezolid (a monoamine oxidase inhibitor) and ritonavir (through inhibition of cytochrome P450 isoenzyme 3A4)

Over-the-counter cough and cold remedies: dextromethorphan

Drugs of abuse: methylenedioxymethamphetamine (MDMA or "ecstasy"), lysergic acid diethylamide (LSD), 5-methoxy-N,N-diisopropyltryptamine ("foxy methoxy"), and Syrian rue (contains harmine and harmaline, both monoamine oxidase inhibitors)

Dietary supplements and herbal products: tryptophan, *Hypericum perforatum* (St. John's wort), and *Panax ginseng* (ginseng)

Other: lithium

Drug interactions associated with severe serotonin syndrome

Zoloft, Prozac, Sarafem, Luvox, Paxil, Celexa, Desyrel, Serzone, Buspar, Anafranil, Effexor, Nardil, Manerix, Marplan, Depakote, Demerol, Duragesic, Sublimaze, Ultram, Talwin, Zofran, Kytril, Reglan, Imitrex, Meridia, Redux, Pondimin, Zyvox, Norvir, Parnate, Tofranil, Remeron

Phenelzine and meperidine

Tranylcypromine and imipramine

Phenelzine and selective serotonin reuptake inhibitors

Table 4–10. Drugs and drug interactions associated with serotonin syndrome *(continued)*

Drug interactions associated with severe serotonin syndrome *(continued)*

Paroxetine and buspirone

Linezolid and citalopram

Moclobemide and selective serotonin reuptake inhibitors

Tramadol, venlafaxine, and mirtazapine

Source. Reprinted from Boyer EW, Shannon M: "The Serotonin Syndrome." *New England Journal of Medicine* 352:1114, 2005. Used with permission.

lar abnormalities and hyperactive (rather than hypoactive) bowel sounds, and skin is diaphoretic and of normal color rather than flushed and dry (Boyer and Shannon 2005).

Treatment of serotonin syndrome involves discontinuation of the offending drugs, supportive care, control of agitation, use of 5-HT$_{2A}$ antagonists, control of autonomic instability, and treatment of hyperthermia (Boyer and Shannon 2005). The most important step in treating serotonin syndrome is discontinuation of all serotonergic drugs (Table 4–10); if this is not done, the syndrome will not resolve. Benzodiazepines can sometimes help to reduce the autonomic component, eliminate excessive muscle activity in mild to moderate cases, and improve survival. Physical restraints should be avoided in the treatment of serotonin syndrome, as straining against restraints can exacerbate muscle breakdown and contribute to hyperthermia.

Specific 5-HT$_{2A}$ antagonists that may be useful in treating serotonin syndrome include cyproheptadine and olanzapine or chlorpromazine. However, given the difficulties in distinguishing serotonin syndrome from NMS (Pies 2005), any use of an antipsychotic for this indication carries considerable risk. NMS must be ruled out before antipsychotic medications are given. Moreover, the doses of medications listed in the next paragraph are not specifically geriatric doses and, because these treatments are unstudied in the geriatric population, it is not clear how doses should be adjusted for use in elders.

Cyproheptadine can be given orally or crushed and given via nasogastric tube at an initial dose of 12 mg followed by 2 mg every 2 hours as long as signs of toxicity continue. The maintenance dose of cyproheptadine is 8 mg every 6 hours. It is not known how these doses should be adjusted for geriatric use. Olanzapine can be administered as Zyprexa Zydis at a dose of 10 mg orally; the geriatric dose may be 5 mg. Chlorpromazine can be administered at a dose of 50–100 mg intramuscularly; the geriatric dose may be 25–50 mg.

The patient's vital signs should be monitored carefully, and antipyretics should not be used initially because fever is used diagnostically. In severe cases, where the patient's fever is very high (>41.1°C), in addition to the interventions listed above, the patient may require sedation and intubation so that a muscle relaxant (paralytic) can be used to eliminate excessive muscle activity (Boyer and Shannon 2005). In such a case, the intensive care unit team will likely choose a nondepolarizing paralytic agent such as vecuronium or rocuronium rather than succinylcholine, because the latter carries a risk of arrhythmia in the context of hyperkalemia (Boyer and Shannon 2005). In extreme cases, hemofiltration may be used. Super high-flux hemofiltration is said to clear myoglobin more effectively than conventional hemofiltration (Naka et al. 2005).

Tyramine Reaction

When certain foods or medications are ingested by patients being treated with nonselective MAOIs, a tyramine reaction can result. This is characterized by a marked rise in blood pressure within minutes to hours, severe occipital headache, flushing, palpitations, retro-orbital pain, nausea, and diaphoresis. The blood pressure elevation may be so severe as to result in intracerebral bleeding. Patients prescribed these medications should be warned not to lie down if they feel any of these symptoms, since this can further elevate blood pressure. It is no longer recommended that patients carry their own supply of chlorpromazine or nifedipine for sublingual use; instead, patients are advised to report to the nearest emergency room. Treatment consists of acidification of the urine, intravenous phentolamine for blood pressure control, and supportive measures.

Weight Gain and Hyperlipidemia

Patients of varying ages treated with fluoxetine and other SSRIs may initially experience a small weight loss (2–4 lb in the first 6 weeks); with fluoxetine, weight loss peaks at 20 weeks. At 6 months, weight begins to be regained, and at 1 year, weight is at least equal to baseline (Sussman and Ginsberg 1998). In fact, weight gains with SSRIs of up to 20–30 lb are commonly reported when these medications are used chronically. It is not known whether these are true gains or only represent returns to predepression baseline weights. Nevertheless, it has been estimated that up to one-third of patients gain substantial weight with chronic SSRI use (Sachs and Guille 1999). Weight gain also is seen in patients treated with TCAs and MAOIs, although this depends partly on the particular drug (Sachs and Guille 1999). Mirtazapine was found to be associated with weight gain, increase in total cholesterol, and at least a transient increase in triglyceride level in one small ($N=50$) controlled study (Nicholas et al. 2003).

There has been debate not only about the amount of weight gain with antidepressants but about the mechanism by which weight gain occurs, since mechanism is closely linked to treatment. Various mechanisms have been proposed, including fluid retention, H_1 receptor blockade, change in glucose metabolism, hypothalamic dysfunction, and increased appetite (Pollack and Rosenbaum 1987). SSRI-related weight gain may be a function of effects on the $5\text{-}HT_{2C}$ receptor, which appears to function as one component of a fat control system (Sussman and Ginsberg 1998). New-onset fluid retention (edema) is an indication for medical consultation; in some cases, this may be the first evidence of an adverse drug effect or interaction.

For antidepressant-treated patients who gain more than 5 lb in the first 4 months of treatment, dietary consultation should be offered. Consideration should be given to a switch to bupropion, which is associated with less weight gain compared with other antidepressants. The patient should be instructed to minimize carbohydrate and fat intake and to exercise regularly as tolerated; however, these may be formidable instructions for many elderly patients who are not able to select menus or mobilize for activity.

In our experience, topiramate can be useful in facilitating weight loss in the elderly patient at a dosage of 50–100 mg/day. However, topiramate does not have FDA-approved labeling for weight loss and can have significant adverse effects in some patients (see Chapter 5). Elderly patients who experience significant weight gain with antidepressant treatment in spite of the measures discussed here should be monitored for development of metabolic syndrome, as detailed in Chapter 3 of this volume, "Antipsychotics."

Antidepressant Treatment of Selected Syndromes and Disorders

Anxiety Disorders

Generalized Anxiety Disorder

Antidepressants are the first line of treatment for generalized anxiety disorder (GAD) for most elderly patients, regardless of whether depression is present (Flint 2005). Citalopram, escitalopram, and venlafaxine are recommended drugs (Flint 2005; Lenox-Smith and Reynolds 2003). A pooled analysis of randomized controlled trials of extended-release venlafaxine for GAD in patients ages ≥60 years concluded that this medication was as safe and effective for this group as for younger patients (Katz et al. 2002), although concerns remained about the use of this drug for old-old patients. Treatment of GAD is discussed further in Chapter 6 of this volume, "Anxiolytic and Sedative-Hypnotic Medications."

Obsessive-Compulsive Disorder

Compulsive behaviors may be seen among elderly patients with schizophrenia or dementia, and obsessional ruminations may be seen among those with depression. Primary OCD is seen less often and usually represents the persistence of illness that developed earlier in life. Little is known from systematic study about the interplay of this disorder with other diseases of old age. Both pharmacologic and behavioral treatments can be used in this population, with SSRIs being the drugs of choice rather than clomipramine. It is recommended that medications be started at half the usual dose and titrated upward as tolerated to clinical effect. No controlled studies of optimal dosage for elderly OCD patients have been performed, but clinical experience suggests that the equivalent of fluoxetine 60 mg/day may be needed for symptom control in many elderly OCD patients. Treatment of OCD is discussed further in Chapter 6.

Panic Disorder

The recommended treatment for panic disorder in elderly patients is an SSRI antidepressant such as citalopram or sertraline (Flint and Gagnon 2003). The potential to induce panic when treatment is initiated imposes a limit on starting dose and titration rate. For example, citalopram could be started at 5–10 mg/day, and if the medication is tolerated, the dosage could be increased after 1 week to 20 mg/day. The medication could be maintained at that dosage for 4–6 weeks; if there is still no significant response, the dosage could be increased in slow increments (Flint and Gagnon 2003). Sertraline could be started at 12.5–25 mg/day, and if the medication is tolerated, the dosage could be increased after 1 week to 50–100 mg/day. The medication could be maintained at that dosage for 4–6 weeks; if there is still no significant response, the dosage could be increased in slow increments to a maximum of 200 mg/day (Flint and Gagnon 2003). A benzodiazepine such as lorazepam may be needed as adjunctive therapy during the initial weeks of treatment, and frequent follow-up during this period is recommended (Flint and Gagnon 2003).

Patients who do not tolerate SSRIs can be treated with venlafaxine, which should also be started at a low dose and titrated slowly. The use of benzodiazepines in the treatment of panic in elders is discussed in Chapter 6.

Posttraumatic Stress Disorder

The first line of pharmacologic treatment for posttraumatic stress disorder (PTSD) is an SSRI antidepressant (Asnis et al. 2004). Appropriate SSRI dosing for PTSD in elderly patients has yet to be established, although clinical experience suggests that fluoxetine up to 60 mg/day or sertraline up to 150 mg/day may be required for optimal effect. Trazodone can be helpful for certain patients, but sedation often limits adequate dosing. Mirtazapine, venlafaxine, and duloxetine may be useful but have been understudied or unstudied among geriatric patients for this indication. Other potential treatments for PTSD in elders are discussed in Chapter 6.

Depressive Disorders

Major Depressive Disorder

The diagnosis of major depression in elderly patients should rely less on neurovegetative symptoms and more on psychological symptoms (hopelessness, helplessness, worthlessness, excessive guilt, feelings of emptiness), anhedonia, social withdrawal, psychomotor agitation/retardation, difficulty making decisions or initiating new projects, downcast affect, and suicidal thinking or recurrent thoughts of death (Alexopoulos et al. 2001). Moreover, our own experience suggests that presentations involving "depression without sadness" or "masked depression" are quite common in geriatrics.

Several rating scales have been developed for the assessment of major depression in the geriatric population. The scales are used to quantify degree of improvement in symptoms with treatment and to determine that remission has occurred. The Geriatric Depression Scale (GDS), reproduced in Figure 4–2, is one of the best established of these scales (Yesavage et al. 1982). The GDS is a self-rated scale with good psychometric properties when used for assessing functionally impaired but cognitively intact patients in primary care settings (Friedman et al. 2005). It remains reliable and valid in assessing patients with mild to moderate cognitive impairment.

The Consensus Guidelines recommend both psychotherapy and pharmacotherapy for major depression in elderly patients (Alexopoulos et al. 2001): for mild depression, antidepressant plus psychotherapy or either modality alone is recommended; for severe depression, antidepressant plus psychotherapy, antidepressant alone, or ECT is recommended. Among antidepressants, SSRIs and venlafaxine XR were given the highest ratings in the Consensus Guidelines (Alexopoulos et al. 2001). (At the time of the survey, duloxetine was not yet marketed.) Dosing and dose titration of these medications are covered in the Specific Drug summaries section at the end of this chapter.

For severe or melancholic depression with failure to thrive, patients are best treated in an inpatient setting where they can be adequately

Geriatric Depression Scale

Please circle the best answer for how you have felt over the past week.

Yes No 1. Are you basically satisfied with your life?
Yes No 2. Have you dropped many of your activities and interests?
Yes No 3. Do you feel that your life is empty?
Yes No 4. Do you often get bored?
Yes No 5. Are you hopeful about the future?
Yes No 6. Are you bothered by thoughts you can't get out of your head?
Yes No 7. Are you in good spirits most of the time?
Yes No 8. Are you afraid that something bad is going to happen to you?
Yes No 9. Do you feel happy most of the time?
Yes No 10. Do you often feel helpless?
Yes No 11. Do you often get restless and fidgety?
Yes No 12. Do you prefer to stay at home rather than going out and doing new things?
Yes No 13. Do you frequently worry about the future?
Yes No 14. Do you feel you have more problems with memory than most?
Yes No 15. Do you think it is wonderful to be alive now?
Yes No 16. Do you often feel downhearted and blue?
Yes No 17. Do you feel pretty worthless the way you are now?
Yes No 18. Do you worry a lot about the past?
Yes No 19. Do you find life very exciting?
Yes No 20. Is it hard for you to get started on new projects?
Yes No 21. Do you feel full of energy?
Yes No 22. Do you feel that your situation is hopeless?
Yes No 23. Do you think that most people are better off than you are?
Yes No 24. Do you frequently get upset over little things?
Yes No 25. Do you frequently feel like crying?
Yes No 26. Do you have trouble concentrating?
Yes No 27. Do you enjoy getting up in the morning?
Yes No 28. Do you prefer to avoid social gatherings?
Yes No 29. Is it easy for you to make decisions?
Yes No 30. Is your mind as clear as it used to be?

"No" answers indicate depression for questions numbered 1, 5, 7, 9, 15, 19, 21, 27, 29, and 30.
"Yes" answers indicate depression for all other questions.

Figure 4–2. Geriatric Depression Scale.

Source. Reprinted from Yesavage JA, Brink TL, Rose TL, et al.: "Development and Validation of a Geriatric Depression Screening Scale: A Preliminary Report." *Journal of Psychiatric Research* 17:37–49, 1982.

nourished and hydrated while treatment proceeds. This is a primary indication for ECT, and this modality should be considered for acute treatment. Alternatively, aggressive antidepressant pharmacotherapy can be undertaken. As the patient becomes more active, closer observation for suicidality is often indicated.

When ECT is used, once depression remits, continuation therapy can proceed with medications. The efficacy and safety of maintenance ECT in the geriatric population have not been adequately studied. Post-ECT patients still require aggressive pharmacotherapy, often with drug combinations or augmentation therapies. Those who are not treated adequately are at high risk of relapse in the 6 months following cessation of ECT (Sackeim et al. 2001).

Minor Depression

Minor depression is defined as a depressive syndrome involving two to four symptoms from the DSM-IV-TR "A" criterion for major depressive episode (depressed mood, sleep problems, anhedonia, psychological symptoms such as excessive or inappropriate guilt, hopelessness, lack of energy, poor concentration, appetite or weight change, psychomotor change, or thoughts of suicide or frequent thoughts of death). In one study, minor depression was found to be less common than major depression in older medical inpatients (McCusker et al. 2005). It has been found to have the same associations as major depression, with variables such as cognitive impairment or history of depression, although correlations are weaker for minor depression (McCusker et al. 2005). Among patients with Alzheimer's disease, minor depression was found in another study to be as prevalent as major depression (Starkstein et al. 2005). Moreover, depression without sadness was more common in minor depression in patients with late-stage Alzheimer's disease (Starkstein et al. 2005). Current recommendations are to initiate treatment for patients with minor depression associated with significant disability or symptoms that pose a risk to the patient (e.g., suicidal ideation). For others, watchful waiting can serve to identify those with persistent symptoms who will require treatment. Paroxetine was shown to be of moderate benefit in a randomized controlled trial of minor depression (and dysthymia) in primary care settings (Williams et al. 2000).

Bipolar Depression

Lithium and valproate remain the mainstays of treatment for bipolar disorder in geriatric patients. For bipolar depression, a number of treatment options exist. These include quetiapine monotherapy, lamotrigine monotherapy, lamotrigine added to an existing mood stabilizer, combinations of the above drugs, olanzapine-fluoxetine as a combination drug, or (in treatment-refractory cases) an antidepressant added to an existing mood stabilizer (Suppes et al. 2005). The magnitude of improvement in depressive symptoms in bipolar I patients appears to be larger for quetiapine monotherapy than for either olanzapine or the combination drug olanzapine-fluoxetine; however, the limitations of cross-study comparisons are substantial, and large-scale studies of elderly bipolar patients are lacking (Calabrese et al. 2005).

Quetiapine can be initiated as described in Chapter 3 of this volume, "Antipsychotics," and lamotrigine as described in Chapter 5 (see Specific Drug summaries). When lamotrigine is added to an existing mood stabilizer to treat breakthrough depression, it is reported to be effective at a dosage of 75–100 mg/day in elderly patients (Robillard and Conn 2002).

There remains controversy as to the actual risk of introducing an antidepressant into the treatment regimen for a patient with bipolar I disorder—even when a mood stabilizer is coadministered—because of the risk of inducing rapid cycling or a switch into mania. A review of randomized controlled trials of antidepressants for short-term treatment of bipolar depression concluded that antidepressants (except for TCAs) were no more likely to induce mania than placebo (Gijsman et al. 2004). Of note, most patients in those trials also were treated with mood stabilizers. Furthermore, none of the studies reviewed were longer than 10 weeks in duration, so conclusions regarding the long-term safety of antidepressants in bipolar populations await further study. When antidepressants are used for bipolar depression, preferred drugs include SSRIs, bupropion, and venlafaxine (Suppes et al. 2005). It is recommended that treatment be limited to the acute phase (induction of remission), usually 6–12 weeks.

Psychotic Depression (Delusional Depression)

Although DSM-IV-TR considers psychotic depression a subtype of major depression, there is some evidence to suggest that psychotic depression is distinct from depression without psychotic features and is a syndrome that often remains true to form from one depressive episode to the next in a given individual (Schatzberg 2003). Psychotic symptoms can be either delusions or hallucinations. Delusions need not be mood-congruent for the diagnosis to be made. Psychotic depression in the elderly is the foremost indication for ECT. If pharmacotherapy is used for acute treatment, an antipsychotic must be used in tandem with the antidepressant (Alexopoulos et al. 2001). When the psychotic symptoms have remitted (either with ECT or with antipsychotic medication), the antidepressant often can be used as sole continuation therapy. There is no consensus as to how long the antipsychotic should be continued (Alexopoulos et al. 2001), although many clinicians attempt to taper and discontinue the antipsychotic after about 2 months of combined treatment. Subsequent relapse of psychotic symptoms after depression has remitted may suggest a schizoaffective process requiring maintenance therapy with an antidepressant-antipsychotic combination.

Dysthymia (Subsyndromal Depression)

Dysthymia is a milder but more chronic depressive illness that is relatively common in the elderly population. It is often misattributed to growing old but in fact may be amenable to combined pharmacotherapy and psychotherapy in many cases (Alexopoulos et al. 2001). An SSRI may be preferred because of a favorable risk-benefit ratio, although there is some evidence that SSRI therapy might not successfully maintain remission if the patient has "atypical" symptoms, as discussed below (McGrath et al. 2000). The latency to antidepressant effect in dysthymia may be considerably longer than for major depression (Albert and Ebert 1996).

Atypical Depression

Atypical depression, a variant of major depression, is characterized by neurovegetative symptoms of reversed polarity, including hypersomnia, hyperphagia with weight gain, psychomotor retardation, mood reactivity, and in some cases, sensitivity to interpersonal rejection. Phobic symptoms can be present, as can a subjective sense of fatigue or heaviness in the limbs ("leaden paralysis"). This disorder does occur in elderly patients, although probably not as commonly as in younger cohorts. In general, atypical depression is more responsive to MAOIs than to TCAs. While anecdotal reports and clinical experience suggest that SSRIs are useful for inducing remission of symptoms in atypical depression, they might not be as effective as MAOIs in maintaining remission over time (McGrath et al. 2000).

Bereavement-Related Depression

It is not uncommon to encounter elderly patients who still grieve the death of a loved one (usually a spouse or a child) many years after the loss. These patients often meet criteria for major depression, and careful history suggests that symptoms have been present since the loss. The question of when and with which patients to intervene using pharmacotherapy is important, since these patients may suffer an added burden of excessive guilt, preoccupation with worthlessness, persistent thoughts of suicide (American Psychiatric Association 2000), and social isolation. In addition, the length of a depressive episode in part determines treatment responsiveness. In one small, open-label study of a mixed-age group of recently bereaved individuals meeting criteria for major depression, symptoms responded to treatment with sustained-release bupropion (Zisook et al. 2001). The authors noted that antidepressant medication did not interfere with the grieving process but rather facilitated grieving. Patients treated with antidepressants for this indication often benefit as well from psychotherapy to address the grieving process.

Dementia With Depression

The syndromes of dementia and depression are associated in several ways: depression can represent a prodrome to dementia, can occur in the context of an established dementia, or can be associated with reversible cognitive impairment in the "dementia of depression" (Alexopoulos et al. 1993). Psychological symptoms of excessive guilt, low self-esteem or self-loathing, or persistent suicidal ideation are important flags for depression and can help to distinguish depression from uncomplicated dementia in the geriatric population. A scale such as the Cornell Scale for Depression in Dementia can be used to assist in the diagnosis and to quantitate severity (Alexopoulos et al. 1988). This is a 19-item scale with reasonably good psychometric properties that integrates information from patient and caregiver reports with the clinician's direct observations of the patient. A cutoff score of 5 has been found to optimize identification of true-positive cases of depression (Schreiner et al. 2003). The scale is reproduced in Figure 4–3.

Cornell Scale for Depression in Dementia

U = unable to evaluate   0 = absent   1 = mild or intermittent   2 = severe

Ratings should be based on symptoms and signs occurring during the week prior to interview. No score should be given in symptoms result from physical disability or illness.

A. Mood-related signs

1. Anxiety: anxious expression, ruminations, worrying   U 0 1 2

2. Sadness: sad expression, sad voice, tearfulness   U 0 1 2

3. Lack of reactivity to pleasant events   U 0 1 2

4. Irritability: easily annoyed, short-tempered   U 0 1 2

B. Behavioral disturbance

5. Agitation: restlessness, handwringing, hairpulling   U 0 1 2

6. Retardation: slow movement, slow speech, slow   U 0 1 2
reactions

7. Multiple physical complaints (score 0 if gastrointestinal   U 0 1 2
symptoms only)

8. Loss of interest: less involved in usual activities   U 0 1 2
(score only if change occurred acutely, i.e., in less than
1 month)

C. Physical signs

9. Appetite loss: eating less than usual   U 0 1 2

10. Weight loss (score 2 if greater than 5 lb in 1 month)   U 0 1 2

11. Lack of energy: fatigues easily, unable to sustain   U 0 1 2
activities
(score only if change occurred acutely, i.e., in less than
1 month)

Figure 4–3.   Cornell Scale for Depression in Dementia.
Source.   Reprinted from Alexopoulos GS, Abrams RC, Young RC, et al: "Cornell Scale for Depression in Dementia." *Biological Psychiatry* 23:271–284, 1988. Used with permission.

D. Cyclic functions

12. Diurnal variation of mood: symptoms worse   U 0 1 2
    in the morning

13. Difficulty falling asleep: later than usual for this   U 0 1 2
    individual

14. Multiple awakenings during sleep   U 0 1 2

15. Early morning awakening: earlier than usual for this   U 0 1 2
    individual

E. Ideational disturbance

16. Suicide: feels life is not worth living, has suicidal   U 0 1 2
    wishes, or makes suicide attempt

17. Poor self esteem: self-blame, self-depreciation,   U 0 1 2
    feelings of failure

18. Pessimism: anticipation of the worst   U 0 1 2

19. Mood congruent delusions: delusions of poverty,   U 0 1 2
    illness, or loss

Figure 4–4.   Cornell Scale for Depression in Dementia.
(Continued)

In cases of established dementia, patients may meet criteria for major depression or for more minor degrees of depression (see earlier discussion of minor depression). When depressive syndromes are associated with behavioral disturbances, significant improvement can be seen with antidepressant therapy. Elderly patients with dementia should be treated with lower initial antidepressant doses and may respond at lower target doses than those without dementia (Streim et al. 2000). In the case of nonresponse at lower doses, however, the drug should be titrated to the standard dose before concluding the trial. For dementia-associated depression, efficacy and tolerability have been demonstrated for paroxetine (Katona et al. 1998), citalopram (Nyth et al. 1992), and sertraline (Lyketsos et al. 2000).

Seasonal Depression

Little is known about the prevalence of seasonal depression in the elderly population from systematic study, but it may be particularly common among elders in northern climates who are likely to spend more time indoors, and in elderly "shut-ins" who have virtually no outside light exposure (in which case, the depression might not be seasonal). Features of this disorder show a high degree of overlap with those of atypical depression as well as bipolar depression. For mild to moderately severe seasonal depression in outpatients, BLT can be used as the sole intervention. Exposure to a 10,000-lux lamp for 30 minutes every morning is sufficient to maintain normal mood for many patients (Rosenthal 1993). Intervention prior to the usual onset of depressive symptoms is preferred (e.g., in September for those with usual onset in October) (Meesters et al. 1993). Light sessions are continued on a daily basis for a minimum of 2 weeks and may need to be continued for the duration of the low-light season. There are few controlled studies comparing BLT to standard antidepressant therapy in seasonal depression. In our view, for more severe seasonal depression, BLT should be considered an adjunct to other standard antidepressant treatments. For certain patients, a mood stabilizer also may be indicated, since BLT has the potential to induce mania in susceptible individuals. Among patients with Alzheimer's disease, BLT also has been used to treat insomnia and other disturbances of the sleep-wake cycle, such as nighttime agitation (Ancoli-Israel et al. 2003).

Medical Disorders

Cancer and Depression

Depression in the cancer patient takes many forms, depending in part on how long the patient has lived with the disease and the remaining life expectancy. A patient recently diagnosed with cancer may suffer an adjustment reaction and benefit most from intensive supportive or educative psychotherapy. The patient who has lived with cancer for some time may develop major depression; this is thought to occur in 5%–15% of patients (McDaniel et al. 1995). The patient with terminal illness may suffer from treatable depressive symptoms (e.g., apathy, low energy, lack of motivation). In the latter two cases, aggressive treatment is indicated to alleviate suffering, improve compliance with needed treatment, optimize function, and reduce the incidence of suicide; the suicide rate among cancer patients is twice that of the general population (McDaniel et al. 1995).

For elderly patients with cancer and major depression, SSRIs are considered first-line antidepressants, although newer atypical antidepressants have been understudied for this indication (McDaniel et al. 1995). Issues of concern in using medications in this population include anticholinergic effects, nausea, weight loss, and medication interactions (especially with opioids). Specific SSRIs of choice include citalopram, escitalopram, and sertraline because of minimal CYP450 effects. In the experience of the authors, both mirtazapine and venlafaxine are effective as well, and these drugs also have minimal CYP450 effects. For terminally ill patients, there may not be adequate time remaining to experience an antidepressant effect from one of these medications. For these patients, a psychostimulant can be used, and often is effective not only in increasing energy and motivation but in reducing somnolence secondary to opioids required for pain treatment.

Coronary Heart Disease and Depression

Depression is associated with increased risk of CHD, MI, and cardiac death (Roose et al. 2005). Up to half of MI patients experience depression (major depression or subsyndromal depression) postinfarction, and the presence of depression predicts a fourfold increase in mortality in the 6 months postinfarction (Frasure-Smith et al. 1993). Even mild to moderate depression (Beck Depression Inventory score≥10) in post-MI patients predicts mortality within 18 months after the event; the risk is greatest among those with frequent (≥10) premature ventricular complexes per hour, suggesting a possible arrhythmic mechanism (Frasure-Smith et al. 1995).

Depression in CHD patients is treatable, and the initial drugs of choice for this indication are SSRI antidepressants. SSRIs have negligible effects on heart rate, rhythm, rate variability, or interval (QTc) variability, making them safer than other drugs for CHD patients (Roose et al. 1998). In addition, SSRIs may confer the added benefit in the CHD population of normalization of indices of platelet activation and aggregation, thought to be mediated by inhibition of serotonin transport into platelets (Roose 2003; Sauer et al. 2001). In fact, however, the SADHART study, a large, randomized controlled trial of patients with CHD (75% post-MI, 25% unstable angina), found sertraline 50–200 mg/day to be ineffective in treating depression as gauged by score on the Ham-D (Glassman et al. 2002). In addition, although sertraline was found to be safe in terms of adverse effects, it was not associated with a statistically significant reduction in the rate of severe cardiovascular adverse events compared with placebo (14.5% in sertraline group, 22.4% in placebo group) (Glassman et al. 2002). Similarly, the ENRICHD trial, a large, randomized controlled trial of CBT for depression and low perceived social support in CHD patients, found that CBT was not significantly better statistically than placebo in treating depression in CHD patients and was ineffective in influencing mortality or recurrent infarction rates (Berkman et al. 2003).

The newer atypical antidepressants may be effective in the treatment of depression in CHD, but there are concerns about the safety of using any medication with noradrenergic effects. None of the atypical antidepressants have yet been shown to be safe in the CHD population.

Medication-Induced Depression

A number of commonly prescribed medications have been implicated as causes of depression in susceptible patients (Reynolds 1995); a list of these drugs is shown in Table 4–11. The onset of depression often can be linked temporally to the initiation of the offending medication. In such cases, if the medical condition permits and suitable alternative treatments exist, the medication should be withdrawn. If depression persists, antidepressant therapy may be indicated.

For medications that are best continued in spite of incident depression (e.g., a "statin" drug), antidepressant medication may need to be added. Among other benefits, this helps the patient maintain compliance with the cholesterol-lowering agent. For medication such as interferon, prophylactic antidepressant therapy is often begun before the drug is initiated because of the high rate of depression in susceptible individuals.

Parkinson's Disease With Depression

Among patients with Parkinson's disease (PD), an estimated 30%–40% suffer from some form of depression (Weintraub et al. 2005). Incident

Table 4–11. Medications associated with depression

Acyclovir	Fluoroquinolone antibiotics
Amphotericin B	(ciprofloxacin)
Anabolic steroids	Guanethidine
Angiotensin-converting enzyme	H_2-receptor blockers
inhibitors	Interferon-α
Anticonvulsants	Interleukin-2
Asparaginase	Isotretinoin
Baclofen	Levodopa
Barbiturates	Mefloquine
Benzodiazepines	Methyldopa
β-Blockers	Metoclopramide
Bromocriptine	Metrizamide
Calcium channel blockers	Metronidazole
Cholesterol-lowering drugs	Nonsteroidal anti-inflammatory drugs
(statins)	(indomethacin)
Clonidine	Opioids
Corticosteroids	Pergolide
Cycloserine	Procarbazine
Dapsone	Reserpine
Digitalis	Sulfonamides
Disopyramide	Thiazide diuretics
Disulfiram	Topiramate
Estrogen	Vinblastine
Ethionamide	Vincristine

depression in PD is thought to have a bimodal peak, with high frequencies soon after diagnosis and late in the course of the disease (Rickards 2005). Although the diagnosis is made clinically, severity can be gauged using instruments such as the Ham-D or the Montgomery-Åsberg Depression Rating Scale (Rickards 2005). In general, the diagnosis of depression in PD is complicated by a considerable overlap of symptoms between the two diseases; those that can be helpful in parsing out depression are as follows (Rickards 2005):

- Pervasive low mood (for ≥2 weeks) with diurnal variation
- Early-morning awakening
- Pessimism about the world, self, and future that does not correspond to level of disability or previous attributional style
- Suicidal thinking

Neurotransmitter derangements in PD are primarily dopaminergic but also involve serotonergic and noradrenergic systems. Treatments include ECT and antidepressant medication. ECT results in rapid improvement in depressive as well as motor symptoms, but improvement in the latter may be short-lived (Cummings 1992).

There is little controlled research to guide therapy in this area (Ghazi-Noori et al. 2003). A review and meta-analysis concluded that PD patients may benefit less from antidepressant treatment (particularly SSRIs) than elderly patients without PD (Weintraub et al. 2005). None of the studies reviewed used dual-acting agents other than TCAs, and none used dopamine agonists, which have been observed anecdotally to have antidepressant effects in this population.

Thyroid Disease and Depression

Hypothyroidism is highly prevalent in the elderly population, particularly among women, and is associated with depression as well as cognitive slowing, two common presenting complaints in geriatric psychiatry (Laurberg et al. 2005). Hyperthyroidism is much less prevalent and, although it can be associated with depression, it is more likely to be associated with anxiety (panic and generalized anxiety). In general, when depression occurs in the context of clinical thyroid disease, the thyroid disease should be treated; depressive symptoms usually remit spontaneously. When depression is very severe or depressive symptoms do not remit, antidepressant medication may be indicated.

When depression occurs in the context of subclinical thyroid disease, what constitutes appropriate treatment is not so well established. For example, subclinical hypothyroidism (defined by TSH higher than upper limit of reference range, with T_4 and triiodothyronine T_3 in range) may be treated, untreated, or followed in the clinical setting, depending on the clinician. Some experts advocate treatment on the grounds that the signs and symptoms of even mild hypothyroidism are not benign: fatigue, slowed thinking, cold intolerance, dry skin, constipation, weight gain, arthralgia, myalgia, depression, alterations in hair, dyspnea, and edema (Laurberg et al. 2005). With comorbid depression, if subclinical hypothyroidism is not treated, a full response to antidepressant treatment is less likely (Pies 1997a). Others argue against treatment on the grounds that transient hypothyroidism occurs in patients recovering from nonthyroidal illnesses (Laurberg et al. 2005) and that most patients with subclinical hypothyroidism revert to normal TSH values without any intervention (Diez et al. 2005). A recommended algorithm for the management of subclinical hypothyroidism is shown in Figure 4–4 (Col et al. 2004).

Vascular Depression and Poststroke Depression

In cerebrovascular disease as in CHD, the prevalence of depression is high, and the presence of depression not only is a risk factor for stroke (Yamanaka et al. 2005) but predicts higher levels of morbidity and mortality poststroke (Ramasubbu and Patten 2003). The relationship of depression and stroke is bidirectional (Astrom et al. 1993); a 3-year prospective study of stroke patients found that the most important predictors of depression immediately after stroke were left anterior brain lesion, language problems, and living alone, whereas the most important predictor after 12 months was few social contacts outside the family. Other contributors included dependence for activities of daily living and cerebral atrophy (Astrom et al. 1993).

Treatment of depression is important because it affects outcome after a stroke. Although head-to-head studies are lacking, certain medications are recommended for this population, including SSRIs, nortriptyline, and venlafaxine (Robinson et al. 2000). Use of psychostimulants is somewhat controversial, although these medications are recommended on the basis of preliminary studies (Crisostomo et al. 1988; Grade et al. 1998; Sugden and Bourgeois 2004). Bupropion is generally avoided because of seizure risk. Trazodone and amitriptyline are not recommended, as these drugs have been found to slow recovery after stroke (Alexopoulos et al. 1996), possibly because of sedative effects on rehabilitation efforts. When SSRIs are used to treat poststroke depression, those with low to moderate affinity for 5-HTT (citalopram or escitalopram) are preferred because of reduced risk of bleeding poststroke (Ramasubbu 2004).

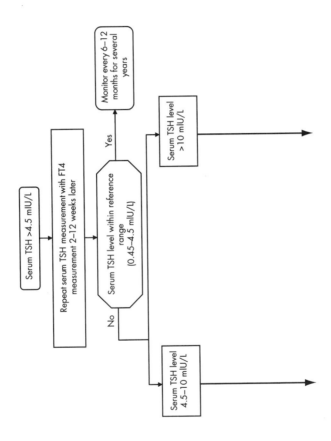

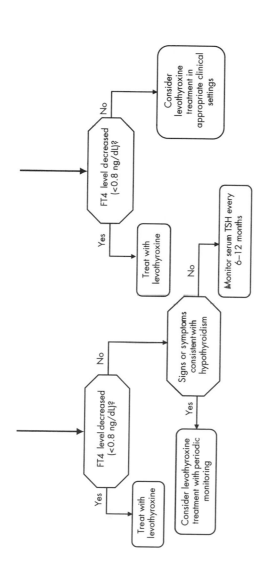

Figure 4–4. Algorithm for workup and management of subclinical hypothyroidism.

Note. FT4 = free thyroxine; TSH = thyroid-stimulating hormone.

Source. Reprinted from Col NF, Surks MI, Daniels GH: "Subclinical Thyroid Disease: Clinical Applications." *The Journal of the American Medical Association* 291:239–243, 2004. Copyright 2004, American Medical Association. Used with permission.

Depression related to chronic ischemic disease rather than stroke (vascular depression) usually has a more insidious onset than poststroke depression. The clinical picture of the patient with vascular depression includes apathy, social isolation, anhedonia, dysfunction in activities of daily living, and cognitive impairment involving mainly executive function and speed of information processing (Steffens and Krishnan 1998). The diagnosis requires the presence of vascular lesions, presumably involving not only subcortical white matter but also subcortical gray matter (basal ganglia) (Steffens et al. 1999). Patients with vascular depression have been shown to exhibit a poorer response to antidepressant treatment with more frequent adverse effects compared to age-matched control patients (Fujikawa et al. 1996). As with treatment of vascular dementia, treatment of vascular depression also involves management of underlying risk factors (e.g., hypertension, hypercholesterolemia, smoking) and use of aspirin and other platelet aggregation inhibitors, as discussed in Chapter 9, "Medications to Treat Dementia and Other Cognitive Disorders."

Chapter Summary

- Elderly patients are at chronic risk of undertreatment for depression because of low expectations regarding recovery and fears about aggressive pharmacotherapy and electroconvulsive therapy (ECT).
- "Psychological" symptoms of excessive guilt, low self-esteem or self-loathing, and persistent suicidal ideation are important flags for depression and can help to distinguish depression from uncomplicated dementia in the geriatric population.
- Potential drug interactions with antidepressants are numerous and include both pharmacokinetic and pharmacodynamic mechanisms.
- Although there is a great deal of between-individual variability in time to effect, in general, a minimum of 6 weeks of antidepressant treatment at a therapeutic dose should be undertaken in an elderly patient before a declaration of "no response" is made for that trial.
- For continuation as well as maintenance therapy, full acute doses of antidepressant medication are recommended, as is continuation of any adjunctive treatment such as lithium.
- ECT is well tolerated in the elderly, even in patients with dementia.
- Over time, tolerance develops to certain adverse effects of antidepressants (sedation, dizziness, and gastrointestinal distress) but not to others (orthostasis, cardiac rhythm disturbances, or delirium).
- All tricyclic antidepressants (TCAs) affect cardiac conduction and are relatively contraindicated in patients with ischemic heart disease, preexisting bundle branch block, or intraventricular conduction delay.
- Both hyponatremia and syndrome of inappropriate antidiuretic hormone have been associated with selective serotonin reuptake inhibitor (SSRI) use in elderly patients.
- The association of SSRIs with bleeding is apparently dose dependent and is greatest for SSRIs with high serotonin transporter affinity, such as fluoxetine, paroxetine, and sertraline.
- The increased risk of falls with SSRIs and TCAs appears to be dose dependent.

References

Abrams R: Relapse of depression after electroconvulsive therapy. JAMA 285:3087; author reply 3088–3089, 2001

Albert R, Ebert D: Full efficacy of SSRI treatment in refractory dysthymia is achieved only after 16 weeks. J Clin Psychiatry 57:176, 1996

Alexopoulos GS: The treatment of depressed demented patients. J Clin Psychiatry 57 (suppl 14):14–20, 1996

Alexopoulos GS, Abrams RC, Young RC, et al: Cornell Scale for Depression in Dementia. Biol Psychiatry 23:271–284, 1988

Alexopoulos GS, Meyers BS, Young RC, et al: The course of geriatric depression with "reversible dementia": a controlled study. Am J Psychiatry 150:1693–1699, 1993

Alexopoulos GS, Meyers BS, Young RC, et al: Recovery in geriatric depression. Arch Gen Psychiatry 53:305–312, 1996

Alexopoulos GS, Katz IR, Reynolds CF, et al: Pharmacotherapy of depression in older patients: a summary of the expert consensus guidelines. J Psychiatr Pract 7:361–376, 2001

American Psychiatric Association: Diagnostic and Statistical Manual of Mental Disorders, 4th Edition, Text Revision. Washington, DC, American Psychiatric Association, 2000

Ancoli-Israel S, Gehrman P, Martin JL, et al: Increased light exposure consolidates sleep and strengthens circadian rhythms in severe Alzheimer's disease patients. Behav Sleep Med 1:22–36, 2003

Anderson IM: Selective serotonin reuptake inhibitors versus tricyclic antidepressants: a meta-analysis of efficacy and tolerability. J Affect Disord 58:19–36, 2000

Asnis GM, Kohn SR, Henderson M, et al: SSRIs versus non-SSRIs in post-traumatic stress disorder: an update with recommendations. Drugs 64:383–404, 2004

Astrom M, Adolfsson R, Asplund K: Major depression in stroke patients. A 3-year longitudinal study. Stroke 24:976–982, 1993

Barak Y, Olmer A, Aizenberg D: Antidepressants reduce the risk of suicide among elderly depressed patients. Neuropsychopharmacology 31:178–181, 2006

Beers MH, Berkow R: The Merck Manual of Geriatrics, 3rd Edition. Whitehouse Station, NJ, Merck Research Laboratories, 2000

Berkman LF, Blumenthal J, Burg M, et al: Effects of treating depression and low perceived social support on clinical events after myocardial infarction: the Enhancing Recovery in Coronary Heart Disease Patients (ENRICHD) Randomized Trial. JAMA 289:3106–3116, 2003

Blumenthal JA, Babyak MA, Moore KA, et al: Effects of exercise training on older patients with major depression. Arch Intern Med 159:2349–2356, 1999

Boyer EW, Shannon M: The serotonin syndrome. N Engl J Med 352:1112–1120, 2005

Bruce ML, Ten Have TR, Reynolds CF, et al: Reducing suicidal ideation and depressive symptoms in depressed older primary care patients. JAMA 291:1081–1091, 2004

Calabrese JR, Elhaj O, Gajwani P, et al: Clinical highlights in bipolar depression: focus on atypical antipsychotics. J Clin Psychiatry 66 (suppl 5):26–33, 2005

Col NF, Surks MI, Daniels GH: Subclinical thyroid disease: clinical applications. JAMA 291:239–243, 2004

Cole JO, Bodkin JA: Antidepressant drug side effects. J Clin Psychiatry 51(suppl):21–26, 1990

Crisostomo EA, Duncan PW, Propst M, et al: Evidence that amphetamine with physical therapy promotes recovery of motor function in stroke patients. Ann Neurol 23:94–97, 1988

Cummings JL: Depression and Parkinson's disease: a review. Am J Psychiatry 149:443–454, 1992

Dalton SO, Johansen C, Mellemkjaer L, et al: Use of selective serotonin reuptake inhibitors and risk of upper gastrointestinal tract bleeding. Arch Intern Med 163:59–64, 2003

de Abajo FJ, Rodriguez LA, Montero D: Association between selective serotonin reuptake inhibitors and upper gastrointestinal bleeding: population based case-control study. BMJ 319:1106–1109, 1999

DeBattista C, Solvason HB, Poirier J, et al: A prospective trial of bupropion SR augmentation of partial and non-responders to serotonergic antidepressants. J Clin Psychopharmacol 23:27–30, 2003

DeBattista C, Lembke A, Solvason HB, et al: A prospective trial of modafinil as an adjunctive treatment of major depression. J Clin Psychopharmacol 24:87–90, 2004

de Boer RA, van Dijk TH, Holman ND, et al: QT interval prolongation after sertraline overdose: a case report. BMC Emerg Med 5:5, 2005

Delgado PL, McGahuey CA, Moreno FA, et al: Treatment strategies for depression and sexual dysfunction. J Clin Psychiatry Monograph 17:15–21, 1999

Dietch JT, Fine M: The effect of nortriptyline in elderly patients with cardiac conduction disease. J Clin Psychiatry 51:65–67, 1990

Diez JJ, Iglesias P, Burman KD: Spontaneous normalization of thyrotropin concentrations in patients with subclinical hypothyroidism. J Clin Endocrinol Metab 90:4124–4127, 2005

Ensrud KE, Blackwell T, Mangione CM, et al: Central nervous system active medications and risk for fractures in older women. Arch Intern Med 163:949–957, 2003

Fabian TJ, Amico JA, Kroboth PD, et al: Paroxetine-induced hyponatremia in older adults. Arch Intern Med 164:327–332, 2004

Fava M, Borus JS, Alpert JE, et al: Folate, vitamin B12, and homocysteine in major depressive disorder. Am J Psychiatry 154:426–428, 1997

Fava M, Alpert J, Nierenberg A, et al: Double-blind study of high-dose fluoxetine versus lithium or desipramine augmentation of fluoxetine in partial responders and nonresponders to fluoxetine. J Clin Psychopharmacol 22:379–387, 2002

Fava M, Thase ME, DeBattista C: A multicenter, placebo-controlled study of modafinil augmentation in partial responders to selective serotonin reuptake inhibitors with persistent fatigue and sleepiness. J Clin Psychiatry 66:85–93, 2005

Fawcett J, Barkin RL: A meta-analysis of eight randomized, double-blind, controlled clinical trials of mirtazapine for the treatment of patients with major depression and symptoms of anxiety. J Clin Psychiatry 59:123–127, 1998

Fernandez F, Adams F, Holmes FV, et al: Methylphenidate for depressive disorders in cancer patients. Psychosomatics 28:455–461, 1987

Flint AJ: Recent developments in geriatric psychopharmacotherapy. Can J Psychiatry 39:S9–S18, 1994

Flint AJ: Pharmacologic treatment of depression in late life. CMAJ 157:1061–1067, 1997

Flint AJ: Generalised anxiety disorder in elderly patients. Drugs Aging 22:101–114, 2005

Flint AJ, Gagnon N: Diagnosis and management of panic disorder in older patients. Drugs Aging 20:881–891, 2003

Flint AJ, Rifat SL: The effect of sequential antidepressant treatment on geriatric depression. J Affect Disord 36:95–105, 1996

Flint AJ, Rifat SL: Maintenance treatment for recurrent depression in late life. Am J Geriatr Psychiatry 8:112–116, 2000

Folstein MF, Folstein SE, McHugh PR: "Mini-mental state". A practical method for grading the cognitive state of patients for the clinician. J Psychiatr Res 12:189–198, 1975

Frasure-Smith N, Lesperance F, Talajic M: Depression following myocardial infarction. JAMA 270:1819–1825, 1993

Frasure-Smith N, Lesperance F, Talajic M: Depression and 18-month prognosis after myocardial infarction. Circulation 91:999–1005, 1995

Fregni F, Santos CM, Myczkowski ML, et al: Repetitive transcranial magnetic stimulation is as effective as fluoxetine in the treatment of depression in patients with Parkinson's disease. J Neurol Neurosurg Psychiatry 75:1171–1174, 2004

Friedman B, Heisel MJ, Delavan RL: Psychometric properties of the 15-item Geriatric Depression Scale in functionally impaired, cognitively intact, community-dwelling elderly primary care patients. J Am Geriatr Soc 53:1570–1576, 2005

Frommer DA, Kulig KW, Marx JA, et al: Tricyclic antidepressant overdose: a review. JAMA 257:521–526, 1987

Fujikawa T, Yokota N, Muraoka M, et al: Response of patients with major depression and silent cerebral infarction to antidepressant drug therapy, with emphasis on central nervous system adverse reactions. Stroke 27:2040–2042, 1996

Fuller MA, Sajatovic M: Drug Information Handbook for Psychiatry, 5th Edition. Hudson, OH, Lexi-Comp Inc., 2005

Furlan PM, Kallan MJ, Ten Have T, et al: Cognitive and psychomotor effects of paroxetine and sertraline in healthy elderly volunteers. Am J Geriatr Psychiatry 9:429–438, 2001

Gershon AA, Dannon PN, Grunhaus L: Transcranial magnetic stimulation in the treatment of depression. Am J Psychiatry 160:835–845, 2003

Ghazi-Noori TH, Chung KHO, Deane H, et al: Therapies for depression in Parkinson's disease. Cochrane Database of Systematic Reviews, Issue 2, Article No: CD003465. DOI: 10.1002/14651858.CD003465, 2003

Gijsman HJ, Geddes JR, Rendell JM, et al: Antidepressants for bipolar depression: a systematic review of randomized, controlled trials. Am J Psychiatry 161:1537–1547, 2004

Glassman AH, Preud'homme XA: Review of the cardiovascular effects of heterocyclic antidepressants. J Clin Psychiatry 54(suppl):16–22, 1993

Glassman AH, Roose SP: Risks of antidepressants in the elderly: tricyclic antidepressants and arrhythmia-revising risks. Gerontology 40 (suppl 1):15–20, 1994

Glassman AH, Roose SP, Bigger JT: The safety of tricyclic antidepressants in cardiac patients. JAMA 269:2673–2675, 1993

Glassman AH, O'Connor CM, Califf RM, et al: Sertraline treatment of major depression in patients with acute MI or unstable angina. JAMA 288:701–709, 2002

Goldman DP, Joyce GF, Escarce JJ, et al: Pharmacy benefits and the use of drugs by the chronically ill. JAMA 291:2344–2350, 2004

Goldstein DJ, Lu Y, Detke MJ, et al: Duloxetine in the treatment of depression: a double-blind placebo-controlled comparison with paroxetine. J Clin Psychopharmacol 24:389–399, 2004

Grade C, Redford B, Chrostowski J, et al: Methylphenidate in early poststroke recovery: a double-blind, placebo-controlled study. Arch Phys Med Rehabil 79:1047–1050, 1998

Halper JP, Mann JJ: Cardiovascular effects of antidepressant medications. Br J Psychiatry 153 (suppl 3):87–98, 1988

Harnett DS: The difficult-to-treat psychiatric patient with comorbid medical illness, in The Difficult-to-Treat Psychiatric Patient. Edited by Dewan MJ, Pies RW. Washington, DC, American Psychiatric Publishing, 2001, pp 325–357

Heard K, Cain BS, Dart RC, et al: Tricyclic antidepressants directly depress human myocardial mechanical function independent of effects on the conduction system. Acad Emerg Med 8:1122–1127, 2001

Heeren TJ, Derksen P, van Heycop Ten Ham BF, et al: Treatment, outcome and predictors of response in elderly depressed in-patients. Br J Psychiatry 170:436–440, 1997

Hirschfeld RMA, Schatzberg AF: Long-term management of depression. Am J Med 97 (suppl 6A):33S–38S, 1994

Hussein S, Kaufman BM: Bradycardia associated with fluoxetine in an elderly patient with sick sinus syndrome (letter). Postgrad Med J 70:56, 1994

Isacsson G, Holmgren P, Ahlner J: Selective serotonin reuptake inhibitor antidepressants and the risk of suicide: a controlled forensic database study of 14,857 suicides. Acta Psychiatr Scand 111:286–290, 2005

Isbister GK, Bowe SJ, Dawson A, et al: Relative toxicity of selective serotonin reuptake inhibitors (SSRIs) in overdose. J Toxicol Clin Toxicol 42:277–285, 2004

Katona CLE, Hunter BN, Bray J: A double-blind comparison of the efficacy and safety of paroxetine and imipramine in the treatment of depression with dementia. Int J Geriatr Psychiatry 13:100–108, 1998

Katz IR, Reynolds CF, Alexopoulos GS, et al: Venlafaxine ER as a treatment for generalized anxiety disorder in older adults: pooled analysis of five randomized placebo-controlled clinical trials. J Am Geriatr Soc 50:18–25, 2002

Kelly CA, Dhaun N, Laing WJ, et al: Comparative toxicity of citalopram and the newer antidepressants after overdose. J Toxicol Clin Toxicol 42:67–71, 2004

Kitanaka I, Ross RJ, Cutler NR, et al: Altered hydroxydesipramine concentrations in elderly depressed patients. Clin Pharmacol Ther 31:51–55, 1982

Konig SA, Elger CE, Vassella F, et al: Recommendations for blood studies and clinical monitoring in early detection of valproate-associated liver failure. Nervenarzt 69:835–840, 1998

LaFrance WC, Lauterbach EC, Coffey CE, et al: The use of herbal alternative medicines in neuropsychiatry. J Neuropsychiatry Clin Neurosci 12:177–192, 2000

Laurberg P, Andersen S, Pedersen IB, et al: Hypothyroidism in the elderly: pathophysiology, diagnosis and treatment. Drugs Aging 22:23–38, 2005

Lejoyeux M, Rouillon F, Leon E, et al: The serotonin syndrome: review of the literature and description of an original study. Encephale 21:537–543, 1995

Lenox-Smith AJ, Reynolds A: A double-blind, randomised, placebo-controlled study of venlafaxine XL in patients with generalised anxiety disorder in primary care. Br J Gen Practice 53:772–777, 2003

Leon AC, Keller MB, Warshaw MG, et al: Prospective study of fluoxetine treatment and suicidal behavior in affectively ill subjects. Am J Psychiatry 156:195–201, 1999

Lyketsos CG, Sheppard J-ME, Steele CD, et al: Randomized, placebo-controlled, double-blind clinical trial of sertraline in the treatment of depression complicating Alzheimer's disease: initial results from the Depression in Alzheimer's Disease study. Am J Psychiatry 157:1686–1689, 2000

Mamdani MM, Parikh SV, Austin PC, et al: Use of antidepressants among elderly subjects: trends and contributing factors. Am J Psychiatry 157:360–367, 2000

Manly DT, Oakley SP, Bloch RM: Electroconvulsive therapy in old-old patients. Am J Geriatr Psychiatry 8:232–236, 2000

Martin-Facklam M, Rieger K, Riedel K-D, et al: Undeclared exposure to St. John's wort in hospitalized patients. Br J Clin Pharmacol 58:437–441, 2004

McCusker J, Cole M, Dufouil C, et al: The prevalence and correlates of major and minor depression in older medical inpatients. J Am Geriatr Soc 53:1344–1353, 2005

McDaniel JS, Musselman DL, Porter MR, et al: Depression in patients with cancer. Arch Gen Psychiatry 52:89–99, 1995

McEvoy GK, Snow EK, Kester L, et al: AHFS Drug Information. Bethesda, MD, American Society of Health-System Pharmacists, 2006

McGrath PJ, Stewart JW, Petkova E, et al: Predictors of relapse during fluoxetine continuation or maintenance treatment of major depression. J Clin Psychiatry 61:518–524, 2000

McIntyre RS, O'Donovan C: The human cost of not achieving full remission in depression. Can J Psychiatry 49 (suppl 1):10S–16S, 2004

Meesters Y, Jansen JHC, Beersma DGM, et al: Early light treatment can prevent an emerging winter depression from developing into a full-blown depression. J Affect Disord 29:41–47, 1993

Montejo AL, Llorca G, Izquierdo JA, et al: Incidence of sexual dysfunction associated with antidepressant agents: a prospective multicenter study of 1022 outpatients. J Clin Psychiatry 62 (suppl 3):10–21, 2001

Murphy GM, Kremer C, Rodrigues H, et al: The apolipoprotein E ε4 allele and antidepressant efficacy in cognitively intact elderly depressed patients. Biol Psychiatry 54:665–673, 2003a

Murphy GM, Kremer C, Rodrigues HE, et al: Pharmacogenetics of antidepressant medication intolerance. Am J Psychiatry 160:1830–1835, 2003b

Naka T, Jones D, Baldwin I, et al: Myoglobin clearance by super high-flux hemofiltration in a case of severe rhabdomyolysis: a case report. Crit Care 9:R90–R95, 2005

Nelson JC: Combined drug treatment strategies for major depression. Psychiatr Ann 28:197–203, 1998

Nelson JC, Mazure CM, Jatlow PI: Characteristics of desipramine-refractory depression. J Clin Psychiatry 55:12–19, 1994

Nelson JC, Mazure CM, Jatlow PI: Desipramine treatment of major depression in patients over 75 years of age. J Clin Psychopharmacol 15:99–105, 1995

Nicholas LM, Ford AL, Esposito SM, et al: The effects of mirtazapine on plasma lipid profiles in healthy subjects. J Clin Psychiatry 64:883–889, 2003

Nurnberg HG, Hensley PL, Gelenberg AJ, et al: Treatment of antidepressant-associated sexual dysfunction with sildenafil. JAMA 289:56–64, 2003

Nyth AL, Gottfries CG, Lyby K, et al: A controlled multicenter clinical study of citalopram and placebo in elderly depressed patients with and without concomitant dementia. Acta Psychiatr Scand 86:138–145, 1992

Oslin DW, Ten Have TR, Streim JE, et al: Probing the safety of medications in the frail elderly: evidence from a randomized clinical trial of sertraline and venlafaxine in depressed nursing home residents. J Clin Psychiatry 64:875–882, 2003

Pereira J, Bruera E: Depression with psychomotor retardation: diagnostic challenges and the use of psychostimulants. J Palliat Med 4:15–21, 2001

Pies R: The diagnosis and treatment of subclinical hypothyroid states in depressed patients. Gen Hosp Psychiatry 19:344–354, 1997a

Pies RW: Must we now consider SSRIs neuroleptics? J Clin Psychopharmacol 17:443–445, 1997b

Pies RW: Handbook of Essential Psychopharmacology, 2nd Edition. Washington, DC, American Psychiatric Publishing, 2005

Piscitelli SC, Burstein AH, Chaitt D, et al: Indinavir concentrations and St. John's wort. Lancet 355:547–548, 2000

Pollack MH, Rosenbaum JF: Management of antidepressant-induced side effects: a practical guide for the clinician. J Clin Psychiatry 48:3–8, 1987

Pollock BG, Everett G, Perel JM: Comparative cardiotoxicity of nortriptyline and its isomeric 10-hydroxymetabolites. Neuropsychopharmacology 6:1–10, 1992

Pollock BG, Perel JM, Paradis CF, et al: Metabolic and physiologic consequences of nortriptyline treatment in the elderly. Psychopharmacol Bull 30:145–150, 1994

Quitkin FM, Petkova E, McGrath PJ, et al: When should a trial of fluoxetine for major depression be declared failed? Am J Psychiatry 160:734–740, 2003

Ramasubbu R: Cerebrovascular effects of selective serotonin reuptake inhibitors: a systematic review. J Clin Psychiatry 65:1642–1653, 2004

Ramasubbu R, Patten SB: Effect of depression on stroke morbidity and mortality. Can J Psychiatry 48:250–257, 2003

Ray WA, Meredith S, Thapa PB, et al: Cyclic antidepressants and the risk of sudden cardiac death. Clin Pharmacol Ther 75:234–241, 2004

Reynolds CF 3rd: Recognition and differentiation of elderly depression in the clinical setting. Geriatrics 50 (suppl 1):S6–S15, 1995

Reynolds CF 3rd, Perel JM, Frank E, et al: Three-year outcomes of maintenance nortriptyline treatment in late-life depression: a study of two fixed plasma levels. Am J Psychiatry 156:1177–1181, 1999

Richelson E: Interactions of antidepressants with neurotransmitter transporters and receptors and their clinical relevance. J Clin Psychiatry 64 (suppl 13):5–12, 2003

Rickards H: Depression in neurological disorders: Parkinson's disease, multiple sclerosis, and stroke. J Neurol Neurosurg Psychiatry 76 (suppl 1):48–52, 2005

Roberts RL, Joyce PR, Mulder RT, et al: A common P-glycoprotein polymorphism is associated with nortriptyline-induced postural hypotension in patients treated for major depression. Pharmacogenomics J 2:191–196, 2002

Robillard M, Conn DK: Lamotrigine use in geriatric patients with bipolar depression. Can J Psychiatry 47:767–770, 2002

Robinson RG, Schultz SK, Castillo C, et al: Nortriptyline versus fluoxetine in the treatment of depression and in short-term recovery after stroke: a placebo-controlled, double-blind study. Am J Psychiatry 157:351–359, 2000

Roose SP: Treatment of depression in patients with heart disease. Biol Psychiatry 54:262–268, 2003

Roose SP, Dalack GW: Treating the depressed patient with cardiovascular problems. J Clin Psychiatry 53(suppl):25–31, 1992

Roose SP, Glassman AH: Antidepressant choice in the patient with cardiac disease: lessons from the Cardiac Arrhythmia Suppression Trial (CAST) studies. J Clin Psychiatry 55 (suppl A):83–87, 1994

Roose SP, Suthers KM: Antidepressant response in late-life depression. J Clin Psychiatry 59 (suppl 10):4–8, 1998

Roose SP, Laghrissi-Thode F, Kennedy JS, et al: Comparison of paroxetine and nortriptyline in depressed patients with ischemic heart disease. JAMA 279:287–291, 1998

Roose SP, Sackeim HA, Krishnan KR, et al: Antidepressant pharmacotherapy in the treatment of depression in the very old: a randomized, placebo-controlled trial. Am J Psychiatry 161:2050–2059, 2004

Roose SP, Glassman AH, Seidman SN: Relationship between depression and other medical illnesses. JAMA 286:1687–1690, 2005

Rosenbaum JF, Fava M, Hoog SL, et al: Selective serotonin reuptake inhibitor discontinuation syndrome: a randomized clinical trial. Biol Psychiatry 44:77–87, 1998

Rosenthal NE: Diagnosis and treatment of seasonal affective disorder. JAMA 270:2717–2720, 1993

Rouillon F, Gorwood P: The use of lithium to augment antidepressant medication. J Clin Psychiatry 59 (suppl 5):32–39, 1998

Ruschitzka F, Meier PJ, Turina M, et al: Acute heart transplant rejection due to St. John's wort. Lancet 355:548–549, 2000

Sachs GS, Guille C: Weight gain associated with use of psychotropic medications. J Clin Psychiatry 60 (suppl 21):16–19, 1999

Sackeim HA, Haskett RF, Mulsant BH, et al: Continuation pharmacotherapy in the prevention of relapse following electroconvulsive therapy. JAMA 285:1299–1307, 2001

Sauer WH, Berlin JA, Kimmel SE: Selective serotonin reuptake inhibitors and myocardial infarction. Circulation 104:1894–1898, 2001

Schatzberg AF: New approaches to managing psychotic depression. J Clin Psychiatry 64 (suppl 1):19–23, 2003

Schneider LS, Cooper TB, Staples FR, et al: Prediction of individual dosage of nortriptyline in depressed elderly outpatients. J Clin Psychopharmacol 7:311–314, 1987

Schneider LS, Cooper TB, Suckow RF, et al: Relationship of hydroxynortriptyline to nortriptyline concentration and creatinine clearance in depressed elderly outpatients. J Clin Psychopharmacol 10:333–337, 1990

Schreiner AS, Hayakawa H, Morimoto T, et al: Screening for late-life depression: cut-off scores for the Geriatric Depression Scale and the Cornell Scale for Depression in Dementia among Japanese subjects. Int J Geriatr Psychiatry 18:498–505, 2003

Semla TP, Beizer JL, Higbee MD: Geriatric Dosage Handbook, 11th Edition. Hudson, OH, Lexi-Comp Inc., 2006

Sheline YI, Freedland KE, Carney RM: How safe are serotonin reuptake inhibitors for depression in patients with coronary heart disease? Am J Med 102:54–59, 1997

Singhal AB, Caviness VS, Begleiter AF, et al: Cerebral vasoconstriction and stroke after use of serotonergic drugs. Neurology 58:130–133, 2002

Skolnick P: Beyond monoamine-based therapies: clues to new approaches. J Clin Psychiatry 63 (suppl 2):19–23, 2002

Spier SA, Frontera MA: Unexpected deaths in depressed medical inpatients treated with fluoxetine. J Clin Psychiatry 52:377–382, 1991

Starkstein SE, Jorge RE, Mizrahi R, et al: The construct of minor and major depression in Alzheimer's disease. Am J Psychiatry 162:2086–2093, 2005

Steffens DC, Krishnan KRR: Structural neuroimaging and mood disorders: recent findings, implications for classification and future directions. Biol Psychiatry 43:705–712, 1998

Steffens DC, Helms MJ, Krishnan KRR, et al: Cerebrovascular disease and depression symptoms in the Cardiovascular Health Study. Stroke 30:2159–2166, 1999

Steffens DC, Skoog I, Norton MC, et al: Prevalence of depression and its treatment in an elderly population: the Cache County study. Arch Gen Psychiatry 57:601–607, 2000

Stein G, Bernadt M: Lithium augmentation therapy in tricyclic-resistant depression: a controlled trial using lithium in low and normal doses. Br J Psychiatry 162:634–640, 1993

Stevinson C, Ernst E: Can St. John's wort trigger psychoses? Int J Clin Pharmacol Ther 42:473–480, 2004

Stoudemire A: New antidepressant drugs and the treatment of depression in the medically ill patient. Psychiatr Clin North Am 19:495–514, 1996

Streim JE, Oslin DW, Katz IR, et al: Drug treatment of depression in frail elderly nursing home residents. Am J Geriatr Psychiatry 8:150–159, 2000

Sugden SG, Bourgeois JA: Modafinil monotherapy in poststroke depression. Psychosomatics 45:80–81, 2004

Suppes T, Dennehy EB, Hirschfeld RMA, et al: The Texas implementation of medication algorithms: update to the algorithms for treatment of bipolar I disorder. J Clin Psychiatry 66:870–886, 2005

Sussman N, Ginsberg D: Rethinking side effects of the selective serotonin reuptake inhibitors: sexual dysfunction and weight gain. Psychiatr Ann 28:89–97, 1998

Tan RS, Bransgrove L: Drugs and orthostatic hypotension in the elderly, part II: reversing orthostatic hypotension with drug treatment. Clinical Geriatrics 6:38–44, 1998

Thapa PB, Gideon P, Cost TW, et al: Antidepressants and the risk of falls among nursing home residents. N Engl J Med 339:875–882, 1998

Thase ME: Therapeutic alternatives for difficult-to-treat depression: a narrative review of the state of the evidence. CNS Spectr 9:808–821, 2004

Trick L, Stanley N, Rigney U, et al: A double-blind, randomized, 26-week study comparing the cognitive and psychomotor effects and efficacy of 75 mg (37.5 mg b.i.d.) venlafaxine and 75 mg (25 mg mane, 50 mg nocte) dothiepin in elderly patients with moderate major depression being treated in general practice. J Psychopharmacol 18:205–214, 2004

Tulloch IF, Johnson AM: The pharmacologic profile of paroxetine, a new selective serotonin reuptake inhibitor. J Clin Psychiatry 53(suppl):7–12, 1992

UK ECT Review Group: Efficacy and safety of electroconvulsive therapy in depressive disorders: a systematic review and meta-analysis. Lancet 361:799–808, 2003

Van der Wurff FB, Stek ML, Hoogendijk WL, et al: Electroconvulsive therapy for the depressed elderly. The Cochrane Database of Systematic, Issue 2, Article No: CD003593. DOI: 003510.001002/14651858.CD14003593, 2003

van Walraven C, Mamdani MM, Wells PS, et al: Inhibition of serotonin reuptake by antidepressants and upper gastrointestinal bleeding in elderly patients: retrospective cohort study. BMJ 323:655–658, 2001

Vieweg WV, Wood MA: Tricyclic antidepressants, QT interval prolongation, and torsade de pointes. Psychosomatics 45:371–377, 2004

Wang PS, Schneeweiss S, Brookhart MA, et al: Suboptimal antidepressant use in the elderly. J Clin Psychopharmacol 25:118–126, 2005

Weintraub D, Morales KH, Moberg PJ, et al: Antidepressant studies in Parkinson's disease: a review and meta-analysis. Mov Disord 20:1161–1169, 2005

Whyte EM, Basinski J, Farhi P, et al: Geriatric depression treatment in nonresponders to selective serotonin reuptake inhibitors. J Clin Psychiatry 65:1634–1641, 2004

Williams JWJ, Barrett J, Oxman T, et al: Treatment of dysthymia and minor depression in primary care: a randomized controlled trial in older adults. JAMA 284:1519–1526, 2000

Wilson S, Argyropoulos S: Antidepressants and sleep: a qualitative review of the literature. Drugs 65:927–947, 2005

Yamanaka G, Otsuka K, Hotta N, et al: Depressive mood is independently related to stroke and cardiovascular events in a community. Biomed Pharmacother 59 (suppl 1):S31–S39, 2005

Yesavage JA, Brink TL, Rose TL, et al: Development and validation of a geriatric depression screening scale: a preliminary report. J Psychiatr Res 17:37–49, 1982

Young RC, Alexopoulos GS, Dhar AK, et al: Plasma 10-hydroxynortriptyline and renal function in elderly depressives. Biol Psychiatry 22:1283–1287, 1987

Zisook S, Shuchter SR, Pedrelli P, et al: Bupropion sustained release for bereavement: results of an open trial. J Clin Psychiatry 62:227–230, 2001

Generic name	bupropion
Trade name	Wellbutrin, Wellbutrin SR, Wellbutrin XL (generic available for immediate-release form)
Class	Atypical
Half-life	About 30 hours (longer for metabolites)
Mechanism of action	Not fully understood; probably dopaminergic and/or noradrenergic
Available preparations	Tablets: 75, 100 mg SR tablets: 100, 150, 200 mg XL tablets: 150, 300 mg
Starting dose	37.5–75 mg/day SR: 100 mg/day
Titration	Increase by 37.5 mg (or 75 mg) every 3–4 days SR: increase by 100 mg after 3–4 days
Typical daily dose	150 mg (2–3 divided doses separated by 6 hours) SR: 100 mg bid XL: 150 mg
Dose range	75–225 mg/day SR: 100–300 mg/day
Therapeutic serum level	Not established, although levels > 40 ng/mL may be poorly tolerated

237

Comments: Bupropion is understudied in the geriatric population even though adverse-effect profile is relatively favorable (lack of cardiovascular effects, cognitive effects, anticholinergic effects, sedation, or weight gain). Well absorbed orally. Peak levels in 3 hours for immediate release and 5 hours for extended release (healthy adults). Metabolized primarily by CYP2B6 enzyme. Three active metabolites: hydroxy-bupropion, erythro-hydro-bupropion, and threo-hydro-bupropion; metabolite levels may be much higher than parent drug, and high metabolite levels are associated with poor response and psychotic symptoms. Bupropion itself is a potent CYP2D6 inhibitor. Clearance decreased in elderly and in those with renal or hepatic insufficiency, so lower doses are used. *Important drug interactions:* Additive effects with other drugs that lower the seizure threshold; increased toxicity of bupropion or metabolites with levodopa, MAOIs, cimetidine, CYP2B6 inhibitors (see Table 2–2); hypertension with nicotine patch; altered hemostasis or international normalized ratio (INR) with warfarin. *Relatively common adverse effects:* Dizziness, anxiety, agitation, dry mouth, insomnia, headache, nausea, constipation or diarrhea, and tremor. *Less common but serious effects:* Hypertension, chest pain, cardiac arrhythmias, syncope, confusion, and seizures.

Generic name	citalopram
Trade name	Celexa (generic available)
Class	Selective serotonin reuptake inhibitor
Half-life	35–90 hours
Mechanism of action	Highly selective serotonin reuptake inhibition
Available preparations	Tablets: 10, 20, 40 mg Oral solution: 10 mg/5 mL
Starting dose	10–20 mg/day
Titration	Increase by 10 mg after 7 days Maintain at 20 mg (target dose) for 3–4 weeks, with further titration as needed and tolerated
Typical daily dose	20 mg
Dose range	10–40 mg/day
Therapeutic serum level	Not established

Comments: A first-line drug in elderly patients because of favorable side-effect profile and relative lack of significant drug interactions. Rapidly absorbed, unaffected by food. Highly linear kinetics. Peak levels in 4 hours. About 80% protein bound. Extensively metabolized by CYP3A4, C19, and 2D6 enzymes. Parent drug shows no significant CYP inhibition, but desmethyl metabolite might be a weak CYP2D6 inhibitor. Clearance decreased in elderly and in those with liver disease and to a lesser extent in those with renal disease. Half-life significantly prolonged in elderly patients and those with liver disease. *Relatively common adverse effects:* Nausea, vomiting, dry mouth, headache, somnolence, insomnia, increased sweating, tremor, diarrhea, and sexual dysfunction. *Less common but serious adverse effects:* Abnormal bleeding (especially upper gastrointestinal tract) and SIADH.

Generic name	desipramine
Trade name	Norpramin (generic available)
Class	Tricyclic
Half-life	12–57 hours (varies directly with age)
Mechanism of action	Norepinephrine and (weak) serotonin reuptake inhibition
Available preparations	Tablets: 10, 25, 50, 75, 100, 150 mg
Starting dose	25 mg/day
Titration	Increase by 25 mg every 7 days
Typical daily dose	100 mg (can be given in one dose after initial titration)
Dose range	25–150 mg
Therapeutic serum level	> 115 ng/mL at steady state for geriatric patients (possible toxicity > 300 ng/mL)

Comments: Not a drug of choice for elderly patients, primarily because of cardiovascular effects. Well absorbed orally, with peak concentrations in 4–6 hours. About 90% protein bound. Substrate for CYP2D6. Hydroxylation yields the active metabolite 2-hydroxy-desipramine, which is excreted intact by the kidney. Mean elimination half-life in elders is more than twice that in younger patients. Numerous drug interactions, both pharmacokinetic and pharmacodynamic. *Adverse effects:* Serotonin syndrome with reported deaths in combination with linezolid and MAOIs. Increased anticoagulant effect with warfarin. Additional adverse effects include significant cardiotoxicity (avoid or use with caution in patients with history of MI, stroke, tachycardia, or cardiac conduction abnormality), orthostasis, hypotension or hypertension, anticholinergic effects (e.g., urinary retention, precipitation of angle closure in glaucoma, constipation), tremor, agitation, and insomnia. (Note that list is not complete.)

Generic name	dextroamphetamine
Trade name	Dexedrine, DextroStat (generics available)
Class	Psychostimulant
Half-life	7–34 hours
Mechanism of action	Blocks reuptake of dopamine and norepinephrine; causes release of catecholamines; inhibits monoamine oxidase
Available preparations	Tablets: 5, 10 mg XR capsules: 5, 10, 15 mg
Starting dose	2.5 mg qam (with breakfast)
Titration	Increase by 2.5–5 mg every 2–3 days
Typical daily dose	5 mg bid (with breakfast and lunch)
Dose range	2.5–10 mg bid
Therapeutic serum level	Not applicable

Comments: Useful in medically ill, depressed elders needing urgent intervention for whom ECT is not an option. Anecdotal report of use for 2–3 weeks as an "accelerator" to bridge the period of antidepressant latency. As a sole antidepressant, efficacy is established for several months' use, but not for longer periods. Well absorbed orally; not affected by food. Onset in 2–3 hours, with a duration of 4–24 hours. Extensively metabolized in liver; substrate for CYP2D6. Removed by dialysis. Contraindicated in patients with severe vascular or cardiovascular disease, hypertension, hyperthyroidism, diabetes, glaucoma, drug abuse, significant agitation, or untreated psychosis. *Drug interactions:* Potentially significant drug interaction with MAOIs, not often seen clinically. *Adverse effects:* Tachycardia, hypertension, restlessness, dizziness, insomnia, tremor, headache, psychotic symptoms, aggression, diarrhea, nausea/vomiting, constipation, anorexia, and blurred vision.

Generic name	duloxetine
Trade name	Cymbalta
Class	Atypical
Half-life	12 hours (8–17 hours)
Mechanism of action	Serotonin and norepinephrine reuptake inhibitor
Available preparations	Capsules: 20, 30, 60 mg (contain enteric-coated pellets)
Starting dose	20 mg/day
Titration	Increase by 20 mg after 7 days
Typical daily dose	20 mg bid
Dose range	20–60 mg/day (40–60 mg doses divided bid)
Therapeutic serum level	Not established

Comments: Little is known about the efficacy and safety of duloxetine in the geriatric population. Recently, a warning was issued regarding aggravation of preexisting liver disease. Duloxetine received an FDA-approved labeling for depression and diabetic neuropathic pain and is under investigation for treatment of stress urinary incontinence. There is no evidence for a unique spectrum of efficacy or faster onset of action compared with other antidepressants. Well absorbed orally. Drug is contained in enteric-coated pellets inside a non-enteric-coated capsule. Capsules should not be chewed or divided; contents should not be sprinkled in juice. Medications or conditions that increase stomach pH could affect absorption. Pellets do not dissolve until they reach a part of the GI tract where pH > 5.5. There is a 2-hour delay in absorption after ingestion. Peak levels in 6 hours. More than 90% protein bound, to albumin and α_1-acid glycoprotein. Metabolized via CYP1A2 and 2D6 to inactive metabolites. Moderately inhibits CYP2D6. Clearance decreases by 1% per year between 25 and 75 years. Not recommended for patients with end-stage renal disease or hepatic insufficiency. *Drug interactions:* Risk of scrotonin syndrome when used with other serotonergic medications (e.g., buspirone, linezolid, MAOIs, meperidine, nefazodone, SSRIs, TCAs, sibutramine, tramadol, trazodone, venlafaxine). Expected interactions with CYP1A2 and 2D6 inhibitors and inducers. (See Table 2–2.) *Relatively common adverse effects:* Nausea, dry mouth, constipation, poor appetite, diarrhea, headache, insomnia, somnolence, fatigue, diaphoresis, and dizziness. *Less common but serious adverse effects:* Hypertension, oropharyngeal edema, seizures, cardiac conduction and rhythm disturbances, and thrombocytopenia. Flu-like discontinuation syndrome on abrupt withdrawal.

Generic name	fluoxetine
Trade name	Prozac, Sarafem (generic available), Prozac Weekly
Class	Selective serotonin reuptake inhibitor
Half-life	Fluoxetine: 5 days Norfluoxetine: 13 days
Mechanism of action	Selective serotonin reuptake inhibition
Available preparations	Capsules: 10, 20 mg Tablets: 10, 20 mg Delayed-release capsule: 90 mg Liquid concentrate: 20 mg/5 mL
Starting dose	10 mg (depression and OCD) 5 mg (panic disorder)
Titration	In treating depression or OCD, increase dose to 20 mg after 1–2 weeks. Maintain there for 3–4 weeks before further dose increases, then only if response is partial In treating panic disorder, increase dose to 10 mg after 1–2 weeks, then to 20 mg after 1–2 weeks as tolerated. Maintain there for 6 weeks before further dose increases (if needed) to maximum dose of 30 mg
Typical daily dose	20 mg
Dose range	5–40 mg for depression 5–40 mg for panic disorder 20–60 mg for OCD
Therapeutic serum level	Not established

Comments: A second-line drug in elderly patients, although side effects may limit use and prolonged half-life is associated with accumulation of parent drug and metabolite on repeated dosing. Minimal age-related pharmacokinetic changes. Well absorbed orally, with peak levels in 4–8 hours. Food slows absorption. 95% protein bound. Extensively metabolized in the liver by CYP2C9, 2C19, 2D6, and 3A4 isoenzymes. Potent inhibitor of CYP2D6 and 2C19; also inhibits other isoenzymes. (See Table 4–3.) Norfluoxetine is an active metabolite. More than 4 weeks to steady state or washout for fluoxetine, 8–10 weeks for norfluoxetine; risk of drug interactions continues long after drug has been stopped. Nonlinear kinetics. The dose concentration is the same in elderly as in younger patients. *Drug interactions:* These are numerous (see Table 4–5) and include serotonin syndrome with MAOIs and other drugs listed in Table 4–10, and EPS with coadministered antipsychotics. *Adverse effects:* Nausea, vomiting, diarrhea, insomnia, nervousness, restlessness, agitation, anxiety, light-headedness, drowsiness, fatigue, headache, tremor, initial weight loss (especially in those over 75 years and underweight to begin with), possible long-term weight gain, hyponatremia and SIADH, and increased risk of bleeding (upper GI and intraoperative) compounded by coadministration of NSAIDs, aspirin, and probably warfarin.

Generic name	methylphenidate
Trade name (selected)	Concerta, Ritalin, Methylin, Metadate
Class	Psychostimulant
Half-life	2–7 hours
Mechanism of action	Blocks dopamine reuptake; stimulates cerebral cortex and subcortical structures
Available preparations	XR capsules: 10, 20, 30, 40 mg Oral solution: 5 mg/5mL, 10 mg/5mL Tablets: 5, 10, 20 mg Chewable tablets: 2.5, 5, 10 mg (grape flavor) SR tablets: 20 mg XR tablets: 10, 20 mg (and others)
Starting dose	2.5 mg qam (with breakfast)
Titration	Increase by 2.5–5 mg every 2–3 days
Typical daily dose	5 mg bid (with breakfast and lunch)
Dose range	2.5–10 mg bid
Therapeutic serum level	Not established

Comments: Useful in medically ill, depressed elders needing urgent intervention for whom ECT is not an option. Anecdotal report of use for 2–3 weeks as an "accelerator" to bridge period of antidepressant latency. As a sole antidepressant, efficacy is not well established in long-term use. Absorption is slow and incomplete from GI tract. For immediate-release, peak effect is within 2 hours; duration 3–6 hours. For sustained-release, peak effect is within 4–7 hours; duration 8 hours. Metabolized in liver via hydroxylation. Substrate of CYP2D6; also weakly inhibits 2D6. Eliminated in urine and bile. Contraindicated in patients with marked anxiety, tension, or agitation; in those with Tourette's syndrome or glaucoma; and in combination with MAOIs (or following their discontinuation). Significant drug interactions with warfarin, TCAs. *Adverse effects:* Restlessness, behavioral disturbances, hallucinations, slurred speech, ataxia, vertigo, Tourette's syndrome, mania, hepatotoxicity, rash, rhabdomyolysis, and physical dependence with withdrawal symptoms upon discontinuation.

Generic name	mirtazapine
Trade name	Remeron, Remeron SolTab (generics available)
Class	Tetracyclic
Half-life	31–39 hours
Mechanism of action	Noradrenergic and specific (postsynaptic) serotonergic antagonism; also interferes with α_2 receptors (both auto- and heteroceptors), leading to increased presynaptic outflow of norepinephrine and serotonin.
Available preparations	Tablets: 15, 30, 45 mg Orally disintegrating tablets: 15, 30, 45 mg
Starting dose	7.5 mg/day (evening)
Titration	Increase by 7.5–15 mg every 1–2 weeks
Typical daily dose	30 mg (evening)
Dose range	7.5–45 mg/day
Therapeutic serum level	Not established

Comments: Understudied in elderly patients. Rapidly and completely absorbed orally, with peak levels in 2 hours; not affected by food. 85% protein bound. Extensively metabolized in liver via CYP1A2, 2D6, and 3A4 enzymes. Clearance reduced in elders (especially males) and in patients with hepatic or renal dysfunction. Anecdotally, lower doses more sedating than higher doses, possibly because of relative predominance of histaminergic (vs. noradrenergic) effects at lower doses. *Drug interactions:* Substrates, inhibitors, and inducers of CYP isoenzymes noted above (see Table 2–2), reduced antihypertensive effect with clonidine, additive sedative effects with other CNS depressants, and potential for serotonin syndrome with other serotonergic drugs. *Common adverse effects (>10%):* Somnolence, increased appetite with weight gain, increased serum cholesterol, constipation, dry mouth. *Less common adverse effects (1%–10%):* Hypertension, edema, dizziness, increased serum triglycerides, weakness, flu-like symptoms. *Uncommon but severe adverse effects:* Agranulocytosis, neutropenia, dehydration, orthostasis, abnormalities in liver function test results.

Generic name	modafinil
Trade name	Provigil
Class	Stimulant
Half-life	15 hours; may be longer in elderly
Mechanism of action	Unknown
Available preparations	Tablets: 100, 200 mg
Starting dose	50–100 mg qam
Titration	Increase by 50–100 mg after 4–7 days
Typical daily dose	200 mg qam
Dose range	50–200 mg qam
Therapeutic serum level	Not established

Comments: Efficacy and safety in the elderly not established. Reported anecdotally to increase wakefulness and activity in elderly patients with excessive daytime somnolence. Potential use as an accelerator in the initial stage of antidepressant treatment unstudied in the elderly. Peak levels in 2–4 hours. Food delays absorption but does not affect bioavailability. About 60% protein bound, primarily to albumin. Metabolized in the liver by multiple pathways. Substrate of CYP3A4. Strong inhibitor of CYP2C19. (See Table 2–2.) Excreted in urine, mostly as metabolites. Drug interactions: Complex and incompletely characterized CYP450 interactions; concentrations of TCAs or SSRIs could be increased in patients deficient in CYP2D6 activity, since 2C19 is a secondary metabolic pathway inhibited by modafinil; others. Common adverse effects (>10%): Headache and nausea. Less common adverse effects (1%–10%): Hypertension, chest pain, nervousness, anxiety, insomnia, dizziness, diarrhea, dyspepsia, dry mouth, anorexia, and back pain. Has been reported to be associated with mania and psychosis. Use not recommended in patients with history of angina, cardiac ischemia, recent MI, left ventricular hypertrophy, or mitral valve prolapse.

Generic name	nefazodone
Trade name	(generic only)
Class	Phenylpiperazine
Half-life	2–4 hours (metabolites persist longer)
Mechanism of action	5-HT_2 antagonism, serotonin and norepinephrine reuptake inhibition, α_1 antagonism
Available preparations	Tablets: 50, 100, 150, 200, 250 mg
Starting dose	25–50 mg bid
Titration	Increase by 50–100 mg/day every 1–2 weeks as tolerated
Typical daily dose	100 mg bid
Dose range	50–400 mg/day total
Therapeutic serum level	Not established

Comments: Usefulness in elderly limited by significant adverse effects and drug interactions. Food delays absorption and insignificantly lowers maximum concentration. Significant first-pass metabolism. Nonlinear kinetics. Peak concentrations in 30 minutes. Metabolized in liver via CYP3A4 and 2D6. Three active metabolites are mCPP, triazolodione, and hydroxy-nefazodone. Potent CYP3A4 inhibitor. (See Table 2–2.) Dose-to-concentration ratio different for elderly patients compared with younger patients, so dosing guidelines adjusted as noted above. Lower doses used in hepatic disease. Drug interactions: Numerous, some serious. Common adverse effects (>10%): Headache, drowsiness, insomnia, agitation, dizziness, dry mouth, nausea, constipation, and weakness. Less common adverse effects (1%–10%): Bradycardia, hypotension, edema, orthostasis, vasodilation, confusion, ataxia, tremor, vomiting, diarrhea, increased appetite, urinary retention, blurred vision, and others. Uncommon but serious adverse effects: Hepatic failure, seizures, leukopenia, thrombocytopenia, atrioventricular block, and Stevens-Johnson syndrome. Onset of hepatic injury in patients who develop hepatic failure usually 2 weeks to 6 months after drug initiation.

Generic name	nortriptyline
Trade name	Pamelor (generic available)
Class	Tricyclic
Half-life	37–45 hours in elderly
Mechanism of action	Norepinephrine and serotonin reuptake inhibition
Available preparations	Capsules: 10, 25, 50, 75 mg Liquid concentrate: 10 mg/5 mL
Starting dose	10–25 mg/day
Titration	Increase by 10 mg (or 25 mg) every 7 days
Typical daily dose	50 mg
Dose range	10–100 mg
Therapeutic serum level	50–150 ng/mL

Comments: Substantial evidence for efficacy in severe or melancholic depression in elderly patients, but not a drug of choice because of adverse effects, particularly cardiac effects. About 95% protein bound. Significant first-pass metabolism. Peak levels in about 8 hours. Substrate for CYP2D6 enzyme; also inhibits 2D6. Active metabolite 10-hydroxy-nortriptyline excreted intact by the kidney. Metabolite may accumulate to toxic levels in patients with renal insufficiency. In general, a target dose of 1 mg/kg is adequate for patients ages 60–80 years. Drug interactions are numerous (Table 4–6). Warnings about use in patients with ischemic heart disease or preexisting cardiac conduction abnormalities (bundle branch block or intraventricular conduction delay) because of slowing of cardiac conduction. *Adverse effects:* Orthostasis, hypertension, MI, ataxia, EPS, seizures, glucose dysregulation, SIADH, sexual dysfunction, dry mouth, anorexia, constipation, nausea, vomiting, diarrhea, weight gain (or loss), urinary retention, impotence, blood dyscrasias, increased levels in liver function test values, paresthesias, and mydriasis.

Generic name	paroxetine
Trade name	Paxil, Paxil CR (generic available for immediate-release form)
Class	Selective serotonin reuptake inhibitor
Half-life	31 hours (13–92 hours)
Mechanism of action	Selective serotonin reuptake inhibition; also has prominent noradrenergic effects; more anticholinergic than other SSRIs
Available preparations	Tablets: 10, 20, 30, 40 mg Liquid suspension: 10 mg/5 mL Controlled-release (CR) tablets: 12.5, 25, 37.5 mg
Starting dose	10 mg CR: 12.5 mg
Titration	Increase to 20 mg after 1–2 weeks; maintain for 3–4 weeks before further dose increases, then increase only if partial response is seen CR: increase to 25 mg after 1–2 weeks
Typical daily dose	20 mg CR: 25 mg
Dose range	5–40 mg (to 60 mg for OCD) CR: 12.5–50 mg
Therapeutic serum level	Not established

Comments: A second-line drug for the treatment of elderly patients. Well absorbed orally. For immediate-release form, peak concentration in 7–8 hours; dinnertime administration may avoid daytime drowsiness. Metabolized in liver via CYP2D6; no active metabolites. Strongly inhibits CYP2D6 and 2B6; also inhibits 1A2, 2C9, 2C19, and 3A4. Higher plasma levels achieved in elders compared to younger patients because of reduced clearance. Higher levels also in renal and hepatic disease. Nonlinear kinetics with longer duration of therapy or higher doses. Drug interactions are numerous (Table 4–5). *Common adverse effects (>10%):* Headache, somnolence, dizziness, insomnia, dry mouth, constipation, diarrhea, ejaculatory disturbances, weakness, and diaphoresis. *Less common adverse effects (1%–10%):* Orthostasis, palpitations, vasodilation, anxiety, agitation, anorexia, dyspepsia, vomiting, taste perversion, flatulence, frequency in urination, impotence, tremor, paresthesia, myalgia, myopathy, blurred vision. *Uncommon but serious adverse effects:* Hyponatremia, SIADH, abnormal bleeding, blood dyscrasias, serotonin syndrome in combination with other serotonergic drugs, and others. Withdrawal syndrome common with abrupt discontinuation.

Generic name	sertraline
Trade name	Zoloft
Class	Selective serotonin reuptake inhibitor
Half-life	36 hours in elderly
Mechanism of action	Selective serotonin reuptake inhibition; also has significant dopaminergic effects
Available preparations	Tablets: 25, 50, 100 mg Oral solution: 20 mg/mL
Starting dose	12.5–25 mg/day
Titration	Increase by 12.5–25 mg every 2–3 days as tolerated
Typical daily dose	50–100 mg
Dose range	25–200 mg/day (may be higher in OCD)
Therapeutic serum level	Not established

Comments: A first-line drug for treatment of depression in elderly patients. Slowly but well absorbed orally, with peak concentrations in 4.5–8.4 hours. Food increases rate and extent of absorption, so drug must be given consistently with respect to meals. Extensive first-pass metabolism. 98% protein bound. Metabolized in the liver by multiple CYP isoenzymes; also inhibits multiple isoenzymes and glucuronidation, although not strongly. Principal metabolite (*N*-desmethyl-sertraline) relatively inactive. Clearance reduced by 40% in elderly. Numerous potential drug interactions (Table 4–5), although relatively weak CYP450 effects make this a preferred drug. *Common adverse effects (>10%):* Insomnia, somnolence, dizziness, headache, fatigue, dry mouth, diarrhea, nausea, and ejaculatory disturbances. *Less common adverse effects (1%–10%):* Palpitations, anxiety, agitation, constipation, anorexia, dyspepsia, flatulence, vomiting, weight gain, micturition disorders, tremor, paresthesia, abnormal vision, tinnitus, and diaphoresis. *Uncommon but serious adverse effects:* Hyponatremia, SIADH, abnormal bleeding, blood dyscrasias, serotonin syndrome in combination with other serotonergic drugs, and others. Withdrawal syndrome may be seen with abrupt discontinuation.

Generic name	St. John's wort
Trade name	(various)
Class	Herbal
Half-life	16–36 hours
Mechanism of action	Serotonin reuptake inhibition, MAO inhibition
Available preparations	Capsules: 150, 300 mg
Starting dose	
Titration	
Typical daily dose	300 mg tid
Dose range	300 mg bid to 300 mg tid
Therapeutic serum level	Not applicable

Comments: Not a drug of choice in elderly patients because of significant drug interactions and side effect of spontaneous bleeding. Available over the counter. As with other herbal preparations, concerns have been raised about product content and purity. Steady state in 4 days; onset of antidepressant effect after several weeks. Inducer of CYP3A4 enzyme and P-glycoprotein expression, so has significant interactions with antivirals (including indinavir), immunosuppressants (including cyclosporine), anticoagulants, and antiarrhythmics. *Adverse effects:* Spontaneous bleeding (subarachnoid hemorrhage, subdural hematoma), photosensitivity, GI symptoms, allergic reactions, fatigue, dizziness, xerostomia, and induction of mania.

Generic name	trazodone
Trade name	Desyrel (generic available)
Class	Atypical
Half-life	11.6 hours
Mechanism of action	Parent drug antagonizes 5-HT$_{2A/2C}$ receptors mCPP metabolite agonist at 5-HT$_{1C}$, antagonist at α_2 Significant α_1 and histamine blockade
Available preparations	Tablets: 50, 100, 150, 300 mg
Starting dose	25 mg qhs
Titration	Increase by 25 mg every 3–5 days, as tolerated
Typical daily dose	Insomnia: 25–50 mg qhs Depression: 75–150 mg/day (qhs or divided up to tid)
Dose range	12.5–400 mg/day (higher doses divided)
Therapeutic serum level	Not established

Comments: Used mainly as a hypnotic; use as an antidepressant limited by sedation and orthostasis. Onset of sedative effect in 20–30 minutes; peaks at 30 minutes. Absorption delayed by food (up to 2.5 hours). 85%–95% protein bound. Greatly increased volume of distribution in obese patients, resulting in prolonged half-life. Extensively metabolized in the liver via CYP3A4; mCPP is an active metabolite that may be anxiogenic for some patients. CYP2D6 inhibitor. Reduced clearance in elderly men necessitates dose reduction with chronic administration. Minimal anticholinergic effects. *Drug interactions:* Expected interactions due to CYP3A4 and 2D6 effects, serotonin syndrome with other serotonergic agents, additive hypotensive effects with low-potency antipsychotics. *Adverse effects:* Orthostasis (α_1 effect), ventricular irritability (premature ventricular contractions, possible ventricular tachycardia), sedation, dizziness, gait instability, mild cognitive impairment, seizures, weight gain, priapism, headache, dry mouth, edema, nausea, and diarrhea.

Generic Name	venlafaxine
Trade name	Effexor, Effexor XR
Class	Atypical
Half-life	5 hours O-desmethyl-venlafaxine: 11 hours XR: 15 hours
Mechanism of action	Serotonin and norepinephrine reuptake inhibition (dopamine reuptake inhibition at doses >350 mg/day)
Available preparations	IR tablets: 25, 37.5, 50, 75, 100 mg XR capsules: 37.5, 75, 150 mg
Starting dose	IR: 25 mg bid XR: 37.5 mg/day
Titration	IR: Increase by 25 mg every 4–7 days as tolerated to 25 mg tid; if response is inadequate after 3 weeks at this dose, increase slowly to 50 mg tid; if response is still inadequate after 3 more weeks, increase slowly to 75 mg tid XR: Increase to 75 mg (target dose) after 4–7 days; may need to increase to 150 mg or 225 mg if response is inadequate
Typical daily dose	IR: 50 mg tid XR: 150 mg (given at the same time every day; swallowed whole)
Dose range	IR: 150–225 mg (divided bid to tid) XR: 150–225 mg (one daily dose)
Therapeutic serum level	Not established

Comments: A second-line drug for treatment of depression in elderly patients. Indicated for depression, poststroke depression, and GAD (XR form). XR form appears superior to IR form in tolerability. Age has little effect on pharmacokinetics, except for potential accumulation of metabolite with decreased renal function. Well absorbed orally, with peak levels in 2–3 hours. About 30% protein bound. Metabolized in the liver via CYP2D6; major metabolite is *O*-desmethyl-venlafaxine, which is active and has the same adverse-effect profile as the parent compound. Weak inhibitor of several CYP isoenzymes. Wide interindividual variation in dose-concentration ratios. Dose adjustments needed for mild to moderate renal dysfunction (decrease by 25%) and hepatic dysfunction (decrease by 50%). Not readily dialyzed. *Drug interactions:* Serotonin syndrome with other serotonergic agents, clozapine (increased clozapine levels), haloperidol (increased venlafaxine levels), indinavir (reduced indinavir levels), warfarin (possibly increased INR), various interactions with CYP2D6 and 3A4 inhibitors/inducers. *Common adverse effects (>10%):* Headache, somnolence, dizziness, insomnia, nervousness, nausea, dry mouth, constipation, anorexia, abnormal ejaculation/orgasm, weakness, and diaphoresis. *Less common adverse effects (1%–10%):* Dose-related hypertension (3% with doses <100 mg/day; up to 13% with doses >300 mg/day), diarrhea, vomiting, impotence, tremor. *Uncommon but serious adverse effects:* Abnormal bleeding, blood dyscrasias, exfoliative dermatitis, cardiac arrhythmias, hyponatremia/SIADH, others.

5

Mood Stabilizers

Introduction

The population of elderly patients with bipolar disorder is among the most heterogeneous in clinical psychiatric practice. These patients differ in age at onset of bipolar disease, access to appropriate treatment, genetic loading for other psychopathologies, access to alcohol and other drugs of abuse, comorbid medical conditions, and psychosocial histories. They also differ in number, severity, and polarity of mood episodes. Although the presenting signs and symptoms of mania, hypomania, mixed states, and depression are similar in elders as compared with younger patients, the response to treatment is highly variable in this population. Some patients benefit from usual treatments, but incomplete response to medication is not uncommon (Young 2005).

Elders with bipolar disorder account for 5%–19% of patients presenting for acute care at geriatric psychiatry services (Young 2005). They are predominantly female (69%) (Depp and Jeste 2004). Most have extensive medical comorbidity (Kilbourne et al. 2005), often involving cerebrovascular risk factors, including hypertension (Sajatovic et al. 2005a) and diabetes (Depp and Jeste 2004). In fact, there is some evidence that late-onset bipolar disease (mania) may represent a different pathogenetic mechanism, involving a primarily vascular etiology (Cassidy and Carroll 2002). Consistent with these observations, neuroimaging studies commonly reveal atrophy (often involving ventricular enlargement) and cerebrovascular lesions (Depp and Jeste 2004). More than half of patients exhibit cognitive impairment of sufficient magnitude to be detected by bedside screening instruments, such as the Mini-Mental State Examination, Executive Interview, and Mattis Dementia Rating Scale (Gildengers et al. 2004). For most, functional impairment appears to be less than what would be seen in patients with schizophrenia but more than that seen in those with unipolar depression (Depp and Jeste 2004).

Secondary mania can occur in patients with no history of mood disorder and in association with medications, cancer, and metabolic dysfunction such as hyperthyroidism, among other conditions. This observation, originally made by Krauthammer and Klerman (1978), suggests that mania is a syndrome with multiple causes, unlikely to be explained by a unitary etiologic hypothesis. As noted in a later section, the index of suspicion for secondary mania should be high for any elderly patient presenting as manic, particularly if this is the first episode.

In pharmacologic treatment of elderly patients with bipolar disorder, considerations of tolerability and safety of medications are as important as those of efficacy. Many of these patients will have some history of treatment with first-line drugs, such that a careful and critical review of benefits, side effects, blood levels, coadministered drugs, and actual adherence will be essential in determining an individualized approach to treatment (Young 2005).

Given current evidence, first-line drugs for the treatment of bipolar mania in elderly patients include lithium and valproate (Young 2005). Carbamazepine, although commonly prescribed for this indication (Sajatovic et al. 2005b), should be viewed as a second-line treatment with potentially problematic drug interactions and adverse effects. First-line drugs for the treatment of bipolar depression in this population include lithium and lamotrigine. Lamotrigine also may have a role in the treatment of patients with rapid-cycling illness.

More limited data suggest that atypical antipsychotics—quetiapine, olanzapine, risperidone, aripiprazole, and ziprasidone—may be useful for elderly patients with bipolar disorder (Bowden 2005; Dunner 2005a; Keck 2005; Sajatovic et al. 2005b). The recent U.S. Food and Drug Administration (FDA) advisory regarding increased mortality in elderly patients treated with these drugs coupled with findings from the CATIE

Table 5–1. DSM-IV-TR codes for conditions treated with mood stabilizers

296.xx	Bipolar I disorder
296.89	Bipolar II disorder
301.13	Cyclothymic disorder
296.80	Bipolar disorder not otherwise specified
293.83	Mood disorder due to a general medical condition
29x.xx	Substance-induced mood disorder
296.90	Mood disorder not otherwise specified
295.70	Schizoaffective disorder, bipolar type

study suggests that caution is warranted in the use of these drugs (Lieberman 2005). These risks notwithstanding, the atypical antipsychotics remain an important therapeutic option in treating bipolar disorder, both as monotherapies and as adjunctive agents.

A number of newer anticonvulsant medications have been investigated as potential treatments for bipolar disorder. Oxcarbazepine appears to have a spectrum of efficacy similar to that of carbamazepine, as well as a better tolerability profile (Hirschfeld and Kasper 2004). Gabapentin and topiramate have shown poor efficacy as mood stabilizers. Studies of levetiracetam and zonisamide are still under way. Benzodiazepines are commonly used as adjunctive agents in elderly patients with bipolar mania to treat symptoms of insomnia, anxiety, and agitation. This use has not been studied in any systematic fashion.

DSM-IV-TR diagnoses that may represent indications for the use of mood stabilizers are shown in Table 5–1. The use of anticonvulsant mood stabilizers to treat various pain syndromes, movement disorders, anxiety disorders, and alcohol and sedative withdrawal is discussed in other relevant chapters.

Pharmacology

Mood stabilizers are listed in Table 5–2. In addition to the "classic" medications such as lithium and valproate, the table includes newer anticonvulsants

Table 5–2. Selected mood stabilizers: preparations

Generic name	Trade name	Available preparations				
		Tablets (mg)	Capsules (mg)	SR/CR/XR tablets/ capsules (mg)	Oral solution (concentrate, suspension, or elixir)	Injectable form
aripiprazole	Abilify	5, 10, 15, 20, 30			1 mg/mL	
carbamazepine	Carbatrol, Epital, Equetro, Tegretol, Tegretol XR	200, 300, 400 Chewable: 100	100, 200, 300	100, 200, 300, 400	100 mg/5mL	
lamotrigine	Lamictal	25, 100, 150, 200 Chewable: 2, 5, 25				
levetiracetam	Keppra	250, 500, 750			100 mg/mL	
lithium	Eskalith CR, Eskalith, Lithobid	300	150, 300, 600	300, 450	300 mg/5mL	
olanzapine	Zyprexa Zyprexa Zydis Zyprexa IM	2.5, 5, 7.5, 10, 15, 20 5, 10, 15, 20				10 mg
oxcarbazepine	Trileptal	150, 300, 600			300 mg/5mL	
quetiapine	Seroquel	25, 50, 100, 200, 300, 400				

Table 5–2. Selected mood stabilizers: preparations *(continued)*

| Generic name | Trade name | Available preparations | | | | |
		Tablets (mg)	Capsules (mg)	SR/CR/XR tablets/ capsules (mg)	Oral solution (concentrate, suspension, or elixir)	Injectable form
risperidone	Risperdal	0.25, 0.5, 1, 2, 3, 4			1 mg/mL	
	Risperdal M-Tabs	0.5, 1, 2				
	Risperdal Consta					Long-acting: 25, 37.5, 50 mg
topiramate	Topamax	25, 50, 100, 200	Sprinkles: 15, 25			
valproate	Depacon, Depakene, Depakote Delayed Release, Depakote ER, Depakote Sprinkles		250 Sprinkles: 125	Depakote: 125, 250, 500 ER: 250, 500	250 mg/5 mL	100 mg/mL
ziprasidone	Geodon		20, 40, 60, 80 mg			20 mg
zonisamide	Zonegran		25, 50, 100			

Note. CR=controlled-release; IM=intramuscular; SR=sustained-release; XR=extended-release.

under investigation and atypical antipsychotics. Detailed pharmacology of the latter class of drugs is discussed in Chapter 3, "Antipsychotics."

Known metabolic pathways for drugs discussed in this chapter are listed in Table 5–3. Given the substantial differences in the chemical nature and neurotransmitter effects of these various agents, what they have in common is of interest because it may shed light on the neurobiology of bipolar disorder itself. Current hypotheses relate to actions at voltage-gated sodium channels (Stahl 2004), regulation of glutamatergically mediated synaptic plasticity (Du et al. 2004), and effects on the phosphoinositol cycle.

Lithium

Aging significantly alters lithium pharmacokinetics. Although absorption is relatively unchanged, distribution and clearance are both affected. The volume of distribution decreases with aging because of a relative decrease in total body water and an increase in adipose tissue, as discussed in Chapter 2 of this volume, "Basic Psychopharmacology and Aging." Clearance decreases in proportion to decreases in glomerular filtration. The elimination half-life of lithium in elderly individuals is in the range of 28–36 hours compared with 24 hours for nonelderly individuals (Sajatovic et al. 2005a). Diseases that are more prevalent in old age, such as congestive heart failure and renal insufficiency, are associated with further reductions in lithium clearance. Many hypotheses have been advanced regarding lithium's mechanism of action. Recent investigations have focused on down-regulation of α-amino-3-hydroxy-5-methyl-4-isoxazolepropionic acid (AMPA) GluR1 synaptic expression in the hippocampus after prolonged lithium treatment with therapeutically relevant concentrations (Du et al. 2004), with hypothesized effects on neuronal plasticity.

Valproate

Valproate is rapidly absorbed orally; the controlled-release form (Depakote) is designed to slow this process. Absorption can also be delayed by food. Valproate is highly protein bound, and in elders with low albumin levels, its free fraction is increased. This could result in overdosing because where the free fraction is high, the measured total level of drug underestimates the amount of drug available to act on the target organ (as noted in Chapter 2).

Distribution of valproate is rapid; the drug reaches the central nervous system within minutes, and peak serum concentrations are achieved in 1–4 hours (3–5 hours with Depakote). Valproate is extensively metabolized, primarily via glucuronidation and mitochondrial β-oxidation but also by a variety of cytochrome P450 (CYP450) enzymes (representing minor routes). Some metabolites are active. Clearance of valproate is reduced by 39% in elderly patients, necessitating lower initial doses and more conservative titration. Valproate increases availability of γ-aminobutyric acid (GABA) and has other effects in down-regulation of AMPA GluR1 synaptic expression, which affects plasticity, but its mechanism of action has not been fully elucidated (Du et al. 2004).

Lamotrigine

Lamotrigine is rapidly and completely absorbed when taken orally, and this process is unaffected by food. Peak concentration is achieved in plasma in 1.4–4.8 hours. The drug is metabolized via glucuronidation (a substrate of uridine 5'-diphosphate glucuronosyltransferase [UGT] 1A4) to an inactive metabolite. It is primarily renally excreted, and because of reduced renal clearance with aging, drug exposure is increased in elders by more than 50%. There is some evidence of autoinduction, with half-life decreased by 25% over time. The mechanism by which this drug exerts antidepressant effects and influences rapid cycling is not completely known. Lamotrigine modulates release of the excitatory amino acids glutamate and aspartate by blocking presynaptic voltage-sensitive sodium channels (McEvoy et al. 2006).

Carbamazepine

Absorption of carbamazepine is slow; peak levels occur unpredictably after 4–8 hours. Of note, this drug is a substrate for the P-glycoprotein pump (discussed in Chapter 2). Carbamazepine is 85% bioavailable and highly protein bound. It is metabolized in the liver via CYP3A4 to an active epoxide metabolite that may be neurotoxic in high concentrations. The drug's half-life changes with multiple dosing because of autoinduction effects. Also because of autoinduction, the drug level may drop after 2–4 weeks, requiring upward dose adjustment. Clearance of carbamazepine is reduced by 23% in the elderly. Carbamazepine is a signifi-

Table 5–3. Mood stabilizers and agents under investigation as mood stabilizers: known metabolic pathways

Drug	Metabolic pathways	Enzyme(s) inhibited	Enzyme(s) induced
Aripiprazole	CYP2D6, 3A4	None known	None known
Carbamazepine	CYP3A4, 2C8, 2C9, 1A2, phase II	None known	CYP3A4, 1A2, 2C19
Gabapentin	Excreted in urine unchanged	None known	None known
Lamotrigine	UGTs; excreted in urine unchanged	None known	UGTs (mild, autoinduction)
Levetiracetam	Non-P450 phase I hydrolysis	None known	None known
Lithium	Not metabolized	None	None
Olanzapine	CYP1A2, 2D6, UGT1A4, ?other UGTs, ?FMO$_3$	None known	None known
Oxcarbazepine	CYP3A4	CYP2C19	CYP3A4[a]
Quetiapine	CYP3A4, sulfation	None known	None known
Risperidone	CYP2D6, 3A4	CYP2D6[a]	None known
Topiramate	70% excreted in urine unchanged; phase I, phase II	CYP2C19[a]	None known; decreases ethinyl estradiol levels

Table 5–3. Mood stabilizers and agents under investigation as mood stabilizers: known metabolic pathways *(continued)*

Drug	Metabolic pathways	Enzyme(s) inhibited	Enzyme(s) induced
Valproate	Complex: CYP2C9, 2C19, 2A6, phase II	CYP2D6, 2C9, UGTs, epoxide hydroxylase	None known; indirect evidence of CYP2C9, 2C19, and phase II
Ziprasidone	Aldehyde oxidase, CYP3A4, 1A2	None known	None known
Zonisamide	Acetylation, sulfonation, CYP3A4	None known	None known

Note. Bold type indicates potent induction. CYP = cytochrome P450; UGT = uridine 5'-diphosphate glucuronosyltransferase.
[a]Moderate.
Source. Adapted from Cozza et al. 2003.

cant inducer of CYP3A4 and CYP2C19 and is associated with variably decreased concentrations of psychotropic and cardiac medications, as well as other drugs. Pharmacodynamic actions of carbamazepine are numerous and resemble those of phenytoin, primarily involving inhibition of synaptic transmission. Other actions include sedative, anticholinergic, muscle relaxant, and antiarrhythmic effects (McEvoy et al. 2006).

Details regarding the pharmacology of newer anticonvulsant drugs in use or under investigation for bipolar disorder may be found in the Specific Drug summaries at the end of this chapter.

Drug Interactions

With only a few exceptions, the newer drugs under investigation for the treatment of bipolar disorder appear to be superior to lithium and carbamazepine (and valproate, to a lesser extent) in terms of the number and severity of drug interactions. Lithium has important interactions not only with medications but also with dietary modifications influencing salt concentrations (especially sodium chloride). A dietary change as simple as the initiation of a low-salt regimen can result in raised serum lithium levels. The combination of lithium with haloperidol and other antipsychotic drugs has been reported to be neurotoxic, although it is often used safely in practice; at least some case reports showing lithium-antipsychotic neurotoxicity involved excessive lithium doses or blood levels.

Carbamazepine has been called "the great inducer" because of its capacity to induce CYP3A4 and CYP2C19 and thereby speed the metabolism of a number of other drugs. In addition, because carbamazepine itself is metabolized by a single isoenzyme (CYP3A4), the drug is more susceptible to inhibition by agents such as antifungals, grapefruit juice, or nefazodone. Valproate has fewer problematic interactions than carbamazepine because it is metabolized via several CYP450 pathways as well as noncytochrome mitochondrial pathways. The combination of valproate with carbamazepine, however, may be associated with complex interactions. Drug interactions are summarized for lithium in Table 5–4, valproate in Table 5–5, lamotrigine in Table 5–6, and carbamazepine in Table 5–7.

Table 5–4. Lithium drug interactions

Added agent	Potential interaction	Clinical management
ACE inhibitors (enalapril, captopril, lisinopril)	Increased lithium serum levels due to decreased clearance	Monitor lithium levels during treatment with ACE inhibitor.
Acetazolamide	Decreased lithium level due to increased renal excretion	Monitor lithium level closely with this combination.
Calcium channel blockers (verapamil, diltiazem)	Increased risk of cardiac toxicity and/or neurotoxicity (ataxia, tremors, nausea, vomiting, diarrhea, tinnitus)	Avoid combination if possible.
Carbamazepine	Increased neurotoxic effect despite therapeutic lithium and carbamazepine levels (mechanism unknown)	This combination is usually well tolerated; toxicity may be more likely in patients with medical illness or previous history of lithium neurotoxicity. Monitor carefully for clinical signs or symptoms when this combination is used.
COX-2 inhibitors (only celecoxib still marketed at this writing)	Increased lithium serum levels due to decreased clearance	Monitor lithium levels during and after discontinuation of COX-2 inhibitors.

Table 5–4.   Lithium drug interactions (continued)

Added agent	Potential interaction	Clinical management
Fluoxetine, fluvoxamine, and other SSRIs	Increased serum lithium levels and/or lithium toxicity occasionally reported; tremor common; neurotoxicity may progress to ataxia, serotonin syndrome, or confusion Fluvoxamine may provoke hyperpyrexia or seizures when combined with lithium, perhaps as part of serotonin syndrome	Consider lithium dose reduction, change to different SSRI, or change to nonserotonergic antidepressant (e.g., bupropion).
Haloperidol, other antipsychotics	Reported increased neurotoxic effects despite therapeutic lithium levels; similar to neuroleptic malignant syndrome (confusion, rigidity)	It is not clear whether haloperidol is more likely than other neuroleptics to interact in this way with lithium; any antipsychotic may increase EPS associated with lithium and vice versa. Dosage reduction of one or both agents is indicated.
Methyldopa	Increased lithium level or increased lithium toxicity without change in level	Avoid combination.
Metronidazole	Increased lithium level due to decreased renal clearance	Monitor lithium levels closely during treatment.

Table 5–4. Lithium drug interactions (*continued*)

Added agent	Potential interaction	Clinical management
NSAIDs	Increased lithium level, perhaps due to NSAID effect on renal prostaglandin synthesis	Monitor lithium levels closely and use sulindac if NSAID must be used; consider alternative to NSAID.
Theophylline	Decreased lithium level due to increased renal excretion	Monitor lithium level closely with this combination.
Thiazide diuretics	Increased serum lithium level due to decreased renal lithium clearance; possible lithium toxicity	50% reduction in lithium dose indicated with use of hydrochlorothiazide, 50 mg/day. Consider use of furosemide instead.
Tricyclic antidepressants (TCAs)	A few reports of combination of lithium and TCA (amitriptyline, imipramine, possibly others) leading to increased likelihood of seizures, tremor, and cardiac toxicity	This combination is usually well tolerated and may be good strategy for refractory unipolar depression. Monitor for signs and symptoms of neurotoxicity and consider reduced lithium dose if neurotoxicity is present. ECG is prudent with this combination.
Topiramate	Increased lithium level	Monitor lithium levels closely with this combination.

Note. ACE=angiotensin-converting enzyme; COX-2=cyclooxygenase-2; ECG=electrocardiogram; EPS=extrapyramidal side effects; NSAID = non-steroidal anti-inflammatory drug; SSRI=selective serotonin reuptake inhibitor.
Source. Adapted from Pies 2005.

Table 5–5.   Valproate drug interactions

Added agent	Potential interaction	Clinical management
Aspirin, naproxen	Aspirin and naproxen may displace valproate from its binding sites on plasma proteins, resulting in difficulty interpreting total valproate levels. Aspirin also inhibits valproate metabolism. Some clinical evidence suggests aspirin/valproate toxicity.	Use nonaspirin pain relievers with valproate if possible, or reduce valproate dose if aspirin is required.
Bupropion	Bupropion concentration unaffected, but increased hydroxy-bupropion level	Consider reduction of bupropion dose if signs of toxicity develop.
Carbamazepine	Carbamazepine reduces valproate levels but increases levels of 2-propyl-4-pentenoic acid metabolite, which is hepatotoxic.	May need to monitor liver function more closely; adjust one or both anticonvulsant doses and follow levels periodically.
Chlorpromazine (possibly other antipsychotics)	Increased valproate levels due to competitive inhibition of metabolism	Monitor valproate levels closely when valproate and phenothiazines are used concomitantly; haloperidol may not have this effect on valproate.
Cimetidine	Increased valproate levels due to decreased clearance	Use ranitidine or famotidine with valproate.

Table 5–5. Valproate drug interactions *(continued)*

Added agent	Potential interaction	Clinical management
Fluoxetine	Increased valproate levels via inhibition of hepatic metabolism	Monitor valproate levels and adjust dose.
Lamotrigine	Modest decrease in valproate levels (±25%) after addition of lamotrigine in healthy volunteers; no change in valproate steady-state levels in clinical trials; however, lamotrigine levels will rise in presence of valproate	Addition of valproate to lamotrigine is not usually recommended in routine cases. If lamotrigine must be added to valproate in an elderly patient, start at a low dose and titrate slowly; monitor closely for rash.
	Increased risk of rash, which may be serious	
Magnesium/Aluminum hydroxide antacids	Increased valproate levels	Adjust dosage of valproate if side effects occur.
Phenobarbital	Increased phenobarbital levels	Reduce phenobarbital dose.
Topiramate	Slightly decreased levels of both drugs	Monitor valproate blood levels.

Source.   Adapted from Pies 2005.

Table 5–6.   Lamotrigine drug interactions

Added agent	Potential interaction	Clinical management
Carbamazepine/ Oxcarbazepine	Decreased lamotrigine levels with CBZ, less so with oxcarbazepine; possibly increased production of neurotoxic CBZ-epoxide metabolite (conflicting reports); some reports of toxicity when lamotrigine is added to CBZ, probably due to pharmacodynamic interaction	Carefully monitor combined use of CBZ and lamotrigine, using lower than usual doses of one or both agents. Toxicity is more likely when lamotrigine is added to CBZ if initial CBZ level > 8 µg/mL; reduction of CBZ dose often reduces toxicity. Oxcarbazepine plus lamotrigine may be safe (based on anecdotal reports).
Phenytoin, phenobarbital, primidone	Decreased lamotrigine levels	Adjust lamotrigine dosage accordingly.
Sertraline (possibly other SSRIs)	Inhibition of glucuronidation may increase lamotrigine levels substantially.	Adjust lamotrigine dosage accordingly.
Topiramate	No major pharmacokinetic interactions	Watch for pharmacodynamic interactions (e.g., increased sedation, cognitive problems).
Valproate	Addition of adjunctive valproate leads to increased lamotrigine half-life (from about 25 to 70 hours) and blood levels due to valproate inhibition of glucuronidation and may lead to neurotoxicity and increased incidence of Stevens-Johnson syndrome.	Slow titration of lamotrigine dose is necessary; monitor more closely for any report of rash.

Note.   CBZ=carbamazepine; SSRI=selective serotonin reuptake inhibitor.   *Source.*   Adapted from Pies 2005.

Table 5–7. Carbamazepine drug interactions

Added agent	Potential interaction	Clinical management
Anticoagulants	Increased metabolism of anticoagulants; may reduce their effects	Adjustment of warfarin (Coumadin) dose may be necessary when CBZ is coadministered (or dose is changed or CBZ is discontinued).
Antifungals (azoles)	Increased level of CBZ via CYP3A4 inhibition	Monitor level of CBZ and reduce dose as needed while antifungal is in use.
Aripiprazole	Increased clearance of aripiprazole through hepatic induction	Manufacturer recommends doubling the dose of aripiprazole; clinical monitoring is recommended.
Bupropion	Possibly decreased plasma levels of bupropion with greatly increased levels of hydroxy-bupropion; may lead to toxicity in some patients	If bupropion is used with CBZ, obtain plasma levels of both bupropion and its metabolite; watch for signs of confusion or psychosis secondary to very high hydroxy-bupropion levels.
Calcium channel blockers	Increased CBZ levels and neurotoxicity, probably due to inhibition of CYP3A4; additive cardiac effects	Seems to occur with use of verapamil or diltiazem, but not nifedipine, which is the calcium channel blocker of choice in this context
Cimetidine	Transient increase in CBZ levels, with possible increase in CBZ side effects during first 3–5 days of treatment	When possible, use ranitidine, famotidine, or other antacid in patients taking CBZ.

Table 5–7. Carbamazepine drug interactions *(continued)*

Added agent	Potential interaction	Clinical management
Clozapine, haloperidol (possibly other antipsychotics)	Induced metabolism of clozapine and haloperidol, which reduces levels of both agents; reduction of haloperidol may be clinically significant in some cases (reduction of antipsychotic effect in some cases, but not all)	Monitor clinical response when CBZ and antipsychotic are coadministered.
		Monitor clozapine or other antipsychotic levels; consider dose increase when CBZ is coadministered; if CBZ is discontinued, may need to reduce antipsychotic dose
	Theoretically, increased risk of agranulocytosis when CBZ is used with clozapine	Consider switch to oxcarbazepine if clinically appropriate (although oxcarbazepine may induce CYP3A4 and inhibit CYP2C9).
Grapefruit juice	Increased CBZ level because of CYP3A4 inhibition	Monitor CBZ levels according to usual recommendation and educate patient regarding interaction.
Isoniazid (INH)	Increased CBZ level and toxicity; and possible increased risk of INH-induced hepatotoxicity	Monitor CBZ levels, LFT values carefully with this combination.
Lamotrigine	Increased clearance, reduced blood levels of lamotrigine through induction of glucuronidation; possibly increased production of neurotoxic CBZ-epoxide metabolite (conflicting reports)	Dose of lamotrigine may need to be increased. Oxcarbazepine might be alternative, but can reduce lamotrigine levels by about 30%

Table 5–7. Carbamazepine drug interactions *(continued)*

Added agent	Potential interaction	Clinical management
Macrolide antibiotics (erythromycin, clarithromycin, troleandomycin)	CBZ toxicity, probably due to inhibition of CYP3A4 by macrolides	May be more likely with larger doses of macrolides; if possible, use a different class of antibiotic. Monitor CBZ levels and clinical signs of weakness, lethargy, and ataxia, among others. Use azithromycin or dirithromycin (less CYP3A4 inhibition).
Monoamine oxidase inhibitors (MAOIs)	Potential for hypertensive crisis	Avoid coadministration of CBZ with MAOIs.
Nefazodone	Complex interaction; CBZ induces CYP3A4 while nefazodone inhibits CYP3A4; may result in decreased level of nefazodone and increased level of CBZ	Avoid coadministration of CBZ with nefazodone if possible.
Phenobarbital, primidone	Reduced CBZ levels via enhanced hepatic metabolism; apparently no loss of seizure control	Monitor CBZ levels.
Phenytoin	Reduced CBZ levels via enhanced hepatic metabolism of CBZ; effect of CBZ on phenytoin highly variable	Monitor CBZ and phenytoin levels.

Table 5–7.   Carbamazepine drug interactions *(continued)*

Added agent	Potential interaction	Clinical management
Protease inhibitors (indinavir, ritonavir)	Increased CBZ levels via CYP3A4 inhibition	Monitor CBZ levels and adjust CBZ dose as indicated.
Selective serotonin reuptake inhibitors (SSRIs)	Studies inconsistent, but possible impairment of CBZ metabolism by fluoxetine and perhaps other SSRIs (e.g., fluvoxamine), leading to CBZ toxicity and/or serotonin syndrome	Monitor CBZ levels closely when SSRI (especially fluoxetine or fluvoxamine) is used concomitantly; in theory, nefazodone may also increase CBZ levels via inhibition of CYP3A4.
Tricyclic antidepressants	Additive sedation, cardiac conduction effects; high doses of CBZ associated with anticholinergic side effects, which may be additive	Use caution in dosing; check ECG; monitor for dry mouth, urinary retention, and tachycardia.
Valproate	Increased ratio of CBZ epoxide to CBZ via inhibition of epoxide hydroxylase (possible neurotoxicity); displacement of CBZ from plasma binding proteins; CBZ reduces valproate levels but increases levels of 2-propyl-4-pentenoic acid metabolite, which is hepatotoxic and teratogenic	If CBZ and valproate are used together, monitor levels of both closely. Obtain level of CBZ epoxide if possible and closely monitor patient for signs of neurotoxicity. Check LFT values more frequently than with either agent alone.

Note.   CBZ=carbamazepine; CYP=cytochrome P450; ECG=electrocardiogram; LFT=liver function test.
Source.   Adapted from Pies 2005.

Efficacy

Most of what is known about the efficacy of mood stabilizers in the geriatric population has been extrapolated from studies performed in younger cohorts. This approach is limited by the pharmacologic differences between these groups (as discussed in Chapter 2) and further complicated by heterogeneity in the geriatric population itself. Thus, although effective medications do exist for bipolar disorder, elders treated for acute episodes often have incomplete response and go on to have further episodes (Young 2005).

Lithium is often effective in treating acute mania in elderly patients (Chen et al. 1999; Foster 1992; Shulman et al. 1987), although certain subgroups of bipolar patients tend to be less responsive to this medication. These groups include patients with depressive or mixed mania; patients with an episode sequence pattern of depressed-manic-well interval (as opposed to manic-depressed-well interval); those with more than three prior episodes before prophylaxis, those with no family history of bipolar disorder, and those with a history of substance abuse, head injury, or other complicating medical condition (Post et al. 1998). Valproate and possibly other anticonvulsants may be more effective for certain of these patients. For example, valproate is probably superior to lithium for mixed episodes: valproate has greatest efficacy in elders when levels are in the range of 65–90 μg/mL (Chen et al. 1999).

For the depressed phase of bipolar illness, effective drugs include lithium, lamotrigine, and quetiapine (Calabrese et al. 1999, 2005). Lamotrigine also has prophylactic efficacy in rapid cycling and in preventing depressive relapse (Calabrese et al. 2000). In general, the addition of an atypical antipsychotic to a mood stabilizer may substantially increase the likelihood of response in acute mania (Dunner 2005b). Although the combination drug fluoxetine-olanzapine has FDA-approved labeling for bipolar depression, it is not necessarily recommended for use in elderly patients because fluoxetine is not a first-line drug for this population (as discussed in Chapter 4, "Antidepressants," in this volume) and because the lowest available dose of the drug is too high for many geriatric patients.

Clinical Use

Initial Evaluation and Baseline Laboratory Studies

For the elderly patient who presents in an obviously manic state that is not secondary to medical or neurologic causes (i.e., is primary), the issue of bipolarity is already settled; although unipolar mania does exist, it is rarely encountered. For the elderly patient who presents in a depressed state, the question of bipolarity should be considered as early as possible. Clinical experience suggests that unless specific questions are asked to elicit a history of mania or hypomania, the diagnosis can be missed. An instrument such as the Mood Disorder Questionnaire (Figure 5–1) can be helpful in this task. Corroborating history from a family member, caregiver, or friend is often necessary to establish a bipolar diagnosis with any certainty, particularly if manic episodes are remote.

The index of suspicion for secondary mania should be high for any elderly patient presenting as manic, particularly if this is the first episode. As suggested by Krauthammer and Klerman (1978) in their seminal paper, possible etiologies of secondary mania are numerous and include medications as listed in Table 5–8 and medical conditions as listed in Table 5–9.

The diagnostic evaluation involves not only the clinical examination but also specific laboratory testing. The workup should include the following elements: vital signs (including orthostatic), physical and neurologic examination, cognitive screening, complete blood count (CBC) with platelets, basic chemistries (including blood urea nitrogen [BUN], creatinine, sodium, potassium, calcium, and magnesium); liver function tests (LFTs; aspartate transaminase [AST], alanine transaminase [ALT], and alkaline phosphatase); creatinine clearance (usually calculated), thyroid function tests; and electrocardiogram (ECG). Neuroimaging (brain magnetic resonance imaging [MRI] or computed tomography) may be indicated in many cases. For women being considered for lithium treatment, consideration should also be given to checking thyroid autoantibodies, since those with thyroid autoimmunity are at higher risk for the development of hypothyroidism on lithium (Kupka et al. 2002). Correction of hypothyroidism and electrolyte derangements may be essential for optimal response to mood stabilizers and for stabilization of rapid cycling.

Mood Disorder Questionnaire

1. Has there ever been a period of time when you were not your usual self and...

   ...you felt so good or so hyper that other people thought you were not your normal self or you were so hyper that you got into trouble?   Yes   No

   ...you were so irritable that you shouted at people or started fights or arguments?   Yes   No

   ...you felt much more confident than usual?   Yes   No

   ...you got much less sleep than usual and found you didn't really miss it?   Yes   No

   ...you were much more talkative or spoke faster than usual?   Yes   No

   ...thoughts raced through your head or you couldn't slow down your mind?   Yes   No

   ...you were so easily distracted by things around you that you had trouble concentrating or staying on track?   Yes   No

   ...you had much more energy than usual?   Yes   No

   ...you were much more active or did many more things than usual?   Yes   No

   ...you were much more social or outgoing than usual; for example, you telephoned friends in the middle of the night?   Yes   No

   ...you were much more interested in sex than usual?   Yes   No

   ...you did things that were unusual for you or that other people might have thought were excessive, foolish, or risky?   Yes   No

   ...spending money got you or your family into trouble?   Yes   No

2. If you checked YES to more than one of the above, have several of these ever happened during the same period of time?   Yes   No

3. How much of a problem did any of these cause you —like being unable to work; having family, money, or legal troubles; getting into arguments or fights?   No problem   Minor problem   Moderate problem   Serious problem

Figure 5–1. Mood Disorder Questionnaire.

Source. Reprinted from Hirschfeld RM, Williams JB, Spitzer RL, et al: "Development and Validation of a Screening Instrument for Bipolar Spectrum Disorder: The Mood Disorder Questionnaire." *American Journal of Psychiatry* 157:1873–1875, 2000. Used with permission.

Table 5-8.   Causes of secondary mania: medications

Alprazolam	Corticotropin (ACTH)	Pergolide
Amantadine	Cyclobenzaprine	Prednisone
Amphetamines	Cyproheptadine	Procainamide
Anabolic steroids	Decongestants	Procarbazine
Antidepressants	(phenylephrine)	Procyclidine
Baclofen	Dextromethorphan	Propafenone
Beclomethasone	Disulfiram	Ranitidine
Bronchodilators	Dronabinol	St. John's wort
Bromocriptine	Enalapril	Sympathomimetics
Buspirone	Indomethacin	Thyroid supplements
Captopril	Iproniazid	Tolmetin
Cimetidine	Isoniazid	Trazodone
Corticosteroids/	Levodopa	Triazolam
Corticosteroid	Methylphenidate	Yohimbine
withdrawal	Metoclopramide	Zidovudine
	Metrizamide	

Choice of Drug and Initial Treatment

Practice guidelines for the treatment of bipolar disorder specific to elderly patients have yet to be published. Guidelines for the adult population can be used with some modification (Hirschfeld 2000; Suppes et al. 2005; Yatham 2005). For the geriatric patient with mania, initial monotherapy with lithium or valproate coupled with discontinuation of antidepressants is recommended. For mixed mania, valproate would be preferred. Use of an atypical antipsychotic as primary treatment for a manic episode may be considered in less severely ill patients (Hirschfeld 2000). Initial therapy should be monitored for several weeks (if possible) before deciding that augmentation or switching is needed (Young 2005). Nonresponse should prompt a switch of medication, and partial response should prompt the addition of another mood stabilizer or an atypical antipsychotic (Young 2005).

Table 5–9. Selected causes of secondary mania: medical conditions

Brain aneurysm	Hyperthyroidism
Brain tumor	Influenza
Cerebrovascular lesions (especially in the right hemisphere)	Multiple sclerosis
	Niacin deficiency
Cryptococcal meningitis/encephalitis	Parkinson's disease
Cushing's syndrome	Polycythemia
Dementia (including Alzheimer's disease and vascular dementia)	Postencephalitic syndrome
	Rickettsial diseases
Epilepsy (including complex-partial seizures)	Syphilis
	Thalamotomy
Hemodialysis	Traumatic brain injury
Herpes simplex encephalitis	Uremia
HIV encephalopathy	Viral meningitis/encephalitis
Hydrocephalus	Vitamin B_{12} deficiency

For the geriatric patient with bipolar depression, initial monotherapy with lithium or lamotrigine should be tried. If one of these medications is not effective or not tolerated, a switch to the other could be tried. If this is ineffective or poorly tolerated, an atypical antipsychotic could be tried as monotherapy or as add-on therapy. If this also proves ineffective, consideration should be given to the use of an antidepressant medication in combination with a mood stabilizer or electroconvulsive therapy (ECT). The use of an antidepressant introduces the risk of a switch into mania.

When an antipsychotic medication is considered for the treatment of an elderly bipolar patient, risk versus benefit should be carefully weighed, in view of the recent FDA advisory warning regarding increased mortality with atypical antipsychotics and emerging data regarding the risks of conventional agents (Wang et al. 2005). These issues are discussed more fully in Chapter 3. In general, atypical agents are considered to be superior to conventional drugs in treating bipolar illness and have

FDA-approved labeling for this indication. In view of findings from the CATIE study regarding weight gain and other metabolic effects of olanzapine (Lieberman et al. 2005) and potentially serious adverse effects of clozapine, preferred atypical drugs include aripiprazole, quetiapine, and risperidone. Inadequate data are available for the geriatric population to recommend ziprasidone for this indication.

For elderly patients with treatment-refractory mania or depression or for those with depression associated with suicidality or inadequate nutritional intake, ECT should be considered (Young 2005). Rapid symptom remission can be seen with ECT after as few as four to six treatments. Follow-up treatment with a mood stabilizer may be sufficient to maintain remission, although some patients may require maintenance ECT.

For the treatment of secondary mania, when mood-stabilizing medication is necessary, anticonvulsants such as valproate or carbamazepine should be used in preference to lithium. For the treatment of patients with bipolar depression or rapid cycling who have seizures, lamotrigine could be used to treat both conditions (Pugh et al. 2004; Sajatovic et al. 2005a).

Alternative Formulations

Valproate is available as a capsule (Depakene), a capsule containing coated particles (Depakote Sprinkles), a delayed-release tablet (Depakote), an extended-release tablet (Depakote ER), an oral solution (Depakene Syrup), and an injectable form (Depacon). Depakote and Depakote Sprinkles may be less irritating to the gastrointestinal (GI) tract than the Depakene formulations. Compared with the delayed-release Depakote tablet, Sprinkles yield steadier serum levels, with reduced peak-level side effects (McEvoy et al. 2006). The new extended-release formulation shares this property and is now available in 250-mg as well as 500-mg tablets and so may find greater use in the geriatric population. The intravenous formulation has not been systematically studied in elderly patients but appeared to be safe and effective at initial doses of 125–250 mg administered two times a day in a small case series (Regenold and Prasad 2001).

In our experience, the preferred preparation of lithium for use in elderly patients is the immediate-release tablet because it provides an adequately low trough level when the drug is administered once daily. The slow-release formulation of lithium may be useful for patients who do not develop tolerance to certain side effects related to peak drug levels (nausea or tremor), but actually may be associated with worsening of diarrhea. The citrate formulation can be used to initiate lithium at very low doses (e.g., <75 mg), for patients unable to swallow tablets, and for those with prominent GI side effects.

Dose and Dose Titration

Lithium should be started in elderly patients at 75–150 mg in a single nightly dose. The dose should be increased by 75–150 mg every 4–7 days. For "young-old" patients (patients <75 years of age) without concomitant medical disease or dementia who are adequately monitored, increments could be as high as 300 mg every 4 days. Serum lithium levels should be checked at steady state (approximately 7 days after a dose change) from 8–12 hours after the last dose is administered. For reasons noted below relating to renal protection, lithium should generally be given as a single nightly dose (Plenge et al. 1982). When side effects necessitate splitting the dose during the early phase of treatment, the dose should generally be consolidated to a once-nightly schedule as soon as possible after therapy is initiated. Every-other-day dosing is not recommended because of reduced prophylactic efficacy and compliance problems (Jensen et al. 1995). In the presence of certain diseases (e.g., dementia) or coarse brain injury (e.g., stroke), more conservative lithium dosing may be necessary (Young 2005), with correspondingly lower lithium levels attained.

Valproate should be started in the geriatric patient at a dosage of 125 mg/day to 250 mg two times a day. If the patient tolerates initial dosing, the dose should be increased by 125–250 mg every 3–5 days, as tolerated. Although splitting the dose results in reduced peak-level side effects, the pharmacokinetics of valproate allow single daily dosing at bedtime. In the hospitalized manic patient, initial dosing could be higher, at least in the young-old patient. In one study of oral loading with extended-release divalproex (30 mg/kg/day), 2 of 14 patients were geriatric (ages 64 and 67 years) (Miller et al. 2005). Both patients were administered an initial dose of 2,000 mg of extended-release divalproex, and both achieved therapeutic drug levels by day 3 that remained stable at steady state; neither reported side effects (Miller et al. 2005).

Dose and dose titration of other mood stabilizers are discussed in the Specific Drug summaries at the end of this chapter.

Course of Response

Time to response has not been studied in exclusively geriatric samples. In patients of varying ages, the response to lithium or valproate in acute mania occurs in as little as several days to as long as 2 weeks or more, depending on initial dose and rapidity of titration. The antidepressant response to lithium usually takes longer, on the order of 6–8 weeks (American Psychiatric Association 2002). For elderly patients, longer latencies to response may be seen.

Monitoring Treatment

Elderly patients treated with mood stabilizers require ongoing monitoring of efficacy, adverse effects, drug levels, and specific laboratory parameters. In addition, with combination treatment (e.g., a mood stabilizer with an antipsychotic or a benzodiazepine), the need for each drug should be regularly reassessed. Drug levels should be routinely monitored for lithium, valproate, and carbamazepine. Levels should be checked after the drug has reached steady state and drawn as trough levels (i.e., just before the morning dose, with dosing two times a day, or 8–12 hours after the last dose, with dosing one time a day). Drug levels should be obtained after initiating therapy, after any change in dose, after other medications that could affect levels are started or changed, or at any sign of toxicity. Levels should also be checked at regular intervals during maintenance treatment. For newer anticonvulsants used as mood stabilizers (e.g., oxcarbazepine), drug levels may prove useful but are not yet established in bipolar management.

For lithium, steady state is reached after 5–7 days. What constitutes an optimal serum lithium level for the elderly patient is somewhat controversial; we recommend a target serum level in the range of 0.4–1.0 mEq/L for acute treatment as well as maintenance therapy, with the exact level depending on individual clinical response and tolerability. A trough level should be drawn as described in the paragraph above even when single nightly doses of short-acting lithium are used (as is recommended for elderly patients). This 12-hour level is approximately the same as for twice-daily dosing, since the half-life of lithium in elders is greater than 36 hours. An instant blood test is now available to check lithium levels at the point-of-care using whole blood obtained by a fingerstick. The test has been found reliable in comparison to levels obtained by venipuncture (Glazer et al. 2004).

Lithium dosing may require downward adjustment as the patient ages. Dosage reductions also are indicated whenever there is a change in renal function, electrolyte imbalance (particularly with sodium), severe diarrhea, or dehydration. As noted in Table 5–4, concurrent treatment with medications such as angiotensin-converting enzyme inhibitors or nonsteroidal anti-inflammatory drugs also may necessitate lowering of the lithium dose. If a decline in renal function or significant polyuria occurs during lithium treatment, creatinine clearance should be measured or calculated (see Chapter 2) and compared with baseline, and urine osmolality or specific gravity should be obtained to rule out diabetes insipidus.

Frequency of follow-up for elderly lithium-treated patients is not well established. We recommend that lithium levels be obtained (fingerstick or venipuncture) every 1–2 weeks during the first 2 months of therapy, and every 3 months thereafter. Serum BUN and creatinine should be checked periodically (e.g., every 1–3 months), as should serum thyroid-stimulating hormone (TSH) (e.g., every 4–6 months). For any complication of therapy (including coadministered interacting medication), more frequent monitoring may be required.

For valproate, steady state is achieved after 3–4 days. Target serum levels for acute mania in the geriatric patient are in the range of 65–90 μg/mL (Chen et al. 1999), usually achieved with dosages in the 750–1,500 mg/day range. During the first 2 months of therapy, we recommend that patients have serum valproate level checks every 1–2 weeks and monthly checks of CBC with platelets and LFTs. During long-term therapy, we suggest checking serum valproate levels every 3 months, and CBC with platelets and LFT values every 6 months.

Serum level monitoring is more complicated for carbamazepine because the half-life changes with autoinduction. In general, trough levels should be checked 5 days after a dose change, and rechecked to ensure that the level has stabilized (usually after several months). Target levels are not well established. Anecdotal support exists for a carbamazepine level in the acutely manic geriatric patient of 4–8 μg/mL, although some patients require higher levels. During the first 2 months of therapy with carbamazepine, we recommend serum carbamazepine level checks every 1–2 weeks, and CBC and LFT values monthly. During long-term therapy, we suggest checking serum carbamazepine levels every 3 months, and CBC and LFT values every 4–6 months. An ECG should be obtained when the therapeutic level of carbamazepine has been reached; if a disturbance of cardiac conduction is detected, the dose should be reduced or the medication withdrawn (Kasarskis et al. 1992). Serum sodium should also be checked periodically, because of the risk of hyponatremia and syndrome of inappropriate antidiuretic hormone (SIADH) (Eastham et al. 1998). Although not widely employed clinically, saliva samples could at least theoretically be used to determine levels of carbamazepine (Grim et al. 2003) as well as other anticonvulsants (Grim et al. 2003; Jones et al. 2005).

Duration of Treatment

The medications used to treat acute mania or bipolar depression should be continued for 6–12 months after remission. If remission is sustained at that time, a slow discontinuation of adjunctive medications (e.g., atypical antipsychotics) could be attempted with close monitoring (Young 2005). For most elderly patients with primary bipolar disorder, long-term treatment with a mood stabilizer should be considered. This is particularly true for patients with frequent manic episodes (every 12 months or less) or any serious episode requiring hospitalization. Some patients with early-onset disease will experience cycle acceleration later in life, and morbidity is greatly minimized with appropriate prophylaxis.

For mania that is secondary to medical conditions or medication treatment, a different treatment algorithm should be used; when the offending medication can be withdrawn or the medical condition treated, the mania often subsides. At that time, mood stabilizers should be tapered and discontinued, since maintenance treatment is not needed. In cases where definitive treatment is not possible (e.g., completed right hemisphere stroke), maintenance mood stabilization therapy may be needed.

Managing Treatment Resistance

Initial treatment will be inadequate, either completely or partially, for a substantial subgroup of elderly bipolar patients. Treatment algorithms developed for the adult population such as those published by the Texas Consensus Conference Panel (Suppes et al. 2005) and the Canadian Network for Mood and Anxiety Treatments (Yatham et al. 2005) should then be consulted for evidence-based recommendations regarding the next stage or step of treatment.

Discontinuation of Mood Stabilizers

Abrupt discontinuation of lithium therapy is associated with increased risk of early relapse (Suppes et al. 1991), so lithium is best tapered over a period of at least 2–4 weeks (Faedda et al. 1993). Although not specifically studied in geriatric patients, discontinuation of other mood stabilizers is most safely done by slow taper as well, over a period of several weeks.

Management of Overdose or Overmedication

In the elderly patient treated with a mood stabilizer, toxic effects can occur with inadvertent overmedication, even with levels in the "therapeutic" range, as well as with acute overdose. With lithium, toxicity at therapeutic levels may be associated with rapid dosage escalation, coadministration of other psychotropics (antipsychotics, antidepressants, or anticonvulsants), preexisting electroencephalogram (EEG) abnormalities, or structural brain disease (Bell et al. 1993; Emilien and Maloteaux 1996). In addition, any derangement associated with reduction of the glomerular filtration rate will cause an increase in lithium levels and potential toxicity. Other potential causes of toxicity include dehydration and reduction of sodium levels through dietary restriction and severe diarrhea.

Signs and symptoms of lithium intoxication can be GI, neuropsychiatric, cardiac, renal, or systemic. Neuropsychiatric signs include impaired cognition, lethargy, weakness, hyperreflexia, coarse tremor and other abnormal movements, dysarthria, rigidity, ataxia, delirium, seizures, and coma (Bell et al. 1993). Characteristic EEG abnormalities are seen (Ghadirian and Lehmann 1980). A syndrome of disinhibition and giddiness that resembles mania can occur. Cardiac dysrhythmias (e.g., bradycardia), hypotension, renal failure, and fever can also be seen in the lithium-toxic patient (Jefferson 1991).

The goal of treatment in lithium toxicity is to minimize exposure. This can be accomplished by discontinuation of lithium and initiation of gastric lavage, provision of continuous gastric suction, and restoration of normal fluid and electrolyte balance (Jefferson 1991). Administration of the ion exchange resin Kayexalate may be helpful. Except for the mildest cases, patients should be admitted to the hospital. Clinical examination should be conducted and lithium levels should be checked serially and frequently. Hemodialysis should be used for severe lithium intoxication (with coma, seizures, respiratory failure, or progressive deterioration), very high serum levels, rising serum levels, or impaired renal excretion (Jaeger et al. 1993). In general, chronic lithium toxicity or acute-on-chronic toxicity is more severe than acute toxicity (Jaeger et al. 1993).

Clinical recovery after lithium intoxication may take several weeks, with neurologic symptoms persisting long after lithium levels have normalized. Depending on the severity and duration of the toxic episode, a patient may demonstrate irreversible neurologic injury, with dysarthria, nystagmus, ataxia, and intention tremor being most characteristic (Apte and Langston 1983; Donaldson and Cunningham 1983; Schou 1984).

Valproate overdose may result in somnolence, heart block, coma, and hepatic or pancreatic toxicity, and has been associated with fatalities (McEvoy et al. 2006). Treatment is supportive, with an emphasis on maintaining adequate urine output. The effectiveness of gastric lavage or emesis is limited for immediate-release valproate because the drug is so rapidly absorbed, but it may be of value for the delayed-release form if the time since ingestion is short enough (McEvoy et al. 2006). Hemodialysis can remove significant amounts of valproate from the system. Naloxone can reverse central nervous system depressant effects of valproate but has been reported to increase the risk of seizure in some cases (McEvoy et al. 2006).

Carbamazepine overdose may produce GI, neurologic, and systemic signs. Anticholinergic effects may be associated with urinary retention. Treatment consists of emesis induction or gastric lavage as well as general supportive therapy. The patient's ECG should be monitored for dysrhythmias (McEvoy et al. 2006).

Symptoms of lamotrigine overdose may include ataxia, nystagmus, increased frequency of seizures, depressed level of consciousness (including coma), and intraventricular conduction delay (McEvoy et al. 2006).

Emesis and gastric lavage are recommended, particularly for recent inges-
tions, since lamotrigine is rapidly absorbed. Only about 20% of the drug
is removed during a 4-hour hemodialysis session.

Few data are available regarding other new anticonvulsants. In one reported case involving a nonelderly patient who took a 4-g dose of topiramate (serum level of 18.9 mg/L), no medical complications were noted
(Smith et al. 2001). In another reported case involving a nonelderly patient who took an overdose of levetiracetam, symptoms included sedation,
respiratory depression, and diminished deep tendon reflexes; recovery was
rapid with only supportive care (Barrueto et al. 2002).

Adverse Effects

Much of what is known about adverse effects of anticonvulsant mood-
stabilizing medications comes from the literature regarding use in the
treatment of epilepsy. Few data are available regarding the frequency of
adverse effects in bipolar patients, particularly the elderly.

Lithium

Adverse effects of lithium that may be particularly frequent or problematic in elderly patients include cognitive impairment, drowsiness, fatigue,
ataxia, tremor, cerebellar dysfunction, urinary incontinence, polyuria,
constipation, excessive thirst, increased urinary frequency, increase in fasting blood glucose, weight gain, worsening of chronic skin conditions
(e.g., psoriasis), worsening arthritis, and peripheral edema (Chacko et al.
1987; Sajatovic et al. 2005b). Many of these effects—including cognitive
impairment—are dose and level dependent.

Whether lithium treatment causes structural (e.g., glomerular)
changes in the kidney remains controversial, at least with regard to long-
term treatment (Bendz et al. 1994; Conte et al. 1989; Hetmar et al.
1989). Episodes of lithium toxicity as well as multiple daily dosing may
represent risks for renal injury; both should be avoided as far as possible
(Hetmar et al. 1991). The rationale for use of once-daily dosing of regular lithium is that the trough level achieved is sufficiently low to allow the
kidneys to recover before the next dose (Plenge et al. 1982). A separate
problem is that lithium impairs the ability of the kidneys to concentrate

urine in about one-third of elderly patients. The resultant polyuria, which may be manifested as urinary incontinence, is also reduced with single daily dosing. When polyuria remains problematic, the diuretic amiloride can be used; this medication paradoxically causes a reduction in urine volume in the polyuric patient (Price and Heninger 1994). More rarely, lithium treatment is associated with nephrogenic diabetes insipidus, with huge urine volumes and unquenchable thirst. This syndrome may reverse when lithium is discontinued, but the authors have seen a number of cases in which symptoms were persistent.

Cardiac effects of lithium include ECG changes, conduction changes, and dysrhythmias (Steckler 1994). T-wave depression on ECGs that is benign and reversible occurs in 20%–30% of lithium-treated patients (McEvoy et al. 2006). Sinus bradycardia, sinoatrial block, atrioventricular block, junctional rhythms, and ventricular premature depolarizations also occur, although less commonly. Sinus node dysfunction most often occurs in those with preexisting cardiac disease and in those taking blocking medications such as digoxin, calcium channel blockers, or propranolol (Steckler 1994). Ventricular arrhythmias may be precipitated or aggravated by lithium, even at therapeutic levels (Tilkian et al. 1976).

Neuropsychiatric effects of lithium are frequently reported by elderly patients with serum levels in the therapeutic range and particularly by patients with underlying structural brain disease (Bell et al. 1993). Effects include fatigue, weakness, hand tremor, memory problems, dysarthria, balance problems, ataxia, neuromuscular irritability (fasciculations and twitching), lack of coordination, and nystagmus. In general, tolerance to these neuropsychiatric symptoms does not develop, but they may improve with reduction in dose, albeit slowly in some cases. When lithium is discontinued because of the development of delirium or cerebellar dysfunction, symptoms can persist for weeks after serum levels are undetectable (Nambudiri et al. 1991). In cases of more severe toxicity, irreversible cerebellar signs (ataxia and dysarthria) can occur (Kores and Lader 1997).

Among other effects, lithium is associated with reduced bone mineral content because of reduced uptake of magnesium, calcium, and phosphate (Ghose 1977). Associated abnormalities include elevated serum calcium and magnesium levels, and elevated muscle magnesium and phosphate levels. The clinical significance of these findings in elderly patients is not known.

Approximately half of lithium-treated patients gain weight—an average of about 10–20 pounds with chronic treatment (Price and Heninger 1994). Hypothyroidism that occurs in 6% of elderly lithium-treated patients may be managed with exogenous thyroid supplementation (Shulman et al. 2005). Alopecia may also be reported, possibly more commonly among elders.

Valproate

The most common side effects of valproate are gastrointestinal: dyspepsia, nausea, and vomiting (McEvoy et al. 2006). These effects are usually transient and can be minimized by giving the medication with food, by using the enteric-coated formulation divalproex sodium (Depakote), and by starting at a low dose and titrating slowly. Increased appetite and weight gain are also common. Many other GI side effects have been reported, including fecal incontinence. Hepatotoxicity is rare, idiosyncratic, and unrelated to dose. Sedation is commonly seen upon initiation of therapy, with tolerance developing to this effect over 1–2 weeks. Tremor also may be seen. One underappreciated but potentially serious side effect of valproate is skeletal muscle weakness, which can interfere with the patient's ability to transfer, stand, and walk without assistance. Other adverse effects of valproate include parkinsonism (especially tremor), alopecia, elevated ammonia level, thrombocytopenia, rash, and SIADH. When the ammonia level becomes elevated with valproate use, the patient may exhibit asterixis and confusion or delirium and require discontinuation of the medication and initiation of lactulose to lower the ammonia level.

Carbamazepine

The most common adverse effects of carbamazepine are dizziness, drowsiness, nausea, skin reactions, and asthenia. Cognitive effects may be particularly problematic in elders (Sajatovic et al. 2005b). The most serious adverse effects—hematologic, cardiac, and gastrointestinal—make carbamazepine the last choice among mood stabilizers in the treatment of elderly patients. This medication is in rare cases (1 in 200,000) associated with aplastic anemia, with an unquantified incidence in elders. Cardiac effects include bradycardia, exacerbation of existing sinus node dysfunction, and slowed atrioventricular node and His' bundle conduction (Steckler 1994). Cardiac effects are especially common in elderly women and may be seen at therapeutic or only modestly elevated carbamazepine serum levels (Kasarskis et al. 1992). GI effects include significant elevations in LFT values (AST, ALT, and γ-glutamyltransferase), which may in rare cases be associated with hepatic insufficiency or failure. Neuropsychiatric effects of carbamazepine include confusion, disorientation, sedation, dizziness, unsteadiness, ataxia, diplopia, lassitude, and weakness. Various dermatologic reactions may be seen, including Stevens-Johnson syndrome. Impaired water excretion with hyponatremia (SIADH) can occur with carbamazepine and is more common in geriatric patients than in younger patients.

Oxcarbazepine

Oxcarbazepine is related to carbamazepine but is metabolized by reduction to a monohydroxy derivative rather than to carbamazepine's toxic epoxide metabolite; its adverse-effect profile is therefore more benign. For the most part, adverse effects in elders are similar to those in younger populations: GI effects, dizziness, somnolence, and fatigue. In addition, however, elderly patients have a high rate (25%) of hyponatremia on oxcarbazepine that usually is asymptomatic (Dunner 2005b) but in severe cases may present as altered mental status. Hyponatremia is a cause for discontinuation of oxcarbazepine in 3.8% of elderly patients, compared with 0.7% of younger patients (Kutluay et al. 2003).

Lamotrigine

Common adverse effects of lamotrigine among patients with epilepsy include dizziness, ataxia, somnolence, headache, diplopia, blurred vision, nausea, vomiting, and rash. Other side effects include insomnia, incoordination, tremor, impairment in memory and concentration, constipation, and arthralgia. Among patients with bipolar disorder, the only adverse effect that is consistently found more frequently with treated patients than with placebo is headache. Benign rash is seen in 8.3% of treated patients (Calabrese et al. 2002). The rash has no particular distinguishing features, but it may uncommonly herald the onset of Stevens-Johnson syndrome or toxic epidermal necrolysis, for which fatalities have been reported. The risk of rash is increased by coadministration of valproate, by exceeding initial dosing recommendations, or especially by exceeding dose escalation recommendations.

Levetiracetam

In one study of elderly patients administered levetiracetam for epilepsy, 19.2% of subjects stopped the drug because of adverse effects. Most common were dizziness, somnolence, confusion, and (in those over 80 years of age) accidental injury (Ferrendelli et al. 2003).

System-Specific Adverse Effects

Cardiovascular Effects

Cardiovascular effects are found primarily with lithium and carbamazepine and are discussed above under individual agents.

Dermatologic Effects

Both lamotrigine and carbamazepine have been associated with a syndrome first manifested as a nonspecific rash that can progress to Stevens-Johnson syndrome or toxic epidermal necrolysis—potentially fatal syndromes. In fact, the risk of serious rash appears to be minimal among adults treated with lamotrigine and is further minimized by slow initial titration of dose and avoiding the combination of lamotrigine and valproate (Calabrese et al. 2002). When a rash does develop with any of these medications, serious systemic signs and fever may be present (Dunner 2005b). In these cases, the drug should be discontinued and the rash evaluated. If the rash is judged to be secondary to one of the medications, that medication should not be restarted (Dunner 2005b).

Lithium can exacerbate psoriasis, acne, and folliculitis. Although all may limit treatment, lithium exacerbation of psoriasis is potentially very serious, necessitating hospitalization for treatment with intravenous steroids in some cases. Lithium is also associated with the de novo development of rash as well as with hair loss and edema (Gitlin et al. 1989).

Alopecia is a side effect of a number of different psychotropic drugs. Hair loss associated with long-term use of mood stabilizers occurs with lithium in 12%–19%, with valproate in up to 12% of patients (although this is apparently dose dependent, and at higher concentrations has been reported in up to 28%), and with carbamazepine in up to 6% of patients

(Mercke et al. 2000). In addition to hair loss, change in hair structure and/or color can occur. Stopping the offending medication usually results in complete hair regrowth (Mercke et al. 2000). Mineral supplementation (e.g., with zinc and selenium) to counter hair loss in patients who continue medication has been suggested, but the efficacy of supplementation is not known.

Endocrine Effects

Among other thyroid effects, lithium inhibits release of thyroxine and triiodothyronine, resulting in decreased circulating levels of these hormones and a feedback increase in TSH (McEvoy et al. 2006). Approximately 6% of geriatric patients undergoing long-term treatment with lithium develop either hypothyroidism (Shulman et al. 2005). Lithium-induced hypothyroidism develops more often in women. Symptoms can include fatigue, weight gain, hair loss, coarse skin, hoarse voice, pretibial edema, sensitivity to cold, dementia and depression. Hypothyroidism usually comes on insidiously and, once developed, is associated with resistance to mood-stabilizing treatment. Treatment options include discontinuation of lithium or initiation of thyroid hormone replacement. Lithium-associated goiters develop more often in men, usually 1–2 years after treatment is initiated. Much less commonly, lithium may be associated with hyperthyroidism (Oakley et al. 2000).

Certain bipolar patients appear to be at risk of having or developing glucose dysregulation (McIntyre et al. 2005). Several factors contribute to this problem, with medication-induced weight gain, other medication effects, and excessive carbohydrate intake all having some role.

Gastrointestinal Effects

Initiation of lithium may be associated with mild, reversible GI side effects (McEvoy et al. 2006). These include nausea, anorexia, epigastric bloating, diarrhea, vomiting, and abdominal pain—symptoms that usually resolve during continued therapy. Persistent effects may be associated with high peak serum concentrations and can be reduced by lowering the dose, giving the drug with food, or switching to a different preparation (capsule or tablet). When diarrhea is a problem, some patients benefit from a switch to the citrate preparation, since this symptom can be worsened by the use of slow-release preparations.

Lamotrigine use may be associated with nausea and vomiting, effects that are dose-related, and thus more common among epilepsy patients than bipolar patients (Marken and Pies 2006). Other GI effects of lamotrigine include diarrhea, dyspepsia, abdominal pain, and hepatic failure (which is rare). GI effects of carbamazepine, gabapentin, and valproate are specifically discussed for each drug in "Adverse Effects" above.

Hematologic Effects

Carbamazepine is commonly associated with leukopenia and thrombocytopenia, dose-dependent phenomena associated at times with a rapid rate of dose escalation. For white cells, the reduction from baseline for patients of varying ages is on the order of 15%–20%. Usually, this cytopenia plateaus after several weeks and does not presage an aplastic episode (Gerner and Stanton 1992). Much more rarely, carbamazepine and other anticonvulsants may be associated with agranulocytosis and aplastic anemia (1 in 200,000 cases). If the white blood cell count falls to 3,000, the dose of carbamazepine or other anticonvulsant should be reduced and the CBC should be monitored weekly. If it falls to 2,500 or less, the drug should be discontinued and restarted only after the cell count exceeds 3,000 after several weeks (Gerner and Stanton 1992).

The risk of leukopenia with valproate is an order of magnitude less than with carbamazepine and about the same as with antidepressants (Tohen et al. 1995). The guidelines outlined above for carbamazepine-associated leukopenia apply as well to valproate. Thrombocytopenia is relatively common with valproate treatment, especially among elderly patients, but most often is not clinically significant. The patient with low or declining platelet count should be monitored for bruising or bleeding, and serial platelet counts should be obtained.

Lithium is commonly associated with a mild to moderate leukocytosis involving mature neutrophils, and this laboratory finding should not be mistaken for infection or a more serious blood dyscrasia. Although leukocytosis can counter clozapine-induced leukopenia, the addition of lithium to clozapine does not prevent the development of agranulocytosis.

Hepatic Effects

Early in treatment, both carbamazepine and valproate can produce elevations in LFT values (AST and ALT) (Gerner and Stanton 1992). These findings usually do not presage severe disease. If AST and ALT values are less than three times baseline values and alkaline phosphatase and bilirubin are normal, the patient should be monitored with weekly LFTs. When values plateau, longer testing intervals are permitted. If LFT values rise to more than three times baseline (or more than twice the upper limit of normal), the drug should be discontinued or appropriate consultation obtained (Gerner and Stanton 1992). Another warning sign is elevation in either alkaline phosphatase or bilirubin; these laboratory abnormalities indicate that the anticonvulsant should be held, if not discontinued. Prothrombin time can also help determine functional hepatic effects. No laboratory test, however, should take precedence over clinical observations of malaise, nausea, anorexia, or jaundice, which can indicate significant hepatotoxicity and often precede changes in LFT values. Because preexisting liver disease predisposes to hepatotoxicity, patients with any evidence of hepatic dysfunction are best treated with mood stabilizers other than carbamazepine or valproate.

Neuropsychiatric Effects

Sedation is an effect common to all mood stabilizers except lamotrigine (which is activating) and possibly topiramate and zonisamide (which have mixed sedating/activating effects). Sedation is most prominent upon initiation of therapy or after a dose increase. For most patients, tolerance to this effect develops over 1–2 weeks; in some cases, however, dose reduction is required.

All medications used to treat bipolar disorder have cognitive effects, although the agents differ in terms of severity of these effects, and at least one drug (lamotrigine) appears to be associated with cognitive improvement (Aldenkamp et al. 2003; Khan et al. 2004). Cognitive effects attributed to lithium include poor concentration, memory impairment, word-finding difficulty, cognitive dulling, and mental slowness (Gitlin et al. 1989; Lund et al. 1982). These effects can be seen during the early phases of treatment and even at low doses. They can continue during long-term treatment and can persist for a period of time after lithium is discontinued. In some cases, however, lowering the lithium dose can result in cognitive improvement. It is worth noting that the extent to which cognitive decline may be attributable to long-term bipolar illness itself is not known.

In general, cognitive effects of valproate and carbamazepine are fewer than those of lithium, occurring mostly in the realm of psychomotor slowing (Aldenkamp et al. 2003). This is apparent fairly early in treatment, usually by the time steady-state levels are achieved. Among newer agents, lamotrigine is associated with the least cognitive impairment, while topiramate and zonisamide appear to be associated with the greatest impairment (Dunner 2005b; Martin et al. 1999; Sajatovic et al. 2005b).

Patients with subjective complaints of cognitive impairment should be evaluated clinically. Because actual impairment might be too subtle to be detected by screening measures, referral for neuropsychologic testing may be necessary. If impairment is confirmed, the dose of offending medication should be reduced, if possible. In addition, TSH should be checked to determine whether hypothyroidism might be contributing in lithium-treated patients. If no improvement is noted with dose reduction, the medication should be stopped and another substituted. Lamotrigine may be of particular use in this context (Dunner 2005b).

Motor effects of mood stabilizers are not uncommon in geriatric patients. With lithium treatment, hand tremor occurs in up to 50% of patients of varying ages (McEvoy et al. 2006). The tremor is described as a distal resting/intention tremor that is less coarse than a parkinsonian tremor. This tremor diminishes with time for many patients, but severe cases can be treated with dose reduction and/or administration of a β-blocker such as propranolol up to 40 mg/day in divided doses. A similar tremor can be seen with valproate, carbamazepine, lamotrigine, and topiramate and is treated in the same way as for lithium. In addition, worsening of preexisting Parkinson's disease and de novo appearance of parkinsonism have been reported with lithium therapy (Mirchandani and Young 1993).

Other motor effects of lithium include cerebellar dysfunction (ataxia, incoordination, dysarthria, nystagmus), weakness, and myoclonus (Gitlin et al. 1989). As discussed earlier, valproate has been associated with skeletal muscle weakness, which is severe at times. Carbamazepine has been associated with ataxia. Topiramate has been associated with an incidence of paresthesias >10% (Semla et al. 2006). Although paresthesias may be tolerated by patients who have been informed in advance about the possibility of their occurrence, their development may necessitate drug discontinuation in other patients. It has been speculated that paresthesias may be an effect of topiramate's carbonic anhydrase inhibition.

The development of seizures is a rare complication of mood stabilizer therapy, since most agents are anticonvulsants and are associated with seizure development only at toxic levels. The one exception to this is lithium, which can be associated with generalized seizures if the patient is clinically toxic, regardless of serum level (McEvoy et al. 2006). Usually, seizures resolve when lithium is withheld and resumed at a lower dosage.

Renal Effects

Effects of lithium on the kidney are discussed in an earlier section, "Adverse Effects."

Weight Gain

Obesity is a prevalent and significant problem in patients with bipolar disorder, whether or not these patients are treated with a medication associated with weight gain (Dunner 2005b). Obesity appears to be associated with a number of factors, including excessive carbohydrate consumption, low levels of exercise, comorbid binge eating disorder, frequent depressive episodes, and medication treatment (Keck and McElroy 2003). Medications that cause weight gain can of course only be expected to worsen weight problems. When weight gain occurs, it can be significant within weeks and continue throughout treatment (at least for 8 months in one study involving valproate) (Biton et al. 2001).

Counseling and referral to weight management programs where indicated are an important part of early management (Keck and McElroy 2003). When weight gain occurs, lowering the dose of medication may not help. It may be necessary to select drugs on the basis of their propensity to cause weight gain: high propensity with lithium, valproate, clozapine, and olanzapine; low propensity with lamotrigine and oxcarbazepine (Dunner 2005b). Topiramate and zonisamide are actually associated with weight loss, but the role of these drugs in treating elders with bipolar disorder is not yet clear. In addition, the use of topiramate as a weight loss agent in elderly patients appears risky in view of its generally poor tolerability. As noted in Chapter 3, other strategies to minimize weight gain may be necessary when atypical antipsychotics are used.

Treatment of Selected Disorders and Syndromes

Bipolar Mania

Earlier sections of this chapter have noted the similarity of presenting signs and symptoms of mania in geriatric patients to those of nongeriatric patients, and the fact that current evidence suggests that the same treatment algorithms can be used for elders, with a few modifications. The algorithm for treatment of hypomania, mania, or mixed episodes in patients with bipolar I disorder from the Texas Consensus Conference Panel on Medication Treatment of Bipolar Disorder is reproduced as Figure 5–2.

For the geriatric patient with mania, the initial use of monotherapy with a mood stabilizer (lithium or valproate) coupled with discontinuation of antidepressants is recommended. Initial therapy should be monitored for several weeks (if possible) before deciding that augmentation or switching is needed (Young 2005). Nonresponse should prompt a switch of medication, and partial response should prompt the addition of another mood stabilizer or an atypical antipsychotic (Young 2005). ECT (algorithm stage 4) is a viable treatment option in elderly patients, with demonstrated efficacy in mania.

Bipolar Mixed State

The algorithm shown in Figure 5–2 also applies to mixed episodes, in which manic and depressed features are present simultaneously. These presentations are seen more frequently in elderly patients than in younger patients, and valproate is preferred to lithium for this indication. ECT is also effective for mixed states, but a longer course of ECT may be required for mixed states than for manic or depressed states (Devanand et al. 2000).

Bipolar Depression

The algorithm for treatment of acute depressive episodes in patients with bipolar I disorder from the Texas Consensus Conference Panel on Medication Treatment of Bipolar Disorder is reproduced as Figure 5–3. For

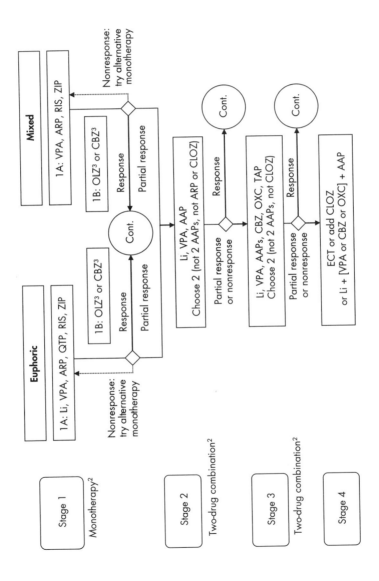

Figure 5–2. Algorithm for treatment of acute hypomanic/manic/mixed episodes in patients with bipolar disorder.[1]

Note. AAP=atypical antipsychotic; ARP=aripiprazole; CBZ=carbamazepine; CLOZ=clozapine; Cont.=continuation; ECT=electroconvulsive therapy; Li=lithium; OLZ=olanzapine; OXC=oxcarbazepine; QTP=quetiapine; RIS=risperidone; TAP=typical antipsychotic; VPA=valproate; ZIP=ziprasidone.

[1]It is appropriate to try more than one combination at a given level. New trials from each stage can be labeled Stage 2 (1), Stage 2 (2), etc.

[2]Use targeted adjunctive treatment as necessary before moving to next stage: agitation/aggression—clonidine, sedatives; insomnia—hypnotics; anxiety—benzodiazepines, gabapentin.

[3]Safety and other concerns led to placement of OLZ and CBZ as alternate first-stage choices.

Source. Reprinted from Suppes T, Dennehy EB, Hirschfeld RMA, et al: "The Texas Implementation of Medication Algorithms: Update to the Algorithms for Treatment of Bipolar I Disorder." *Journal of Clinical Psychiatry* 66:870–886, 2005. Used with permission.

elderly patients, monotherapy should be attempted for the initial step, using either lithium or lamotrigine. If one of these medications is not effective or not tolerated, a switch to the other could be tried. If the switch to the other is ineffective or poorly tolerated, an atypical antipsychotic could be tried as monotherapy or as add-on therapy. If this also proves ineffective, consideration should be given to the use of an antidepressant medication in combination with a mood stabilizer or ECT. Suggested antidepressants for this indication for elderly patients include bupropion, citalopram, and escitalopram. Venlafaxine may be particularly risky in terms of a switch to mania. As noted in an earlier section, the olanzapine/ fluoxetine combination drug is not recommended for elders.

An antidepressant used for bipolar depression should generally be tapered and discontinued after 2–6 months, depending on the duration and severity of the depressive episode and on previous clinical response to this maneuver; some patients may relapse rapidly (Altshuler et al. 2003). For the geriatric bipolar patient already taking lithium who presents with major depression, the possibility that the patient is hypothyroid should be considered, and a serum TSH level should be obtained.

When psychotic symptoms (delusions or hallucinations) accompany a bipolar-depressed or bipolar-manic episode, adjunctive antipsychotic medication or ECT may be necessary. Generally, the antipsychotic should be tapered and withdrawn when the acute episode is fully treated, from 2–6 months after psychotic symptoms are in remission.

Rapid Cycling

DSM-IV-TR defines rapid cycling as four or more episodes of mood disturbance in 12 months that meet criteria for a major depressive, manic, mixed, or hypomanic episode. The episodes must be demarcated by a 2-month period of remission or by a switch of polarity. There is evidence that once rapid cycling is established (whether spontaneous or induced), it can become a stable rhythm for many years in a substantial proportion of patients (Koukopoulos et al. 2003). In other patients, the rapid-cycling pattern may wax and wane over the years. There is a preponderance of women among rapid cyclers, possibly related to the link between rapid cycling and hypothyroidism (Coryell 2005). Rapid cycling may also be associated with antidepressant use.

It is not known whether rapid cycling is more or less common in elders, presents differently, or responds differently to treatment in this population (Depp and Jeste 2004). However, some bipolar patients do show a pattern of cycle acceleration with aging, sometimes attributed to the hypothesized "kindling" phenomenon (Post 2004).

The first step in pharmacotherapy for rapid-cycling bipolar illness is discontinuation of antidepressant medication. First-line treatment is lamotrigine monotherapy (Ernst and Goldberg 2003), but other medications may be effective. In elder patients, as in younger patients, it is the depressive symptoms that often prove most difficult to control (Coryell 2005).

Bipolar II Disorder

In elderly patients, as in nonelderly patients, the longitudinal course of bipolar II disorder is dominated by depressive symptoms. Symptom severity is primarily in the minor or subsyndromal range, with occasional major depressive episodes and rare hypomanias or mixed episodes (Judd et al. 2003). The hypomania often goes undetected, such that the condition is often misdiagnosed as unipolar depression. The use of a mood questionnaire such as the Bipolar Spectrum Diagnostic Scale can help in eliciting a history of hypomania and appears to be more sensitive than the Mood Disorder Questionnaire in the detection of bipolar II disorder (Ghaemi et al. 2005). For bipolar II depression in elderly patients, lamotrigine appears to be a reasonable choice of drug. Other options include a first-line mood stabilizer in combination with an antidepressant, or possibly pramipexole (Yatham 2005). Hypomania usually responds to monotherapy with a first-line mood stabilizer (lithium or valproate).

Bipolar Disorder Prophylaxis and Maintenance

The algorithm for maintenance treatment of bipolar disorder in which the most recent episode was hypomanic, manic, or mixed from the Texas Consensus Conference Panel on Medication Treatment of Bipolar Disorder is reproduced as Table 5–10. The algorithm for maintenance treatment in which the most recent episode was depressed is reproduced as Table 5–11. For elderly patients, the preference in maintenance treatment is for monotherapy whenever possible.

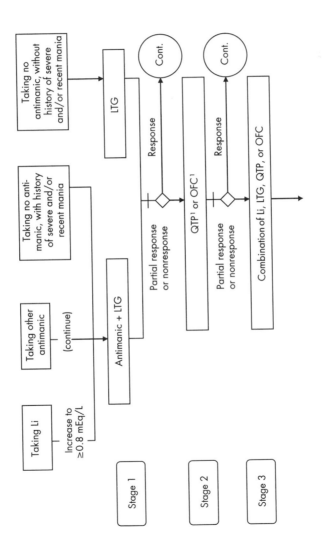

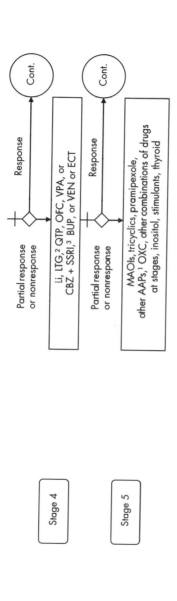

Figure 5–3. Algorithm for treatment of acute depressive episodes in patients with bipolar disorder.

Note. AAP = atypical antipsychotic; BUP = bupropion; CBZ = carbamazepine; Cont. = continuation; ECT = electroconvulsive therapy; Li = lithium; LTG = lamotrigine; MAOI = monoamine oxidase inhibitor; OFC = olanzapine-fluoxetine combination; OXC = oxcarbazepine; QTP = quetiapine; SSRI = selective serotonin reuptake inhibitor; VEN = venlafaxine; VPA = valproate.

[1]Note safety issue described in text.

[2]Lamotrigine has limited antimanic efficacy and, in combination with an antidepressant, may require the addition of an antimanic.

[3]SSRIs include citalopram, escitalopram, fluoxetine, paroxetine, sertraline, and fluvoxamine.

Source. Reprinted from Suppes T, Dennehy EB, Hirschfeld RMA, et al: "The Texas Implementation of Medication Algorithms: Update to the Algorithms for Treatment of Bipolar I Disorder." *Journal of Clinical Psychiatry* 66:870–886, 2005. Used with permission.

Table 5–10. Guidelines for maintenance treatment: most recent episode hypomanic, manic, or mixed

It is an option to remain on well-tolerated, effective, acute-phase treatments. Available evidence supports the options presented for the prevention of new episodes or maintenance treatment.

Level

I	Patients with frequent, recent, or severe mania	Lithium or valproate
	Patients without frequent, recent, or severe mania	Lithium, valproate, or lamotrigine
	Alternative	Olanzapine[a]
II	Aripiprazole[b]	
III	Carbamazepine or clozapine[a]	
IV	Quetiapine,[b] risperidone,[b] or ziprasidone[b]	
V	Typical antipsychotics,[a] oxcarbazepine,[b] electroconvulsive therapy	

[a] Safety issues warrant careful consideration of this option for potential long-term use.
[b] Relatively limited information is currently available on this agent for long-term use.
Source. From Suppes T, Dennehy EB, Hirschfeld RMA, et al: "The Texas Implementation of Medication Algorithms: Update to the Algorithms for Treatment of Bipolar I Disorder." *Journal of Clinical Psychiatry* 66:870–886, 2005. Used with permission.

Schizoaffective Disorder

Treatment of schizoaffective disorder in elderly patients has been focused on the use of atypical antipsychotic agents, although anticonvulsant mood stabilizers may be useful (see Chapter 3).

Secondary Mania

The diagnostic evaluation for secondary mania is discussed in an earlier section, and causes of secondary mania are listed in Table 5–8 (medications) and Table 5–9 (medical conditions). In general, secondary mania is more likely in an elderly patient who has a first episode in late life, has cerebrovascular disease, has no family history of mood disorder, responds poorly to lithium or becomes toxic at low lithium levels, or has been

Table 5–11. Guidelines for maintenance treatment: most recent episode depressed

It is an option to remain on well-tolerated, effective, acute-phase treatments. Available evidence supports the options presented for maintenance treatment.

Level		
I	Patients with recent and/or severe history of mania	Lamotrigine combined with antimanic agent
	All other patients	Lamotrigine monotherapy
II	Lithium	
III	Combination of an antimanic and antidepressant that has been effective in the past, including olanzapine-fluoxetine combination[a]	
IV	Valproate, carbamazepine, aripiprazole,[b] clozapine,[a] olanzapine,[a] quetiapine,[b] risperidone,[b] ziprasidone[b]	
V	Typical antipsychotics,[a] oxcarbazepine,[b] electroconvulsive therapy	

[a]Safety issues warrant careful consideration of this option for potential long-term use.
[b]Relatively limited information is currently available on this agent for long-term use.
Source. From Suppes T, Dennehy EB, Hirschfeld RMA, et al: "The Texas Implementation of Medication Algorithms: Update to the Algorithms for Treatment of Bipolar I Disorder." *Journal of Clinical Psychiatry* 66:870–886, 2005. Used with permission.

treated with a mania-inducing medication such as an antidepressant (Young and Klerman 1992). It is generally believed that secondary mania is characterized by more irritable mood and less grandiosity than primary mania and that cognitive dysfunction is more common in secondary mania (Carroll et al. 1996; Das and Khanna 1993).

The treatment of secondary mania primarily involves discontinuation of the offending medication or treatment of the underlying medical condition. When this has been accomplished in a timely and effective way, most deficits generally resolve (Brooks and Hoblyn 2005). When mood-stabilizing medication is needed, an anticonvulsant such as valproate should be used in preference to lithium. In some cases, this medication should be continued for a period of weeks to months while the underlying medical condition is treated, but in other cases, where definitive treatment is not possible (e.g., completed right hemisphere stroke), longer-term therapy may be required.

Chapter Summary

- First-line drugs for the treatment of bipolar mania in elderly patients include lithium and valproate.
- First-line drugs for the treatment of bipolar depression in this population include lithium and lamotrigine.
- Electroconvulsive (ECT) is effective for the treatment of geriatric mania and results in rapid remission of symptoms, typically after four to six treatments.
- For elderly patients with treatment-refractory mania or depression, or for depressed states associated with suicidality or inadequate nutritional intake, ECT should be considered.
- Preferred atypical antipsychotics for the treatment of elderly patients with bipolar disorder include aripiprazole, quetiapine, and risperidone.
- Target serum lithium levels in the range of 0.4–1.0 mEq/L should be used for acute treatment and for maintenance therapy of bipolar disorder, with the exact level depending on individual clinical response and tolerability.
- For valproate, target serum levels for acute mania in the geriatric patient should be in the range of 65–90 µg/mL.
- For most elderly patients with primary bipolar disorder, long-term treatment with a mood stabilizer is recommended.
- The first step in pharmacotherapy for rapid-cycling bipolar illness is discontinuation of antidepressant medication.
- Secondary mania is more likely in an elderly patient who has a first episode in late life, has cerebrovascular disease, has no family history of mood disorder, responds poorly to lithium or becomes toxic at low lithium levels, or has been treated with a mania-inducing medication such as an antidepressant.
- The treatment of secondary mania primarily involves discontinuation of the offending medication or treatment of the underlying medical condition.

References

Aldenkamp AP, De Krom M, Reijs R: Newer antiepileptic drugs and cognitive issues. Epilepsia 44 (suppl 4):21–29, 2003

Altshuler L, Suppes T, Black D, et al: Impact of antidepressant discontinuation after acute bipolar depression remission on rates of depressive relapse at 1-year follow-up. Am J Psychiatry 160:1252–1262, 2003

American Psychiatric Association: Practice guideline for the treatment of patients with bipolar disorder (revision). Am J Psychiatry 159 (suppl 4):1–50, 2002

Apte SN, Langston JW: Permanent neurological deficits due to lithium toxicity. Ann Neurol 13:453–455, 1983

Barrueto F, Williams K, Howland MA, et al: A case of levetiracetam (Keppra) poisoning with clinical and toxokinetic data. J Toxicol Clin Toxicol 40:881–884, 2002

Bell AJ, Cole A, Eccleston D, et al: Lithium neurotoxicity at normal therapeutic levels. Br J Psychiatry 162:689–692, 1993

Bendz H, Aurell M, Balldin J, et al: Kidney damage in long-term lithium patients: a cross-sectional study of patients with 15 years or more on lithium. Nephrol Dial Transplant 9:1250–1254, 1994

Biton V, Mirza W, Montouris G, et al: Weight change associated with valproate and lamotrigine monotherapy in patients with epilepsy. Neurology 56:172–177, 2001

Bowden CL: Atypical antipsychotic augmentation of mood stabilizer therapy in bipolar disorder. J Clin Psychiatry 66 (suppl 3):12–19, 2005

Brooks JO, Hoblyn JC: Secondary mania in older adults. Am J Psychiatry 162:2033–2038, 2005

Calabrese JR, Bowden CL, Sachs GS, et al: A double-blind placebo-controlled study of lamotrigine monotherapy in outpatients with bipolar I depression. J Clin Psychiatry 60:79–88, 1999

Calabrese JR, Suppes T, Bowden CL, et al: A double-blind, placebo-controlled, prophylaxis study of lamotrigine in rapid-cycling bipolar disorder. J Clin Psychiatry 61:841–850, 2000

Calabrese JR, Sullivan JR, Bowden CL, et al: Rash in multicenter trials of lamotrigine in mood disorders: clinical relevance and management. J Clin Psychiatry 63:1012–1019, 2002

Calabrese JR, Keck PE Jr, Macfadden W, et al: A randomized, double-blind, placebo-controlled trial of quetiapine in the treatment of bipolar I or II depression. Am J Psychiatry 162:1351–1360, 2005

Carroll BT, Goforth HW, Kennedy JC, et al: Mania due to general medical conditions: frequency, treatment, and cost. Int J Psychiatry Med 26:5–13, 1996

Cassidy F, Carroll B: Vascular risk factors in late onset mania. Psychol Med 32:359–362, 2002

Chacko RC, Marsh BJ, Marmion J, et al: Lithium side effects in elderly bipolar outpatients. Hillside J Clin Psychiatry 9:79–88, 1987

Chen ST, Altshuler LL, Melnyk KA, et al: Efficacy of lithium vs. valproate in the treatment of mania in the elderly: a retrospective study. J Clin Psychiatry 60:181–186, 1999

Conte G, Vazzola A, Sacchetti E: Renal function in chronic lithium-treated patients. Acta Psychiatr Scand 79:503–504, 1989

Coryell W: Rapid cycling bipolar disorder: clinical characteristics and treatment options. CNS Drugs 19:557–569, 2005

Das A, Khanna R: Organic manic syndrome: causative factors, phenomenology and immediate outcome. J Affect Disord 27:147–153, 1993

Depp CA, Jeste DV: Bipolar disorder in older adults: a critical review. Bipolar Disord 6:343–367, 2004

Devanand DP, Polanco P, Cruz R, et al: The efficacy of ECT in mixed affective states. J ECT 16:32–37, 2000

Donaldson IM, Cunningham J: Persisting neurologic sequelae of lithium carbonate therapy. Arch Neurol 40:747–751, 1983

Du J, Gray NA, Galke CA, et al: Modulation of synaptic plasticity by antimanic agents: the role of AMPA glutamate receptor subunit 1 synaptic expression. J Neurosci 24:6578–6589, 2004

Dunner DL: Atypical antipsychotics: efficacy across bipolar disorder subpopulations. J Clin Psychiatry 66 (suppl 30):20–27, 2005a

Dunner DL: Safety and tolerability of emerging pharmacological treatments for bipolar disorder. Bipolar Disord 7:307–325, 2005b

Eastham JH, Jeste DV, Young RC: Assessment and treatment of bipolar disorder in the elderly. Drugs Aging 12:205–224, 1998

Emilien G, Maloteaux JM: Lithium neurotoxicity at low therapeutic doses: hypotheses for causes and mechanism of action following a retrospective analysis of published case reports. Acta Neurol Belg 96:281–293, 1996

Ernst CL, Goldberg JF: Antidepressant properties of anticonvulsant drugs for bipolar disorder. J Clin Psychopharmacol 23:182–192, 2003

Faedda GL, Tondo L, Baldessarini RJ, et al: Outcome after rapid vs. gradual discontinuation of lithium treatment in bipolar disorders. Arch Gen Psychiatry 50:448–455, 1993

Ferrendelli JA, French J, Leppik I, et al: Use of levetiracetam in a population of patients aged 65 years and older: a subset analysis of the KEEPER trial. Epilepsy Behav 4:702–709, 2003

Foster JR: Use of lithium in elderly psychiatric patients: a review of the literature. Lithium 3:77–93, 1992

Gerner RH, Stanton A: Algorithm for patient management of acute manic states: lithium, valproate, or carbamazepine? J Clin Psychopharmacol 12:57S–63S, 1992

Ghadirian AM, Lehmann HE: Neurological side effects of lithium: organic brain syndrome, seizures, extrapyramidal side effects, and EEG changes. Comp Psychiatry 21:327–335, 1980

Ghaemi SN, Miller CJ, Berv DA, et al: Sensitivity and specificity of a new bipolar spectrum diagnostic scale. J Affect Disord 84:273–277, 2005

Ghose K: Lithium salts: therapeutic and unwanted effects. Br J Hosp Med 18:578–583, 1977

Gildengers AG, Butters MA, Seligman K, et al: Cognitive functioning in late-life bipolar disorder. Am J Psychiatry 161:736–738, 2004

Gitlin MJ, Cochran SD, Jamison KR: Maintenance lithium treatment: side effects and compliance. J Clin Psychiatry 50:127–131, 1989

Glazer WM, Sonnenberg JG, Reinstein MJ, et al: A novel, point-of-care test for lithium levels: description and reliability. J Clin Psychiatry 65:652–655, 2004

Grim SA, Ryan M, Miles MV, et al: Correlation of levetiracetam concentrations between serum and saliva. Ther Drug Monit 25:61–66, 2003

Hetmar O, Brun C, Ladefoged J, et al: Long-term effects of lithium on the kidney: functional-morphological correlations. J Psychiatr Res 23:285–297, 1989

Hetmar O, Povlsen UJ, Ladefoged J, et al: Lithium: long-term effects on the kidney. A prospective follow-up study ten years after kidney biopsy. Br J Psychiatry 158:53–58, 1991

Hirschfeld RM: Practice guideline for the treatment of patients with bipolar disorder, in American Psychiatric Association Practice Guidelines for the Treatment of Psychiatric Disorders. Edited by McIntyre RS. Washington, DC, American Psychiatric Association, 2000, pp 497–562

Hirschfeld RM, Kasper S: A review of the evidence for carbamazepine and oxcarbazepine in the treatment of bipolar disorder. Int J Neuropsychopharmacol 7:507–522, 2004

Jaeger A, Sauder P, Kopferschmitt J, et al: When should dialysis be performed in lithium poisoning? a kinetic study in 14 cases of lithium poisoning. J Toxicol Clin Toxicol 31:429–447, 1993

Jefferson JW: Lithium poisoning. Emergency Care Quarterly 7(1):18–28, 1991

Jensen HV, Plenge P, Mellerup ET, et al: Lithium prophylaxis of manic-depressive disorder: daily lithium dosing schedule versus every second day. Acta Psychiatr Scand 92:69–74, 1995

Jones MD, Ryan M, Miles MV, et al: Stability of salivary concentrations of the newer antiepileptic drugs in the postal system. Ther Drug Monit 27:576–579, 2005

Judd LL, Akiskal HS, Schettler PJ, et al: A prospective investigation of the natural history of the long-term weekly symptomatic status of bipolar II disorder. Arch Gen Psychiatry 60:261–269, 2003

Kasarskis EJ, Kuo C-S, Berger R, et al: Carbamazepine-induced cardiac dysfunction. Arch Intern Med 152:186–191, 1992

Keck PE, McElroy SL: Bipolar disorder, obesity, and pharmacotherapy-associated weight gain. J Clin Psychiatry 64:1426–1435, 2003

Keck PE Jr: Bipolar depression: a new role for atypical antipsychotics? Bipolar Disorder 7 (suppl 4):34–40, 2005

Khan A, Ginsberg LD, Asnis GM, et al: Effect of lamotrigine on cognitive complaints in patients with bipolar I disorder. J Clin Psychiatry 65:1483–1490, 2004

Kilbourne AM, Cornelius JR, Han X, et al: General-medical conditions in older patients with serious mental illness. Am J Geriatr Psychiatry 13:250–254, 2005

Kores B, Lader MH: Irreversible lithium neurotoxicity: an overview. Clin Neuropharmacol 20:283–299, 1997

Koukopoulos A, Sani G, Koukopoulos AE, et al: Duration and stability of the rapid-cycling course: a long-term personal follow-up of 109 patients. J Affect Disord 73:75–85, 2003

Krauthammer C, Klerman GL: Secondary mania: manic syndromes associated with antecedent physical illness or drugs. Arch Gen Psychiatry 35:1333–1339, 1978

Kupka RW, Nolen WA, Post RM, et al: High rate of autoimmune thyroiditis in bipolar disorder: lack of association with lithium exposure. Biol Psychiatry 51:305–311, 2002

Kutluay E, McCague K, D'Souza J, et al: Safety and tolerability of oxcarbazepine in elderly patients with epilepsy. Epilepsy Behav 4:175–180, 2003

Lieberman JA, Stroup TS, McEvoy JP, et al: Effectiveness of antipsychotic drugs in patients with chronic schizophrenia. N Engl J Med 353:1209–1223, 2005

Lund Y, Nissen M, Rafaelsen OJ: Long-term lithium treatment and psychological functions. Acta Psychiatr Scand 65:233–244, 1982

Marken PA, Pies RW: Emerging treatments for bipolar disorder: safety and adverse effect profiles. Ann Pharmacother 40:1–10, 2006

Martin R, Kuzniecky R, Ho S, et al: Cognitive effects of topiramate, gabapentin, and lamotrigine in healthy young adults. Neurology 52:321–327, 1999

McEvoy GK, Snow EK, Kester L, et al: AHFS Drug Information. Bethesda, MD, American Society of Health-System Pharmacists, 2006

McIntyre RS, Konarski JZ, Misener VL, et al: Bipolar disorder and diabetes mellitus: epidemiology, etiology, and treatment implications. Ann Clin Psychiatry 17:83–93, 2005

Mercke Y, Sheng H, Khan T, et al: Hair loss in psychopharmacology. Ann Clin Psychiatry 12:35–42, 2000

Miller BP, Perry W, Moutier CY, et al: Rapid oral loading of extended release divalproex in patients with acute mania. Gen Hosp Psychiatry 27:218–221, 2005

Mirchandani IC, Young RC: Management of mania in the elderly: an update. Ann Clin Psychiatry 5:67–77, 1993

Nambudiri DE, Meyers BS, Young RC: Delayed recovery from lithium neurotoxicity. J Geriatr Psychiatry Neurol 4:40–43, 1991

Oakley PW, Dawson AH, Whyte IM: Lithium: thyroid effects and altered renal handling. J Toxicol Clin Toxicol 38:333–337, 2000

Pies RW: Handbook of Essential Psychopharmacology, 2nd Edition. Washington, DC, American Psychiatric Publishing, 2005

Plenge P, Mellerup ET, Bolwig TG, et al: Lithium treatment: does the kidney prefer one daily dose instead of two? Acta Psychiatr Scand 66:121–128, 1982

Post RM: Neurobiology of seizures and behavioral abnormalities. Epilepsia 45 (suppl 2):5–14, 2004

Post RM, Frye MA, Denicoff KD, et al: Beyond lithium in the treatment of bipolar illness. Neuropsychopharmacology 19:206–219, 1998

Price LH, Heninger GR: Lithium in the treatment of mood disorders. N Engl J Med 331:591–598, 1994

Pugh MJ, Cramer J, Knoefel J, et al: Potentially inappropriate antiepileptic drugs for elderly patients with epilepsy. J Am Geriatr Soc 52:417–422, 2004

Regenold WT, Prasad M: Uses of intravenous valproate in geriatric psychiatry. Am J Geriatr Psychiatry 9:306–308, 2001

Sajatovic M, Bingham R, Campbell EA, et al: Bipolar disorder in older adult inpatients. J Nerv Ment Disord 193:417–419, 2005a

Sajatovic M, Madhusoodanan S, Coconcea N: Managing bipolar disorder in the elderly: defining the role of newer agents. Drugs Aging 22:39–54, 2005b

Schou M: Long-lasting neurological sequelae after lithium intoxication. Acta Psychiatr Scand 70:594–602, 1984

Semla TP, Beizer JL, Higbee MD: Geriatric Dosage Handbook, 11th Edition. Hudson, OH, Lexi-Comp Inc., 2006

Shulman KI, Mackenzie S, Hardy B: The clinical use of lithium carbonate in old age: a review. Prog Neuropsychopharmacol Biol Psychiatry 11:159–164, 1987

Shulman KI, Sykora K, Gill SS, et al: New thyroxine treatment in older adults beginning lithium therapy: implications for clinical practice. Am J Geriatr Psychiatry 13:299–304, 2005

Smith AG, Brauer HR, Catalano G, et al: Topiramate overdose: a case report and literature review. Epilepsy Behav 2:603–607, 2001

Stahl SM: Anticonvulsants as mood stabilizers and adjuncts to antipsychotics: valproate, lamotrigine, carbamazepine, and oxcarbazepine and actions at voltage-gated sodium channels. J Clin Psychiatry 65:738–739, 2004

Steckler TL: Lithium- and carbamazepine-associated sinus node dysfunction: nine-year experience in a psychiatric hospital. J Clin Psychopharmacol 14:336–339, 1994

Suppes T, Baldessarini RJ, Faedda GL, et al: Risk of recurrence following discontinuation of lithium treatment in bipolar disorder. Arch Gen Psychiatry 48:1082–1088, 1991

Suppes T, Dennehy EB, Hirschfeld RMA, et al: The Texas Implementation of Medication Algorithms: update to the algorithms for treatment of bipolar I disorder. J Clin Psychiatry 66:870–886, 2005

Tilkian AG, Schroeder JS, Kao J, et al: Effect of lithium on cardiovascular performance: report on extended ambulatory monitoring and exercise testing before and during lithium therapy. Am J Cardiol 38:701–708, 1976

Tohen M, Castillo J, Baldessarini RJ, et al: Blood dyscrasias with carbamazepine and valproate: a pharmacoepidemiological study of 2,228 patients at risk. Am J Psychiatry 152:413–418, 1995

Wang PS, Schneeweiss S, Avorn J, et al: Risk of death in elderly users of conventional vs. atypical antipsychotic medications. N Engl J Med 353:2335–2341, 2005

Yatham LN: Diagnosis and management of patients with bipolar II disorder. J Clin Psychiatry 66 (suppl 1):13–17, 2005

Yatham LN, Kennedy SH, O'Donovan C, et al: Canadian Network for Mood and Anxiety Treatments (CANMAT) guidelines for the management of patients with bipolar disorder: consensus and controversies. Bipolar Disord 7 (suppl 3):5–69, 2005

Young RC: Evidence-based pharmacological treatment of geriatric bipolar disorder. Psychiatr Clin North Am 28:837–869, 2005

Young RC, Klerman GL: Mania in late life: focus on age at onset. Am J Psychiatry 149:867–876, 1992

Generic name	carbamazepine
Trade name	Tegretol, Tegretol XR, Carbatrol, Epital, Equetro (generics available, except for extended-release [XR])
Class	Anticonvulsant (structurally related to TCAs)
Half-life	Initial: 18–55 hours; multiple dosing: 12–17 hours Epoxide metabolite: 25–43 hours
Mechanism of action	Not fully known; multiple pharmacodynamic effects
Available preparations	Tablets: 100, 200, 300, 400 mg Chewable tablet: 100 mg XR tablets: 100, 200, 400 mg XR capsules: 100, 200, 300 mg Oral suspension: 100 mg/5 mL
Starting dose	100 mg bid
Titration	Increase by 100–200 mg every 3–5 days as tolerated
Typical daily dose	300 mg bid
Dose range	200–800 mg/day (divided bid)
Therapeutic serum level	Bipolar disorder: 4–12 μg/mL

Comments: Second-line agent for bipolar mania in the elderly because of adverse effects and drug interactions. Absorption of this drug is slow; peak levels occur unpredictably at 4–8 hours. Substrate for P-glycoprotein pump. Bioavailability 85%. Highly protein bound. Metabolized in the liver via CYP3A4 to an active epoxide metabolite, which is responsible for many of the drug's adverse effects. Half-life changes with multiple dosing because of autoinduction effects. Also because of autoinduction, drug levels may drop after 2–4 weeks, requiring upward dose adjustments. Excreted mostly in urine, also in feces. Clearance reduced by 23% in the elderly. Kinetics in general are nonlinear (increase in dose does not necessarily result in proportionate increase in serum level). Carbamazepine is a significant inducer of CYP3A4 and CYP2C19 and is associated with variably decreased concentrations of psychotropic, cardiac, and other drugs. Pharmacodynamic actions are numerous and resemble those of phenytoin, primarily involving inhibition of synaptic transmission. Other actions include sedative, anticholinergic, muscle relaxant, and antiarrhythmic effects. *Drug interactions:* Numerous; see Table 5–7. Warnings regarding the use of carbamazepine in patients with cardiac damage, hepatic disease, renal disease, or any history of adverse hematologic reaction to any drug. *Adverse effects:* Cardiac arrhythmias, atrioventricular (AV) block, bradycardia, chest pain, congestive heart failure, edema, hypertension, hypotension, syncope, amnesia, ataxia, depression, dizziness, fatigue, headache, slurred speech, somnolence, pruritis, exfoliative dermatitis (see text), hyponatremia, SIADH, anorexia, constipation, diarrhea, nausea, vomiting, dry mouth, urinary frequency, increased urinary retention, renal failure, various blood dyscrasias (including agranulocytosis), abnormal LFT values, hepatitis, hepatic failure, weakness, blurred vision, and tinnitus.

Generic name	lamotrigine
Trade name	Lamictal
Class	Anticonvulsant
Half-life	31 hours
Mechanism of action	Inhibits release of excitatory neurotransmitters by blocking presynaptic sodium channels
Available preparations	Tablets: 25, 100, 150, 200 mg Chewable dispersible tablets: 2, 5, 25 mg
Starting dose	12.5 mg/day
Titration	Increase by 12.5–25 mg every 2 weeks
Typical daily dose	50 mg bid
Dose range	100–300 mg/day
Therapeutic serum level	Not established

Comments: A first-line drug for the treatment of bipolar depression and for maintenance treatment of bipolar I and bipolar II disorders. Less effect on manic than depressive episodes. Wide therapeutic index. Rapidly and completely absorbed when taken orally, unaffected by food. Peak concentration is achieved in plasma in 1.4–4.8 hours. Bioavailability 98%. 55% protein bound. Metabolized in the liver, primarily via glucuronidation; substrate of UGT1A4. Major metabolite is inactive. Linear kinetics are observed, but kinetics are affected by aging. In elders, drug exposure is increased by 55% and clearance reduced by 37%. There is some evidence of autoinduction, with half-life decreased by 25% over time. Predominantly renally excreted. Half-life increased in renal insufficiency. Clearance 25% lower in non-Caucasians. The mechanism by which this drug exerts antidepressant effects and influences rapid cycling is not completely known. Lamotrigine modulates release of the excitatory amino acids glutamate and aspartate by blocking presynaptic, voltage-sensitive sodium channels. Does not activate CYP450 enzymes, but lamotrigine levels are affected by carbamazepine and valproate. Elimination half-life of lamotrigine more than doubled by coadministration of valproate. Avoid abrupt discontinuation when stopping therapy. Warning regarding skin rash, which uncommonly may progress to Stevens-Johnson syndrome or toxic epidermal necrolysis. *Drug interactions:* See Table 5–6. *Common adverse effects (> 10%):* In patients with epilepsy, these include headache, dizziness, ataxia, somnolence, nausea, diplopia, and blurred vision. *Less common adverse effects (1%–10%):* Peripheral edema, incoordination, insomnia, vomiting, and diarrhea (among others). *Uncommon but serious adverse effects:* Blood dyscrasias (agranulocytosis, anemia, leukopenia, thrombocytopenia), acute renal failure, angina, apnea, dysphagia, hepatitis, hypertension, orthostasis, stroke, and suicidal ideation (among others).

Generic name	levetiracetam
Trade name	Keppra
Class	Anticonvulsant
Half-life	10–11 hours in elderly
Mechanism of action	Not completely known; multiple pharmacodynamic actions
Available preparations	Tablets: 250, 500, 750 mg Oral solution: 100 mg/mL
Starting dose	250–500 mg bid
Titration	Increase every 3–7 days by 250–500 mg/dose
Typical daily dose	3,000 mg (divided bid)
Dose range	1,000–4,000 mg/day (divided bid)
Therapeutic serum level	Not established for bipolar disorder

Comments: Role in treating bipolar disorder not yet established. Rapidly absorbed, with peak concentration in about 1 hour. Food slows absorption. Bioavailabiliyt 100%. Not metabolized in the liver, but hydrolyzed in the blood to inactive metabolites. Excreted mostly in urine. Dose adjustment needed in moderate to severe renal impairment. *Drug interactions:* No known pharmacokinetic drug interactions, but pharmacodynamic interactions described with carbamazepine and topiramate and expected with other GABA-ergic drugs. *Most common adverse effects in elders:* Dizziness, somnolence, confusion, and accidental injury. *Common adverse effects (>10%):* In general adult population with epilepsy, effects include behavioral symptoms (e.g., agitation, aggression, emotional lability), somnolence, headache, hostility, vomiting, anorexia, weakness, and cough. *Less common but potentially serious adverse effects:* Diarrhea, blood dyscrasias, and suicidality.

Generic name	lithium
Trade name	Eskalith, Eskalith CR, Lithobid
Class	Salt
Half-life	28–36 hours in elderly
Mechanism of action	Not fully known; see text
Available preparations	Tablets: 300 mg CR tablets: 450 mg SR tablets: 300 mg Capsules: 150, 300, 600 mg Syrup: 300 mg/5 mL
Starting dose	75–150 mg/day
Titration	Increase by 75–150 mg every 4–7 days, as tolerated
Typical daily dose	300–900 mg
Dose range	150–1,800 mg/day
Therapeutic serum level	0.4–1.0 mEq/L

Comments: First-line drug in the treatment of all phases of bipolar disorder. Aging significantly alters lithium pharmacokinetics. Although absorption is relatively unchanged, distribution and clearance are both affected. Peak plasma concentrations 1–2 hours after an oral dose. Peak brain concentrations up to 24 hours later, so neurotoxic effects can be delayed. The volume of distribution decreases with aging because of a relative decrease in total body water and increase in adipose tissue, as discussed in Chapter 2. Lithium is not metabolized and has no CYP450 interactions. Clearance decreases in proportion to decrease in glomerular filtration. Reduced clearance is exacerbated by renal insufficiency, dehydration, change in salt intake, extra-renal salt loss, and use of diuretic drugs. Blood level of lithium may not be equivalent to brain level. Lithium alters distribution and kinetics of other important ions (sodium, potassium, calcium, and magnesium). *Drug interactions:* See Table 5–4. Warnings regarding the use of this drug in patients with preexisting thyroid disease, mild to moderate renal impairment, or mild to moderate cardiovascular disease. *Adverse effects:* Cardiac arrhythmias, hypotension, sinus node dysfunction, bradycardia, syncope, edema, ECG changes, dizziness, seizures, sedation, fatigue, psychomotor retardation, alopecia, exacerbation of psoriasis, hypothyroidism, goiter, diabetes insipidus, nausea, vomiting, diarrhea, dry mouth, weight gain, polyuria, urinary incontinence, leukocytosis, tremor, ataxia, nystagmus, and blurred vision. Chronic therapy results in diminished renal concentrating ability, which usually (but not always) resolves with discontinuation of the drug. Single daily dosing of immediate-release drug should be used for chronic treatment to minimize effects on the kidney.

Generic name	oxcarbazepine
Trade name	Trileptal
Class	Anticonvulsant (carbamazepine derivative)
Half-life	1–5 hours (parent drug; longer in elders) 7–20 hours (10-hydroxy metabolite; longer in elders)
Mechanism of action	Not completely known; blocks voltage-sensitive sodium and calcium channels
Available preparations	Tablets: 150, 300, 600 mg Oral suspension: 300 mg/5mL
Starting dose	150 mg bid
Titration	Increase by 300 mg/day at 7-day intervals, at minimum
Typical daily dose	300 mg bid
Dose range	300–1,200 mg/day (divided bid)
Therapeutic serum level	Not established for bipolar disorder

Comments: May have a role like that of carbamazepine in existing treatment algorithms. Rapidly absorbed, unaffected by food. 86%–99% protein bound. Rapidly reduced in the liver to the active 10-hydroxy metabolite. Also a substrate of CYP3A4, inhibitor of CYP2C19, and inducer of CYP3A4. Autoinduction is not significant. Maximum plasma concentrations 30%–60% higher in geriatric patients, mostly due to decreased clearance. Elimination half-life increased in elderly. Dose adjustment required in renal impairment (creatinine clearance < 30 mL/min). Drug interactions: Additive effects with other central nervous system depressants, theophylline may antagonize drug's effect, headache with concurrent use of zidovudine. Reportedly well tolerated by elders as an anticonvulsant. Hyponatremia in up to 25% of elders; SIADH can occur (increased risk when given with diuretics). Other common adverse effects (> 10%): Dizziness, somnolence, headache, ataxia, fatigue, vertigo, vomiting, nausea, abdominal pain, abnormal gait, tremor, diplopia, nystagmus, abnormal vision. Less common adverse effects (1%–10%): Nervousness, diarrhea, weakness. Uncommon but serious adverse effects: Allergic skin reactions (including Stevens-Johnson Syndrome and toxic epidermal necrolysis) and blood dyscrasias.

Generic name	valproate
Trade name	Depacon, Depakene, Depakote Delayed Release, Depakote ER, Depakote Sprinkles
Class	Anticonvulsant (carboxylic acid derivative)
Half-life	9–16 hours in adults
Mechanism of action	Multiple GABA-related actions
Available preparations	DR tablets: 125, 250, 500 mg ER tablets: 250, 500 mg Capsules: 250 mg Capsules with sprinkles: 125 mg Syrup: 250 mg/ 5 mL Injectable: 100 mg/mL
Starting dose	125–250 mg/day to bid
Titration	Increase by 125–250 mg/day every 3–5 days, as tolerated
Typical daily dose	500–1,000 mg (divided bid)
Dose range	250–1,500 mg/day (divided bid)
Therapeutic serum level	65–90 μg/mL

Comments: A first-choice drug for mood stabilization in elderly patients. In plasma, all formulations (including enteric-coated, syrup, and sprinkles) exist as valproate. Rapidly absorbed orally; the controlled-release form (Depakote) designed to slow this process (2–4 hours with Depakote). Absorption also delayed by food. High bioavailability (low first-pass metabolism). Highly protein bound. Increased free fraction (by 44%) in elders. Distribution is rapid; reaches the central nervous system within minutes. Peak serum concentrations in 1–4 hours (3–5 hours with Depakote). Extensively metabolized in the liver, primarily via glucuronidation and mitochondrial β-oxidation, but also by a variety of CYP450 enzymes (minor routes). Some metabolites are active. Nonlinear kinetics of dose with total drug concentration, but linear with unbound drug concentration. Eliminated in urine, 30%–50% as glucuronide conjugate. Clearance is reduced by 39% in elderly. Valproate increases availability of GABA and has other effects in down-regulating AMPA GluR1 synaptic expression (affecting plasticity). *Drug interactions:* See Table 5–5. Warnings regarding hepatic failure, pancreatitis, and hyperammonemia with this drug. *Common adverse effects (>10%):* Somnolence, dizziness, insomnia, nervousness, alopecia, nausea, diarrhea, vomiting, abdominal pain, dyspepsia, anorexia, thrombocytopenia, tremor, weakness, and dyspnea. *Less common adverse effects (1%–10%):* Hypertension, tachycardia, edema, chest pain, amnesia, depression, anxiety, confusion, bruising, rash, pancreatitis, weight gain, urinary frequency, urinary incontinence, increased liver transaminases, abnormal gait, incoordination, myalgia, blurred vision, nystagmus, tinnitus, thrombocytopenia, and abnormal bleeding. *Uncommon but serious adverse effects:* Blood dyscrasias, hepatotoxicity, pancreatitis, and SIADH. Hepatotoxicity is rare, idiosyncratic, and unrelated to dose.

6

Anxiolytic and Sedative-Hypnotic Medications

Introduction

The attempt to organize chapters of this book along lines of medication classes has necessarily resulted in overlap among certain chapters in the discussion of relevant disorders, none so much as the current chapter with Chapter 4 of this volume, "Antidepressants." As mentioned in that chapter, many of the most important treatments in current practice for anxiety disorders are actually antidepressant medications. Thus, the lumping of anxiety and sleep/activity disorders in the present chapter bears the mark of historical artifact. In past practice, benzodiazepines were a mainstay of therapy for many of the conditions discussed here; in current practice, the treatment algorithms for anxiety disorders and sleep/activity disorders in elderly patients have substantially diverged. However, medications in the pharmacologic class that is the focus of this chapter—the benzodiazepines—have some role even today in the treatment of many of the disorders discussed here. In certain cases, that role is small (e.g., in bridging selective serotonin reuptake inhibitor [SSRI] initiation in the patient with panic disorder), and in other cases more substantial (e.g., treatment of catatonia).

Primary anxiety disorders generally have a lower incidence and prevalence in the elderly than in younger cohorts (Hybels and Blazer 2003). Among community-dwelling elders, pure generalized anxiety disorder

(GAD) has a reported period prevalence of about 1% (Flint 2005) and panic disorder less than 0.5% (Flint and Gagnon 2003; Hybels and Blazer 2003). As in younger populations, anxiety disorders in older patients are more common in women. Most elders with panic disorder (Flint and Gagnon 2003) and half of those with GAD (Flint 2005) report onset earlier in life with persistence of symptoms into old age. Anxiety as a symptom is very commonly seen among elders and is often transient or situation dependent; in some patients, however, it can be persistent even though the patient may not meet DSM-defined criteria for any of the anxiety disorders.

When anxiety disorders are encountered in the elderly, they are often comorbid with other conditions, particularly depressive disorders (Flint 2005; Flint and Gagnon 2003) or particular medical conditions. GAD in the patient with stroke or Parkinson's disease, for example, is most often seen with major depression (Flint 2005). Panic disorder has been found to be comorbid with alcohol dependence and somatization disorder (Mohlman et al. 2004). In addition, panic attacks are more common among elderly women with certain medical conditions (e.g., migraine, emphysema, and cardiovascular disease) (Smoller et al. 2003) and among elders treated with certain medications, such as theophylline. Agoraphobia in elders has been observed to result from physical illness or a traumatic event such as a mugging rather than from panic attacks (Flint and Gagnon 2003). Symptoms of anxiety are often present in patients with dementia and also correlated with comorbid depression in this population (Flint 2005). In fact, the distinction between anxiety and agitation in patients with dementia is not clear, and there has been no validation of the various anxiety disorder diagnoses in this population.

Little is known about the epidemiology of posttraumatic stress disorder (PTSD), obsessive-compulsive disorder (OCD), and phobic disorders in the elderly population. PTSD with onset in earlier life can become symptomatic again in late life (Murray 2005) or can result from a different type of trauma in old age, such as a serious fall.

Sleep complaints are common among elderly patients, and use of hypnotic medications generally increases in older age, particularly among women. Old age itself is associated with decreased amounts of slow-wave sleep as well as disruption in sleep continuity (Reynolds et al. 1999). Since disease also may contribute to sleep disruption, the elderly patient presenting with a sleep complaint should be evaluated for conditions requiring specific treatment. These include psychiatric disorders such as mood disorders, anxiety disorders, panic disorder, psychosis, and alcoholism, among others. In addition, specific sleep disorders such as sleep apnea and periodic limb movements of sleep (PLMS) become more prevalent with aging (Reynolds et al. 1999), so symptoms suggestive of these conditions should be flagged for follow-up study. Medical conditions that can cause or contribute to sleep disruption include nocturnal cardiac ischemia, other forms of heart disease, gastroesophageal reflux disease, obesity, pain and stiffness from arthritis, diabetes, stroke, and lung disease, among others (Foley et al. 2004). If these conditions are not addressed, symptomatic treatment of insomnia either may be unsuccessful or may actually exacerbate the problem.

The sleep problem most often encountered in geriatrics is insomnia, although certain patient populations (e.g., those with Parkinson's disease) may report more difficulty with excessive daytime sleepiness. In older patients, insomnia is often reported as a chronic problem, with complications that include hypnotic dependence, self-medication with alcohol, depression, diminished quality of life, earlier placement in long-term-care facilities (Reynolds et al. 1999), falls, cognitive decline, and disruption of caregiver sleep (McCall 2004). When the evaluation described in the preceding paragraph has been completed and treatable contributors to insomnia have been addressed, symptomatic treatment can proceed. Optimally, this is initiated using measures to improve sleep hygiene rather than pharmacotherapy, as discussed in a later section.

Of all anxiolytic and sedative drugs, none is so controversial in geriatrics as the class of benzodiazepines. These medications are effective, have a wide therapeutic index, and are associated with few significant drug interactions. There are, however, several ways that benzodiazepines can be misused in geriatric prescribing: the amount prescribed or taken can be too much or too little, the specific drug selected can be inappropriate, the duration of treatment can be too long, patient selection can be inappropriate, diagnosis can be wrong, target symptoms can be so ill-defined that the end point of treatment is unclear, or follow-up for dosage adjustment and monitoring for adverse effects can be inadequate (Burch 1990).

Excessive doses of benzodiazepines can be associated with serious adverse effects, including falls, motor vehicle accidents, and cognitive impairment. Inadequate doses can be associated with persistent anxiety symptoms or between-dose withdrawal. Benzodiazepines with long elimination half-lives, such as diazepam, accumulate in fatty tissues with repeated dosing and can lead to toxic effects. Inappropriately prolonged duration can come about, for example, when treatment intended for acute hospitalization is continued after discharge.

Patient selection for benzodiazepine therapy should take into account any history of alcoholism or other substance abuse. Clinical experience suggests that non–substance abusers usually adopt a pattern of benzodiazepine use that is not consistent with abuse. This pattern of "medical use" involves physician supervision of the treatment of a recognized clinical condition with the goal of restoring normal function. For many of these patients, tolerance to anxiolytic effects does not develop over time, so escalation of dose does not occur. In contrast, substance abusers appear more likely to adopt a nonmedical or a "recreational use" pattern, which involves escalation of dose over time (Farnsworth 1990). What might underlie this pattern in an elderly patient is not clear, but certain of the same behaviors seen in younger substance-dependent individuals (e.g., taking more than is prescribed, running out of medication early) are seen in this population as well.

Pharmacokinetics

Drugs covered in this chapter include benzodiazepines, nonbenzodiazepine hypnotics (also called nonbenzodiazepine benzodiazepine receptor agonists [NBRAs] in some texts), and several other medications affecting γ-aminobutyric acid (GABA) function (buspirone, gabapentin) and used as hypnotics (ramelteon, trazodone). Available preparations for each of these drugs are listed in Table 6–1. Relative potency values also are listed for the benzodiazepines and nonbenzodiazepine hypnotics. The pharmacology of benzodiazepines and nonbenzodiazepine hypnotics will be discussed here. The pharmacology of other individual drugs is covered in the Specific Drug summary section at the end of this chapter. Table 6–2 summarizes pharmacokinetic data for benzodiazepines and nonbenzodiazepine hypnotics.

Although aging itself is associated with altered pharmacokinetics of benzodiazepines, these processes can be further altered by smoking, disease, and coadministration of other drugs (Greenblatt et al. 1991a; Thompson et al. 1983). Benzodiazepines are well absorbed, with absorption enhanced by alcohol and delayed by antacids or food. When a faster effect is desired (as with initial insomnia), oral medication should be taken on an empty stomach, and a drug with a relatively rapid onset of action should be selected. All of the nonbenzodiazepine hypnotics have a relatively rapid onset; in fact, onset may be so rapid that the drugs should only be taken after the patient physically is in bed for the night. Note that with intramuscular use, lorazepam and midazolam are rapidly and completely absorbed, while diazepam and chlordiazepoxide are not (McEvoy et al. 2006).

All benzodiazepines are lipophilic, and with the exception of alprazolam, their volume of distribution increases with age. The most lipophilic drugs (e.g., diazepam) have a short duration of effect with single dosing because of rapid redistribution to adipose tissue (Greenblatt 1991). With multiple dosing, redistribution is reduced and duration of effect is prolonged. Less lipophilic drugs (e.g., lorazepam) have a longer duration of effect with single dosing and a smaller change in duration of effect with multiple dosing because of limited tissue distribution (Greenblatt and Shader 1978; Greenblatt et al. 1977).

Benzodiazepines can be divided into two groups on the basis of metabolic pathway:

- Those that are *oxidatively metabolized,* including alprazolam, chlordiazepoxide, clorazepate, diazepam, flurazepam, halazepam, quazepam, and prazepam. Most of these drugs have active metabolites. As shown in Table 6–2, metabolites have half-lives of 100 hours or more, so these drugs are very long-acting. In general, drugs in this group are not recommended for use in elderly patients.
- Those that are *conjugated (undergo glucuronidation),* including lorazepam, oxazepam, and temazepam. These drugs have no active metabolites. Lorazepam and oxazepam have half-lives of <24 hours, while temazepam's half-life is up to 40 hours. Lorazepam and oxazepam are recommended for the treatment of elderly patients for whom benzodiazepines are indicated.

Table 6–1. Selected anxiolytic and sedative-hypnotic preparations

Generic name	Trade name	Relative potency	Tablets (mg)	Capsules (mg)	SR/CR/XR capsules (mg)	Oral solution (concentrate, suspension, or elixir)	Injectable form
alprazolam	Xanax, Xanax XR, Niravam, Alprazolam Intensol, generic for Xanax	1	0.25, 0.5, 1, 2 OD: 0.25, 0.5, 1, 2		0.5, 1, 2, 3	1 mg/mL	
buspirone	BuSpar, generic	N/A	5, 7.5, 10, 15, 30				
chlordiazepoxide[a]	Librium, generic	25		5, 10, 25			100 mg
clonazepam	Klonopin, generic	0.5–1	0.5, 1, 2 OD: 0.125, 0.25, 0.5, 1, 2				
diazepam[a,b]	Diazepam Intensol, Valium, generic	10	2, 5, 10			5 mg/mL 5 mg/5 mL	5 mg/mL
eszopiclone	Lunesta	2	1, 2, 3				
lorazepam	Ativan, Lorazepam Intensol, generic	2	0.5, 1, 2			2 mg/mL	2 mg/mL 4 mg/mL

Table 6–1.   Selected anxiolytic and sedative-hypnotic preparations *(continued)*

Generic name	Trade name	Relative potency	Tablets (mg)	Capsules (mg)	SR/CR/XR capsules (mg)	Oral solution (concentrate, suspension, or elixir)	Injectable form
oxazepam	Serax, generic	30	15	10, 15, 30			
ramelteon	Rozerem	N/A	8				
temazepam	Restoril, generic	20		7.5, 15, 30			
zaleplon	Sonata	10		5, 10			
zolpidem	Ambien, Ambien CR	10		5, 10	6.25, 12.5		

Note.   CR=controlled-release; OD=orally disintegrating; SR=sustained-release; XR=extended-release.
[a]Not recommended for elderly patients, for reasons noted in text.
[b]Also available in rectal gel form in 2.5, 5. 10, 15, and 25 mg.

Table 6–2.   Pharmacokinetics of benzodiazepines and nonbenzodiazepine hypnotics

Drug	Onset of effect	Peak level (hours)	Major active metabolite	Parent half-life (hours)	Metabolite[a] half-life (hours)
Benzodiazepines					
alprazolam	Intermediate	1–2	No	12–15	—
chlordiazepoxide	Intermediate	2–4	Yes	5–30	24–96
clonazepam	Intermediate	1–2	No	18–50	—
clorazepate	Rapid	1–2	Yes	Not significant	50–100
diazepam	Rapid	0.5–2	Yes	20–80	50–100
estazolam	Slow	2	No	10–24	—
flurazepam	Rapid	0.5–2	Yes	Not significant	40–114
lorazepam	Intermediate	1–6	No	10–20	—
midazolam	Rapid	0.4–0.7[b]	No	2–5	—
oxazepam	Slow	2–4	No	5–20	—
quazepam	Intermediate	2	Yes	25–41	28–114
temazepam	Slow	2–3	No	10–40	—
triazolam	Intermediate	1	No	2.3	—

Table 6–2. Pharmacokinetics of benzodiazepines and nonbenzodiazepine hypnotics *(continued)*

Drug	Onset of effect	Peak level (hours)	Major active metabolite	Parent half-life (hours)	Metabolite[a] half-life (hours)
Nonbenzodiazepine hypnotics					
eszopiclone	Intermediate	1	No	9	—
ramelteon	Intermediate	0.5–1.5	No	1–2.6	—
zaleplon	Intermediate	1	No	1–2	—
zolpidem	Intermediate	2.2	No	2–2.6 (longer in elderly)	—

Note. Rapid=15 minutes; Intermediate=15–30 minutes; Slow=30–60 minutes.
[a]Significant metabolite.
[b]Intravenous only.
Source. Adapted from Semla TP, Beizer JL, Higbee MD: *Geriatric Dosage Handbook,* 11th Edition. Hudson, OH, Lexi-Comp Inc., 2006; Fuller MA, Sajatovic M: *Drug Information Handbook for Psychiatry,* 5th Edition. Hudson, OH, Lexi-Comp Inc., 2005. Used with permission.

Clearance of oxidatively metabolized benzodiazepines is reduced in old age, particularly among men (Greenblatt et al. 1991a). Reduced clearance is associated with increased half-life, which may be associated with significant daytime sedation and psychomotor impairment in the absence of dosing adjustments (Greenblatt 1991). Clearance of conjugated benzodiazepines is relatively unaffected by age (Greenblatt et al. 1991a). Table 6–3 shows metabolic pathways for benzodiazepines, nonbenzodiazepine hypnotics, and other selected sedatives.

Pharmacodynamics and Mechanisms of Action

For reasons that are not fully understood, elderly patients appear to demonstrate a greater pharmacodynamic sensitivity to benzodiazepines at a given concentration at the receptor than nonelderly patients (Greenblatt et al. 1991b). In addition, clinical experience suggests that structural brain disease (e.g., dementia, traumatic brain injury, stroke) can be associated with similarly increased sensitivity.

Benzodiazepines act as classic agonists at the $GABA_A$-benzodiazepine receptor complex (Greenblatt 1992) located predominantly on postsynaptic neurons in the cerebral cortex, cerebellar cortex, and limbic regions (Bone et al. 1995). This receptor complex contains binding sites for barbiturates, neurosteroids, and several nonbenzodiazepine hypnotics, including zolpidem, zaleplon, zopiclone, and eszopiclone, in addition to benzodiazepines. All these agents act at least in part as GABA agonists, causing an influx of negatively charged chloride ions into the neuron, leading to hyperpolarization of the neuron and a decreased rate of firing.

The $GABA_A$ receptor consists of five subunits in a rosette formation, usually comprising two α subunits, two β subunits, and one γ subunit. The subunits have variant forms, such as α_1, α_2, and so on. GABA itself binds to the β subunit of the $GABA_A$ receptor. Benzodiazepines bind to the major binding cleft defined by the interface of the α and γ subunits. All the classic benzodiazepines bind to receptors containing α subunits (either 1, 2, or 3). The nonbenzodiazepine hypnotics zolpidem and zaleplon also bind to the benzodiazepine site on the $GABA_A$ receptor, but these drugs bind with high affinity only to receptors containing

Table 6–3.   Benzodiazepines and related drugs: known metabolic pathways

Drug	Metabolic pathways
Benzodiazepines	
Alprazolam	CYP3A4, glucuronidation
Clonazepam	CYP3A4, acetylation
Diazepam	CYP2C19, **3A4**, 2B6, 2C9, glucuronidation
Lorazepam	**UGT2B7**, ? other UGTs
Midazolam	**CYP3A4, glucuronidation**
Oxazepam	S-oxazepam: UGT2B15
	R-oxazepam: UGT1A9, UGT2B7
Temazepam	**UGT2B7**, ? other UGTs, CYP2C19, 3A4
Triazolam	**CYP3A4**, glucuronidation
Nonbenzodiazepine sedative-hypnotics	
Buspirone	**CYP3A4**
Eszopiclone	Zopiclone: **CYP2C8, 3A4, excreted through kidneys, lungs, and liver**
Gabapentin	Excreted in urine unchanged
Trazodone	CYP3A4, 2D6
Zaleplon	**Aldehyde oxidase**, CYP3A4
Zolpidem	**CYP3A4**, 1A2, 2C9

Note.   CYP = cytochrome P450; UGT = uridine 5′-diphosphate glucuronosyltransferase. Bold type indicates major pathway.
Source.   Adapted from Cozza et al. 2003.

the α_1 subunit (termed *omega-1 receptors* in the older literature). Eszopiclone also interacts with the benzodiazepine site on the GABA$_A$ receptor, probably binding to specific "microdomains" within the γ subunit (Davies et al. 2000). Since different α subunits are variably expressed in specific brain regions (cortex, brain stem, etc.), these binding differences among agents may have clinical implications in terms of differential amnestic, sedative, and true hypnotic effects (Davies et al. 2000).

The anxiolytic buspirone has no appreciable affinity for the benzodiazepine receptor complex. This drug acts as a serotonin (5-HT) agonist at the presynaptic 5-HT_{1A} receptor but as a partial agonist at the postsynaptic 5-HT_{1A} receptor. Buspirone binding causes down-regulation of 5-HT_2 receptors, similar to the action of antidepressants. Thus, this medication is anxiolytic at usual doses and possibly antidepressant at higher doses (Ninan and Muntasser 2004). Buspirone also has complex dopaminergic effects that are not fully characterized (McEvoy et al. 2006). The recently approved nonbenzodiazepine hypnotic ramelteon binds selectively to melatonin type 1 (MT_1) and type 2 (MT_2) receptors, which act on the suprachiasmatic nucleus to regulate circadian rhythms (Roth et al. 2004).

Drug Interactions

Benzodiazepines have little effect on the metabolism of other drugs, but because several of these agents are metabolized primarily by cytochrome P450 (CYP) 3A4, inhibitors and inducers of that isoenzyme may have a significant effect on benzodiazepine metabolism. These include alprazolam, clonazepam, midazolam, and triazolam. In the presence of CYP3A4 inhibitors such as antifungals, antibiotics, nefazodone, fluvoxamine, or grapefruit juice, levels of benzodiazepines can be elevated, as discussed in Chapter 2 of this volume, "Basic Psychopharmacology and Aging." These elevations can be clinically important; for example, nefazodone is associated with a 34% increase in alprazolam level and a 500% increase in triazolam level (Rickels et al. 1998). Diazepam is also substantially metabolized by CYP3A4, but inhibition of that pathway results in metabolism by the alternative pathway of CYP2C19. In the presence of CYP3A4 inducers such as St. John's wort, carbamazepine, chronic alcohol consumption, or smoking, levels of any of these benzodiazepines can be reduced. Note that benzodiazepines recommended for elders (lorazepam and oxazepam) are not CYP3A4 substrates.

In addition to CYP450 interactions, benzodiazepines have additive sedative effects with other central nervous system (CNS) depressants, including alcohol, opioids, and trazodone. Table 6–4 lists these and other important benzodiazepine drug interactions, and Table 6–5 lists important nonbenzodiazepine hypnotic and ramelteon interactions.

Table 6–4. Benzodiazepines: drug interactions

Added drugs	Interaction/Effect
Antacids	May alter rate but not extent of absorption of benzodiazepine; may delay onset of effect with single dosing at bedtime for sleep, but does not usually affect multiple-dose (chronic) treatment
Anticholinergics	Additive cognitive impairment with benzodiazepines
Clozapine	Severe sedation, hypotension, respiratory depression with benzodiazepines (see discussion in Chapter 3)
CNS depressants (e.g., alcohol, opioids)	Additive sedation and potential toxicity
CYP3A4 inhibitors	Increased levels of certain benzodiazepines
CYP3A4 inducers	Decreased levels of certain benzodiazepines
CYP2C19 inducers	Potential for decreased level of diazepam
Digoxin	Alprazolam (and possibly diazepam) increase digoxin level, with potential toxicity
Levodopa	Possibly decreased effect of levodopa
Nefazodone	Increased levels of alprazolam, triazolam, and midazolam; substantially increased half-life for alprazolam
SSRI antidepressants	Increased levels of alprazolam and diazepam with fluoxetine or fluvoxamine

Increased levels of alprazolam, triazolam, and midazolam with norfluoxetine

Increased level of diazepam with sertraline

Possibly increased levels of alprazolam, triazolam, and midazolam with sertraline metabolite |
| Tricyclic antidepressants | Increased levels of imipramine and desipramine (not nortriptyline) with alprazolam

Additive psychomotor effects of amitriptyline and benzodiazepines |

Note. CNS = central nervous system; SSRI = selective serotonin reuptake inhibitor.
Source. Adapted from Pies 2005.

Table 6–5.   Nonbenzodiazepine hypnotics: drug interactions

Hypnotic agent	Added drug	Effect on hypnotic level
Zaleplon	Inhibitors of aldehyde oxidase (e.g., cimetidine, hydralazine, methadone) or of CYP3A4	Increased
	Rifampin and other CYP3A4 inducers	Decreased
Zolpidem	Ritonavir, ketoconazole, sertraline, nefazodone, and other CYP3A4 inhibitors	Increased
	Rifampin and other CYP3A4 inducers	Decreased
Zopiclone, eszopiclone[a]	Ritonavir, ketoconazole, sertraline, nefazodone, and other CYP3A4 inhibitors	Increased
	Rifampin and other CYP3A4 inducers	Decreased
Ramelteon	Fluvoxamine, ciprofloxacin, and other CYP1A2, 3A4, 2C9 inhibitors	Increased
	Rifampin	Decreased

[a]Data are preliminary and extrapolated from experience with racemic zopiclone.
Source.   Adapted from Pies 2005.

Indications

DSM-IV-TR codes for anxiety and sleep disorders that affect the geriatric population are shown in Table 6–6. As has been previously noted, the treatments of choice for many of these conditions in the elderly population are not benzodiazepines. Rather, benzodiazepines are most often used in elderly patients for a variety of nonpsychiatric indications, with only some overlap with the classic anxiety and sleep disorders. Actual indications for benzodiazepines in elderly patients are shown in Table 6–7. Treatment approaches for selected conditions are outlined later in this chapter.

Table 6–6.   Anxiety and sleep disorders in elderly patients

Anxiety disorders

293.84	Anxiety disorder due to a general medical condition
***.**	Substance-induced anxiety disorder
300.01	Panic disorder without agoraphobia
300.02	Generalized anxiety disorder
300.21	Panic disorder with agoraphobia
300.22	Agoraphobia without history of panic disorder
300.23	Social phobia
300.29	Specific phobia
300.3	Obsessive-compulsive disorder
308.3	Acute stress disorder
309.81	Posttraumatic stress disorder
300.00	Anxiety disorder not otherwise specified

Sleep disorders

307.42	Primary insomnia
780.59	Breathing-related sleep disorder
780.xx	Sleep disorder due to a general medical condition
***.**	Substance-induced sleep disorder

Efficacy

All benzodiazepines are effective for the short-term treatment of insomnia (Greenblatt 1991); continued long-term efficacy has not been systematically studied. Although head-to-head comparative studies are lacking, it is probably true that all benzodiazepines are equally effective for the treatment of anxiety. For anxiety occurring in the context of panic disorder, alprazolam and clonazepam have been most studied. Buspirone may be effective in the treatment of GAD in a subset of patients but is not effective in panic disorder. Clinical failures with buspirone may relate to its long latency to effect, to inadequate dosage, or to lack of specificity in diagnosis. In addition, it has

Table 6–7.   Indications for benzodiazepines and related drugs in elderly patients

- Anxiety (generalized, panic)
- Insomnia
- Alcohol and sedative withdrawal
- Adjunctive use with mood-stabilizing medication for mania
- Adjunctive use with antipsychotic medication for acute psychosis
- Sedation for brief procedures (bronchoscopy, cardioversion, electroconvulsive therapy, intubation, colonoscopy, etc.)
- Ongoing sedation (e.g., mechanical ventilation)
- Anesthesia induction
- Nausea/Vomiting secondary to cytotoxic therapy (lorazepam)
- Adjunctive use with antidepressant for phantom limb pain (clonazepam)
- Seizures
- Myoclonus
- Akathisia
- Periodic limb movements of sleep
- Restless legs syndrome
- Rapid eye movement sleep behavior disorder
- Tinnitus (alprazolam)

frequently been noted that patients already exposed to benzodiazepines may respond poorly to buspirone, although this is not true in all cases, particularly where the history of benzodiazepine use is remote (DeMartinis et al. 2000). Clinical experience suggests that the nonbenzodiazepine hypnotics are effective in some but not all patients with short-term use. The efficacy of ramelteon in elderly patients has yet to be demonstrated.

Clinical Use

Nonpharmacologic Therapies

Among patients of unselected age, cognitive-behavioral therapy (CBT) is well established as an effective mode of treatment for anxiety disorders. It may be used in conjunction with certain medications, such as antidepressants, but there is some suggestion that cotreatment with benzodiazepines reduces its efficacy (van Balkom et al. 1996). There is also evidence that CBT is not as effective in the treatment of GAD in elderly patients as it is in younger patients (Mohlman 2004). Recommendations as to which nonpharmacologic therapies should be recommended in elders with GAD await further study (Flint 2005).

Anxiety in the hospitalized patient can be reduced substantially through various environmental and psychological interventions. These include increased physical activity, facilitated visits through more flexible visiting hours, familiarization of the setting with personal effects, skillful ventilator weaning, patient education about what to expect from procedures, frequent reassurance, maintenance of consistent staffing, distraction, and relaxation techniques (Bone et al. 1995).

For the treatment of insomnia, various nonpharmacologic modalities can be recommended: regular exercise early in the day (Foley et al. 2004), bright light therapy (Lewy and Sack 1986), CBT (Montgomery and Dennis 2006; Reynolds et al. 1999), and various sleep hygiene measures as noted in Table 6–8. In persistent cases, the clinician may need to work with the patient to restrict time spent in bed, avoid daytime naps, quit smoking, and/or undertake a program of bladder retraining (McCall 2004; Morin et al. 1994; Reynolds et al. 1998).

Choice of Drug

The updated Beers criteria listed in Chapter 1 of this volume, "The Practice of Geriatric Psychopharmacology," contain recommendations regarding drugs to avoid in the class of benzodiazepines. Because of long half-life ($t_{1/2}$) with prolonged sedation and increased risk of falls and fractures, the following medications are *not* recommended in elders: chlordiazepoxide, clorazepate, diazepam, flurazepam, halazepam, and quazepam (Fick et al. 2003). When benzodiazepines are used in elderly patients, small doses of short- or intermediate-acting drugs are preferred. For oral use, recommended drugs include lorazepam and oxazepam. If longer half-life drugs such as clonazepam are prescribed ($t_{1/2} = 18$–50 hours), frequency should be once daily or every other day. For parenteral use, lorazepam is recom-

Table 6–8.   Sleep hygiene measures

• Maintain a regular sleep-wake cycle.

• Avoid caffeine consumption after 12:00 P.M.

• Daily exercise during morning hours.

• Move evening meal to an earlier hour.

• Hot bath before bedtime.

• Small bedtime snack (e.g., hot milk, turkey; avoid chocolate).

• Meditation or relaxation exercise at bedtime.

• Keep bedroom quiet and dark (except for night-light).

mended. Clinical experience suggests that midazolam, because of its short half-life, may be associated with recurrence of anxiety or agitation within hours of administration. In general, oral or intravenous administration is preferred to intramuscular administration because the latter is painful and with some drugs is associated with erratic absorption. In addition to necessitating much lower doses, intravenous administration requires more careful patient monitoring for adverse effects such as respiratory depression. In special cases, such as with oncology patients who are unable to swallow, other means of benzodiazepine administration (rectal, sublingual, or orally disintegrating forms) may be needed. Other anxiolytic and sedative-hypnotic agents recommended for the treatment of elderly patients with specific syndromes are discussed later in this chapter.

The nonbenzodiazepine hypnotics eszopiclone, zaleplon, and zolpidem are often used in preference to benzodiazepines for short-term pharmacologic treatment of insomnia in the geriatric patient. All of these drugs are generally effective in reducing sleep latency (time to fall asleep) and lack the undesired effect of reducing slow-wave (Stage IV) sleep common to the benzodiazepines (Hemmeter et al. 2000; Uchimura et al. 2006). In one comparative study of zolpidem and zaleplon versus placebo in elderly patients, zolpidem was associated with a decreased number of awakenings after sleep onset and more consistent improvement in total sleep time compared to zaleplon (Ancoli-Israel et al. 1999). In the only study of chronic use of these agents performed to date, eszopiclone was found to improve sleep maintenance (decreased number of awakenings and time spent awake after sleep onset) over 6 months, with no evidence of tolerance to these effects (Krystal et al. 2003).

Another option for treatment of insomnia in elders is the selective melatonin receptor agonist ramelteon, which recently received U.S. Food and Drug Administration (FDA)–approved labeling for this indication. In addition, clinical experience suggests that several other drugs that are used off-label can be effective for insomnia, including trazodone and gabapentin.

Antipsychotic medication is used for patients with anxiety or insomnia seen in the context of psychosis with positive symptoms (delusions or hallucinations). Antipsychotics are *not* recommended for the treatment of anxiety or insomnia in nonpsychotic elderly patients. In addition, a number of other drugs used historically for anxiety or insomnia are currently not recommended, including diphenhydramine, chloral hydrate, barbiturates, meprobamate (Miltown), ethchlorvynol (Placidyl), glutethimide (Doriden), and methyprylon (Noludar) ("Hypnotic Drugs," *The Medical Letter*, August 7, 2000).

Over-the-counter antihistamines such as diphenhydramine (Benadryl, Nytol, and others) and doxylamine (Unisom and others) are sold as sleep aids and are still used by a substantial number of well-intentioned but poorly informed elders. These drugs are not recommended for elderly patients for several reasons. Antihistamines may help with initiation of sleep, but they work poorly to maintain sleep. In addition, they are associated with the development of tolerance within days to weeks (Monane 1992). Side effects include anticholinergic effects (constipation, urinary retention, visual blurring, memory impairment, delirium), daytime sedation, and impairment of driving performance. Diphenhydramine is also a potent inhibitor of CYP2D6 and thus can increase the risk of drug interactions (Lessard et al. 2001).

Chloral hydrate has a very low therapeutic index, with fatalities reported after doses as small as 4 g (The Medical Letter, August 7, 2000). This drug is also associated with gastric irritation and interacts with the metabolism of warfarin. In addition, tolerance may develop to its hypnotic effects within 2 weeks, and physical dependence may develop with continued use of the drug. Withdrawal is associated with nightmares and significant insomnia. At present, chloral hydrate should be used only for patients who do not respond to recommended drugs for insomnia and for premedication prior to sleep electroencephalogram (EEG) in doses of 125–500 mg.

Barbiturates and related sedatives are not recommended in elders for several reasons. These drugs are associated with serious side effects, significant drug interactions because of their role as CYP450 enzyme inducers, high physical dependence and abuse liability, low therapeutic index, high lethality in overdose, and seizures, nightmares, and insomnia on withdrawal (Thompson et al. 1983).

Patient Education and Informed Consent

Informed consent should be obtained before a benzodiazepine is prescribed for an elderly patient, with risks detailed (including physical dependence), the plan for frequency and duration of use discussed, and potential rebound or discontinuation symptoms explained. In particular, elderly patients who drive should understand that driving while taking these medications may be hazardous, and in some cases the risk extends to the day after taking a benzodiazepine or related drug for sleep.

Baseline Labs and Studies

For any patient presenting for the first time with GAD, panic disorder, severe anxiety as an isolated symptom, or insomnia, consideration should be given to medical disorders or medications as possible causes. Table 6–9 lists medical conditions and medications that can cause anxiety in elderly patients.

Any suspicion that one of these factors might be causing or contributing to symptoms should prompt appropriate diagnostic testing or discontinuation of the offending drug, if possible. Recommended laboratory studies for routine workup for GAD include a complete blood count, fasting glucose, calcium, vitamin B_{12}, red blood cell folate, thyroid-stimulating hormone, and electrocardiogram (ECG) (Flint 2005). Recommended laboratory studies for a routine workup for panic disorder include a complete blood count, fasting glucose, calcium, thyroid panel, and ECG (Flint and Gagnon 2003). Depending on the patient's particular symptoms, further testing may be indicated, such as an EEG to evaluate possible complex partial seizures. In addition, patients treated with medications such as theophylline should have levels drawn to determine whether toxicity may be implicated.

Table 6–9.   Causes of secondary anxiety in elderly patients

Medical conditions	Medications and drugs
Angina	Albuterol
Asthma	Alcohol withdrawal
Benign prostatic hypertrophy	Amphetamines
Cardiac arrhythmia (supraventricular tachycardia)	Antiarrhythmics (e.g., quinidine)
	Antibiotics (dyspepsia)
Chronic obstructive pulmonary disease (hypoxia)	Anticholinergics
	Antidepressants
Congestive heart failure	Caffeine
Dementia	Diuretics (restless legs)
Depression	L-Dopa
Hemolytic anemia	Methyldopa
Hyperthyroidism	Methysergide
Hypoglycemia	Neuroleptics (akathisia)
Hypothyroidism, hypoparathyroidism	Nicotine
Hypovolemia	Nicotine withdrawal
Left ventricular failure	Phenytoin
Neoplasm	Steroids (adrenal and gonadal)
Pain	Sympathomimetics (theophylline)
Parkinson's disease ("off" phase)	Thyroid hormone
Pheochromocytoma	
Pneumonia	
Pneumothorax	
Pulmonary embolism	
Seizures (complex partial)	
Substance abuse	

In addition to a review of prescribed and over-the-counter medications, it is important to obtain a history of past or current abuse of alcohol and other drugs. As noted above, the problem of abuse of prescribed benzodiazepines with dose escalation over time is largely limited to patients with a substance abuse history. In addition, current use of alcohol can have additive sedative effects with those of prescribed benzodiazepines, and this may represent a danger for vulnerable elderly patients. A decision as to whether anxiety or insomnia should be treated pharmacologically will depend on a weighing of risk relative to benefit. Nonbenzodiazepine and non-pharmacologic treatment options provide alternatives, as outlined earlier.

Dose and Dose Titration

The updated Beers criteria contain several specific recommendations regarding recommended maximum geriatric doses for several benzodiazepines: lorazepam, 3 mg/day; oxazepam, 60 mg/day; alprazolam, 2 mg/day; temazepam, 15 mg/day; and triazolam, 0.25 mg/day (Fick et al. 2003). As with the prescription of other psychotropic medications to elderly patients, the rule in using benzodiazepines and other sedatives is to start at the lowest end of the therapeutic dose range and to increase the dose slowly, usually every few days (Shader and Greenblatt 1993). With oral benzodiazepines, anxiolytic, muscle relaxant, and anticonvulsant effects may be observed after the first dose; effects may then increase until steady state is attained. Most elderly patients respond to low doses of these medications. Because some medications require full doses for therapeutic effect, however, it is important to continue titrating until target symptoms are under control, while monitoring for side effects. When a longer-acting drug is used, there may eventually be a need to decrease the dose or change to a less frequent schedule to avoid toxicity.

When antidepressants are used to treat primary anxiety disorders in elderly patients, *very low* starting doses and *very slow* titration are often necessary to minimize anxiogenic side effects. This may be especially true for SSRI antidepressants.

Duration of Treatment

The length of time that medication treatment is continued for an anxiety disorder in an elderly patient depends on the specific disorder being treated, on whether it is comorbid with depression or secondary to a treatable medical condition, and on which class of medication is used for treatment. For example, early-onset GAD may require lifelong treatment, while late-onset GAD with comorbid depression may be treated according to guidelines governing depression (Flint 2005). For late-onset GAD without depression, some experts recommend treatment for 1 year after remission of symptoms (Flint 2005). For symptomatic anxiety in the context of a medical disorder such as hyperthyroidism, treatment with a benzodiazepine can be continued until the underlying condition is treated, and then gradually withdrawn.

For panic disorder, initial treatment may consist of both an SSRI or venlafaxine and a benzodiazepine, with the latter continued only for 1–2 weeks as the antidepressant dose is titrated. The SSRI should then be continued for a period of 6 months to 1 year, with shorter times possible in cases where CBT or another therapy has been used in tandem with medication.

In the treatment of insomnia, it is recommended that benzodiazepines and related drugs be used for 1–2 weeks and that the need for this medication then be reassessed. If insomnia persists at 2 weeks, a comorbid psychiatric or medical condition should be considered, as discussed below. Some patients do benefit from an extension to 4 weeks of treatment, but it is best if the medication is taken only intermittently (e.g., fewer than four times per week). The efficacy of intermittent, longer-term use of nonbenzodiazepine hypnotics has been demonstrated (Perlis et al. 2004). In fact, in a mostly nongeriatric sample, eszopiclone was found to be effective over 6 months of nightly treatment (Krystal et al. 2003), and it is possible that long-term nightly efficacy applies to the other selective $GABA_A$ agonists as well. Long-term efficacy of ramelteon is not known.

Discontinuation of Anxiolytics and Sedative-Hypnotics

Except in cases of toxicity, benzodiazepines and nonbenzodiazepine hypnotics should be tapered very gradually to avoid discontinuation symptoms, which may include significant rebound anxiety and insomnia. Even with gradual tapering, some patients will be unable to tolerate medication withdrawal and may require indefinite treatment. Pretreatment with imipramine has been reported as effective in facilitating a successful benzodiazepine taper among patients with GAD (Rickels et al. 2000) but not panic disorder (Rynn et al. 2003). Even for GAD, however, this would not be a recommended strategy in elderly patients. Clinical experience suggests that alprazolam tapering may be particularly difficult for patients with panic disorder, with characteristic symptoms including confusion, delirium, heightened sensory perception, dysosmia, paresthesias, muscle cramps, muscle twitching, blurred vision, diarrhea, decreased appetite, and weight loss (Pecknold 1993). Symptoms of benzodiazepine discontinuation are observed to peak during the last week of tapering and first week of complete abstinence (Pecknold 1993). When these difficulties with tapering are encountered with a short-acting drug such as alprazolam, it may be advisable to attempt a switch to a longer-acting agent, with subsequent taper of that drug. Success with chlordiazepoxide but not clonazepam has been reported with this method, possibly due to incomplete cross-dependence with the latter agent and alprazolam (Closser and Brower 1994).

Monitoring Treatment

Response to anxiolytic and sedative-hypnotic drugs should be monitored clinically, by changes in target signs and symptoms and development of adverse effects. The only drug for which meaningful serum levels might be drawn is alprazolam. In the treatment of panic disorder, alprazolam levels between 20 and 40 ng/mL are associated with therapeutic response in nongeriatric patients with spontaneous panic attacks (Greenblatt et al. 1993). Therapeutic levels for geriatric patients have not been established.

Elderly patients who require chronic treatment with benzodiazepines or nonbenzodiazepine hypnotics should be evaluated at least every 3–6 months to assess cognitive and psychomotor function. Escalation of benzodiazepine dosage over time or concomitant excessive alcohol consumption should be understood as serious evidence of misuse. Anecdotal experience suggests that older patients treated with benzodiazepines chronically may begin to develop symptoms of toxicity as they reach old age, presumably a function of altered drug clearance. For this reason, it is important to reassess the need for treatment at regular intervals and to adjust the dose downward as indicated.

It is not yet clear what monitoring might be required for long-term use of ramelteon. In general, the drug is believed to have a benign adverse-effect profile.

Anxiolytic and Sedative-Hypnotic Overdose

In general, fatal overdose with an oral benzodiazepine is rare unless the medication is ingested with alcohol or another CNS depressant (Martin and Chan 1986). Among benzodiazepines, oxazepam may be one of the safest in overdose (Buckley et al. 1995). Least safe may be temazepam, as gauged by death rates per million prescriptions (Buckley et al. 1995), or alprazolam, as gauged by longer hospital stays, more admissions to the intensive care unit (ICU), more use of flumazenil, and lower Glasgow Coma Scale scores with this medication compared with other benzodiazepines taken in overdose (Isbister et al. 2004). Nonbenzodiazepine hypnotics appear to be as toxic as benzodiazepines in overdose and as often fatal (Reith et al. 2003).

Symptoms of serious benzodiazepine toxicity include extreme sedation, respiratory depression, falls, immobility, restlessness, incontinence, confusion, delirium, and coma (Buckley et al. 1995; Fancourt and Castleden 1986). A benzodiazepine antagonist such as flumazenil can be used to reverse toxicity through competitive inhibition (Bone et al. 1995). Because sleep induction requires 60% benzodiazepine receptor occupancy, sedation and anticonvulsant effects require 30%–50% occupancy, and anxiolysis requires only 20% occupancy, flumazenil can usually reverse sedation without affecting anxiolysis or anticonvulsant effects (Bone et al. 1995). Flumazenil does not reverse respiratory depressant effects of benzodiazepines.

Issues of Tolerance and Abuse

Tolerance involves a change in receptor sensitivity with continued drug exposure (Miller et al. 1988), which is manifested clinically as reduced effect from a constant drug dose. There is no good evidence that tolerance develops to anxiolytic or hypnotic effects of benzodiazepines or nonbenzodiazepine hypnotics, even with chronic use (Dubovsky 1990; Farnsworth 1990; Hollister et al. 1993; van Steveninck et al. 1997). Tolerance has been shown to develop to most adverse effects of these drugs, including daytime sedation, but not to amnestic effects (Hollister et al. 1993). How long it takes for tolerance to develop depends on the half-life of the particular benzodiazepine, as well as the specific effect in question (Byrnes et al. 1993).

Abuse denotes nontherapeutic use of a medication, involving deliberate overuse despite contrary warnings. There is no evidence that medical use of benzodiazepines is a precursor of abuse in patients not already predisposed by a history of alcohol or substance abuse (Ciraulo et al. 1997; Shader and Greenblatt 1993). This is also true for chronic use of these medications (Geiselmann and Linden 1991). For patients with such a history, however, use of benzodiazepines is fraught with problems such as rekindling of craving, coingestion of alcohol with the prescribed medication, and increased risk of motor vehicle accidents (Graham et al. 1992); similar problems could be anticipated with the nonbenzodiazepine hypnotics (Gericke and Ludolph 1994). Benzodiazepines with a fast onset of action—alprazolam, diazepam, and lorazepam—are thought to have higher abuse potential (and greater street value) because of the rapid "kick" associated with ingestion (Griffiths and Wolf 1990). These issues are discussed more fully in Chapter 7 of this volume, "Treatment of Substance-Related Disorders."

Dependence and Withdrawal

Physical dependence is defined by the appearance of an objective withdrawal syndrome after a drug is discontinued. The risk of physical dependence increases with increases in dose and duration of therapy (Kruse 1990; Shader and Greenblatt 1993), but it is clear that dependence on benzodiazepines can occur at usual therapeutic doses (Shader and Greenblatt 1993) and after as little as 2 weeks of treatment (Ayd 1994). There is no evidence that some benzodiazepines are more likely than others to produce physical dependence.

Discontinuation of benzodiazepines can result in *recurrence* of symptoms; in *rebound* symptoms, in which symptoms are more intense than they were to begin with; or in *withdrawal* symptoms, in which physical effects of reduced GABA neurotransmission are seen. At times, these phenomena are difficult to distinguish. In general, however, interruption of therapeutic doses of benzodiazepines is associated with rebound symptoms, while interruption of high doses is associated with withdrawal symptoms (Pourmotabbed et al. 1996). Rebound symptoms include anxiety, restlessness, dysphoria, anorexia, and insomnia (Jerkovich and Preskorn 1987); in elderly patients, disorientation and confusion can be prominent

(Foy et al. 1986; Kruse 1990). Withdrawal symptoms can include fever, tachycardia, postural hypotension, headache, sweating, photosensitivity, sensory distortion, delirium, tremor, myoclonus, and seizures (Fancourt and Castleden 1986); catatonia has also been reported in elderly patients (Rosebush and Mazurek 1996). In medically compromised elders, severe withdrawal can be life threatening.

How early withdrawal or other discontinuation symptoms develop depends on the half-life of the discontinued drug. In nongeriatric patients, withdrawal reactions peak at 2 days for short-half-life (<6 hours) agents and 4–7 days for long-half-life agents (Rickels et al. 1990).

Symptoms of withdrawal are best avoided, by a slow taper of benzodiazepines, especially shorter-acting agents. Most patients tolerate a taper of 10%–25% of the total dose each week, although the last few dose decrements might require longer intervals (Schweizer et al. 1990; Shader and Greenblatt 1993). Patients unable to tolerate dose reductions may benefit from one of the following: carbamazepine, 200–800 mg/day, with a plasma level of approximately 6 μg/mL (Schweizer et al. 1991); gabapentin, 300–900 mg/day; propranolol for autonomic symptoms; or a switch to a longer-acting agent and subsequent taper of that agent.

Rebound insomnia that usually lasts 1–2 nights may occur after discontinuation of benzodiazepines of short (<6 hours) or intermediate (6–24 hours) half-life (Roth and Roehrs 1992). This syndrome is dose-related and can be prevented by the use of the lowest effective dose of benzodiazepine (Roth and Roehrs 1992). It probably also occurs with long-half-life benzodiazepines but is less intense and more delayed in onset.

Adverse Effects

The most common adverse effects of benzodiazepines and nonbenzodiazepine hypnotics are drowsiness, fatigue, memory impairment, weakness, and incoordination. The severity of these effects is dependent on dose, and the clinical impact is greater for frail elderly individuals than for younger patients. As the dose increases, the risk of extreme sedation, weakness, confusion, depression, and ataxia increases. Among elderly patients treated with benzodiazepines, there is a significantly increased risk of falls, particularly in the first week after therapy is initiated (Ray et al. 2000), as well as motor vehicle accidents involving personal injury (Hemmelgarn et al. 1997). Data are conflicting with regard to the relationship of drug half-life to risk of falls (Cumming and Le Couteur 2003; Ray et al. 2000). This risk may relate specifically to benzodiazepines that undergo oxidative metabolism (Cumming and Le Couteur 2003). In patients over the age of 85 years), although benzodiazepine use is not associated with increased all-cause mortality, it is associated with increased mortality related to fractures (Vinkers et al. 2003).

The most common adverse effects of nonbenzodiazepine hypnotics are headache, somnolence, dizziness, light-headedness, amnesia, and gastrointestinal disturbance (nausea, diarrhea, constipation). Less common but serious adverse effects include chest pain, edema, syncope, cardiac rhythm disturbances, confusional states, and hallucinations. Adverse effects of individual agents are listed in the Specific Drug summaries at the end of the chapter.

Cognitive Effects

Amnesia may be regarded as a main (intended) effect of sedative-hypnotic therapy (as in sedation for ventilated ICU patients or for brief medical procedures) or as an undesired side effect. Amnestic effects of benzodiazepines include impairment of information acquisition, impairment of consolidation and storage of memory, or both (Greenblatt 1992). The magnitude of the amnestic effects of benzodiazepines depends on drug dose, plasma concentration, and the time of information presentation relative to the time of dosing (Greenblatt 1992). Elders appear to be more sensitive to amnestic effects, even with single-dose administration (Pomara et al. 1989; Satzger et al. 1990). Amnestic effects may be more marked in heavy alcohol drinkers (Ashton 1995). Explicit memory is more affected by sedatives than implicit memory.

Among patients with dementia, use of benzodiazepines can be associated with exacerbation of cognitive deficits in multiple domains. Even in patients without dementia, chronic therapy with benzodiazepines also may be associated with deficits in sustained attention and visuospatial impairment that are insidious and not recognized by the patient (Ashton 1995; Ayd

1994). The benzodiazepine-treated elder with amnesia along with other cognitive impairments may meet diagnostic criteria for dementia, which may turn out to be reversible upon taper and discontinuation of the benzodiazepine. The nonbenzodiazepine hypnotics have effects similar to the benzodiazepines in terms of amnesia and confusion at higher doses and levels.

In general, the nonbenzodiazepine hypnotics may be associated with fewer amnestic and other cognitive effects than benzodiazepines because of their selectivity in binding, as discussed earlier (Terzano et al. 2003). In addition, it may be that zaleplon, with its ultrashort half-life, is the least likely of these drugs to have residual (next-day) cognitive effects (Barbera and Shapiro 2005). Buspirone also appears to have little amnestic effect (Lawlor et al. 1992).

Hemodynamic Effects

Benzodiazepines can be associated with hypotension and slowing of the heart rate, particularly when combined with medications, such as opioids (Bone et al. 1995). These effects are less marked with benzodiazepines than with barbiturates. In combination with clozapine, benzodiazepines can be associated with cardiorespiratory collapse. Specific guidelines regarding coadministration of these medications appear in Chapter 3 of this volume, "Antipsychotics." Effects of nonbenzodiazepine hypnotics on heart rate and blood pressure appear to be minimal (Terzano et al. 2003). Zaleplon has an uncommon association with bundle branch block and ventricular tachycardia (Semla et al. 2006).

Psychiatric Effects

Confusion or delirium is a relatively common sequela when benzodiazepines are administered to medically compromised elders (e.g., to control agitation in the hospital). Increased anxiety, panic attacks, agitation, or irritability can be seen with once-daily dosing of short-half-life agents (e.g., alprazolam for insomnia) and is likely due to rebound effects (Martinez-Cano and Vela-Bueno 1993). Exacerbation of depression can be seen with benzodiazepines, possibly as function of sedation, but is also likely mediated by other neurotransmitter effects. Alprazolam at higher doses may have some antidepressant effect, making discontinuation more difficult for a subset of treated patients.

Elderly patients with dementia, brain injury, or mental retardation who are administered benzodiazepines may exhibit behavioral disturbances (aggressiveness, irritability, agitation, hyperactivity), sometimes referred to as *paradoxical reactions*. These may be more severe during the initiation of therapy and may abate with continuation of therapy. The mechanism underlying this phenomenon remains unexplained; there is no evidence from controlled studies that benzodiazepines directly impair impulse control or lead to aggression in individuals without structural brain disease (Shader and Greenblatt 1993).

Psychiatric effects of nonbenzodiazepine hypnotics are uncommon (Semla et al. 2006). Hallucinations and confusional states may be seen with zaleplon and zolpidem, possibly related to high levels resulting from coadministered drugs that inhibit metabolism via CYP3A4 (Terzano et al. 2003).

Psychomotor Impairment

All benzodiazepines have the capacity to produce impairment in performance (Greenblatt 1992), including abilities critical to safe driving such as reaction time, tracking, hand-eye coordination, and judgment. With short-acting agents used at very low doses, impairment may be minimal in the "young-old" patient (<75 years of age). With long-half-life agents used nightly, effects may persist throughout the following day, ultimately resulting in daytime impairment (Fancourt and Castleden 1986; Woo et al. 1991). Agents with a half-life of more than 24 hours confer a 45% increased risk of motor vehicle accident with injury in the first 7 days of use (Hemmelgarn et al. 1997). Some degree of increased risk for falls and accidents persists as long as these drugs are taken. There is currently no evidence for clinically significant psychomotor impairment with appropriate use of any of the newer nonbenzodiazepine hypnotics (Terzano et al. 2003).

Respiratory Effects

When used as sedative-hypnotics, benzodiazepines may be associated with collapse of the oropharyngeal musculature during nocturnal respiration, similar to the effect of alcohol. This could further exacerbate breathing difficulties in patients with obstructive sleep apnea. Benzodiazepines are best avoided in patients with sleep apnea, whether obstructive or central in origin.

Respiratory depression, which can occur in any patient, is more likely to occur with high doses of benzodiazepine administered intravenously. Midazolam reportedly causes more respiratory depression than diazepam, and lorazepam causes the least (Bone et al. 1995). When respiratory depression does occur with benzodiazepines, it is rapid in onset, usually of brief duration, and exacerbated by coadministration of opioids (Bone et al. 1995). Respiratory depression induced by benzodiazepines is not reversed by flumazenil administration.

Respiratory effects have not been reported with recommended doses of nonbenzodiazepine hypnotics (Terzano et al. 2003). Similarly, ramelteon has not been associated with adverse respiratory effects.

Sedative Effects

All benzodiazepines have the capacity to produce dose- and concentration-dependent sedation, which can manifest as tiredness, drowsiness, weakness, trouble concentrating, decreased visual accommodation, slowed thought, ataxia, balance problems (Shader and Greenblatt 1993), dysarthria, diplopia, vertigo, and confusion (Ashton 1995). Tolerance to these effects usually develops within the first 2 weeks of treatment (Ayd 1994; Shader and Greenblatt 1993), but sedation is persistent in some cases.

Residual (next-day) sedation is a potential side effect of nonbenzodiazepine hypnotics in geriatric patients, but is possibly less likely with zaleplon because of its very short half-life (Terzano et al. 2003).

Sensorimotor Effects

Sensorimotor side effects of benzodiazepines and other sedatives include weakness, postural sway, ataxia, dysarthria, and incoordination (Swift et al. 1984). Preexisting deficits can be unmasked or exacerbated by even minimal sedation (Thal et al. 1996). In addition, benzodiazepines, like many other drugs, may impair recovery after stroke (Goldstein 1995) and are associated with an increased risk of falls. Among elderly benzodiazepine users, the risk of falls is highest in the first 7 days after the drug is initiated. Excessive doses and a rapid rate of dose increases are both associated with a greater risk of falls (Fick et al. 2003; Ray et al. 2000).

Whether drugs with longer half-lives confer greater risk is controversial. With nonbenzodiazepine hypnotics, incoordination and falls are uncommon but may occur, possibly associated with CYP3A4 inhibition (Terzano et al. 2003).

Treatment of Selected Syndromes and Disorders

Alcohol and Sedative Withdrawal

Alcohol and sedative withdrawal are primary indications for the use of benzodiazepines in elderly as in younger patients. This use is discussed in Chapter 7.

Anxiety Disorders

Agoraphobia

In elderly patients, apparent agoraphobia can result from depression, apathy, onset of dementia, or a combination of these conditions; therefore, a careful diagnostic evaluation is indicated to rule out these other disorders. As noted in an earlier section, true agoraphobia in elders starts more often with medical illness or trauma than with panic. There is no evidence that pharmacologic therapy is effective for this condition. The treatment of choice is in vivo exposure and gradual desensitization (Flint and Gagnon 2003).

Anxiety in Dementia

When anxiety occurs in the patient with dementia, it usually takes the form of anxious mood or generalized anxiety rather than panic. Often, the behavioral manifestation of anxiety in this population is agitation. Anxiety may be associated with depression (Flint and Gagnon 2003) and may be effectively treated with antidepressants. For acute anxiety in the patient with dementia, behavioral and/or environmental approaches should be tried first. If anxiety persists or escalates, several pharmacologic options exist: SSRI antidepressants, lorazepam, oxazepam, trazodone, buspirone, and gabapentin. Nonbenzodiazepines are preferred. SSRI doses for anxiolysis are generally low (e.g., sertraline, 12.5–25 mg, or fluoxetine, 5–10 mg suspension or capsule). Buspirone can be used at dosages ranging from 5 mg two times a day to 20 mg three times a day. Gabapentin can be used at dosages ranging from 300–2,400 mg/day divided three times a day (Hawkins et al. 2000; Herrmann et al. 2000; Roane et al. 2000). For all of these agents, a trial of at least 12 weeks is needed to determine efficacy. In cases where no response is seen, a switch to another agent is indicated.

Anxiety in Depression

In elderly patients, anxiety is often associated with depressive illness, particularly major depression (Flint 2005; Flint and Gagnon 2003). Antidepressant medication effectively treats anxiety along with other depressive signs and symptoms. Use of an anxiolytic alone for treatment of depression with anxiety is associated with a poor outcome (Flint 2005). When an antidepressant is initiated for patients with depression and panic attacks, slow titration is necessary. A subset of these patients will require a benzodiazepine for the first 1–2 weeks of treatment. SSRIs and venlafaxine are known to have good anxiolytic efficacy. Other novel antidepressants (mirtazapine and duloxetine) also may be effective anxiolytics (Dunner et al. 2003; Gambi et al. 2005).

Anxiety Secondary to Medical Illness

Symptomatic anxiety may occur in a number of medical conditions, as listed in Table 6–9. In particular, anxiety is often seen among patients with breathing difficulties from lung or head/neck cancer, chronic obstructive pulmonary disease (COPD), or asthma. Among patients with COPD, for example, GAD is found in 10%–15.8% and panic disorder in 32%–37% (Periyakoil et al. 2005). For generalized anxiety in patients with COPD or sleep apnea, SSRIs or buspirone may be useful because these medications do not depress the respiratory drive or cause sedation or cognitive impairment (Flint 2005). For panic anxiety in this population, SSRI antidepressants may be used (Smoller 1996; Smoller et al. 1998). For patients with terminal lung disease, dyspnea becomes the focus of a treatment algorithm involving first the correction of physical causes of dyspnea (hypoxia, anemia, bronchospasm) and then symptomatic management with opioids along with pharmacotherapy for anxiety using antidepressants (sertraline, venlafaxine) and/or benzodiazepines (Periyakoil et al. 2005).

In patients with Parkinson's disease, anxiety may be especially prominent during "off" periods and seems to be more prevalent among those with left-sided symptoms (right brain involvement) (Walsh and Bennett 2001). Neither the relationship of anxiety symptoms to medications used to treat parkinsonism nor the optimal pharmacologic treatment of anxiety in Parkinson's disease is known (Richard 2005). Management involves lowering antiparkinsonian medication to the lowest effective dose and adding antidepressant medication such as an SSRI. Benzodiazepines may actually worsen Parkinson's disease in some cases. The GABA agonist effect of benzodiazepines reduces dopaminergic outflow in the basal ganglia and may thus interfere with the effects of levodopa (Yosselson-Superstine and Lipman 1982).

Catatonia

Catatonia is a syndrome involving motor abnormalities and mental status changes that can occur in the context of medical or neurologic disease or severe psychiatric disease such as major depression or schizophrenia. In a manner analogous to delirium, the diagnosis of catatonia suggests the presence of an underlying disease and an obligation on the part of the clinician to make an accurate and rapid diagnosis and to provide definitive treatment for that condition. While that workup is ongoing, however, the elderly patient with catatonia may require symptomatic treatment: a benzodiazepine "challenge" test, a trial of benzodiazepine administration, may be useful in confirming the diagnosis. Clinical experience suggests that catatonia may mimic other syndromes, particularly in the medical setting, and is often misdiagnosed.

The neurobiology of catatonia is incompletely understood but likely involves abnormalities in the GABAergic and dopaminergic systems, among others (Fink and Taylor 2003). It can be classified generally into retarded, excited, and malignant types, the latter including neuroleptic malignant syndrome (discussed in Chapter 3) and serotonin syndrome (discussed in Chapter 4). Cardinal signs of catatonia include mutism, immobility or excessive motor activity, negativism, posturing, stereotypy, and echophenomena (echopraxia, echolalia). Optimally, diagnosis should be made using a standardized instrument such as the Catatonia Rating Scale, shown in Figure 6–1 (Bush et al. 1996).

Catatonia Rating Scale

- Use the presence or absence of items 1–14 for screening
- Use the 0–3 scale for items 1–23 to rate severity

1. Excitement
Extreme hyperactivity, constant motor unrest that is apparently nonpurposeful. Not to be attributed to akathisia or goal-directed agitation.
0 = Absent
1 = Excessive motion, intermittent
2 = Constant motion, hyperkinetic without rest periods
3 = Severe excitement, frenzied motor activity

2. Immobility/Stupor
Extreme hypoactivity, immobility. Minimally responsive to stimuli.
0 = Absent
1 = Sits abnormally still, may interact briefly
2 = Virtually no interaction with external world
3 = Stuporous, not responsive to painful stimuli

3. Mutism
Verbally unresponsive or minimally responsive.
0 = Absent
1 = Verbally unresponsive to most questions; incomprehensible whisper
2 = Speaks less than 20 words/5 minutes
3 = No speech

4. Staring
Fixed gaze, little or no visual scanning of environment, decreased blinking.
0 = Absent
1 = Poor eye contact. Gazes less than 20 seconds between shifting of attention; decreased blinking
2 = Gaze held longer than 20 seconds; occasionally shifts attention
3 = Fixed gaze, nonreactive

5. Posturing/Catalepsy
Maintains posture(s), including mundane (e.g., sitting or standing for long periods without reacting).
0 = Absent
1 = Less than 1 minute
2 = Greater than 1 minute, less than 15 minutes
3 = Bizarre posture, or mundane maintained more than 15 minutes

Figure 6–1. Catatonia Rating Scale.
Source. Adapted from Bush G, Fink M, Petrides G, et al: "Catatonia, I: Rating Scale and Standardized Examination." *Acta Psychiatrica Scandinavica* 93:129–136, 1996. Used with permission.

6. Grimacing
Maintenance of odd facial expressions.
0 = Absent
1 = Less than 10 seconds
2 = Less than 1 minute
3 = Bizarre expression(s) or maintained more than 1 minute

7. Echopraxia/Echolalia
Mimicking of examiner's movements/speech.
0 = Absent
1 = Occasional
2 = Frequent
3 = Continuous

8. Stereotypy
Repetitive, non-goal-directed motor activity (e.g., finger play; repeatedly touching, patting, or rubbing self).
0 = Absent
1 = Occasional
2 = Frequent
3 = Continuous

9. Mannerisms
Odd, purposeful movements (hopping or walking tiptoe, saluting passers by, exaggerated caricatures of mundane movements).
0 = Absent
1 = Occasional
2 = Frequent
3 = Continuous

10. Verbigeration
Repetition of phrases or sentences.
0 = Absent
1 = Occasional
2 = Frequent, difficult to interrupt
3 = Continuous

11. Rigidity
Maintenance of a rigid position despite efforts to be moved. (Exclude if cogwheeling or tremor are present.)
0 = Absent
1 = Mild resistance
2 = Moderate
3 = Severe, cannot be repostured

Figure 6–1. Catatonia Rating Scale. *(Continued)*

12. Negativism
Apparently motiveless resistance to instructions or attempts to move/examine patient. Contrary behavior, does the opposite of instruction.
0 = Absent
1 = Mild resistance and/or occasionally contrary
2 = Moderate resistance and/or frequently contrary
3 = Severe resistance and/or continually contrary

13. Waxy flexibility
During re-posturing of patient, patient offers initial resistance before allowing himself to be repositioned. (Like bending a warm candle.)
0 = Absent
1 = Present

14. Withdrawal
Refusal to eat, drink, and/or make eye contact.
0 = Absent
1 = Minimal oral intake for less than 1 day
2 = Minimal oral intake for more than 1 day
3 = No oral intake for 1 day or more

15. Impulsivity
Patient suddenly engages in inappropriate behavior (e.g., runs down hallway, starts screaming, or takes off clothes) without provocation. Afterwards, cannot explain.
0 = Absent
1 = Occasional
2 = Frequent
3 = Constant or not redirectable

16. Automatic obedience
Exaggerated cooperation with examiner's request, or repeated movements that are requested once.
0 = Absent
1 = Occasional
2 = Frequent
3 = Continuous

17. Passive obedience (mitgehen)
Raising arm in response to light pressure of finger, despite instructions to the contrary.
0 = Absent
3 = Present

Figure 6–1. Catatonia Rating Scale. *(Continued)*

18. Negativism (gegenhalten)
Resistance to passive movement that is proportional to strength of the stimulus; response seems automatic rather than willful.
0 = Absent
3 = Present

19. Ambitendency
Patient appears stuck in indecisive, hesitant motor movements.
0 = Absent
3 = Present

20. Grasp reflex
Stroke open palm of patient with two extended fingers of examiner's hand. Automatic closure of patient's hand.
0 = Absent
3 = Present

21. Perseveration
Repeatedly returns to the same topic or persists with same movements.
0 = Absent
3 = Present

22. Combativeness
Usually in an undirected manner, without explanation.
0 = Absent
1 = Occasionally strikes out, low potential for injury
2 = Strikes out frequently, moderate potential for injury
3 = Danger to others

23. Autonomic abnormality
Circle: temperature, blood pressure, pulse rate, respiratory rate, inappropriate sweating
0 = Absent
1 = Abnormality of one parameter (exclude pre-existing hypertension)
2 = Abnormality of two parameters
3 = Abnormality of three or more parameters

Figure 6–1.   Catatonia Rating Scale. *(Continued)*

In addition to definitive treatment of the underlying condition, symptomatic treatment is needed to maintain basic bodily functions, including adequate hydration and nourishment, and to decrease morbidity from immobility (deconditioning, deep vein thromboses, etc.). Catatonia can be treated with benzodiazepines and/or electroconvulsive therapy

(ECT). Clinical experience suggests that the response of elderly patients to benzodiazepines may not be as robust as that of younger catatonic patients. ECT is an important treatment option for catatonia in the elderly population; although controlled studies for this indication are lacking, substantial clinical experience supports its use (Suzuki et al. 2003). The benzodiazepine of choice for diagnostic challenge and for treatment of catatonia is lorazepam, based on its availability in intravenous and intramuscular formulations, relatively rapid onset of action, and other favorable pharmacokinetic properties. The following algorithm for lorazepam use in catatonia is recommended (Fink and Taylor 2003):

1. Score the Catatonia Rating Scale.
2. Administer 1- to 2-mg intravenous test dose of lorazepam.
3. Score the Catatonia Rating Scale.
4. At 20- to 30-minute intervals, repeat dose of intravenous lorazepam and score the Catatonia Rating Scale up to a total lorazepam dose of 10 mg, administered over several hours.
5. If significant improvement is seen, calculate how much lorazepam was given.
6. Give that amount of lorazepam daily intravenously in divided doses until definitive treatment corrects the underlying problem and/or the syndrome resolves.
7. Anticipate the need for ECT.

Generalized Anxiety Disorder

When symptoms suggestive of GAD occur secondary to a medical condition or medication as shown in Table 6–9, treatment is of course first directed toward the underlying cause. In these cases, the anxiety disorder may be short-lived, depending on successful treatment of the disease or withdrawal of the offending medication. Idiopathic GAD is more persistent and affects quality of life to the same degree as major depression and more so than either myocardial infarction or type 2 diabetes (Wetherell et al. 2004). When GAD occurs as an idiopathic disorder, several treatment options exist. Antidepressants are the first line of treatment for GAD for most elderly patients, regardless of whether depression is present (Flint

2005). Paroxetine, escitalopram, and venlafaxine all have FDA-approved labeling for GAD in adults. For treatment of elderly patients, preferred drugs include escitalopram, citalopram, and venlafaxine (Flint 2005; Lenox-Smith and Reynolds 2003), for reasons noted in an earlier section. Benzodiazepines have a more limited role for treatment of GAD in elderly patients (Flint 2005). If benzodiazepines are used, lorazepam and oxazepam are recommended (Flint 2005). Other options include buspirone in the benzodiazepine-naive patient, and possibly pregabalin, an agent that appears to act through binding to calcium channels (Feltner et al. 2003).

Obsessive-Compulsive Disorder

Among elderly patients, compulsive behaviors are sometimes seen in those with schizophrenia or dementia, and obsessional rumination among those with depression. Primary OCD usually represents the persistence of illness that developed earlier in life. Contrary to a commonly held belief, hoarding among elders is less likely a manifestation of OCD than of schizophrenia or dementia (Grisham et al. 2005; Wu and Watson 2005).

Recommended treatments for OCD in elderly patients include behavior therapy (exposure and response prevention) and pharmacologic therapy. SSRI antidepressants are preferred to clomipramine because of adverse effects of the latter. No controlled studies of optimal dosage of SSRIs for elderly OCD patients have been performed, but clinical experience suggests that the equivalent of fluoxetine 60 mg/day may be needed for symptom control in many patients. Neither benzodiazepines nor buspirone has a role in the treatment of OCD.

Panic Disorder

The population of elders with panic anxiety appears to be a heterogeneous one, comprised of those with panic symptoms secondary to various medical conditions and medications and a small group with idiopathic panic disorder persisting into old age. Clinical experience suggests that CBT is a well-accepted and effective mode of treatment for elderly patients with idiopathic panic disorder.

The recommended pharmacologic treatment for panic disorder in elderly patients is an SSRI antidepressant such as citalopram or sertraline (Flint and Gagnon 2003). Venlafaxine, which received FDA-approved labeling for panic disorder in 2005, provides another option. The potential to induce panic when treatment is initiated with an antidepressant imposes a limit on starting dose and titration rate. For example, citalopram could be started at 5–10 mg/day, and if the medication is tolerated at that level, the dosage could be increased after 1 week to 20 mg/day. The medication could be maintained at that dosage for 4–6 weeks. If there is still no significant response, the dosage could be increased in slow increments to a maximum dosage of 30–40 mg/day (Flint and Gagnon 2003). Sertraline could be started at 12.5–25 mg/day, and if the medication is tolerated at that level, the dosage could be increased after 1 week to 50–100 mg/day. The medication could be maintained at that dosage for 4–6 weeks. If there is still no significant response, the dosage could be increased in slow increments to a maximum of 200 mg/day (Flint and Gagnon 2003). A benzodiazepine such as lorazepam may be needed as adjunctive therapy during the initial weeks of treatment, and frequent follow-up during this period is recommended (Flint and Gagnon 2003). Patients who do not respond to or do not tolerate SSRIs may be treated with venlafaxine; buspirone is not effective for the treatment of panic. Clinical experience suggests that when venlafaxine is used, the optimal dosage may be ≤150 mg/day, since noradrenergic effects become more prominent at higher doses. Based on limited data, tiagabine—a selective GABA reuptake inhibitor—may be useful for panic with agoraphobia in adult patients (Zwanger et al. 2001), although this medication carries some risk of seizure in nonepileptic populations.

In selected older patients, benzodiazepines may be a necessary and appropriate therapy for panic anxiety, in spite of dependence issues and adverse effects discussed elsewhere. The frequent association of panic with alcohol dependence complicates this use. Although alprazolam and clonazepam have been best studied for this indication (Rosenbaum et al. 1997), these are not necessarily recommended drugs in elderly patients. Either lorazepam or oxazepam could be used, with dosing described in the Specific Drug summaries at the end of this chapter.

After 6–12 months of panic symptom remission, an attempt could be made to taper (slowly) and discontinue medications (Flint and Gagnon 2003). Patients also treated with CBT may do well with such a taper. Others may experience a recrudescence of panic symptoms and require reinstatement of medications, at least for a period of time before another slow taper is attempted. Some will require lifelong treatment.

Posttraumatic Stress Disorder

PTSD in the elderly population has not been systematically studied, but anecdotal experience offers some guidance. When the disorder has onset earlier in life, it can manifest again in later years (Murray 2005). Elderly patients with PTSD present with more somatic symptoms than do younger patients (Owens et al. 2005). In addition, PTSD diagnosis is complicated in many older patients by medical comorbidities or cognitive deficits.

In older as in younger patients, the treatment of choice for PTSD is CBT. The first line of pharmacologic treatment is an SSRI antidepressant (Asnis et al. 2004). Appropriate SSRI dosing for PTSD in elderly patients has yet to be established, although clinical experience suggests that fluoxetine up to 60 mg/day or sertraline up to 200 mg/day may be required for optimal effect. Trazodone can be helpful for certain patients, but sedation often limits adequate dosing. Mirtazapine, venlafaxine, and duloxetine may be useful, but these medications have been understudied or unstudied among geriatric patients for this indication. In nongeriatric populations, mood-stabilizing anticonvulsants such as valproate, topiramate, gabapentin, carbamazepine, and lamotrigine have been used to treat patients with PTSD together with prominent impulsivity and anger (Asnis et al. 2004). The required duration of treatment with any of these agents is not established. Benzodiazepines have little role in PTSD treatment and may be problematic for PTSD patients with comorbid substance abuse. For PTSD-associated nightmares, the adrenergic antagonist prazosin titrated to 5 mg/day was found to be helpful in one case series (Raskind et al. 2000); clonidine, guanfacine (Horrigan and Barnhill 1996), and cyproheptadine have also been reported to be useful.

Sedation in the ICU Patient

The elderly ICU patient exhibiting motor restlessness (agitation) should be evaluated to determine precipitating factors, including delirium, alcohol withdrawal, and pain (among other possibilities), and specific treatment should be implemented to correct any of these underlying conditions. Specific treatment itself may be adequate to control agitation, but symptomatic treatment of agitation is often required in this setting. A significant degree of underlying anxiety occurs in an estimated 70%–87% of ICU patients (Bone et al. 1995) and is a particular problem for patients on ventilators and intra-aortic balloon pumps. Nonpharmacologic measures to minimize anxiety and agitation in this patient population are discussed in an earlier section.

Appropriate pharmacologic care for overly anxious or agitated patients in the ICU includes standing doses of a parenteral benzodiazepine (along with analgesic medications as indicated) that are sufficient to sedate, keep calm, and induce amnesia. The use of antipsychotic medication such as haloperidol or quetiapine in this setting is now controversial, in view of the recently issued FDA advisory regarding increased mortality among elderly patients treated with atypical antipsychotics and similar concerns raised about conventional antipsychotics (Wang et al. 2005). The possibility that haloperidol actually reduces mortality in mechanically ventilated ICU patients has been raised by another study (Milbrandt et al. 2005), leaving the issue far from settled.

A great deal of anecdotal evidence supports the use of a combination of intravenous lorazepam, hydromorphone, and haloperidol to maintain calm in the ICU patient (Jacobi et al. 2002). The goal for sedation should be a Riker Sedation-Agitation Scale score of 2–4, with 4 being ideal. The Riker scale is reproduced as Table 6–10 (Riker et al. 1999). The goal for analgesia should be to make pain tolerable for the patient and not interfere with medical care. Pain assessment is discussed more fully in Chapter 10 of this volume, "Analgesic Medications." The goal for symptomatic treatment of delirium or psychosis should be that the patient not be agitated or actively hallucinating and that psychotic symptoms not interfere with care. Delirium treatment is discussed more fully in Chapter 3 and Chapter 8, "Treatment of Movement Disorders."

Social Phobia

Although not specifically studied in elders, CBT may be useful in the treatment of social phobia (social anxiety disorder) in this population as it may be in younger patients. Medications with FDA-approved labeling for social phobia include paroxetine, sertraline, and venlafaxine. Alternatively, clonazepam (Otto et al. 2000) or gabapentin (Pande et al. 1999)

Table 6–10. Riker Sedation-Agitation Scale

Score	Description	Definition
7	Dangerous agitation	Pulling at endotracheal tube (ETT), trying to remove catheters, climbing over bed rail, striking at staff, thrashing side to side
6	Very agitated	Does not calm despite frequent verbal reminding of limits, requires physical restraints, biting ETT
5	Agitated	Anxious or mildly agitated, attempting to sit up, calms down to verbal instructions
4	Calm and cooperative	Calm, awakens easily, follows commands
3	Sedated	Difficult to arouse, awakens to verbal stimuli or gentle shaking but drifts off again, follows simple commands
2	Very sedated	Arouses to physical stimuli but does not communicate or follow commands, may move spontaneously
1	Unarousable	Minimal or no response to noxious stimuli, does not communicate or follow commands

Source. Reprinted from Riker RR, Picard JT, Fraser GL: "Prospective Evaluation of the Sedation-Agitation Scale for Adult Critically Ill Patients." *Critical Care Medicine* 27:1325–1329, 1999. Used with permission.

could be used. Buspirone has been found ineffective for this indication in at least one study (van Vliet et al. 1997).

Sleep Disorders

Insomnia

Transient insomnia is a common complaint in the general population of elders and often warrants little more than reassurance of the patient and/ or caregiver. When insomnia becomes persistent and daytime performance is affected, however, a diagnostic workup may be indicated. A sleep diary can be recommended. This is a 1- to 2-week log of time in bed (including naps), quality of sleep, time of exercise, and time of ingestion of meals, alcohol, caffeine, and nicotine. This information helps to identify appropriate sleep hygiene recommendations and other nonpharmacologic interventions.

Early in the evaluation, potential medical conditions that could be contributing to insomnia should be considered and current medication lists should be reviewed. Common causes of insomnia are listed in Table 6–11 (Doghramji 2001). It should be noted that an overnight sleep laboratory (polysomnography) study is indicated only if sleep apnea, abnormal limb movements, or other abnormal events in sleep are suspected, or if the patient fails to respond to behavioral interventions, medications, or medication changes (listed below). Sleep apnea might be suspected if the patient's sleeping partner or another observer reports heavy snoring or periods when breathing stops during sleep, and the level of suspicion might be raised by the presence of comorbid depression or hypertension. Similarly, periodic limb movements or unusual behaviors such as fighting while asleep may be reported by a sleeping partner.

Treatment of insomnia begins with sleep hygiene measures and other nonpharmacologic therapies, such as timed exposure to bright light, as discussed in an earlier section. The first step in pharmacotherapy for insomnia is to discontinue currently ineffective treatments. As noted earlier, sedating antihistamines have little value in maintaining sleep through the night and may be associated with delirium and other anticholinergic side effects. Prescription hypnotics also should be tapered and discontinued. If insomnia persists (e.g., longer than 2 weeks) after the prescription hypnotic has been stopped and sleep hygiene measures have been implemented, another hypnotic could be considered.

For transient or short-term insomnia (<3 weeks) in elderly patients, any of the following drugs could be used (taken at bedtime): zolpidem, 5 mg; zaleplon, 10 mg; eszopiclone, 1–2 mg; gabapentin, 100–300 mg; mirtazapine, 7.5 mg; trazodone, 25 mg; nortriptyline, 10 mg; or temazepam, 15 mg. Although clinical experience is limited to date, ramelteon 8 mg qhs may be a recommended drug for elders. Drugs *not* recommended for insomnia in this population include diphenhydramine, chloral hydrate, and barbiturates and related sedatives (*The Medical Letter,* August 7, 2000).

Table 6–11.   Selected causes of insomnia in the elderly

Medical

Nonprescription drugs

Caffeine

Diet pills (e.g., those including pseudoephedrine, ephedrine, or phenylpropanolamine)

Nicotine

Prescription drugs

β-Blockers

Theophylline

Albuterol

Quinidine

Stimulants (dextroamphetamine, methylphenidate, bupropion)

Decongestants (pseudoephedrine, ephedrine, phenylpropanolamine)

Thyroid preparations

Corticosteroids

Certain SSRIs (e.g., fluoxetine)

Monoamine oxidase inhibitors

Methyldopa

Phenytoin

Chemotherapy

Benzodiazepines

Medical conditions

Primary sleep disorders

Pain

Drug/Alcohol intoxication or withdrawal

Thyrotoxicosis

Dyspnea (any cause)

Neurologic disease (Parkinson's, Alzheimer's)

Acute and chronic medical illnesses (arthritis, cardiovascular disease, gastrointestinal disease, asthma, COPD)

Table 6–11. Selected causes of insomnia in the elderly *(continued)*

Psychological

Depression

Anxiety

Stress

Bedtime worrying

Conditioning (associating bed with wakefulness)

Mania/Hypomania

Environmental

Temperature (bedroom too hot or cold)

Noise

Food, exercise, caffeine, or alcohol before bedtime

Jet lag

Shift work

Daytime napping

Note. COPD = chronic obstructive pulmonary disease; SSRI = selective serotonin reuptake inhibitor.
Source. Adapted from Doghramji PP: "Detection of Insomnia in Primary Care." *Journal of Clinical Psychiatry* 62 (suppl 10):18–26, 2001. Used with permission.

The same agents may be used for treatment of chronic insomnia, although the use of benzodiazepines for this purpose is more controversial. Some clinicians recommend their use only intermittently (three to four times a week), in patients who are closely followed and for whom a nonpharmacologic plan also is in place (Monane 1992; Perlis et al. 2004). Although many patients experiencing insomnia report continued long-term effectiveness of benzodiazepines, there are few controlled studies of these drugs in chronic insomnia.

Periodic Limb Movements of Sleep
PLMS involve complex involuntary limb movements occurring at regular intervals and associated with arousal from sleep. The syndrome is more prevalent in old age, and there is a large overlap with restless legs

syndrome (discussed in Chapter 8). In addition, systemic conditions associated with neuropathy such as anemia, vitamin B_{12} deficiency, and diabetes may be linked to these abnormal movements. Use of medications such as SSRIs and tricyclic antidepressants or withdrawal from sedative-hypnotic medications or opioids also may be associated with PLMS.

Many clinicians initiate treatment with vitamin and mineral supplements (folate, vitamin B_{12}, vitamin C, iron, and magnesium) when either PLMS or restless legs syndrome is diagnosed. Both conditions may be treated with clonazepam, 0.5–1 mg at bedtime. Duration of treatment has not been studied systematically, and some patients reportedly develop tolerance to the arousal-suppressing effect over time, making the treatment ineffective (Nofzinger and Reynolds 1996). In addition, both PLMS and restless legs syndrome can be comorbid with sleep apnea, a condition for which sedatives may be contraindicated. Several case reports involving this particular population suggest that benzodiazepine use is not associated with exacerbation of apnea (Morfis et al. 1997; Nofzinger and Reynolds 1996), but these data are not adequate for the practice to be recommended as safe. For PLMS patients treated with a tricyclic or SSRI antidepressant, a switch to mirtazapine may be helpful. Movements also can be suppressed and sleep facilitated with the dopamine agonist ropinirole, 0.5 mg at bedtime (Saletu et al. 2000), or levodopa, which is started at 25/100 mg and titrated to effect (Nofzinger and Reynolds 1996). When short-acting levodopa is associated with worsening of leg movements during the day, the medication is given more than once daily and/or in sustained-release form (Brown 1997).

Rapid Eye Movement Sleep Behavior Disorder

Under normal circumstances, skeletal muscle atonia dampens movement during rapid eye movement (REM) sleep. In individuals with REM sleep behavior disorder, atonia is incomplete and dreams may be acted out physically. This disorder can be primary or can be associated with dementia (e.g., dementia with Lewy bodies), Parkinson's disease, olivopontocerebellar degeneration, Guillain-Barré syndrome, or subarachnoid hemorrhage (Brown 1997). Elderly patients with loss of REM sleep atonia are at risk for nighttime falls. In elders, one treatment that may be helpful for REM sleep behavior disorder is clonazepam, 0.5–1 mg at bedtime. The patient's sleep environment should be made safer by a padding of the bed and removal of sharp objects (Brown 1997). Antidepressant medications may be useful by virtue of REM-suppressing effects; clinical experience suggests that mirtazapine may be particularly useful because of its additional sedating effects.

Chapter Summary

- When anxiety disorders are encountered in the elderly, they are often comorbid with other conditions, particularly depressive disorders or particular medical conditions.
- Antidepressants are the pharmacologic treatment of choice for most elderly patients with anxiety symptoms and disorders.
- Patient selection for benzodiazepine therapy should take into account any history of alcoholism or other substance abuse.
- When benzodiazepines are used to treat anxiety in elderly patients, lorazepam and oxazepam are recommended.
- Significant drug interactions involving benzodiazepines are mediated primarily by the CYP3A4 enzyme system.
- Older patients treated with benzodiazepines chronically may begin to develop symptoms of toxicity as they reach old age, presumably a function of altered drug clearance.
- Most patients tolerate a taper of 10%–25% of the total dose of benzodiazepine each week, although the last few dose decrements might require longer intervals.
- Among elderly patients treated with benzodiazepines, there is a significantly increased risk of falls (particularly in the first week after therapy is initiated) as well as motor vehicle accidents involving personal injury.
- A number of medications are available for treatment of insomnia in elderly patients, some labeled for insomnia (eszopiclone, zaleplon, zolpidem, ramelteon, and temazepam) and some off-label (gabapentin, mirtazapine, trazodone, and nortriptyline).
- Drugs *not* recommended for insomnia in the elderly patient include chloral hydrate, diphenhydramine, long-acting benzodiazepines, and barbiturates and related sedative-hypnotics.

References

Ancoli-Israel S, Walsh JK, Mangano RM, et al: Zaleplon, a novel nonbenzodiazepine hypnotic, effectively treats insomnia in elderly patients without causing rebound effects. Prim Care Companion J Clin Psychiatry 1:114–120, 1999

Ashton H: Toxicity and adverse consequences of benzodiazepine use. Psychiatr Ann 25:158–165, 1995

Asnis GM, Kohn SR, Henderson M, et al: SSRIs versus non-SSRIs in post-traumatic stress disorder: an update with recommendations. Drugs 64:383–404, 2004

Ayd FJ: Prescribing anxiolytics and hypnotics for the elderly. Psychiatr Ann 24:91–97, 1994

Barbera J, Shapiro C: Benefit-risk assessment of zaleplon in the treatment of insomnia. Drug Saf 28:301–318, 2005

Bone RC, Hayden WR, Levine RL, et al: Recognition, assessment, and treatment of anxiety in the critical care patient. Dis Mon 41:293–359, 1995

Brown LK: Sleep and sleep disorders in the elderly. Nursing Home Medicine 5:346–353, 1997

Buckley NA, Dawson AH, Whyte IM, et al: Relative toxicity of benzodiazepines in overdose. BMJ 310:219–221, 1995

Burch EA Jr: Use and misuse of benzodiazepines in the elderly. Psychiatr Med 8:97–105, 1990

Bush G, Fink M, Petrides G, et al: Catatonia, I: rating scale and standardized examination. Acta Psychiatr Scand 93:129–136, 1996

Byrnes JJ, Miller LG, Greenblatt DJ, et al: Chronic benzodiazepine administration, XII: anticonvulsant cross-tolerance but distinct neurochemical effects of alprazolam and lorazepam. Psychopharmacology (Berl) 111:91–95, 1993

Ciraulo DA, Barnhill JG, Ciraulo AM, et al: Alterations in pharmacodynamics of anxiolytics in abstinent alcoholic men: subjective responses, abuse liability, and electroencephalographic effects of alprazolam, diazepam, and buspirone. J Clin Pharmacol 37:64–73, 1997

Closser MH, Brower KJ: Treatment of alprazolam withdrawal with chlordiazepoxide substitution and taper. J Subst Abuse Treat 11:319–323, 1994

Cumming RG, Le Couteur DG: Benzodiazepines and risk of hip fractures in older people: a review of the evidence. CNS Drugs 17:825–837, 2003

Davies M, Newell JG, Derry JM, et al: Characterization of the interaction of zopiclone with gamma-aminobutyric acid type A receptors. Mol Pharmacol 58:756–762, 2000

DeMartinis N, Rynn M, Rickels K, et al: Prior benzodiazepine use and buspirone response in the treatment of generalized anxiety disorder. J Clin Psychiatry 61:91–94, 2000

Doghramji PP: Detection of insomnia in primary care. J Clin Psychiatry 62 (suppl 10):18–26, 2001

Dubovsky SL: Generalized anxiety disorder: new concepts and psychopharmacologic therapies. J Clin Psychiatry 51 (suppl 1):3–10, 1990

Dunner DL, Goldstein DJ, Mallinckrodt C, et al: Duloxetine in the treatment of anxiety symptoms associated with depression. Depress Anxiety 18:53–61, 2003

Fancourt G, Castleden M: The use of benzodiazepines with particular reference to the elderly. Br J Hosp Med 35:321–326, 1986

Farnsworth MG: Benzodiazepine abuse and dependence: misconceptions and facts. J Fam Pract 31:393–400, 1990

Feltner DE, Crockatt JG, Dubovsky SJ, et al: A randomized, double-blind, placebo-controlled, fixed-dose, multicenter study of pregabalin in patients with generalized anxiety disorder. J Clin Psychopharmacol 23:240–249, 2003

Fick DM, Cooper JW, Wade WE, et al: Updating the Beers criteria for potentially inappropriate medication use in older adults. Arch Intern Med 163:2716–2724, 2003

Fink M, Taylor MA: Catatonia: A Clinician's Guide to Diagnosis and Treatment. New York, Cambridge University Press, 2003

Flint AJ: Generalised anxiety disorder in elderly patients: epidemiology, diagnosis and treatment options. Drugs Aging 22:101–114, 2005

Flint AJ, Gagnon N: Diagnosis and management of panic disorder in older patients. Drugs Aging 20:881–891, 2003

Foley D, Ancoli-Israel S, Britz P, et al: Sleep disturbances and chronic disease in older adults: results of the 2003 National Sleep Foundation Sleep in America Survey. J Psychosom Res 56:497–502, 2004

Foy A, Drinkwater V, March S, et al: Confusion after admission to hospital in elderly patients using benzodiazepines. Br Med J (Clin Res Ed) 293:1072, 1986

Gambi F, De Berardis D, Campanella D, et al: Mirtazapine treatment of generalized anxiety disorder: a fixed dose, open label study. J Psychopharmacol 19:483–487, 2005

Geiselmann B, Linden M: Prescription and intake patterns in long-term and ultra-long-term benzodiazepine treatment in primary care practice. Pharmacopsychiatry 24:55–61, 1991

Gericke CA, Ludolph AC: Chronic abuse of zolpidem (letter). JAMA 272:1721–1722, 1994

Goldstein LB: Common drugs may influence motor recovery after stroke. The Sygen In Acute Stroke Study Investigators. Neurology 45:865–871, 1995

Graham AV, Parran TV, Jaen CR: Physician failure to record alcohol use history when prescribing benzodiazepines. J Subst Abuse 4:179–185, 1992

Greenblatt DJ: Benzodiazepine hypnotics: sorting the pharmacokinetic facts. J Clin Psychiatry 52 (suppl 9):4–10, 1991

Greenblatt DJ: Pharmacology of benzodiazepine hypnotics. J Clin Psychiatry 53 (suppl 6):7–13, 1992

Greenblatt DJ, Shader RI: Prazepam and lorazepam, two new benzodiazepines. N Engl J Med 299:1342–1344, 1978

Greenblatt DJ, Comer WH, Elliott HW, et al: Clinical pharmacokinetics of lorazepam, III: intravenous injection: preliminary results. J Clin Pharmacol 17:490–494, 1977

Greenblatt DJ, Harmatz JS, Shader RI: Clinical pharmacokinetics of anxiolytics and hypnotics in the elderly. Therapeutic considerations (Part I). Clin Pharmacokinet 21:165–177, 1991a

Greenblatt DJ, Harmatz JS, Shader RI: Clinical pharmacokinetics of anxiolytics and hypnotics in the elderly. Therapeutic considerations (Part II). Clin Pharmacokinet 21:262–273, 1991b

Greenblatt DJ, Harmatz JS, Shader RI: Plasma alprazolam concentrations. Arch Gen Psychiatry 50:715–722, 1993

Griffiths RR, Wolf B: Relative abuse liability of different benzodiazepines in drug abusers. J Clin Psychopharmacol 10:237–243, 1990

Grisham JR, Brown TA, Liverant GI, et al: The distinctiveness of compulsive hoarding from obsessive-compulsive disorder. J Anxiety Disord 19:767–769, 2005

Hawkins JW, Tinklenberg JR, Sheikh JI, et al: A retrospective chart review of gabapentin for the treatment of aggressive and agitated behavior in patients with dementias. Am J Geriatr Psychiatry 8:221–225, 2000

Hemmelgarn B, Suissa S, Huang A, et al: Benzodiazepine use and the risk of motor vehicle crash in the elderly. JAMA 278:27–31, 1997

Hemmeter U, Muller M, Bischof R, et al: Effect of zopiclone and temazepam on sleep EEG parameters, psychomotor and memory functions in healthy elderly volunteers. Psychopharmacology (Berl) 147:384–396, 2000

Herrmann N, Lanctot K, Myszak M: Effectiveness of gabapentin for the treatment of behavioral disorders in dementia. J Clin Psychopharmacol 20:90–93, 2000

Hollister LE, Muller-Oerlinghausen B, Rickels K, et al: Clinical uses of benzodiazepines. J Clin Psychopharmacol 13:1S–169S, 1993

Horrigan JP, Barnhill LJ: The suppression of nightmares with guanfacine (letter). J Clin Psychiatry 57:371, 1996

Hybels CF, Blazer DG: Epidemiology of late-life mental disorders. Clin Geriatr Med 19:663–696, 2003

Isbister GK, O'Regan L, Sibbritt D, et al: Alprazolam is relatively more toxic than other benzodiazepines in overdose. Br J Clin Pharmacol 58:88–95, 2004

Jacobi J, Fraser GL, Coursin DB, et al: Clinical practice guidelines for the sustained use of sedatives and analgesics in the critically ill adult. Crit Care Med 30:119–141, 2002

Jerkovich GS, Preskorn SH: Failure of buspirone to protect against lorazepam withdrawal symptoms (letter). JAMA 258:204–205, 1987

Kruse WHH: Problems and pitfalls in the use of benzodiazepines in the elderly. Drug Saf 5:328–344, 1990

Krystal AD, Walsh JK, Laska E, et al: Sustained efficacy of eszopiclone over 6 months of nightly treatment: results of a randomized, double-blind, placebo-controlled study in adults with chronic insomnia. Sleep 26:793–799, 2003

Lawlor BA, Hill JL, Radcliffe JL, et al: A single oral dose challenge of buspirone does not affect memory processes in older volunteers. Biol Psychiatry 32:101–103, 1992

Lenox-Smith AJ, Reynolds A: A double-blind, randomised, placebo-controlled study of venlafaxine XL in patients with generalised anxiety disorder in primary care. Br J Gen Practice 53:772–777, 2003

Lessard E, Yessine MA, Hamelin BA, et al: Diphenhydramine alters the disposition of venlafaxine through inhibition of CYP2D6 activity in humans. J Clin Psychopharmacol 21:175–184, 2001

Lewy AJ, Sack RL: Light therapy and psychiatry. Proc Soc Exp Biol Med 183:11–18, 1986

Martin CD, Chan SC: Distribution of temazepam in body fluids and tissues in lethal overdose. J Anal Toxicol 10:77–78, 1986

Martinez-Cano H, Vela-Bueno A: Daytime consumption of triazolam. Acta Psychiatr Scand 88:286–288, 1993

McCall WV: Sleep in the elderly: burden, diagnosis, and treatment. Prim Care Companion J Clin Psychiatry 6:9–20, 2004

McEvoy GK, Snow EK, Kester L, et al: AHFS Drug Information. Bethesda, MD, American Society of Health-System Pharmacists, 2006

Milbrandt EB, Kersten A, Kong L, et al: Haloperidol use is associated with lower hospital mortality in mechanically ventilated patients. Crit Care Med 33:263–265, 2005

Miller LG, Greenblatt DJ, Barnhill JG, et al: Chronic benzodiazepine administration, I: tolerance is associated with benzodiazepine receptor downregulation and decreased gamma-aminobutyric acid-A receptor function. J Pharmacol Exp Ther 246:170–176, 1988

Mohlman J: Psychosocial treatment of late-life generalized anxiety disorder: current status and future directions. Clin Psychol Rev 24:149–169, 2004

Mohlman J, de Jesus M, Gorenstein EE, et al: Distinguishing generalized anxiety disorder, panic disorder, and mixed anxiety states in older treatment-seeking adults. Anxiety Disord 18:275–290, 2004

Monane M: Insomnia in the elderly. J Clin Psychiatry 53 (suppl 6):23–28, 1992

Montgomery P, Dennis J: Cognitive behavioral interventions for sleep problems in adults aged 60+. The Cochrane Database of Systematic Reviews, Issue 2, Art. No: CD003161. DOI: 003110.001002/14651858.CD14003161, 2006

Morfis L, Schwartz RS, Cistulli PA: REM sleep behaviour disorder: a treatable cause of falls in elderly people. Age Ageing 26:43–44, 1997

Morin CM, Culbert JP, Schwartz SM: Nonpharmacological interventions for insomnia: a meta-analysis of treatment efficacy. Am J Psychiatry 151:1172–1180, 1994

Murray A: Recurrence of post traumatic stress disorder. Nurs Older People 17:24–30, 2005

Ninan PT, Muntasser S: Buspirone and gepirone, in The American Psychiatric Publishing Textbook of Psychopharmacology, 3rd Edition. Edited by Schatzberg AF, Nemeroff CB. Washington, DC, American Psychiatric Publishing, 2004, pp 391–404

Nofzinger EA, Reynolds CF: Sleep impairment and daytime sleepiness in later life. Am J Psychiatry 153:941–943, 1996

Otto MW, Pollack MH, Gould RA, et al: A comparison of the efficacy of clonazepam and cognitive-behavioral group therapy for the treatment of social phobia. J Anxiety Disord 14:345–358, 2000

Owens GP, Baker DG, Kasckow J, et al: Review of assessment and treatment of PTSD among elderly American armed forces veterans. Int J Geriatr Psychiatry 20:1118–1130, 2005

Pande AC, Davidson JR, Jefferson JW, et al: Treatment of social phobia with gabapentin: a placebo-controlled study. J Clin Psychopharmacol 19:341–348, 1999

Pecknold JC: Discontinuation reactions to alprazolam in panic disorder. J Psychiatr Res 27 (suppl 1):155–170, 1993

Periyakoil VS, Skultety K, Sheikh J: Panic, anxiety, and chronic dyspnea. J Palliat Med 8:453–459, 2005

Perlis ML, McCall WV, Krystal AD, et al: Long-term, non-nightly administration of zolpidem in the treatment of patients with primary insomnia. J Clin Psychiatry 65:1128–1137, 2004

Pies RW: Handbook of Essential Psychopharmacology, 2nd Edition. Washington, DC, American Psychiatric Publishing, 2005

Pomara N, Deptula D, Medel M, et al: Effects of diazepam on recall memory: relationship to aging, dose, and duration of treatment. Psychopharmacol Bull 25:144–148, 1989

Pourmotabbed T, McLeod DR, Hoehn-Saric R, et al: Treatment, discontinuation, and psychomotor effects of diazepam in women with generalized anxiety disorder. J Clin Psychopharmacol 16:202–207, 1996

Raskind MA, Dobie DJ, Kanter ED, et al: The alpha1-adrenergic antagonist prazosin ameliorates combat trauma nightmares in veterans with posttraumatic stress disorder: a report of 4 cases. J Clin Psychiatry 61:129–133, 2000

Ray WA, Thapa PB, Gideon P: Benzodiazepines and the risk of falls in nursing home residents. J Am Geriatr Soc 48:682–685, 2000

Reith DM, Fountain J, McDowell R, et al: Comparison of the fatal toxicity index of zopiclone with benzodiazepines. J Toxicol Clin Toxicol 41:975–980, 2003

Reynolds CF, Regestein Q, Nowell PD, et al: Treatment of insomnia in the elderly, in Clinical Geriatric Psychopharmacology, 3rd Edition. Edited by Salzman C. Baltimore, MD, Williams & Wilkins, 1998, pp 395–416

Reynolds CF, Buysse DJ, Kupfer DJ: Treating insomnia in older adults: taking a long-term view. JAMA 281:1034–1035, 1999

Richard IH: Anxiety disorders in Parkinson's disease. Adv Neurol 96:42–55, 2005

Rickels K, Schweizer E, Case WG, et al: Long-term therapeutic use of benzodiazepines, I: effects of abrupt discontinuation. Arch Gen Psychiatry 47:899–907, 1990

Rickels K, Schweizer E, Case WG, et al: Nefazodone in major depression: adjunctive benzodiazepine therapy and tolerability. J Clin Psychopharmacol 18:145–153, 1998

Rickels K, DeMartinis N, Garcia-Espana F, et al: Imipramine and buspirone in treatment of patients with generalized anxiety disorder who are discontinuing long-term benzodiazepine therapy. Am J Psychiatry 157:1973–1979, 2000

Riker RR, Picard JT, Fraser GL: Prospective evaluation of the Sedation-Agitation Scale for adult critically ill patients. Crit Care Med 27:1325–1329, 1999

Roane DM, Feinberg TE, Meckler L, et al: Treatment of dementia-associated agitation with gabapentin. J Neuropsychiatry Clin Neurosci 12:40–43, 2000

Rosebush PI, Mazurek MF: Catatonia after benzodiazepine withdrawal. J Clin Psychopharmacol 16:315–319, 1996

Rosenbaum JF, Moroz G, Bowden CL: Clonazepam in the treatment of panic disorder with or without agoraphobia: a dose-response study of efficacy, safety, and discontinuance. J Clin Psychopharmacol 17:390–400, 1997

Roth T, Roehrs TA: Issues in the use of benzodiazepine therapy. J Clin Psychiatry 53 (suppl 6):14–18, 1992

Roth T, Stubbs C, Walsh JK: Ramelteon (TAK-375), a selective MT1/MT2-receptor agonist, reduces latency to persistent sleep in a model of transient insomnia related to a novel sleep environment. Sleep 28:303–307, 2004

Rynn M, Garcia-Espana F, Greenblatt DJ, et al: Imipramine and buspirone in patients with panic disorder who are discontinuing long-term benzodiazepine therapy. J Clin Psychopharmacol 23:505–508, 2003

Saletu B, Gruber G, Saletu M, et al: Sleep laboratory studies in restless legs syndrome patients as compared with normals and acute effects of ropinirole, I: findings on objective and subjective sleep and awakening quality. Neuropsychobiology 41:181–189, 2000

Satzger W, Engel RR, Ferguson E, et al: Effects of single doses of alpidem, lorazepam, and placebo on memory and attention in healthy young and elderly volunteers. Pharmacopsychiatry 23:114–119, 1990

Schweizer E, Rickels K, Case WG, et al: Long-term therapeutic use of benzodiazepines. Arch Gen Psychiatry 47:908–915, 1990

Schweizer E, Rickels K, Case WG, et al: Carbamazepine treatment in patients discontinuing long-term benzodiazepine therapy. Arch Gen Psychiatry 48:448–452, 1991

Semla TP, Beizer JL, Higbee MD: Geriatric Dosage Handbook, 11th Edition. Hudson, OH, Lexi-Comp Inc., 2006

Shader RI, Greenblatt DJ: Use of benzodiazepines in anxiety disorders. N Engl J Med 328:1398–1405, 1993

Smoller JW: Panic-anxiety in patients with respiratory disease. American Society of Clinical Psychopharmacology Progress Notes 7:4–5, 1996

Smoller JW, Pollack MH, Systrom D, et al: Sertraline effects on dyspnea in patients with obstructive airways disease. Psychosomatics 39:24–29, 1998

Smoller JW, Pollack MH, Wassertheil-Smoller S, et al: Prevalence and correlates of panic attacks in postmenopausal women: results from an ancillary study to the Women's Health Initiative. Arch Intern Med 163:2041–2050, 2003

Suzuki K, Awata S, Matsuoka H: Short-term effect of ECT in middle-aged and elderly patients with intractable catatonic schizophrenia. J ECT 19:73–80, 2003

Swift CG, Swift MR, Hamley J, et al: Side-effect "tolerance" in elderly long-term recipients of benzodiazepine hypnotics. Age Ageing 13:335–343, 1984

Terzano MG, Rossi M, Palomba V, et al: New drugs for insomnia: comparative tolerability of zopiclone, zolpidem and zaleplon. Drug Saf 26:261–282, 2003

Thal GD, Szabo MD, Lopez-Bresnahan M, et al: Exacerbation or unmasking of focal neurologic deficits by sedatives. Anesthesiology 85:21–25, 1996

Thompson TL Jr, Moran MG, Nies AS: Drug therapy: psychotropic drug use in the elderly (first of two parts). N Engl J Med 308:134–138, 1983

Uchimura N, Nakajima T, Hayashi K, et al: Effect of zolpidem on sleep architecture and its next-morning residual effect in insomniac patients: a randomized crossover comparative study with brotizolam. Prog Neuropsychopharmacol Biol Psychiatry 30:22–29, 2006

van Balkom AJ, de Beurs E, Koele P, et al: Long-term benzodiazepine use is associated with smaller treatment gain in panic disorder with agoraphobia. J Nerv Ment Dis 184:133–135, 1996

van Steveninck AL, Wallnofer AE, Schoemaker RC, et al: A study of the effects of long-term use on individual sensitivity to temazepam and lorazepam in a clinical population. Br J Clin Pharmacol 44:267–275, 1997

van Vliet IM, den Boer JA, Westenberg HG, et al: Clinical effects of buspirone in social phobia: a double-blind placebo-controlled study. J Clin Psychiatry 58:164–168, 1997

Vinkers DJ, Gussekloo J, van der Mast RC, et al: Benzodiazepine use and risk of mortality in individuals aged 85 years or older. JAMA 290:2942–2943, 2003

Walsh K, Bennett G: Parkinson's disease and anxiety. Postgrad Med 77:89–93, 2001

Wang PS, Schneeweiss S, Avorn J, et al: Risk of death in elderly users of conventional vs. atypical antipsychotic medications. N Engl J Med 353:2335–2341, 2005

Wetherell JL, Thorp SR, Patterson TL, et al: Quality of life in geriatric generalized anxiety disorder: a preliminary investigation. J Psychiatr Res 38:305–312, 2004

Woo E, Proulx SM, Greenblatt DJ: Differential side effect profile of triazolam versus flurazepam in elderly patients undergoing rehabilitation therapy. J Clin Pharmacol 31:168–173, 1991

Wu KD, Watson D: Hoarding and its relation to obsessive-compulsive disorder. Behav Res Ther 43:897–921, 2005

Yosselson-Superstine S, Lipman AG: Chlordiazepoxide interaction with levodopa (letter). Ann Intern Med 96:259, 1982

Zwanger P, Baghai TC, Schule C, et al: Tiagabine improves panic and agoraphobia in panic disorder patients. J Clin Psychiatry 62:656–657, 2001

Generic name	alprazolam
Trade name	Xanax, Xanax XR, Niravam, Alprazolam Intensol (generic available for immediate-release [IR] form)
Class	Benzodiazepine
Half-life	12–20 hours
Mechanism of action	Potentiates effects of GABA by binding to $GABA_A$-benzodiazepine receptor complex
Available preparations	IR tablets: 0.25, 0.5, 1, 2 mg XR tablets: 0.5, 1, 2, 3 mg Orally disintegrating tablets: 0.25, 0.5, 1, 2 mg Oral concentrate: 1 mg/mL
Starting dose	IR: 0.125–0.25 mg bid XR: 0.5 mg/day
Titration	IR: increase by 0.125 mg/day every 4–5 days as needed and as tolerated
Typical daily dose	IR: 0.25 mg bid to tid XR: 0.5 mg
Dose range	0.25–2 mg/day (divided bid to tid)
Therapeutic serum level	Not established for elderly (see text)

Comments: Not a first-line drug in elderly patients in spite of short half-life and lack of active metabolites. Interdose anxiety may necessitate tid or qid dosing. Discontinuation is often problematic, requiring a switch to a longer-acting agent or another drug such as carbamazepine. Pharmacokinetics are independent of dose and unchanged during multiple dosing. Rapidly and well absorbed. Protein bound 80%. Metabolized extensively in liver to less active metabolites. Metabolized mainly via CYP3A4. Peak plasma concentration in 1–2 hours. Delayed clearance (prolonged half-life) in elderly men. Withdrawal symptoms occur from 18 hours to 3 days after abrupt discontinuation. *Drug interactions:* Important interactions with CYP3A4 inhibitors and inducers (see Table 2–2), additive effects with other CNS depressants, theophylline antagonizes effects of alprazolam, fluoxetine may increase alprazolam level, alprazolam significantly increases levels of imipramine and desipramine. *Common adverse effects (>10%):* Incoordination, cognitive impairment, depression, drowsiness, fatigue, irritability, light-headedness, sedation, appetite changes, weight loss or gain, constipation, dry mouth, difficulty urinating, and dysarthria. *Less common adverse effects (1%–10%):* Hypotension, confusion, disinhibition, dizziness, hallucinations, seizures, increased salivation, incontinence, abnormal liver function test values, jaundice, arthralgia, ataxia, diplopia, and dyspnea. *Uncommon but serious effects:* Hepatic failure and Stevens-Johnson syndrome.

Generic name	buspirone
Trade name	BuSpar (generic available)
Class	Antianxiety agent
Half-life	2–11 hours
Mechanism of action	5-HT_{1A} receptor agonist (presynaptic), 5-HT_{1A} receptor partial agonist (postsynaptic); down-regulates 5-HT_2; complex dopaminergic effects
Available preparations	Tablets: 5, 7.5, 10, 15, 30 mg
Starting dose	5 mg bid
Titration	Increase by 5 mg/day every 2–3 days
Typical daily dose	10 mg tid
Dose range	5 mg bid to 20 mg tid
Therapeutic serum level	Not established

Comments: A first-line drug for generalized anxiety (but not panic) among elderly patients because of a favorable adverse-effect profile; not associated with psychomotor or cognitive impairment, dependence, withdrawal, abuse, or interaction with alcohol. Prior treatment with benzodiazepines, especially recent treatment, may be associated with reduced effectiveness of buspirone. Pharmacokinetics are not related to age or gender, but considerable between-individual variation is seen. Extensive first-pass metabolism. Food may decrease absorption, but may also decrease hepatic extraction, thus increasing bioavailability. 95% protein bound. Metabolized in the liver mainly by CYP3A4 oxidation. Peak serum concentration in 40–60 minutes. Long latency to primary effect; may see some decrease in anxiety after 1 week, but full effect may take up to 6 weeks. Not effective when used prn. Not recommended for use in patients with severe hepatic or renal impairment. Not dialyzable. When changing from a benzodiazepine to buspirone, add buspirone; administer both for 2–4 weeks before starting benzodiazepine taper. No cross-tolerance with benzodiazepines. When buspirone is discontinued, an extended taper is not necessary. *Drug interactions:* CYP3A4 inhibitors and inducers (see Table 2–2), diltiazem and verapamil increase buspirone concentrations, increased blood pressure when given with monoamine oxidase inhibitors (including selegiline and linezolid), increased CNS adverse effects with nefazodone, serotonin syndrome with SSRIs or trazodone, anxiolytic efficacy of buspirone may be lost with SSRIs. Generally well tolerated. *Adverse effects:* Dizziness, drowsiness, extrapyramidal side effects, serotonin syndrome, confusion, nervousness, light-headedness, excitement, anger, hostility, headache, nausea, weakness, paresthesias, incoordination, tremor, blurred vision, and diaphoresis.

Generic name	clonazepam
Trade name	Klonopin (generic available)
Class	Benzodiazepine
Half-life	19–50 hours
Mechanism of action	Potentiates effects of GABA by binding to GABA$_A$-benzodiazepine receptor complex
Available preparations	Tablets: 0.5, 1, 2 mg Orally disintegrating wafer: 0.125, 0.25, 0.5, 1, 2 mg
Starting dose	0.25–0.5 mg/day
Titration	Increase by 0.25–0.5 mg every 4–5 days
Typical daily dose	1–2 mg
Dose range	0.5 mg every other day to 2 mg/day
Therapeutic serum level	Not established

Comments: Not a first-line drug in the elderly because of prolonged half-life and extensive hepatic metabolism. Rapidly and well absorbed orally. 85% protein bound. Onset of action in 20–60 minutes, duration of action 12 hours. Extensively metabolized in the liver to inactive metabolites. Major substrate of CYP3A4. Metabolites excreted as glucuronide or sulfate conjugates. Contraindicated in patients with significant hepatic impairment. Use with caution in patients with renal impairment, respiratory disease, or impaired gag reflex. Additive effects with alcohol and other CNS depressants; increased risk of falls. *Other drug interactions:* CYP3A4 inducers and inhibitors (see Table 2–2), increased clonazepam level with disulfiram, clonazepam possibly diminishes effect of levodopa, theophylline diminishes effect of clonazepam, absence seizures when clonazepam and valproate are combined. *Adverse effects:* Amnesia, ataxia, dysarthria, sedation, incoordination, dizziness, depression with suicidality, confusion, hallucinations, emotional lability, paradoxical aggression, insomnia, behavioral problems, anorexia, constipation, dehydration, diarrhea, nausea, dry mouth, dysuria, change in frequency of urination, nocturia, urinary retention, encopresis, blood dyscrasias, increased liver function test scores, weakness, myalgia, blurred vision, and increased respiratory secretions.

Generic name	eszopiclone
Trade name	Lunesta
Class	Nonbenzodiazepine hypnotic
Half-life	9 hours in elderly
Mechanism of action	Potentiates effects of GABA, probably by binding to specific "microdomains" within the γ subunit of the $GABA_A$ receptor
Available preparations	Tablets: 1, 2, 3 mg
Starting dose	1 mg for difficulty falling asleep 2 mg for difficulty staying asleep
Titration	N/A
Typical daily dose	1–2 mg qhs
Dose range	1–2 mg qhs
Therapeutic serum level	Not established

Comments: Rapid onset of action, delayed by food (especially high-fat foods or a heavy meal). Peak plasma level in 1 hour. 52%–59% protein bound. Metabolized in the liver via oxidation and demethylation. Major substrate of CYP3A4, minor of CYP2E1. Two metabolites, one with activity less than parent drug. Excreted in urine, mostly as metabolites. Drug interactions: CYP3A4 inhibitors and inducers (see Table 2–2). With olanzapine, possible decreased psychomotor function. Common adverse effects (> 10%): Headache, unpleasant taste. Less common adverse effects (1%–10%): Chest pain, edema, somnolence, dizziness, dry mouth, and dyspepsia. Uncommon but serious adverse effects: Dysphagia, hepatitis, hypertension, incoordination, and ataxia, among others.

Generic name	gabapentin
Trade name	Neurontin (generic available)
Class	Anticonvulsant structurally related to GABA
Half-life	5–7 hours
Mechanism of action	No direct GABA-agonist effects; may increase GABA levels by inhibiting the GABA transporter
Available preparations	Capsules: 100, 300, 400 mg Tablets: 100, 300, 400, 600, 800 mg Oral solution: 250 mg/5 mL
Starting dose	Sedation: 100 mg every 12 hrs Insomnia: 100 mg qhs
Titration	Sedation: increase by 100 mg every 3–5 days, as tolerated Insomnia: increase to 200 mg on second night and 300 mg on third night, as needed and tolerated
Typical daily dose	Sedation: 100 mg tid Insomnia: 300 mg qhs
Dose range	100–1,800 mg/day for anxiolytic effect
Therapeutic serum level	Obtainable, but not used clinically

Comments: Anecdotal experience suggests efficacy of gabapentin for insomnia and anxiety, certain pain syndromes, tremor, and some parkinsonian symptoms in elderly patients; controlled studies not performed to date except in neuropathic pain and social phobia. In proximal small bowel, 50%–60% is absorbed via L-amino transport system. Reduced bioavailability at higher doses because of saturable absorption. Less than 3% protein bound. Not metabolized; excreted in urine as unchanged drug. Clearance declines with age. Dosage adjustment required for renal failure; administered after hemodialysis. Avoid abrupt withdrawal upon discontinuation (seizure risk). *Drug interactions:* Additive effects with other CNS depressants. *Relatively common adverse effects:* Somnolence, dizziness, ataxia, fatigue, peripheral edema, diarrhea, tremor, weakness, nystagmus, and diplopia. Induction of rapid cycling reported in some patients with bipolar disorder. At high doses, asterixis and encephalopathy reported. *Uncommon but serious adverse effect:* Acute renal failure.

Generic name	lorazepam
Trade name	Ativan, Lorazepam Intensol (generic available)
Class	Benzodiazepine
Half-life	10–16 hours
Mechanism of action	Potentiates effects of GABA by binding to $GABA_A$-benzodiazepine receptor complex
Available preparations	Tablets: 0.5, 1, 2 mg Oral concentrate: 2 mg/mL Injectable: 2 or 4 mg/mL
Starting dose	Anxiety: 0.5 mg/day to bid po; 0.25 mg iv bid to tid Insomnia: 0.5–1 mg po hs
Titration	Anxiety: increase by 0.5 mg every 4–5 days, as needed and as tolerated
Typical daily dose	Anxiety: 0.5–1 mg bid to tid Insomnia: 0.5–1 mg hs
Dose range	0.5–4 mg/day
Therapeutic serum level	Obtainable, but not used clinically

Comments: A first-line benzodiazepine for anxiolysis and sedation in elderly patients because of favorable pharmacokinetic profile. Not necessarily recommended for routine use as a hypnotic because some patients report wearing off during the night. Promptly absorbed orally, and reliably absorbed with intramuscular use (not recommended). 85% protein bound. Metabolized by conjugation in the liver; no active metabolites. Excreted in urine. *Drug interactions:* Additive effects with other CNS depressants. *Common adverse effects (> 10%):* Sedation and respiratory depression. *Less common adverse effects (1%–10%):* Hypotension, confusion, dizziness, akathisia, unsteadiness, headache, depression, disorientation, amnesia, weight loss or gain, nausea, change in appetite, weakness, hyperventilation, and apnea. *Uncommon but serious adverse effects:* Blood dyscrasias and polyethylene glycol or propylene glycol poisoning (with prolonged intravenous infusion only).

Generic name	oxazepam
Trade name	Serax (generic available)
Class	Benzodiazepine
Half-life	5–20 hours
Mechanism of action	Potentiates effects of GABA by binding to GABA$_A$-benzodiazepine receptor complex
Available preparations	Capsules: 10, 15, 30 mg Tablets: 15 mg
Starting dose	Anxiety: 10 mg bid to 10 mg tid Insomnia: 10 or 15 mg hs
Titration	Increase by 5–15 mg/day every 4–5 days, as needed and as tolerated
Typical daily dose	Anxiety: 10 mg tid Insomnia: 15 mg hs
Dose range	Anxiety: 10 mg/day to 15 mg tid Insomnia: 10–30 mg hs
Therapeutic serum level	Obtainable, but not used clinically

Comments: A first-line drug in the treatment of elderly patients because of favorable pharmacokinetics. Completely but slowly absorbed orally; therefore it is not useful prn and not useful for initial insomnia unless taken several hours before bedtime. Peak serum concentration in 2–4 hours (faster for tablet than for capsule). 86%–99% protein bound. Metabolized in the liver to inactive compounds, mainly glucuronides. Wide variation in half-life; some individuals with anxiety require at least tid dosing for symptom control. Not dialyzable. *Drug interactions:* Additive effects with other CNS depressants. *Adverse effects:* Edema, drowsiness, ataxia, dizziness, memory impairment, headache, paradoxical excitement, incontinence, blood dyscrasias, jaundice, dysarthria, tremor, diplopia, and syncope (rare).

Generic name	ramelteon
Trade name	Rozerem
Class	Selective MT_1 and MT_2 receptor agonist
Half-life	1–2.6 hours
Mechanism of action	Promotes sleep by acting on the system (involving the MT_1 and MT_2 receptors) involved in maintaining the circadian rhythm underlying the sleep-wake cycle
Available preparations	Tablets: 8 mg
Starting dose	8 mg within 30 minutes of bedtime
Titration	N/A
Typical daily dose	8 mg within 30 minutes of bedtime
Dose range	N/A
Therapeutic serum level	Not established

Comments: A newly approved drug for treatment of insomnia with a unique mechanism of action. Rapidly absorbed, with absorption significantly affected by high-fat foods (it is recommended to avoid giving with a high-fat meal). High first-pass metabolism; bioavailability 1.8%. Protein binding 82%, mostly to albumin. Metabolized in the liver, mostly via CYP1A2 but also via CYP3A4 and CYP2C. One metabolite (M-II) circulates in higher concentration than parent compound, but much less active than parent. Other metabolites inactive. Excreted in urine. *Drug interactions:* Significant interactions with CYP1A2 inhibitors (especially fluvoxamine) and inducers, and also with CYP3A4 and CYP2C inhibitors and inducers (see Table 2–2). *Adverse effects:* Somnolence, dizziness, nausea, fatigue, headache, exacerbation of insomnia, and possibly prolactin elevation.

Generic name	temazepam
Trade name	Restoril (generic available)
Class	Benzodiazepine
Half-life	10–20 hours
Mechanism of action	Potentiates effects of GABA by binding to GABA$_A$-benzodiazepine receptor complex
Available preparations	Capsules: 7.5, 15, 30 mg
Starting dose	7.5 mg po hs
Titration	Increase by 7.5 mg every 4–5 days as needed and as tolerated
Typical daily dose	15 mg po hs (given 1 hour before bedtime)
Dose range	7.5–5 mg hs
Therapeutic serum level	Obtainable, but not used clinically

Comments: Would be a first-line drug for the treatment of insomnia in elderly patients, if not for half-life; although variable, half-life is long enough that some patients experience next-day sedation, particularly at higher doses. Onset of action in 30–60 minutes, peak levels in 1–3 hours. 96% protein bound. Metabolized in the liver to inactive metabolites, primarily via glucuronidation; substrate of UGT2B7. Minor substrate of CYP2B6, 2C8/9, 2C19, and 3A4. Eliminated in the urine. *Drug interactions:* Additive effects with other CNS depressants; theophylline may antagonize benzodiazepine effects. *Less common adverse effects (1%–10%):* Confusion, dizziness, drowsiness, fatigue, anxiety, headache, lethargy, hangover, euphoria, vertigo, diarrhea, dysarthria, weakness, blurred vision, and diaphoresis. *Less common but serious effects:* Ataxia, blood dyscrasias, and paradoxical reactions.

Generic name	trazodone
Trade name	Desyrel (generic available)
Class	Atypical antidepressant
Half-life	11.6 hours
Mechanism of action	Parent drug antagonizes $5\text{-HT}_{2A/2C}$ receptors, mCPP metabolite agonist at 5-HT_{1C}, antagonist at α_2, significant α_1 and histamine blockade
Available preparations	Tablets: 50, 100, 150, 300 mg
Starting dose	25 mg qhs
Titration	Increase by 25 mg every 3–5 days, as tolerated
Typical daily dose	Insomnia: 25–50 mg qhs
Dose range	12.5–100 mg qhs
Therapeutic serum level	Not established

Comments: Widely used in the past as a hypnotic for elderly patients, in spite of problems with orthostasis. Onset of sedative effect in 20–30 minutes; peaks at 30 minutes. Absorption delayed by food (up to 2.5 hours). 85%–95% protein bound. Greatly increased volume of distribution in obese patients, resulting in prolonged half-life. Extensively metabolized in the liver via CYP3A4; mCPP is an active metabolite that may be anxiogenic for some patients. CYP2D6 inhibitor. Reduced clearance in elderly men necessitates dose reduction with chronic administration. Minimal anticholinergic effects. *Drug interactions:* Expected interactions due to CYP3A4 and 2D6 effects, serotonin syndrome with other serotonergic agents, additive hypotensive effects with low-potency antipsychotics. *Adverse effects:* Orthostasis (α_1 effect), ventricular irritability (premature ventricular contractions, possible ventricular tachycardia), sedation, dizziness, gait instability, mild cognitive impairment, seizures, weight gain, priapism, headache, dry mouth, edema, nausea, and diarrhea.

Generic name	zaleplon
Trade name	Sonata
Class	Nonbenzodiazepine hypnotic
Half-life	1 hour
Mechanism of action	Potentiates the effects of GABA by binding to the benzodiazepine site on the $GABA_A$ receptor, with high affinity only for receptors containing the α_1 subunit (formerly termed *omega-1 receptors*).
Available preparations	Capsules: 5, 10 mg
Starting dose	5 mg po qhs (given immediately before bedtime)
Titration	Increase by 5 mg po qhs as needed and as tolerated
Typical daily dose	5 mg po qhs (given immediately before bedtime)
Dose range	5–10 mg po qhs (given immediately before bedtime)
Therapeutic serum level	Not established

Comments: May be useful in reducing sleep latency in elders, but less useful for sleep maintenance overnight because of short duration of action (about 4 hours). Rapidly absorbed, with rapid onset of action. Peak serum levels in 1 hour. Food (especially with high fat content) may delay absorption. Bioavailability 30%. Extensively metabolized, primarily by aldehyde oxidase but also by CYP3A4 to inactive metabolites, mostly excreted in urine. *Drug interactions:* Cimetidine inhibits both aldehyde oxidase and CYP3A4 and can significantly increase zaleplon levels; additive sedative effects with other CNS depressants; zaleplon may potentiate CNS adverse effects of conventional antipsychotics (e.g., thioridazine) and tricyclic antidepressants (e.g., imipramine). *Less common adverse effects (1%–10%):* Chest pain, edema, amnesia, dizziness, hallucinations, light-headedness, incoordination, anorexia, dyspepsia, nausea, constipation, dry mouth, tremor, weakness, and arthralgias. *Uncommon but serious adverse effects:* Angina, ataxia, bundle branch block, ventricular tachycardia, pericardial effusion, syncope, and urinary retention.

Generic name	zolpidem
Trade name	Ambien
Class	Nonbenzodiazepine hypnotic
Half-life	2.6 hours (longer in elderly patients)
Mechanism of action	Potentiates the effects of GABA by binding to the benzodiazepine site on the $GABA_A$ receptor, with high affinity only for receptors containing the α_1 subunit (formerly termed *omega-1 receptors*).
Available preparations	Tablets: 5, 10 mg Controlled-release tablets: 6.25, 12.5 mg
Starting dose	5 mg hs (given immediately before bedtime)
Titration	Increase by 5 mg, as needed and as tolerated
Typical daily dose	5 mg hs (given immediately before bedtime)
Dose range	5–10 mg hs (given immediately before bedtime)
Therapeutic serum level	80–150 ng/mL (not well established)

Comments: May be a drug of choice for the elderly for short-term treatment of insomnia. Pharmacokinetics are affected by age (increased AUC and half-life in elderly) and gender (higher plasma concentrations in women). Rapidly absorbed. First-pass metabolism results in 70% bioavailability. Rapid onset of effect (within 30 minutes), with peak levels in 2.2 hours and duration of action of 6–8 hours; useful to initiate and to maintain sleep. 92% protein bound. Metabolized mostly via CYP3A4, also by CYP1A2, 2C8/9, 2C19, and 2D6 to inactive metabolites. Rapidly eliminated. Dose must be reduced in renal or hepatic disease. Half-life in cirrhosis increased to about 10 hours. *Drug interactions:* Significant, with CYP3A4 inhibitors and inducers (Table 2–2); additive sedative effects with other CNS depressants; rifamycin derivatives may decrease zolpidem levels. On discontinuation, a withdrawal syndrome can occur, with symptoms of tachycardia, tachypnea, anxiety, tremor, sweating, nausea, and abdominal pain. *Less common adverse effects (1%–10%):* Palpitations, headache, dizziness, light-headedness, amnesia, nausea, diarrhea, dry mouth, and constipation. *Less common but serious adverse reactions:* Confusion and falls.

7

Treatment of Substance-Related Disorders

Introduction

In the current cohort of elders, substance abuse and dependence relates mainly to alcohol and tobacco. Currently abused substances in this cohort are mainly alcohol and tobacco. Abuse of drugs such as stimulants and opioids occurs much less commonly, although this pattern may change as the large group of baby boomers grows into old age. In the current cohort of elders, benzodiazepines are the most abused of prescribed medications, an order of magnitude more common than prescribed narcotics (Holroyd and Duryee 1997).

In general, substance-related disorders are classified as either *substance use disorders* (abuse and dependence) or *substance-induced disorders* (e.g., intoxication, withdrawal, cognitive disorders, mood disorders). DSM-IV-TR substance-related disorders are listed in Table 7–1.

Substance abuse is a maladaptive pattern involving harmful consequences of repeated use of alcohol, a drug, or a medication. An elderly alcohol abuser, for example, may meet this criterion by failing to maintain adequate hygiene, suffering repeated falls, failing to seek needed medical care, or alienating children through constant arguments about the consequences of intoxication. *Substance dependence* is a maladaptive pattern involving the development of tolerance, withdrawal symptoms on discontinuation, compulsive use, restriction of activities, and/or continued use despite adverse

Table 7–1. DSM-IV-TR substance-related disorders affecting the elderly

303.90	Alcohol dependence
305.00	Alcohol abuse
303.00	Alcohol intoxication
291.81	Alcohol withdrawal
291.0	Alcohol intoxication delirium
291.0	Alcohol withdrawal delirium
291.2	Alcohol-induced persisting dementia
291.1	Alcohol-induced persisting amnestic disorder
291.x	Alcohol-induced psychotic disorder
.5	with delusions
.3	with hallucinations
291.89	Alcohol-induced disorders:
	Mood disorder
	Anxiety disorder
	Sexual dysfunction
	Sleep disorder
291.9	Alcohol-related disorder not otherwise specified
305.1	Nicotine use disorder
292.0	Nicotine withdrawal
292.9	Nicotine-related disorder
304.00	Opioid dependence
305.50	Opioid abuse
292.89	Opioid intoxication
292.0	Opioid withdrawal
292.81	Opioid intoxication delirium
292.xx	Opioid-induced psychotic disorder
.11	with delusions
.12	with hallucinations
292.84	Opioid-induced mood disorder

Table 7–1. DSM-IV-TR substance-related disorders affecting the elderly *(continued)*

292.89	Opioid-induced sexual dysfunction
292.89	Opioid-induced sleep disorder
292.9	Opioid-related disorder not otherwise specified
304.10	Sedative, hypnotic, or anxiolytic dependence
305.40	Sedative, hypnotic, or anxiolytic abuse
292.89	Sedative, hypnotic, or anxiolytic intoxication
292.0	Sedative, hypnotic, or anxiolytic withdrawal
292.81	Sedative, hypnotic, or anxiolytic intoxication delirium
292.81	Sedative, hypnotic, or anxiolytic withdrawal delirium
292.82	Sedative, hypnotic, or anxiolytic-induced persisting dementia
292.83	Sedative, hypnotic, or anxiolytic-induced persisting amnestic disorder
292.xx	Sedative, hypnotic, or anxiolytic-induced psychotic disorder
.11	with delusions
.12	with hallucinations
292.84	Sedative, hypnotic, or anxiolytic-induced mood disorder
292.89	Sedative, hypnotic, or anxiolytic-induced disorders:
	Anxiety disorder
	Sexual dysfunction
	Sleep disorder
292.9	Sedative, hypnotic, or anxiolytic-related disorder not otherwise specified
304.80	Polysubstance dependence

physical or psychological effects. Applied to alcohol, substance dependence is more commonly known as *alcoholism*. In general, alcohol abuse is more prevalent than alcohol dependence, and problem drinking (not a DSM term) is more prevalent than abuse. Different definitions of *problem drinking* exist; one definition that has been used for older drinkers is as follows: daily drinking of more than two drinks in men or more than one drink in women, or recurrent binge drinking.

As Ciraulo and others have pointed out, the application of the abuse/ dependence criteria to the patient using prescribed medications such as benzodiazepines is problematic (Ciraulo et al. 2005). With these substances, physiologic dependence develops with normal clinical use, and a withdrawal syndrome on abrupt discontinuation would be expected. Moreover, some patients with anxiety disorders adjust the dose of benzodiazepine on their own, depending on the severity of symptoms. Patients who do so responsibly do not warrant a label of addiction (Ciraulo et al. 2005).

Identification of substance abuse or dependence in elders involves a careful and corroborated history, physical and mental status examinations, and laboratory testing drug screens. Elders who present with any of the following should be screened for substance abuse/dependence: trauma or history of recent overdose, respiratory depression, hypotension or hypertension, cardiac arrhythmia, ataxia, seizure(s), psychosis (especially tactile or visual hallucinations), or other mental status changes (Hammett-Stabler et al. 2002).

In the emergency department setting, drug screens need to be done quickly and sent for analysis within 1 hour of the patient's presentation, if possible (Hammett-Stabler et al. 2002). Both serum and urine specimens should be obtained. Serum drug screening is usually performed for ethanol, acetaminophen, and salicylates, the latter being of interest for reasons other than substance abuse screening. Urine drug screening is usually performed for opioids, heroin, methadone, benzodiazepines, cocaine, amphetamines, methamphetamines, and barbiturates. Drugs that are included in the screening vary by laboratory; often, laboratories do not distinguish individual opioids or metabolites but can perform more specific analyses upon request. Assays also are available for currently abused drugs, including cannabis, γ-hydroxybutyrate (GHB), 3,4-methylenedioxymethamphetamine (MDMA or Ecstasy), phencyclidine (PCP), and lysergic acid diethylamide (LSD), but these are complex analyses that are not routinely done (Hammett-Stabler et al. 2002) and are not often indicated in the workup of an elderly patient.

Obtaining a urine specimen from an elderly patient in the emergency department may be complicated by dehydration (requiring hydration first) or urinary incontinence (requiring catheterization). Furthermore, it should be noted that in the case of a very recent ingestion, the drug might not yet appear in urine, and in the case of a very long-acting or highly lip-id-soluble drug identified in urine, the ingestion might not have been recent (Hammett-Stabler et al. 2002). Moreover, false-positive urine test results for amphetamines may be obtained with clinical use of bupropion, desipramine, or conventional antipsychotics such as chlorpromazine (Weintraub and Linder 2000).

Basic Pharmacology of Ethanol

The presence of food in the stomach or the ingestion of food with alcohol has significant pharmacokinetic effects, delaying the time to peak alcohol concentration, lowering the peak concentration itself, and reducing the total amount of alcohol reaching the systemic circulation (Kranzler and Ciraulo 2005). Alcohol in the circulation distributes rapidly to well-perfused tissues such as the brain. As much as 10% of ethanol is excreted unchanged through the respiratory and urinary tracts. Elimination through respiration gives rise to the smell of alcohol on the breath and makes it possible to determine alcohol level using a Breathalyzer (Kranzler and Ciraulo 2005).

Alcohol is metabolized by alcohol dehydrogenase or cytochrome P450 (CYP) 2E1 to acetaldehyde, which is in turn metabolized by aldehyde dehydrogenase to acetic acid, which enters the Krebs cycle. Acetaldehyde is a toxic intermediate that gives rise to flushing reactions and other symptoms. Disulfiram (Antabuse) acts by inhibiting the second step in alcohol metabolism, resulting in buildup of acetaldehyde. CYP2E1 activity is induced by alcohol itself, so it assumes more significance as a metabolic route in heavier drinkers. Functional polymorphisms exist for all enzymes involved in alcohol metabolism, and these may contribute to variability in the risk of developing alcohol dependence and related illnesses (Kranzler and Ciraulo 2005). Significant alterations in serotonin function in chronic alcoholism are likely correlated with alcohol-induced mood and anxiety disorders. It has been hypothesized that low doses of alcohol have positive reinforcing effects by virtue of effects on γ-aminobutyric acid type A ($GABA_A$) receptors and dopamine receptors, whereas higher doses of alcohol (associated with intoxication) are not reinforcing because of antagonism at N-methyl-D-aspartate (NMDA) receptors (Kranzler and Ciraulo 2005).

Alcohol-Related Disorders

Alcohol overuse is the most significant substance abuse problem among the current cohort of elders. During the 1990s, alcohol use disorders among those 65 years of age and older increased from 0.64% to 1.45%, with abuse showing an approximately fivefold increase and dependence showing a small decrease (B.F. Grant et al. 2004a). Rates are higher among clinical populations. When elders (>60 years of age) in the emergency department were studied, current alcohol use disorders were identified in 5.3% of patients (Onen et al. 2005). Rates are also much higher for problem drinking than for abuse or dependence.

Although many different drinking patterns are seen, most elders who drink do so in small amounts on a daily basis. These small amounts may have disproportionately large effects because of age-related pharmacokinetic and pharmacodynamic changes, coprescribed medications, and comorbid illness. Some individuals exhibit either the onset or an acceleration of drinking just after retirement (Giordano and Beckman 1985). This late-onset (after 60 years of age) pattern accounts for approximately one-third of elders with alcohol use disorders, is more common in women, and is thought to reflect problems in coping with life changes (Barrick and Connors 2002). In contrast, those with the early-onset pattern are more likely to have a positive family history of alcohol use disorders and a higher prevalence of comorbid psychiatric conditions (Barrick and Connors 2002). Early-onset individuals may continue established drinking patterns into older age and then come to clinical attention because of developing comorbidities. They are more likely to be male, homeless or living alone, and either never married or separated or divorced (Onen et al. 2005).

Identification of early-onset drinkers or those with advanced alcohol dependence is not difficult; these patients may be brought to the emergency department by police after trauma or because of disorderly conduct. Often, they present with serious comorbidities, such as those listed in Table 7–2. These patients tend to be "young-old" (<75 years of age) with an apparent biologic age greater than chronologic age.

Identification of late-onset drinkers, whose drinking behaviors are only beginning to have medical and psychiatric consequences, may be

Table 7–2. Alcoholism: comorbid medical and psychiatric conditions

Abdominal obesity	Hostility
Aggression	Hygiene problems
Amnesia	Hypercortisolemia
Anemia	Hyperhomocysteinemia
Anxiety	Hypertension
Apathy	Infection
Ataxia	Insomnia
Bruising	Irritability
Cardiomyopathy	Legal problems
Cerebellar degeneration	Malignancy
Cirrhosis	Malnutrition
Dehydration	Medical noncompliance
Delirium	Nausea/Vomiting
Delusions	Neuropathy
Dementia	Osteoporosis
Dental caries	Pancreatitis
Depression	Panic attacks
Electrolyte derangements	Pneumonia
Esophageal varices	Seizures
Falls	Sexual dysfunction
Fractures	Social isolation
Gastritis	Suicidal ideation
Gastrointestinal bleeding	Trauma
Hallucinations	Ulcers
Hepatitis	Wernicke's encephalopathy
Homicidal ideation	

much more difficult. Problem drinking is a covert behavior, often hidden even from close family members. Elders with problem drinking do not necessarily come to clinical attention in the same way that younger drinkers do because in many cases they are not employed and are socially isolated. Among older individuals arrested for driving under the influence of alcohol, most have a lifetime history of alcohol abuse or dependence, and most do not change drinking behavior as a consequence of the arrest (Oslin et al. 1999). Elderly drinkers may present with a cluster of individual comorbidities, as listed in Table 7–2. The list can be used as a review of systems for alcoholism; the more positives, the more likely it becomes that covert alcoholism is an issue.

Alcoholism is principally diagnosed by the individual's history of use, and this may be problematic for elderly patients because they are more likely to deny alcohol use. Several alcoholism screening instruments are used in elderly clinical populations, including the CAGE screening for alcoholism (Buchsbaum et al. 1992), the Alcohol Use Disorders Identification Test (AUDIT) (Bradley et al. 1998), and the Michigan Alcoholism Screening Test—Geriatrics Version (MAST-G). The CAGE Questionnaire has the advantage of brevity but is not well suited to the patient who intends to minimize a drinking problem. The AUDIT does not address many of the problems that particularly plague the alcoholic elder, such as malnutrition or frequent falls. The MAST-G is recommended as a screening instrument and is reproduced as Figure 7–1. Used in a face-to-face encounter with the elder suspected of harmful drinking, this instrument can be therapeutic in helping the patient get past denial of the problem. It is sometimes helpful to obtain the patient's history regarding quantity and frequency of drinking after the MAST-G has been completed, when there may be less of a tendency for the patient to minimize drinking. The Alcohol-Related Problems Survey (ARPS) is another instrument that provides a more detailed inventory of physical and neuropsychiatric problems associated with drinking in elders (Fink et al. 2002).

Laboratory tests that may be useful in confirming recent alcohol consumption include breath analysis, urine alcohol, blood alcohol level (BAL), serum γ-glutamyltransferase (GGT), and percent serum carbohydrate-deficient transferrin (CDT) (Spies et al. 1996). GGT and CDT

Treatment of Substance-Related Disorders 411

have been studied and found useful as markers in mixed-age samples (Gomez et al. 2001; Stranges et al. 2004), but in general they have been found to have better predictive validity in clinical than in community-dwelling populations (Alte et al. 2004; Forsberg et al. 2002). CDT is arguably the most sensitive and specific of these markers (Lesch et al. 1996), but CDT and GGT appear to complement one another, and together the two appear to have better predictive value than either test alone (Schuckit and Tapert 2004) in male drinkers; in females, GGT alone appears to have better predictive value (Chen et al. 2003). GGT elevation is consistent with a history of four or more drinks a day for 4 weeks or more (Schuckit and Tapert 2004). GGT values considered elevated are >35 U/L in men and >30 U/L in women (Schuckit and Tapert 2004). CDT values considered elevated are >20 U/L in men and >26 U/L in women (Schuckit and Tapert 2004). These markers start to normalize within days of drinking cessation and become normal within 2 weeks (Schuckit and Tapert 2004).

Other possible markers of heavy drinking include aspartate transaminase (AST), alanine transaminase (ALT), mean corpuscular volume (MCV), and serum uric acid level. An MCV >91 μm^3 is a relatively good marker; AST >40 U/L in men or >35 U/L in women is a fair marker; ALT >46 in men or >35 in women is a fair marker; uric acid >8.0 mg/dL in men or >6.2 mg/dL in women is a fair marker (Schuckit and Tapert 2004). These markers are not used for confirmation of diagnosis because each can be affected by other comorbid medical conditions (Chang et al. 1990; Mowe and Bohmer 1996; Nyblom et al. 2004).

In recent years, investigators have found that patients with chronic alcoholism have elevated serum total homocysteine levels (Bayerlein et al. 2005; Bleich et al. 2004). Homocysteine is a known neurotoxin with a role in the excitatory cascade involving NMDA receptor activation. High homocysteine levels (>15 $\mu mol/L$) have been linked to alcohol withdrawal seizures (Bayerlein et al. 2005). Although it is possible that chronically elevated homocysteine may be implicated in the neuronal loss (atrophy) seen on neuroimaging studies of patients with alcoholism, this link has yet to be established. It is perhaps relevant that homocysteine levels can be lowered with oral administration of B-complex vitamins, folate in particular, as well as abstinence from alcohol (Bayerlein et al. 2005; Bleich et al. 2004).

412   Clinical Manual of Geriatric Psychopharmacology

Michigan Alcoholism Screening Test—Geriatric Version

1. After drinking; have you ever noticed an increase   Yes   No
   in your heart rate or beating in your chest?

2. When talking with others, do you ever under-   Yes   No
   estimate how much you actually drink?

3. Does alcohol make you sleepy so that you often   Yes   No
   fall asleep in your chair?

4. After a few drinks, have you sometimes not eaten   Yes   No
   or been able to skip a meal because you didn't
   feel hungry?

5. Does having a few drinks help decrease your   Yes   No
   shakiness or tremors?

6. Does alcohol sometimes make it hard for you to   Yes   No
   remember parts of the day or night?

7. Do you have rules for yourself that you won't drink   Yes   No
   before a certain time of the day?

8. Have you lost interest in hobbies and activities you   Yes   No
   used to enjoy?

9. When you wake up in the morning, do you ever   Yes   No
   have trouble remembering part of the night before?

10. Does having a drink help you sleep?   Yes   No

11. Do you hide your alcohol bottles from family   Yes   No
    members?

12. After a social gathering, have you ever felt   Yes   No
    embarrassed because you drank too much?

13. Have you ever been concerned that drinking might   Yes   No
    be harmful to your health?

14. Do you like to end an evening with a nightcap?   Yes   No

15. Did you find your drinking increased after someone   Yes   No
    close to you died?

Figure 7–1.   Michigan Alcoholism Screening Test—Geriatric
Version.

Source.   University of Michigan Alcohol Research Center: "Michigan Alcohol Screening Test (MAST-G)" The Regents of the University of Michigan © 1991. Used with permission.

16. In general, would you prefer to have a few drinks at home rather than go out to social events?   Yes   No

17. Are you drinking more now than in the past?   Yes   No

18. Do you usually take a drink to relax or calm your nerves?   Yes   No

19. Do you drink to take your mind off your problems?   Yes   No

20. Have you ever increased your drinking after experiencing a loss in your life?   Yes   No

21. Do you sometimes drive when you have had too much to drink?   Yes   No

22. Has a doctor or nurse ever said they were worried or concerned about your drinking?   Yes   No

23. Have you ever made rules to manage your drinking?   Yes   No

24. When you feel lonely, does having a drink help?   Yes   No

Scoring: Five or more "yes" responses are indicative of an alcohol problem.

Figure 7–1. Michigan Alcoholism Screening Test–Geriatric Version. *(Continued)*

Cerebellar atrophy and cerebral cortical atrophy that is most prominent frontally are commonly seen on computed tomography (CT) or magnetic resonance imaging (MRI) studies of the head in elderly patients with alcohol use disorders, although these findings are nonspecific (Carlen et al. 1978, 1986; Pfefferbaum et al. 1988). Frontal atrophy may be associated with lack of motivation and social withdrawal, which could be expected to influence the success of alcoholism treatment (Rosse et al. 1997). In addition, frontal atrophy may underlie the poor decision-making abilities of long-standing drinkers.

The prognosis for the alcohol-dependent elder depends in part on the duration of drinking. Those with late-onset alcohol dependence generally have a better prognosis (Gomberg 2004). In elders with long-standing drinking problems, denial may be very entrenched not only in the patient but in the family as well, particularly the spouse. Laboratory abnormalities as objective markers can help in the discussion regarding problem drinking. In long-standing drinkers, readiness to change is likely to be low. In fact, these patients are unlikely to enter treatment voluntarily (Gomberg 2004). Comorbidity with depression is high in this population and contributes to persistence in drinking, greater functional disability, and poorer perceived health (Oslin et al. 1999, 2000). Thus, a convincing argument can be made for the assessment of alcohol use in patients being evaluated for late-life depression (Oslin 2005).

Alcohol Dependence

There is ongoing controversy as to whether treatment for alcohol dependence necessarily involves complete abstinence from alcohol. Some argue that this may be an unachievable goal for the long-standing drinker and advocate an emphasis on day-to-day sobriety. For all patients, nonpharmacologic interventions may be useful in initiating and maintaining abstinence. Physician counseling about alcohol overuse is associated with a significant decrease in alcohol consumption among hospital and clinic patients (Fleming et al. 1999; Moore et al. 1989). Continued abstinence among elders depends on a fairly intensive regimen of regular attendance at programs such as Alcoholics Anonymous or Rational Recovery, an ongoing one-to-one relationship with a supportive family/friend surrogate (usually a sponsor or counselor), regularly scheduled medical and psychiatric follow-up visits, and repeated reinforcement for abstinence. Some elders respond well to group therapy experiences directed toward resocialization as long as they are with age peers who also have a history of alcohol dependence (Gomberg 2004). Family therapy may be used to reduce enabling, deal with conflict, and address poor family dynamics (Gomberg 2004). For homebound elders, identification and education of the supplier of alcohol may be a critical step. Helping the patient and family to identify appropriate medical, dental, and home health services may be useful, as may the arrangement of meals-on-wheels service or participation in senior center activities (Gomberg 2004).

Three medications currently have U.S. Food and Drug Administration (FDA)–approved labeling for treatment of alcohol dependence: naltrexone, acamprosate, and disulfiram. Although most is known about naltrexone, none of these agents have been extensively studied in the geriatric population. Other medications such as ondansetron and topiramate may be useful in some patients, although this claim is based on even more limited evidence. Antidepressants (particularly selective serotonin reuptake inhibitors [SSRIs]) may be helpful for patients with comorbid depression. Table 7–3 summarizes dosing and dose titration for the FDA-approved drugs for treatment of alcohol dependence in the geriatric population.

Naltrexone

Naltrexone is a nonspecific, opioid antagonist that acts by opposing the reinforcing effects of alcohol, suppressing craving, and reducing the chance of continued drinking after a slip (O'Malley et al. 1996; Swift 1998). In one of the only studies of specific pharmacologic treatment for alcohol dependence in older patients, naltrexone was found to be well tolerated and to have a significant effect in preventing relapse (bingeing) in patients who drank after achieving abstinence (Oslin et al. 1997a). Naltrexone should always be administered in conjunction with appropriate nonpharmacologic interventions and should be avoided in patients who are opioid dependent because of the risk of precipitating withdrawal. Side effects are otherwise minimal, and no effect on liver function test values is seen at recommended doses. Naltrexone should be initiated at 25 mg/day in elderly patients, and the dosage should be maintained at that level or increased to 50 mg/day for the duration of treatment (Oslin et al. 1997a).

There is some evidence that a common functional polymorphism in the μ opioid receptor gene (*OPRM1* Asn40Asp) may act as a gatekeeper in the action of naltrexone, affecting an individual's response to the drug (Oslin et al. 2003). The COMBINE Study currently under way is designed to investigate this and other genetic markers relating to addiction and its treatments (Goldman et al. 2005).

In the past, the use of naltrexone was limited by low patient acceptance and poor compliance; the patient who wanted to drink simply stopped taking the medication. For this reason, there has been considerable interest in the development of long-acting injectable forms. One such

Table 7–3. Pharmacologic treatment of alcohol dependence in elderly patients

Drug	Initial dose	Dose titration	Usual therapeutic dose
acamprosate (Campral)	333 mg tid	Increase after 7 days	666 mg tid
disulfiram (Antabuse)	250 mg qd	See Specific Drug summary	125 mg qd (maintenance)
naltrexone (ReVia)	25 mg qd	See Specific Drug summary	50 mg qd

Note. tid = three times a day; qd = once a day.

preparation (Vivitrol, known during trials as Vivitrex) received FDA approval in 2006 and is now available as a monthly injection.

Acamprosate

Acamprosate was approved by the FDA in 2004 and is now marketed in a delayed-release tablet form (Campral). Acamprosate is thought to act by reducing glutamatergic activity and increasing GABAergic activity in the central nervous system (CNS). In addition to its role in treating alcohol dependence, this drug may have a role in treating alcohol withdrawal by protecting against excitotoxic cell death, reducing kindling, and preventing the emergence of negative craving (wanting to drink to avoid withdrawal symptoms) (De Witte et al. 2005). Whether acamprosate has such effects remains to be investigated. When acamprosate is used, it should be started as soon as possible after abstinence has been achieved and continued for 12 months or more, even through relapses (De Witte et al. 2005). This drug promotes continued abstinence and reduces the severity of relapses.

Only 1% of the patients in the initial clinical trials for acamprosate were over 65 years of age, and none was over 75 years of age. The manufacturer recommends against the use of the drug in the geriatric population until more is known about efficacy and safety. Several randomized controlled trials in nongeriatric patients have demonstrated the longer-term effectiveness and safety of this drug in the maintenance of abstinence when it is used as an adjunct to psychosocial therapy (Paille et al. 1995; Whitworth et al. 1996). A pooled analysis of European trials of acamprosate in the nongeriatric population suggested that acamprosate may be more effective when combined with naltrexone or disulfiram (Verheul et al. 2005). Further information regarding clinical use of acamprosate can be found in the Specific Drug summary at the end of this chapter.

Disulfiram

In current practice, disulfiram is used very little in treating the geriatric population because of dangerous adverse effects, particularly in patients who drink during treatment. Disulfiram acts by inhibiting aldehyde dehydrogenase, resulting in accumulation of the toxic intermediate acetaldehyde when alcohol is ingested. The effects vary among individuals and depend on the amount of alcohol that is ingested. Symptoms include flushing (especially of the face and chest), tachycardia, palpitations, hypotension, nausea and vomiting, shortness of breath, sweating, dizziness, blurred vision, and confusion. In severe cases, marked tachycardia or bradycardia, hypotension, myocardial infarction, cardiovascular collapse, heart failure, or seizures may occur (Kranzler and Ciraulo 2005). The more severe reactions are seen with high-dose disulfiram or in patients with preexisting cardiovascular disease. There is no specific antidote. The reaction can occur with certain over-the-counter cough syrups, mouthwashes, and prescribed medications such as metronidazole, tolbutamide, and trimethoprim/sulfamethoxazole (Bactrim).

Compliance problems arise with disulfiram just as they do with oral naltrexone. Patients know that they can stop taking the drug and sometime later start drinking again. Anecdotal experience suggests that supervised administration of disulfiram (which ensures that it is taken) increases its effectiveness, but the risk versus benefit of the drug is always an issue. Fully informed consent is an important component of treatment with this drug, and the process is necessarily lengthy in view of the drug's many warnings, adverse effects, and drug interactions.

When disulfiram is used in elderly patients, the dosage should be maintained at 125–250 mg/day. There is some question as to whether this dose generates a blood level sufficient to produce an alcohol-disulfiram reaction if the patient drinks (Gorelick 1993); the deterrent might actually be the threat of reaction rather than an actual reaction. It appears to be most appropriately used in patients who express the wish to have their abstinence "enforced" by a threat considered substantial. In regular users, disulfiram compliance can be determined by testing urine for the metabolite diethylamine (Fuller and Neiderhiser 1980).

Disulfiram should be avoided in patients with coronary artery disease, preexisting cardiac arrhythmia, cardiomyopathy with chronic congestive heart failure, chronic renal failure, portal hypertension, elevation of liver function test values, cerebrovascular disease, cognitive impairment, peripheral neuropathy, severe pulmonary disease, a history of impulsive behaviors or suicidality, or certain psychotic states. Since disulfiram inhibits the enzyme dopamine-β-hydroxylase, it may be associated with elevation of dopamine levels, resulting in exacerbation of mania or schizophrenia. Dosages above 250 mg/day are associated with higher rates of psychosis, hypertension, and hepatitis. For the patient taking disulfiram, liver function test values should be checked at baseline and every 2–3 weeks thereafter for 2 months, then every 3 months.

Serotonergic Drugs

It has been suggested that SSRI antidepressants may reduce craving and drinking behavior during the first weeks of treatment for alcohol dependence in nongeriatric samples (Gorelick and Paredes 1992; Naranjo et al. 1995; Sellers et al. 1992), but the few available follow-up studies suggest that these effects may not be sustained in all patients (Naranjo et al. 1995). SSRIs have been recommended for the subgroup of patients with low-risk, low-severity (type A) alcoholism (Kranzler and Ciraulo 2005), but it is not clear whether this applies only to those with some degree of comorbid depression. In any event, treatment utilizing SSRIs is best carried out in a structured abstinence program with close follow-up.

One study has demonstrated that ondansetron—a selective 5-HT$_3$ receptor antagonist marketed for treatment of nausea—may be effective at a dosage of 4 μg/kg two times a day in reducing alcohol consumption and increasing abstinence in patients with early-onset alcohol dependence (Johnson et al. 2000). Ondansetron may be effective for the subgroup of patients with high-risk, high-severity (type B) alcoholism, which is characterized by an earlier age at onset (Kranzler and Ciraulo 2005). However, further controlled study is needed before this agent can be recommended in the pharmacotherapy of alcohol dependence.

Early data suggested that buspirone might be useful in reducing alcohol craving. In one controlled 8-week trial of 50 outpatients with mild to moderate alcohol abuse histories, buspirone was associated with reduced craving, reduced anxiety levels, and lower attrition from treatment (Bruno 1989). In general, clinical experience has been that buspirone's effect in reducing alcohol craving and consumption over the long term has been small.

Anticonvulsants

In one randomized controlled trial, topiramate up to 300 mg/day in a nongeriatric cohort was found effective in treating alcohol dependence and improving the quality of life of enrolled subjects (Johnson et al. 2003, 2004). It is not clear how this could be applied to elderly patients, as this medication in general is associated with significant adverse effects, as discussed in Chapter 5 of this volume, "Mood Stabilizers." Other anticonvulsants reported to have some effect in treating alcohol dependence include valproate (Brady et al. 2002), carbamazepine (Mueller et al. 1997), and lamotrigine (Ballasiotes and Skaer 2000), but none of these medications has been studied systematically in the geriatric population for this indication.

Alcohol Intoxication

As a consequence of pharmacokinetic and pharmacodynamic changes noted above, elders may become intoxicated with relatively small amounts of alcohol. Symptoms of intoxication are similar to those seen in younger patients, although falls may be more common in elders. Blackouts—the forgetting of events occurring over several hours while intoxicated, even while consciousness appears normal to observers—can be seen in elders (Rubino 1992). Serious complications of intoxication include coma and death from respiratory depression. When the elderly patient presents in an intoxicated state, his or her BAL can help guide treatment and placement decisions. For example, an alert and nondysarthric patient with a high BAL (e.g., 250 mg percent) is at risk for severe withdrawal because of demonstrated high tolerance (Rubino 1992); such a patient should be monitored closely in a supervised setting.

Alcohol Withdrawal

Chronic alcohol consumption has important effects on a number of neurotransmitter systems (Koob and Le Moal 2001). The glutamatergic system in particular becomes up-regulated with chronic alcohol exposure such that abrupt withdrawal of alcohol is associated with excessive glutamatergic activity (De Witte et al. 2005). This has led to the hypothesis that in this excitotoxic state, neurons may be susceptible to apoptosis (cell death), leading to atrophy in selected brain regions.

The manifestations of alcohol withdrawal in elders are similar to those seen in middle-aged alcoholic individuals but may be more severe and more persistent (Brower 1998). Signs and symptoms may include fever, tachycardia, tachypnea, hypertension, unstable blood pressure, diaphoresis, tremor, hyperreflexia, marked startle response, mydriasis, seizures, headache, disorientation, anxiety, agitation, insomnia, delusions (usually persecutory), perceptual disturbances or hallucinations, and nausea and vomiting. Although DSM-IV-TR refers to any delirium that is secondary to alcohol withdrawal as *delirium tremens,* this latter term also connotes a severe delirious state, often with accompanying seizures. While hallucinations do not distinguish delirium tremens from other alcohol-related disorders, tactile and visual hallucinations are more characteristic of delirium tremens, while auditory hallucinations in the presence of a clear sensorium are more characteristic of alcoholic hallucinosis.

Minor withdrawal symptoms such as tremor and anxiety tend to be seen early, usually 6–12 hours after the last drink. Hallucinations tend to occur after 8–24 hours, seizures after 24 hours, and delirium tremens after 72 hours (Rubino 1992). Delirium tremens may occur earlier in patients with a history of experiencing them. Patients with a history of withdrawal seizures or numerous detoxifications are at increased risk for the development of withdrawal seizures (M.E. Brown et al. 1988). The most sensitive predictor of delirium tremens is a history of heavy daily alcohol use; other predictors include a prior history of delirium tremens or seizures (Cushman 1987), hypertension, and medical comorbidity

(Fiellin et al. 2002). In addition, there has been a report of a possible genetic predisposition to delirium tremens among males with the A9 allele of the dopamine transporter gene (Limosin et al. 2004). In females, this same allele appears to confer instead an increased risk of visual hallucinations (Limosin et al. 2004).

Old age is the most significant factor in the lethality of delirium tremens (Feuerlein and Reiser 1986). Causes of death include cardiac arrhythmias, hypovolemic shock, aspiration pneumonia, hepatic failure, and falls or other accidents. Another significant factor in lethality is the severity of preexisting medical illness or injury (e.g., head trauma) (Wojnar et al. 1999). Since elderly patients experiencing severe withdrawal are at a higher risk of falls and dependence in activities of daily living (Kraemer et al. 1997), they are best treated in a supervised environment.

Severity of the withdrawal syndrome can be evaluated and quantified using a scale such as the revised Clinical Institute Withdrawal Assessment for Alcohol (CIWA-Ar) (J. T. Sullivan et al. 1989), reproduced as Figure 7–2. This instrument scores withdrawal severity in 10 symptom categories: nausea and vomiting, tremor, paroxysmal sweating, anxiety, agitation, tactile disturbance, auditory disturbance, visual disturbance, headache or fullness in head, and orientation or clouding of sensorium. The range of scores in each category is 0–7, except for orientation, for which the range is 0–4. Scores below 8 signify minimal to mild withdrawal; scores from 8 to 15 signify moderate withdrawal; scores above 15 signify severe withdrawal. Higher scores are associated with seizures and delirium tremens. Although the CIWA-Ar is widely used for withdrawal assessment, interrater reliability may be affected by the absence of a complete set of anchor point descriptions, and the score may be elevated by preexisting psychiatric or comorbid medical illnesses. For this reason, clinical judgment is used to determine the need for admission to an intensive care unit (ICU) setting or additional medications for symptom control.

Initial supportive measures that should be used for the treatment of all elderly patients in alcohol withdrawal include hydration, nourishment, and rest in a quiet environment. Parenteral (intramuscular or intravenous) thiamine at 100 mg should be given before any glucose-containing intravenous solution is started, because glucose metabolism utilizes thia-

Clinical Institute Withdrawal Assessment
for Alcohol—Revised

Nausea and vomiting. "Do you feel sick to your stomach? Have you vomited?"
Observation:
0–No nausea and no vomiting
1–Mild nausea with no vomiting
2–
3–
4–Intermittent nausea with dry heaves
5–
6–
7–Constant nausea, frequent dry heaves, and vomiting

Tremor. Ask patient to extend arms and spread fingers apart.
Observation:
0–No tremor
1–Tremor not visible but can be felt, finger to finger
2–
3–
4–Moderate tremor with arms extended
5–
6–
7–Severe tremor, even with arms not extended

Paroxysmal sweats. Observation:
0–No sweat visible
1–Barely perceptible sweating; palms moist
2–
3–
4–Beads of sweat obvious on forehead
5–
6–
7–Drenching sweats

Figure 7–2. Clinical Institute Withrdrawal Assessment for Alcohol Withdrawal–Revised.

Source.   Reprinted from Sullivan JT, Sykora K, Schneiderman J, et al: "Assessment of alcohol withdrawal: the revised Clinical Institute Withdrawal Assessment for Alcohol Scale (CIWA-Ar)." *British Journal of Addiction* 84:1353–1357, 1989.

Anxiety. "Do you feel nervous?" Observation:
0–No anxiety (at ease)
1–Mildly anxious
2–
3–
4–Moderately anxious or guarded, so anxiety is inferred
5–
6–
7–Equivalent to acute panic states as occur in severe delirium or acute schizophrenic reactions

Agitation. Observation:
0–Normal activity
1–Somewhat more than normal activity
2–
3–
4–Moderately fidgety and restless
5–
6–
7–Paces back and forth during most of the interview or constantly thrashes about

Tactile disturbances. "Do you have any itching, pins-and-needles sensations, burning, or numbness, or do you feel like bugs are crawling on or under your skin?" Observation:
0–None
1–Very mild itching, pins-and-needles sensation, burning, or numbness
2–Mild itching, pins-and-needles sensation, burning, or numbness
3–Moderate itching, pins-and-needles sensation, burning, or numbness
4–Moderately severe hallucinations
5–Severe hallucinations
6–Extremely severe hallucinations
7–Continuous hallucinations

Auditory disturbances. "Are you more aware of sounds around you? Are they harsh? Do they frighten you? Are you hearing anything that is disturbing to you? Are you hearing things you know are not there?"

Figure 7–2. Clinical Institute Withrdrawal Assessment for Alcohol Withdrawal–Revised. *(Continued)*

Observation:
0–Not present
1–Very mild harshness or ability to frighten
2–Mild harshness or ability to frighten
3–Moderate harshness or ability to frighten
4–Moderately severe hallucinations
5–Severe hallucinations
6–Extremely severe hallucinations
7–Continuous hallucinations

Visual disturbances. "Does the light appear to be too bright? Is its color different? Does it hurt your eyes? Are you seeing anything that is disturbing to you? Are you seeing things you know are not there?" Observation:
0–Not present
1–Very mild sensitivity
2–Mild sensitivity
3–Moderate sensitivity
4–Moderately severe hallucinations
5–Severe hallucinations
6–Extremely severe hallucinations
7–Continuous hallucinations

Headache, fullness in head. "Does your head feel different? Does it feel like there is a band around your head?" Do not rate for dizziness or lightheadedness; otherwise, rate severity.
0–Not present
1–Very mild
2–Mild
3–Moderate
4–Moderately severe
5–Severe
6–Very severe
7–Extremely severe

Orientation and clouding of sensorium. "What day is this? Where are you? Who am I?" Observation:
0–Oriented and can do serial additions
1–Cannot do serial additions or is uncertain about date
2–Date disorientation by no more than 2 calendar days
3–Date disorientation by more than 2 calendar days
4–Disoriented to place and/or person

Figure 7–2.   Clinical Institute Withrdrawal Assessment for Alcohol Withdrawal–Revised. *(Continued)*

mine and could potentially precipitate Wernicke's encephalopathy in marginally deficient patients. Folate and a multivitamin should also be given, and electrolyte derangements should be corrected. Magnesium repletion is particularly important. Parenteral thiamine at 100 mg/day should be given for at least 3 days (Mayo-Smith et al. 2004) and longer if the patient has cardiovascular signs or neurological signs consistent with Wernicke's encephalopathy (see "Wernicke's Encephalopathy" section later in this chapter). Prescription of one daily intravenous Rally Pack ("banana bag") would meet this requirement and also supply 1 mg of folate, 10 mL of multivitamins, and 2 g of magnesium sulfate in 1 L of 5% dextrose/water or normal saline.

Benzodiazepines are the agents of choice to control the rate of alcohol withdrawal, used either in a fixed-dose regimen or as symptom-triggered therapy. In general, when medication is administered only for a CIWA-Ar score above a threshold of 8–10 (symptom-triggered therapy), less medication is used and the duration of detoxification is shortened (Daeppen et al. 2002). Compared with the fixed-dose strategy, however, symptom-triggered therapy is associated with higher average CIWA-Ar scores for more days (Daeppen et al. 2002), and this could place the frail elder at risk for an adverse medical outcome. Thus, although some clinicians would prefer symptom-triggered therapy for use in nonelderly patients, for elders the use of low, fixed doses of medication may be preferable.

Theoretically, any benzodiazepine could be used to control withdrawal, but pharmacokinetic differences make some agents better choices over others for elderly patients. Lorazepam is often the first-line drug for elders in alcohol withdrawal because it has a relatively rapid onset of action and a moderate duration of effect, it is not oxidatively metabolized and thus can be used for patients with hepatic impairment, it is not highly lipophilic so does not accumulate in the body, and it can be given orally or intravenously (as well as intramuscularly, although intramuscular administration is problematic in elderly patients with reduced muscle mass). Except for intravenous availability, oxazepam has the same advantages. Chlordiazepoxide (Librium) can be used in young-old patients experiencing withdrawal whose hepatic function is intact; in "old-old" (>75 years of age) patients and in those with even moderate degrees of hepatic dysfunction, this drug should be avoided. Chlordiazepoxide has the advantage of a longer half-life, which allows for a smoother withdrawal and possibly greater effectiveness in preventing withdrawal seizures (Mayo-Smith et al. 1997). The disadvantage of the longer half-life in elders is the increased risk of oversedation. As discussed in Chapter 2 of this volume, "Basic Psychopharmacology and Aging," the pharmacodynamic effect of a highly lipid-soluble drug such as diazepam after initial oral or parenteral dosing is more a function of tissue/lipid distribution than elimination half-life. Diazepam may cease to be effective after only a few hours as it moves out of the general circulation into lipid compartments such as adipose tissue.

With lorazepam, the route of administration depends on the clinical status of the patient. Intravenous dosing should be used if the CIWA-Ar score is very high, if the patient is vomiting or too obtunded or delirious to take oral medication, or if the patient is prohibited from taking anything orally (npo) because of medical comorbidities such as pancreatitis or gastrointestinal (GI) bleeding. When the intravenous route is used, doses should be initiated at the lower end of the suggested range and then titrated upward as needed to reduce the rise of hypotension and respiratory depression. Dosing of any of the recommended agents is best individualized, using the dosing guidelines provided in Table 7–4.

For patients with very high CIWA-Ar scores whose agitation cannot be controlled with large doses of benzodiazepines, propofol or pentobarbital sedation can be considered (Mayo-Smith et al. 2004), but this level of intervention requires monitoring in an ICU and the availability of ventilatory support.

Hallucinations (tactile, auditory, and visual), delusions, and psychotic agitation occurring during withdrawal may respond to benzodiazepine treatment alone; however, more severe and persistent psychotic symptoms should be treated with an antipsychotic. Although haloperidol has the best record of efficacy for this indication (at least anecdotally), any antipsychotic could theoretically be used. It should be noted that all antipsychotics carry some risk of lowering the seizure threshold.

Other drugs affecting the GABAergic system also may be useful in treating alcohol withdrawal, although much less is known about these drugs than is known about benzodiazepines in this context. In a nongeriatric sample, a randomized controlled trial of valproate at 500 mg three

Table 7–4.   Pharmacologic treatment of alcohol withdrawal

Drug	Recommended dose	
	Fixed-dose therapy	**Symptom-triggered therapy**
lorazepam (Ativan)	2 mg every 6 hours for 4 doses, then 1 mg every 6 hours for 8 doses Provide additional 2–4 mg every 1–2 hours as needed	2–4 mg every 1–2 hours when CIWA-Ar score is≥8–10
oxazepam (Serax)	30 mg every 6 hours for 4 doses, then 15 mg every 6 hours for 8 doses Provide additional 30–60 mg every 1–2 hours as needed	30–60 mg every 2 hours when CIWA-Ar score is≥8–10
chlordiazepoxide (Librium)	50 mg every 6 hours for 4 doses, then 25 mg every 6 hours for 8 doses Provide additional 50–100 mg every 2 hours as needed	50–100 mg every 2 hours when CIWA-Ar score is≥8–10

Note.   Based on American Society of Addiction Medicine practice guidelines. Per guidelines, adjustment is not needed for elderly patients in general. The only modification made here is that the as-needed schedule is changed from every 1 hour to every 1–2 hours to avoid oversedation. For each individual patient, doses may need to be adjusted upward or downward from the recommended doses. CIWA-Ar=Clinical Institute Withdrawal Assessment for Alcohol–Revised.
Source.   Mayo-Smith MF; Cushman P; Hill AJ, et al: "Pharmacological Management of Alcohol Withdrawal: A Meta-Analysis and Evidence-Based Practice Guideline." *The Journal of the American Medical Association* 278:144–151, 1997. Used with permission.

times a day used with oxazepam in a symptom-triggered protocol demonstrated that the combination resulted in smaller total doses of oxazepam and less frequent progression to higher CIWA-Ar scores (Reoux et al. 2001). Carbamazepine also can be used as an adjunct to a benzodiazepine in a symptom-triggered protocol (Kranzler and Ciraulo 2005). In fact, carbamazepine has been used as an alternative to benzodiazepines for moderate to severe alcohol withdrawal (Butler and Messiha 1986; Malcolm et al. 1989; Stuppaeck et al. 1992), but this use has not been adequately studied in geriatric patients. It is unclear as yet whether gabapentin may be helpful for this indication; anecdotal experience suggests that it is (Bonnet et al. 2003), but one controlled trial found it ineffective (Bonnet et al. 2003).

Although not as useful as monotherapy, a β-blocker could be used as an adjunct to benzodiazepine treatment for withdrawal in selected patients. β-Blockers have been shown to be associated with a more rapid resolution of withdrawal symptoms and a shorter length of hospital stay (Kraus et al. 1985) as well as reduced craving and a lower rate of relapse among outpatients (Horwitz et al. 1989). However, a meta-analysis concluded that they should not be recommended for all patients in withdrawal because of an increased risk of delirium (Mayo-Smith et al. 2004). In addition, β-blockers can cause hypotension and bradycardia and have to be used with caution in patients with asthma, chronic obstructive pulmonary disease (COPD), or cardiomyopathy. β-Blockers could be considered for patients with low CIWA-Ar scores who have persistent hypertension and/or tachycardia. Atenolol could be used initially at a dosage of 25–50 mg/day (titrated to heart rate). Some patients require and tolerate higher dosages (e.g., 100 mg/day).

Alcohol withdrawal seizures are usually of the generalized tonic-clonic type, with a short postictal period. Adequate treatment of alcohol withdrawal with a benzodiazepine prevents the development of seizures. When an alcohol-withdrawal seizure does occur, intravenous administration of 2 mg of lorazepam can decrease the likelihood of recurrence (D'Onofrio et al. 1999). Although phenytoin is not a first-line drug to treat alcohol-withdrawal seizures, it is sometimes administered in the emergency setting when limited history is available regarding the possibility of a preexisting non-alcohol-related seizure disorder.

Alcohol-Induced Persisting Dementia (Alcohol-Related Dementia)

Some alcohol-dependent patients develop global cognitive impairment that persists beyond the period of intoxication and withdrawal (Oslin et al. 1998). Little is known from systematic study about this diagnostic entity, particularly among elderly patients (Nakada and Knight 1984). Reported symptoms include amnesia, disturbance in other cortical functions (e.g., apraxia), and impairment in judgment and abstract thinking. Increased cerebrospinal fluid volume disproportionate to age is found on head CT or MRI in these cases (Pfefferbaum et al. 1993). Among the institutionalized elderly, patients with presumed alcoholic dementia exhibit milder cognitive deficits and are younger than patients with Alzheimer's disease (Carlen et al. 1994). One feature helpful in distinguishing alcoholic dementia from Alzheimer's disease is the presence of a language deficit (*anomia*, or inability to name) in the latter, which is not a prominent feature of alcoholic dementia. In addition, cerebellar atrophy is much more likely to be found in association with alcoholic dementia (Ron 1983), and ataxia and peripheral neuropathy are also more common. These distinctions are highlighted by the proposed criteria for alcohol-related dementia listed in Chapter 9 of this volume, "Medications to Treat Dementia and Other Cognitive Disorders" (Oslin et al. 1998).

It has been suggested that excitotoxic cell death during repeated episodes of alcohol withdrawal might give rise to the atrophy observed in particular areas of the brain in the chronic alcoholic individual. Brain areas most affected include the cerebellum, pons, thalamus, and cortex (particularly frontal), giving rise to observed cognitive and motor impairments (Sullivan 2003a). Since one of the actions of acamprosate is to dampen excitotoxicity, this medication might be expected to have an effect in the prevention of deterioration during the time of drug exposure. In addition, treatment of alcohol-related dementia requires abstinence from alcohol, so acamprosate has a further beneficial effect in promoting abstinence by reducing craving. Other medications that may be useful include memantine (which also dampens excitotoxicity), any drug that promotes abstinence, and possibly cholinesterase inhibitors, as discussed in Chapter 9.

In the patient with alcohol-related cognitive impairment, cognitive function is variably recovered over time with abstinence from alcohol, which may be reflected in improvement in ability to perform activities of daily living (Oslin et al. 1997b). Although the standard on neuropsychiatric units is generally to wait through 2 weeks of abstinence before undertaking neuropsychologic testing (Page and Linden 1974), this period might not actually be long enough; anecdotal experience suggests that recovery in this population takes longer. Even nongeriatric alcohol abusers abstinent 4 weeks may have a subacute syndrome of impairment that resolves with further abstinence (I. Grant et al. 1984). It has been suggested that early improvement might reflect recovery of cortical function, while persistent deficits (e.g., in long-term memory) might reflect permanent injury to the diencephalon (Brandt et al. 1983).

Wernicke's Encephalopathy

Thiamine deficiency associated with alcohol neurotoxicity is thought to underlie Wernicke's encephalopathy, the acute phase of the Wernicke-Korsakoff continuum. *Wernicke's encephalopathy* represents a neurologic emergency manifestation by the clinical triad of confusion, ataxia, and ocular movement abnormalities (nystagmus or ophthalmoplegia) (Rubino 1992). On pathological examination, punctate hemorrhages are seen in the gray matter surrounding the third and fourth ventricles, thalamus, hypothalamus, and mammillary bodies. This midline damage may extend to the midline cerebellum and basal forebrain (Willenbring 1988). Initial treatment for acute thiamine deficiency with neurologic signs consists of parenteral thiamine, glucose, and correction of magnesium deficiency (Nakada and Knight 1984), avoiding carbohydrate loading prior to thiamine administration. Thiamine should be given intravenously or intramuscularly at a dose of 100 mg once daily for 7 days, and this should be followed by 10 mg to be taken orally once daily until recovery is complete (Russell 2005). Improvement in ophthalmoplegia is usually seen within 24 hours (Russell 2005). Patients who do not recover completely with treatment may develop Korsakoff's syndrome (Nakada and Knight 1984). A recent case report suggests that at least some patients with symptoms of Wernicke's encephalopathy that last for months might still benefit from thiamine replacement, with improvement in memory function (Carota and Schnider 2005). For all patients showing signs of Wernicke's encephalopathy, aggressive measures should be undertaken to achieve and maintain abstinence in order to prevent the development of the persisting amnestic disorder. Abstinence may be particularly important for a subset of patients with an abnormality in the transketolase protein that predisposes to more severe neurotoxicity from alcohol (Heap et al. 2002).

Alcohol-Induced Persisting Amnestic Disorder

Untreated or recurrent episodes of Wernicke's encephalopathy provide the pathogenetic link to the persisting amnestic disorder known as *Korsakoff's syndrome*. The cardinal sign of this disorder is persistent anterograde episodic memory loss with preserved semantic memory, intelligence, and learned behavior (Kopelman 1995). Frontal systems also are affected, such that the patient can appear apathetic, disinhibited, perseverative, or confabulatory (Oscar-Berman et al. 2004). Amnesia persists beyond the period of alcohol intoxication and withdrawal.

Patients clinically diagnosed with Korsakoff's syndrome usually are found to have generalized atrophy with enlarged ventricles on neuroimaging study, similar to findings in non-Korsakoff's alcoholic individual. Those with Korsakoff's also have cell loss in anterior diencephalic structures such as the septal nuclei and hypothalamic gray (Jernigan et al. 1991), anterior thalamic nuclei (Harding et al. 2000), and hippocampus (Sullivan 2003b). These more widespread abnormalities are consistent with more severe memory impairment, which in Korsakoff's patients involves verbal as well as visual domains (Salmon and Butters 1985). Even during the Wernicke's phase of the Wernicke-Korsakoff syndrome, degeneration of cholinergic neurons in the nucleus basalis is seen (Cullen et al. 1997), which may account for the observed frontal system dysfunction in patients with this syndrome. The amnestic component of Korsakoff's syndrome is not currently considered treatable, but frontal system dysfunction may respond to cholinesterase inhibitor therapy (Kim et al. 2004). The role of antiglutamatergic drugs remains to be investigated.

Alcohol-Induced Psychotic Disorder

Alcoholic hallucinosis is the acute onset of auditory hallucinations (usually voices) in a clear sensorium in a long-standing heavy drinker. When delusions are present, they are believed to develop secondary to the hallucinations. For some time, this diagnostic entity has been controversial; some experts believe that the cases reported actually represent delirium tremens or are a manifestation of schizophrenia (Glass 1989).

Alcohol-Induced Mood Disorder and Comorbid Alcoholism and Depression

DSM-IV-TR recognizes that alcohol-induced mood disorders may have their onset either during intoxication or during withdrawal. The initial period of withdrawal is often marked by a gradual reduction of dysphoria, anxiety, and insomnia. In some patients, these symptoms persist for weeks to months, a syndrome known as *subacute withdrawal* (Kranzler and Ciraulo 2005). There is no evidence that the use of antidepressant medications during this period improves overall outcome (Kranzler and Ciraulo 2005). In one mixed-age sample, 42% of alcohol-abusing patients were significantly depressed on admission to a treatment unit, but only 6% were still depressed at 4 weeks (S.A. Brown and Schuckit 1988). The biggest change in depressive symptoms was seen in the first 2 weeks. For reasons such as these, the standard of care has been to wait through at least 2 weeks of abstinence from alcohol before treating depression that is mild to moderate in severity.

Nevertheless, it is increasingly recognized that substance use disorders, particularly alcoholism, are highly comorbid with idiopathic mood and anxiety disorders. In the National Epidemiologic Survey on Alcohol and Related Conditions (NESARC) study (involving a mixed-age sample), 41% of those with a current alcohol use disorder who sought treatment had a current mood disorder independent of alcohol use, and 33% had an independent anxiety disorder (B.F. Grant et al. 2004b), making these dualities the most prevalent of psychiatric comorbidities. In the dually diagnosed population, pharmacologic treatment of mood and anxiety disorders may be critical to successful treatment of the alcohol use disorder. Untreated depression may complicate the course of alcoholism and vice versa. Particularly for patients with a history of untreated mood or anxiety disorder predating the development of alcohol abuse, withholding treatment may not be indicated.

Whether treatment commences immediately upon abstinence or after a waiting period, the usual pharmacotherapies are used. Antidepressants are sometimes effective, even if the patient continues to drink (Oslin et al. 2000), although drinking reduces response rates in general. In addition, the combination of antidepressant medication and alcohol is not recommended because of the potential for liver impairment.

Alcohol-Induced Anxiety Disorder and Comorbid Alcoholism and Anxiety

As with mood disorders, DSM-IV-TR recognizes that alcohol-induced anxiety disorders may have their onset during either intoxication or withdrawal. Moreover, anxiety disorders and alcohol use disorders are common comorbidities. In the case of anxiety, the neural substrate is easily understood, since both alcohol and benzodiazepines bind to the $GABA_A$ receptor complex. The problem in treating anxiety disorders in the recidivist alcoholic person is that benzodiazepines (the mainstay of pharmacologic treatment) are cross-tolerant with alcohol and can induce craving in the abstinent alcoholic patient.

For this reason, SSRI antidepressants are often used to treat anxiety disorders in patients with alcohol dependence. The use of SSRIs to treat anxiety disorders is discussed in Chapter 4 of this volume, "Antidepressants."

Benzodiazepines can be used for a subset of patients with an anxiety disorder underlying alcohol dependence and who are carefully selected for their ability to maintain abstinence from alcohol while taking an adequate standing dose of benzodiazepine and their ability to comply with agreed-upon treatment parameters such as dosing frequency. There is some belief that in this particular subset of patients, alcohol was being used as an over-the-counter anxiolytic. When use of benzodiazepines does not escalate over time and the patient continues to function well, therapy is judged successful even when the medication is continued indefinitely. A single source of dispensing should always be used and frequent monitoring is essential (Ciraulo et al. 2003). Notwithstanding the risk of abuse or the interaction of combined alcohol and benzodiazepine, these drugs are much more benign than alcohol when used over the long term. Adverse effects of benzodiazepines in the elderly population are discussed in Chapter 6, "Anxiolytic and Sedative-Hypnotic Medications."

Cerebellar Degeneration

Chronic alcohol abusers may present with a wide-based stance, ataxia, and dysmetria that is more prominent in the lower extremities. On a head CT or MRI, cerebellar atrophy is seen, particularly in the anterior and superior vermis and adjacent folia. It is believed that this syndrome is a further consequence of thiamine deficiency (Rubino 1992). Although there is no specific treatment for this condition, symptoms may improve with abstinence from alcohol (Nakada and Knight 1984).

Nicotine-Related Disorders

Nicotine Use Disorder

Nicotine use disorder (tobacco dependence) is the most common substance-related disorder among elderly individuals in the United States, with an estimated 13.5% of older men and 10.5% of older women currently identified as smokers (Gomberg 2004). Nicotine is a highly addictive substance, and smoking is a highly efficient mechanism for delivery of nicotine into arterial blood and to the brain. When nicotinic receptors are stimulated, neurotransmitters released include dopamine, serotonin, norepinephrine, and endogenous opioids (Oncken and George 2005). Immediate effects include decreased anxiety, increased alertness, and improved concentration (Oncken and George 2005). Since nicotine's half-life is short (on the order of 2 hours), dosing has to be repeated multiple times throughout the day to maintain these effects. Aside from nicotinic pharmacodynamic effects, smoking has pharmacokinetic effects that may be significant because hydrocarbons in cigarette smoke act as inducers of CYP1A2 and CYP3A4 activity, as noted in Chapter 2. This induction has implications for patients either starting or stopping smoking while taking medications that are substrates of CYP1A2, such as clozapine and olanzapine (e.g., drug levels will rise if the patient stops smoking).

It is by now well established that smoking is associated with increased morbidity and mortality in all populations, especially among chronic smokers grown old. Smoking causes heart disease, lung and esophageal cancer, chronic lung disease, and osteoporosis. Smoking is associated with stroke, peripheral vascular disease, pulmonary hypertension, peptic ulcer disease, gastroesophageal reflux disease, bladder cancer, and gastric cancer. In general, older smokers have a lower quality of life than older nonsmokers. Interestingly, however, the incidence of Parkinson's disease appears to be reduced in smokers compared with nonsmokers.

Even in late life, there are definite health benefits to quitting smoking (LaCroix et al. 1991). Elders who stop smoking for 5 years reduce cardiovascular mortality to that of nonsmokers and also reduce their risk of lung cancer. Every year, 10% of elderly smokers are successful in quitting smoking (Salive et al. 1992). Medically based smoking cessation programs are a particularly important intervention in this population.

Pharmacologic treatments for tobacco dependence include nicotine replacement therapies, bupropion, and the nicotinic receptor agonist, varenicline. When used in accordance with prescribing recommendations, these treatments can be used safely in elderly patients.

Nicotine Replacement

In general, nicotine replacement therapies in the form of gum, lozenges, patches, sprays, and inhalers approximately double the rate of quitting smoking compared to placebo (Sofuoglu and Kosten 2004). Effects can be maintained over time. In a mixed-age sample of treatment-refractory tobacco-dependent patients with significant medical comorbidity (e.g., COPD, cardiac disease) who underwent an intensive 2-week inpatient program using the transdermal nicotine patch, 29% were still abstinent after 1 year (Hurt et al. 1992). Aside from the few studies where small numbers of geriatric patients were included, these replacement therapies have not been systematically studied in the elderly population and are not necessarily recommended as safe. In particular, the two forms available by prescription only—intranasal spray and oral inhaler—should be used with caution in elders. In addition, although nicotine replacement products provide lower peak nicotine levels and slower onset compared with cigarette smoking, caution is advised in using these products in patients with coronary artery disease, severe or worsening angina, recent myocardial infarction, uncontrolled hypertension, or serious cardiac dysrhythmia.

Selected nicotine replacement therapies are listed in Table 7–5. When nicotine replacement therapy is initiated, it is important that the patient quit smoking to avoid toxic levels of nicotine.

Although the nicotine content of one cigarette ranges from 6 mg to 11 mg, the actual amount of nicotine delivered by smoking may be only 1–3 mg per cigarette. The amount of nicotine delivered by the transdermal patch, lozenge, or gum varies according to dose used (see Table 7–5). The particular product selected depends primarily on patient preference and to a lesser extent on specific adverse effects. Although it is likely that product combinations (e.g., slow-delivery patch with rapid-delivery lozenge used on an as-needed basis) are more effective in preventing smoking, combinations are not FDA approved and are not recommended in elderly patients until more is known about adverse effects.

Polacrilex gum.   This product is a relatively popular option with smokers that are younger but may be avoided by elders because of problems with teeth or dentures. It is available over the counter in several flavors (original, mint, and orange). For those who prefer this vehicle, the gum is chewed slowly for 20–30 minutes, with intermittent parking of the gum at the buccal mucosa, and then discarded. Peak nicotine concentrations are achieved within 30 minutes. Absorption occurs through the buccal mucosa. The gum has been found to work best when used on a fixed schedule (e.g., every 1–2 hours) rather than prn, and with concomitant behavioral therapy (Oncken and George 2005). Adverse effects include dyspepsia, reflux, and hiccups, all of which can be minimized through more frequent parking of the gum, as described above (Oncken and George 2005).

Lozenge.   The lozenge delivers 25% more nicotine than gum. For the geriatric patient, the product could be taken as follows: one lozenge placed on the tongue every 2 hours for the first 2–4 weeks, then every 4 hours. Most geriatric patients should be treated with the 2-mg lozenge. As with gum, adverse effects include nausea, reflux, and hiccups. It should be noted that the lozenge contains phenylalanine, and the manufacturer recommends caution in its use in frail elders with anxiety, hypertension, or diabetes.

Transdermal patch.   The patch is a preferred method of nicotine delivery in elderly patients because it provides constant delivery of nicotine at a slow rate, has low abuse potential, and is available over the counter.

A recent review of a large database of patients hospitalized for acute coronary syndrome (unstable angina or non–ST-segment myocardial infarction) concluded that the patch was safe for use in this population (Meine et al. 2005). Both 16-hour and 24-hour patches are available; the 16-hour patches should be removed at bedtime and the area wiped clean, and the 24-hour patches should be removed in the morning before the next is applied, and the area wiped clean. Removal of the 24-hour patch at bedtime may be indicated if the patient develops insomnia. In general, patches with smaller doses of nicotine (e.g., 7, 14, or 15 mg) should be used for elderly patients. Higher doses may be tolerated by young-old patients and required for those who smoke more than 10 cigarettes daily. It is important that tobacco use not continue while the patch is in use, or nicotine levels can become toxic. The recommended treatment period is 8 weeks. There is no evidence of significant withdrawal when the patch is discontinued.

Nicotine nasal spray.   This product is available by prescription only. Nicotine is absorbed through the nasal mucosa and has a rapid onset of action. The recommended start dose is one dose per hour (or less in the geriatric patient), in which a dose is one spray to each nostril. This product is contraindicated in patients with nasal polyps, rhinitis, or sinusitis. It is associated with nasal irritation on initial use. This product should be used with caution in elderly patients, considering the paucity of information regarding safety in the geriatric population.

Nicotine inhaler.   This product is available by prescription only. It simulates smoking in that vapors are inhaled from a cartridge. Onset of action is approximately 15 minutes. With 80 deep inhalations over a 20-minute period, 2 mg of nicotine is delivered. Patients use multiple inhalers (up to 16 per day). This product is contraindicated for individuals with asthma. The recommended treatment period is 24 weeks. This product should be used with caution in elderly patients, considering the paucity of information regarding safety in the geriatric population.

Bupropion Sustained-Release

Use of the antidepressant bupropion sustained-release (SR) approximately doubles the quit-smoking rate (Hughes et al. 2004). In conjunction with

Table 7–5. Selected nicotine replacement therapies

Form of nicotine	Trade name	Strength	Amount of nicotine delivered	Time to peak level	Instructions for use	Treatment duration	Initial taper
Chewing gum	Nicorette, generic	2 mg 4 mg	Up to 0.8 mg Up to 1.5 mg	20–30 minutes	Alternate chewing and parking gum for 20 minutes. One piece every 1–2 hours and as needed; not to exceed 24 pieces/day	6 weeks	6 weeks
Lozenge	Commit	2, 4 mg	25% more than gum	20–30 minutes	During initial treatment (weeks 1–6), one lozenge every 1–2 hours; weeks 7–9, one lozenge every 2–4 hours; weeks 10–12, one lozenge every 4–8 hours. Suggested strength for elders is 2 mg Lozenge should not be chewed or swallowed.	6 weeks	6 weeks

Table 7–5. Selected nicotine replacement therapies *(continued)*

Form of nicotine	Trade name	Strength	Amount of nicotine delivered	Time to peak level	Instructions for use	Treatment duration	Initial taper
Transdermal patch	Habitrol, NicoDerm, Nicotrol, generic brand	24-hour patch: 7, 14, 21 mg 16-hour patch: 5, 10, 15 mg	Variable (depends on patch)	8–9 hours	Apply new patch every 24 hours to hairless, clean, dry skin on upper body or arm. Rotate sites. Habitrol or Nicoderm CQ: For healthy young-old patients, starting dose depends on smoking history: ≥10 cigarettes/day—start with 21-mg patch for 4–6 weeks, then 14-mg patch for 2 weeks, then 7-mg patch for 2 weeks. For frail or low-body-weight elders or those with cardiovascular disease, start with 14-mg patch for 4–6 weeks, then 7-mg patch for 2–4 weeks. Nicotrol: One patch daily for 6 weeks (stepped; see package instructions).	4–6 weeks	4 weeks

Source. Adapted from Semla et al. 2006.

behavioral interventions, the drug also reduces withdrawal-related dysphoria and weight gain. In acute nicotine withdrawal, bupropion has similar efficacy to nicotine replacement therapies, and the combination of bupropion with nicotine replacement may be superior to monotherapy (Jorenby et al. 1999), although the safety of this combination has not been specifically studied in elders. Bupropion should be started while the patient is still smoking, and a quit date (usually 1–2 weeks in the future) should be selected. Bupropion SR should be initiated in most elderly patients at a dosage of 100 mg/day; the dosage should be increased to 100 mg two times a day after 4–7 days, as tolerated. SR doses should be separated by 8 hours. Young-old patients may tolerate an initial dose of bupropion SR of 150 mg (Zyban), with a dose increase to 150 mg two times a day after 4–7 days. Bupropion SR should be continued for 7–12 weeks; at 7 weeks, if the patient has made no progress toward quitting, the medication should be discontinued. The goal of therapy is complete cessation of smoking. Ideally, when this is achieved by 12 weeks, the medication is stopped; tapering is not necessary, although the patient should be monitored for the possible emergence of depressive symptoms.

Varenicline

The newly approved varenicline is a partial agonist at the $\alpha 4\beta 2$ nicotinic acetylcholine receptor. It binds with greater affinity than nicotine and blocks nicotine itself from binding. As with nicotine, stimulation of the nicotine receptor leads to the release of dopamine in the nucleus accumbens. Varenicline has been found in several randomized controlled trials to be superior to placebo and to bupropion SR in smoking abstinence rates for periods up to 52 weeks (Gonzales et al. 2006; Jorenby et al. 2006; Tonstad et al. 2006). Although patients up to 75 years of age were eligible to enroll in these trials, the age range of patients studied was not reported and the mean and standard deviation data suggest that the number of geriatric patients was in fact small.

Varenicline is started 1 week before a target quit date. In the studies reported and in the package insert, dosage and dosage titration are as follows: 0.5 mg/day for 3 days, then 0.5 mg two times a day for 4 days, then 1 mg two times a day. The drug is rapidly absorbed through the gastric mucosa, with peak plasma concentration in about 4 hours. It is minimally metabolized and excreted through the kidneys. The drug dosage should be reduced for patients with severe renal impairment. Drug interactions appear to be limited; the most common adverse effects are listed in the Specific Drug summary at the end of this chapter. It should be noted that concomitant use of nicotine replacement therapy with varenicline could be hazardous in elders and that physical dependence may occur.

Nicotine Withdrawal

Nicotine withdrawal is a subjectively unpleasant syndrome, with symptoms of decreased heart rate, insomnia, dysphoria or depressed mood, anxiety, irritability, frustration, restlessness, trouble concentrating, increased eating, and weight gain. Symptoms begin within hours of abstinence, increase over 3–4 days, and then decrease gradually over several weeks (Pbert et al. 2004). This syndrome should be considered in patients with or alcohol dependence who become restless and dysphoric within this time frame after admission to the hospital, and efforts should be made to elicit the smoking history of such a patient if it has not been documented. In this setting, withdrawal can usually be treated with a nicotine patch, as described above.

Abuse and Misuse of Prescribed Drugs

Benzodiazepines

Benzodiazepines and selective $GABA_{A1}$ receptor agonists (zolpidem, zaleplon, and eszopiclone) prescribed for anxiolytic or hypnotic purposes are more likely to be continued long-term by elderly patients—particularly elders with lower educational levels (Mant et al. 1988) who are female and have chronic health problems and high levels of emotional distress (Mellinger et al. 1984)—than by younger cohorts. As in younger patients, long-term use of benzodiazepines in elderly patients is associated with physical dependence. Moreover, elders who use these medications chronically may suffer additional adverse effects such as significant cognitive and motor impairment, which are in turn associated with falls and motor vehicle accidents.

Benzodiazepine Dependence

As discussed in an earlier section, legitimate long-term use of benzodiaz-epines complicates the diagnosis of dependence. The development of physiological dependence is an expected consequence of use of a drug in this class for more than about 2 weeks, so the development of an absti-nence syndrome on abrupt discontinuation is not helpful in determining problematic use (Ciraulo et al. 2005). Like their younger counterparts, elderly patients who take benzodiazepines for treatment of chronic anx-iety and not for the experience of a high usually do not escalate the dose of medication over time. Tolerance does not develop to the anxiolytic ef-fects (Ciraulo et al. 2005). Those who develop psychological dependence are more likely to have a history of substance abuse.

The reinforcing effects of benzodiazepines are less than those of opi-oids, stimulants, and barbiturates (Ciraulo et al. 2005), which is consis-tent with the observation that benzodiazepine administration is associated with decreased activity in the nucleus accumbens rather than increased ac-tivity. The mechanism by which reinforcement occurs with this class of drugs is not completely known but is likely mediated by increased GABA activity and GABA interconnections (Ciraulo et al. 2005). Within the class of benzodiazepines, the medications most likely to induce psycho-logical dependence are those with fast onset (high lipophilicity) and short duration of action (e.g., alprazolam) (Ciraulo et al. 2005). The relative ad-diction potential of selective $GABA_{A1}$ receptor agonists (zolpidem, zale-plon, and eszopiclone) is not yet clear, but the incidence of abuse and dependence among current users appears to be low (Hajak et al. 2003; Soyka et al. 2000).

Long-term use of benzodiazepines in some elderly patients is associ-ated with depression, residual anxiety, cognitive impairment, daytime se-dation, ataxia, falls, and poor physical health (Mellinger et al. 1984; Rodrigo et al. 1988). Chronic benzodiazepine users older than 70 years have a higher frequency of personality pathology, anxiety, and dysthymia than nonusers, but cause and effect is not clear in all cases (Petrovic et al. 2002). Cognitive impairment with benzodiazepines may present as an amnestic syndrome or as a dementia characterized by inattention, mem-ory problems, psychomotor slowing, and incoordination. Unlike alcohol, benzodiazepines are not associated with amnesia or dementia that persists after the medications are stopped. Even when used by elders chronically at high doses, benzodiazepines do not result in brain damage (Ciraulo et al. 2005).

Benzodiazepine Detoxification (Medical Withdrawal)

For older patients treated chronically with therapeutic doses of benzodiazepines, an off-drug trial may be indicated. For these patients, a slow taper (by 10%–25% per week) is indicated. When very short-acting agents such as alprazolam are used, a switch to a longer-acting drug may be required for the taper to proceed. If a switch is made, the dose of the longer-acting drug should be lower than the equivalent dose of the short-acting agent, to avoid overdose (Ciraulo et al. 2005). A subset of patients will be found to do poorly, even with slow withdrawal. These patients are likely to have underlying conditions, such as generalized anxiety disorder, with benefit from chronic treatment that may or may not outweigh the risk. The use of flumazenil is not recommended to expedite withdrawal in elderly patients.

Withdrawal for patients treated long-term with high doses of a benzodiazepine should be accomplished in consultation with the patient's primary care physician and carried out in an inpatient medical setting. The patient should be placed on a cardiac monitor with frequent checks, and vital signs should be taken on a schedule (e.g., every 4 hours). The drug should then be tapered at a rate of 10%–25% per day. If the patient develops fever, tremulousness, or diaphoresis, the dose of drug should be increased again and the patient hydrated and watched more closely until stable. The emergence of new symptoms or a new perceptual disturbance (e.g., tinnitus) can help to identify too-rapid withdrawal and to distinguish it from anxiety (Ciraulo et al. 2005).

Other medications may be useful in facilitating medical withdrawal from benzodiazepines. Propranolol (30–60 mg/day, divided three times a day) may help to attenuate adrenergic signs and symptoms, but cannot be used as sole therapy because it does not prevent seizures. Carbamazepine, valproate, gabapentin, and sedating antidepressants (mirtazapine, paroxetine, and trazodone) also may be useful adjuncts but have not been well studied in elderly patients for this indication. Beyond the period of detox-

ification, medications that can help promote abstinence include buspirone, SSRI antidepressants, and venlafaxine (Ciraulo et al. 2005).

Benzodiazepine Intoxication

Toxicity can be seen with overdose or with therapeutic use of a highly lipophilic drug taken long enough to accumulate in the body. Symptoms
of benzodiazepine intoxication include sedation, respiratory depression,
ataxia, dysarthria, diplopia, and dysphagia. In some patients, "paradoxical" reactions are seen, with symptoms of disinhibition and agitation. Although benzodiazepines are generally among the safest drugs in overdose
among younger patients, the potential for respiratory depression in elders has to be considered, particularly among those with sleep apnea or
COPD. Flumazenil does not reverse benzodiazepine-induced respiratory
depression. Moreover, in contrast to the relative safety of "pure" benzodiazepine overdose, the combination of benzodiazepines in overdose
with alcohol or other medications can be fatal. In addition, benzodiazepines with active metabolites may have a less predictable course in overdose, since recovery from stupor or coma can occur even while serum
levels of active metabolites are still rising (Ciraulo et al. 2005).

Benzodiazepine Withdrawal

When benzodiazepines taken long-term at low doses are abruptly discontinued, both *recurrence* of anxiety and *rebound* of anxiety symptoms
(worse than baseline) can be seen. These symptoms may include headache, sweating, dizziness, tremor, myoclonus, fatigue, dysphoria, irritability, anxiety, fear, insomnia, poor concentration, and various perceptual
abnormalities, including depersonalization and derealization (Ciraulo et
al. 2005). When benzodiazepines taken long-term at high doses are
abruptly discontinued, true withdrawal symptoms may be seen, including
autonomic instability, nausea, anorexia, tinnitus, perceptual distortions,
delirium, delusions, hallucinations, and seizures. Severe benzodiazepine
withdrawal syndromes can be fatal, although rarely. Patients withdrawing
from a combination of alcohol and benzodiazepines can show a later-
onset, longer-lasting withdrawal syndrome characterized by greater autonomic and psychomotor signs than alcohol withdrawal alone (Benzer and
Cushman 1980).

Barbiturates

Although prescription of barbiturates and related sedative-hypnotics has declined with the advent of safer drugs such as the benzodiazepines, there remain elderly patients in the community who have been treated long-term with these medications. As noted in Chapter 6 on sedative-hypnotics, the therapeutic index of barbiturates is narrow, and these drugs have numerous side effects, including respiratory depression and induction of various CYP450 isoenzymes. When an elderly patient taking a barbiturate on a stable regimen is encountered clinically, a decision should be made whether it is feasible to undertake a slow taper and discontinuation of that medication. This taper may need to be done over a period of 3–6 months or more to proceed safely. Unsupervised abrupt withdrawal from barbiturates carries a significant risk of mortality.

Opioids

Opioid Dependence

Most elderly patients who are prescribed opioids for demonstrable pain (e.g., spine pain) do not develop tolerance to analgesic effects over time and do not escalate doses unless painful complications occur (Mahowald et al. 2005). Elders who do develop addiction to prescription opioids often have a prior history of substance abuse. Opioids may be obtained by prescription or from Internet sites offering drugs such as Dilaudid and Vicodin by mail without a prescription. These Internet sites set up, take orders, ship drugs, and close down before being located by federal regulators. The extent to which elders who are denied opioid prescriptions utilize this source is not known.

Elderly patients who misuse prescribed opioids can suffer from all the adverse effects associated with this class of medications, as described in Chapter 10 of this volume, "Analgesic Medications." Treatment consists of detoxification and then close follow-up. Maintenance of the opioid-free state may be extremely difficult in elderly patients with painful comorbid medical conditions. As discussed in Chapter 10, there are other options available to treat chronic pain syndromes in the geriatric population, although for many patients, the best option may be an opioid. Thus, for those elders whose opioid use escalates over time, there may be recurrent questions regarding benefit versus risk of treatment as well as dose adjustment.

Opioid Intoxication

The older patient treated with opioids may present to the emergency department with shallow and slow respiration, bradycardia, hypothermia, and stupor or coma, with miosis (pinpoint pupils) that may change to mydriasis (dilated pupils) with the development of brain anoxia (Schuckit and Segal 2005). This state of overmedication or overdose may occur more often with very potent opioids such as fentanyl (Schuckit and Segal 2005). Naloxone may be useful therapeutically as well as diagnostically in the patient whose recent medication history is unknown. Naloxone should be given at doses starting at 0.4 mg intravenously (or intramuscularly if no intravenous access is established), and some response should be seen within several minutes. The dose can be repeated every 2–3 minutes, titrated to reverse respiratory depression, to a total dose not exceeding 10 mg (Schuckit and Segal 2005). Titration helps to avoid eliciting a severe withdrawal syndrome. Until the administered naloxone is eliminated from the body, only partial suppression of the withdrawal syndrome is possible, and this may require opioid doses high enough to induce respiratory depression (Epstein et al. 2005).

Opioid Withdrawal

A withdrawal syndrome is seen on abrupt discontinuation or rapid dose reduction of opioids. Earliest symptoms include lacrimation, yawning, rhinorrhea, and sweating. These are followed by symptoms of restless sleep, mydriasis, anorexia, gooseflesh, general restlessness, irritability, and tremor. Late symptoms are more severe manifestations of the above, along with tachycardia, abdominal cramping, nausea, vomiting, diarrhea, hypertension, mood lability, depression, muscle spasms, weakness, and bone pain (Epstein et al. 2005). The Clinical Opiate Withdrawal Scale shown in Figure 7–3 can be used to quantify withdrawal severity, in a manner analogous to the CIWA-Ar for alcohol withdrawal. Time to onset and duration of withdrawal symptoms depend on the particular opioid used, as shown in Table 7–6.

Treatment of Opioid Dependence

Options for pharmacologic treatment of opioid dependence have not been specifically studied in the geriatric population. For patients of un-

Clinical Opiate Withdrawal Scale

For each item, circle the number that best describes the patient's symptoms. Rate on just the apparent relationship to opiate withdrawal. For example, if heart rate is increased because the patient was jogging just prior to assessment, the increased pulse rate would not add to the score.

Resting pulse rate: _____beats/minute
Measured after patient is sitting or lying for 1 minute
0   Pulse rate ≤80
1   Pulse rate 81–100
2   Pulse rate 101–120
4   Pulse rate > 120

Sweating:
Over past half-hour not accounted for by room temperature or patient activity
0   No report of chills or flushing
1   Subjective report of chills or flushing
2   Flushed or observable moistness on face
3   Beads of sweat on brow or face
4   Sweat streaming off face

Restlessness:
Observation during assessment
0   Able to sit still
1   Reports difficulty sitting still, but is able to do so
3   Frequent shifting or extraneous movements of legs/arms
5   Unable to sit still for more than a few seconds

Pupil size:
0   Pupils pinned or normal size for room light
1   Pupils possibly larger than normal for room light
2   Pupils moderately dilated
5   Pupils so dilated that only the rim of the iris is visible

Figure 7–3.   Clinical Opiate Withdrawal Scale.
Source.   Wesson DR, Ling W: "The Clinical Opiate Withdrawal Scale (COWS)." *Journal of Psychoactive Drugs* 35:253–259, 2003. Used with permission.

Bone or joint aches:
If patient was having pain previously, only the additional component attributed to opiate withdrawal is scored
0   Not present
1   Mild, diffuse discomfort
2   Patient reports severe diffuse aching of joints and muscles
4   Patient is rubbing joints or muscles and is unable to sit still because of discomfort

Gastrointestinal (GI) upset:
Over the last half-hour
0   No GI symptoms
1   Stomach cramps
2   Nausea or loose stool
3   Vomiting or diarrhea
5   Multiple episodes of diarrhea or vomiting

Tremor:
Observation of outstretched hands
0   No tremor
1   Tremor can be felt, but not observed
2   Slight tremor observable
4   Gross tremor or muscle twitching

Yawning:
Observation during assessment
0   No yawning
1   Yawning once or twice during assessment
2   Yawning three or more times during assessment
4   Yawning several times/minute

Anxiety or irritability:
0   None
1   Patient reports increasing irritability or anxiousness
2   Patient obviously irritable or anxious
4   Patient is so irritable or anxious that participation in the assessment is difficult

Figure 7–3.   Clinical Opiate Withdrawal Scale. *(Continued)*

Gooseflesh skin:
0 Skin is smooth
3 Piloerection of skin can be felt on hairs standing up on arms
5 Prominent piloerection

Runny nose or tearing:
Not accounted for by cold symptoms or allergies
0 Not present
1 Nasal stuffiness or unusually moist eyes
2 Nose running or tearing
4 Nose constantly running or tears streaming down cheeks

Total score: _____
The total score is the sum of all 11 items
Score:
   5–12 Mild withdrawal
 13–24 Moderate withdrawal
 25–36 Moderately severe withdrawal
   >36 Severe withdrawal

Figure 7–3. Clinical Opiate Withdrawal Scale. *(Continued)*

selected age (including a limited number of young-old patients), there is evidence suggesting that potentially useful options include medical withdrawal using clonidine, methadone, or buprenorphine, and replacement therapy using methadone or buprenorphine. Each option should be carried out in tandem with psychosocial treatment (e.g., counseling, group therapy). Twelve-step programs are available in some areas.

Medical withdrawal using clonidine.   Clonidine effectively suppresses autonomic symptoms and for this reason could be expected to reduce the danger of opioid withdrawal in the medically compromised elder. However, clonidine has important adverse effects in elderly patients, some of which may be serious, including bradycardia, atrioventricular block, syncope, hypotension, and orthostasis. In addition, clonidine does not treat withdrawal symptoms of restlessness, insomnia, or drug craving (Epstein et al. 2005). When clonidine is used, a test dose of

Table 7–6.   Onset and duration of opioid withdrawal[a]

Drug	Effects wear off (hours)[b]	Appearance of nonpurposive withdrawal symptoms (hours)	Peak withdrawal effects (hours)	Majority of symptoms over (days)
Meperidine	2–3	4–6	8–12	4–5
Hydromorphone	4–5	4–5	36–72	7–10
Heroin	4[c]	8–12	36–72	7–10
Morphine	4–5	8–12	36–72	7–10
Codeine	4	8–12	36–72	7–10
Methadone	8–12	36–72	96–144	14–21

[a]Times may be prolonged in elderly patients.
[b]Duration may vary with chronic dosing.
[c]Usually taken two to four times per day.
Source.   Reprinted from Collins ED, Kleber HD: "Opioids: Detoxification," in *The American Psychiatric Publishing Textbook of Substance Abuse Treatment,* 3rd Edition. Edited by Galanter M, Kleber HD. Washington, DC, American Psychiatric Publishing, 2004, pp. 267. Used with permission.

0.1 mg should be given first and then vital signs should be checked, including orthostatic blood pressure and pulse. If the patient does not develop significant hypotension or bradycardia, detoxification from a short-acting opioid (e.g., oxycodone) can proceed according to a protocol adapted for the geriatric population such as the following (Epstein et al. 2005):

1. Day 1: clonidine 0.1 mg orally three times a day (range 0.05–0.2 mg three times a day)
2. Day 2: clonidine 0.2 mg three times a day
3. Days 3–6: clonidine 0.3 mg three times a day
4. Days 4–10: decrease clonidine dose by 0.2 mg/day until discontinued

For further information about the use of clonidine, see the Specific Drug summary at the end of this chapter.

Medical withdrawal using methadone.   Methadone is a drug with complex pharmacokinetics. It is highly lipophilic and thus widely distributed. Its duration of action increases substantially with repeated administration. It is extensively metabolized, primarily via CYP3A4. Its renal excretion is dose dependent, and renal reabsorption is dependent on urinary pH. For these and other reasons, there is considerable variability among individuals in levels achieved and in clearance of this drug. Moreover, since the drug's kinetics change over time (with repeated dosing), dose and schedule adjustments are likely to be needed. Since methadone not only shares toxic effects of opioids in general but also has the potential to prolong the QTc (see Chapter 3, "Antipsychotics," this volume), this drug should be used with caution in elderly patients and only with close follow-up.

When methadone is used, detoxification can be accomplished over a week in the hospital or be prolonged for 6 months or more in a methadone clinic. If detoxification is done over a week, not all symptoms of opioid withdrawal will be suppressed. In opioid-tolerant elders, it is recommended that an initial low dose of methadone be used rather than the equivalent dose of the original opioid, since cross-tolerance of methadone with other opioids is incomplete, dosage conversion formulas are imprecise, and variability in kinetics between individuals is large (Mc-Evoy et al. 2006). An initial methadone dose of 10 mg could be given and repeated after several hours if symptoms persist. The total number of milligrams administered to achieve symptom control should then be given as the daily dose, which should be divided in two and given on a twice-daily schedule. When the patient has been stable for 2–3 days, the taper should begin at a rate of 10%–20% per day. Detoxification would thus be completed in 5–10 days. A faster taper can sometimes be accomplished with clonidine, as described earlier, but this combination should be used with extreme caution in elderly patients. Some patients experience exacerbation of withdrawal symptoms while taking methadone at doses below 20 mg, so the taper might require a slower rate (e.g., 3% per week) and thus be completed in the outpatient clinic (Epstein et al. 2005). For further information about the use of methadone, see the Specific Drug summary at the end of this chapter.

Medical withdrawal using buprenorphine.   Buprenorphine is a newly approved drug that acts as a μ opioid partial agonist; it has mild opioid effects itself, but it blocks the effects of full μ agonists. Buprenorphine is currently marketed as Suboxone (buprenorphine plus naloxone) and Subutex (buprenorphine only). The addition of naloxone is designed to prevent diversion of the drug to illicit use. Naloxone is not absorbed with sublingual use, but crushing and injection of the compound results in opioid withdrawal symptoms by virtue of naloxone's effects.

Buprenorphine is classified as a Schedule III drug, so it can be dispensed from an office by a certified clinician for the treatment of opioid dependence and for opioid detoxification. A waiver must be obtained from the Secretary of Health and Human Services for this purpose. To be eligible for a waiver, a physician must either be certified in addiction psychiatry or addiction medicine or complete an 8-hour training course with documented attendance. The training course provides detailed information about buprenorphine pharmacology, patient selection for treatment, induction and maintenance protocols, strategies for integration of psychosocial treatment with pharmacologic treatment, and pain management (both acute and chronic) for patients in maintenance treatment for opioid dependence.

Although this drug is likely to be more acceptable to elderly opioid abusers than methadone, it is associated with higher rates of confusion and drowsiness in this population (Semla et al. 2006). For Suboxone detoxification, recommended inpatient regimens include flexible-dose (4- to 6-day) program and several fixed-dose (3-, 7-, or 10-day) programs. Recommended outpatient regimens include flexible-dose (5- to 8-day) and fixed-dose (20- to 36-day) programs. Doses are not well worked out for elders; these patients are likely to require doses at the lower end of recommended ranges. For further information about the use of buprenorphine, see the Specific Drug summary at the end of this chapter.

Replacement therapy: methadone.   A minority of elderly patients will go on to a replacement therapy program with methadone or buprenorphine. This option is usually a temporizing measure, taken because of patient preference or because active medical or psychiatric issues delay detoxification. Elderly patients can be maintained on methadone for a planned period of time and then undergo a scheduled detoxification when they have met pre-established criteria. When methadone is used at a dosage of 80–120 mg/day, it also produces blockade against the effects of intravenous heroin, hydromorphone, and methadone (Vocci et al. 2005). It is not known how many elders would require or tolerate doses in this range.

Replacement therapy: buprenorphine.   Specific protocols are established for initiation of Suboxone (*induction*) using a timed sequence of dosing along with careful assessment for withdrawal symptoms. If the protocols are not followed and the patient experiences significant withdrawal discomfort, the risk increases for abuse of alcohol or other drugs, or stopping treatment. Protocols are different for induction from short-acting opioids (e.g., morphine, oxycodone, hydrocodone, heroin) versus long-acting opioids (e.g., Oxycontin, MS Contin, methadone). The protocols are made available during required training for certification to dispense buprenorphine.

Chapter Summary

- Elders who present with any of the following should be screened for substance abuse or dependence: trauma or history of recent overdose, respiratory depression, hypotension or hypertension, cardiac arrhythmia, ataxia, seizure(s), psychosis (especially tactile or visual hallucinations), or other mental status changes.
- Alcohol overuse is the most significant substance abuse problem among the current cohort of elders.
- The Michigan Alcoholism Screening Test—Geriatric Version is a recommended screening instrument in the evaluation of the elderly patient who drinks.
- Laboratory tests that may be useful in confirming recent alcohol consumption include breath analysis, urine alcohol, blood alcohol level, serum γ-glutamyltransferase, and carbohydrate-deficient transferrin.
- Three medications currently have U.S. Food and Drug Administration–approved labeling for treatment of alcohol dependence: naltrexone, acamprosate, and disulfiram.
- Tobacco dependence is the most common substance-related disorder among elderly individuals in the United States.
- Elders who stop smoking for 5 years reduce cardiovascular mortality to that of nonsmokers and also reduce their risk of lung cancer.
- Pharmacologic treatments for tobacco dependence in elders include nicotine replacement therapies, bupropion, and varenicline.
- For older patients treated chronically with therapeutic doses of benzodiazepines, a trial off drug may be indicated.
- Withdrawal for patients treated long-term with high doses of a benzodiazepine should be accomplished in consultation with the patient's primary care physician and carried out in an inpatient medical setting.
- Elders who develop addiction to prescription opioids often have a prior history of substance abuse.
- The Clinical Opiate Withdrawal Scale can be used to quantitate opioid withdrawal severity, in a manner analogous to the Clinical Institute Withdrawal Assessment for alcohol withdrawal.

References

Alte D, Luedemann J, Rose H-J, et al: Laboratory markers carbohydrate-deficient transferrin, gamma-glutamyltransferase, and mean corpuscular volume are not useful as screening tools for high-risk drinking in the general population: results from the Study of Health in Pomerania (SHIP). Alcohol Clin Exp Res 28:931–940, 2004

Ballasiotes AA, Skaer TL: Use of lamotrigine in a patient with bipolar disorder and psychiatric comorbidity. Clin Ther 22:1146–1148, 2000

Barrick C, Connors GJ: Relapse prevention and maintaining abstinence in older adults with alcohol-use disorders. Drugs Aging 19:583–594, 2002

Bayerlein K, Hillemacher T, Reulbach U, et al: Alcoholism-associated hyperhomocysteinemia and previous withdrawal seizures. Biol Psychiatry 57:1590–1593, 2005

Benzer D, Cushman P: Alcohol and benzodiazepines: withdrawal syndromes. Alcohol Clin Exp Res 4:243–247, 1980

Bleich S, Bayerlein K, Reulbach U, et al: Homocysteine levels in patients classified according to Lesch's typology. Alcohol Alcohol 39:493–498, 2004

Bonnet U, Banger M, Leweke FM, et al: Treatment of acute alcohol withdrawal with gabapentin: results from a controlled two-center trial. J Clin Psychopharmacol 23:514–519, 2003

Bradley KA, McDonell MB, Bush K, et al: The AUDIT alcohol consumption questions: reliability, validity, and responsiveness to change in older male primary care patients. Alcohol Clin Exp Res 22:1842–1849, 1998

Brady KT, Myrick H, Henderson S, et al: The use of divalproex in alcohol relapse prevention: a pilot study. Drug Alcohol Depend 67:323–330, 2002

Brandt J, Butters N, Ryan C, et al: Cognitive loss and recovery in long-term alcohol abusers. Arch Gen Psychiatry 40:435–442, 1983

Brower KJ: Alcohol withdrawal and aging, in Alcohol Problems and Aging. Edited by Gomberg ESL, Hegedus AM, Zucker RA. Bethesda, MD, U.S. Department of Health and Human Services, 1998, pp 359–372

Brown ME, Anton RF, Malcolm R, et al: Alcohol detoxification and withdrawal seizures: clinical support for a kindling hypothesis. Biol Psychiatry 23:507–514, 1988

Brown SA, Schuckit MA: Changes in depression among abstinent alcoholics. J Stud Alcohol 49:412–417, 1988

Bruno F: Buspirone in the treatment of alcoholic patients. Psychopathology 22 (suppl 1):49–59, 1989

Buchsbaum DG, Buchanan RG, Welsh J, et al: Screening for drinking disorders in the elderly using the CAGE Questionnaire. J Am Geriatr Soc 40:662–665, 1992

Butler D, Messiha FS: Alcohol withdrawal and carbamazepine. Alcohol 3:113–129, 1986

Carlen PL, Wortzman G, Holgate RC, et al: Reversible cerebral atrophy in recently abstinent chronic alcoholics measured by computed tomography scans. Science 200:1076–1078, 1978

Carlen PL, Penn RD, Fornazzari L, et al: Computerized tomographic scan assessment of alcoholic brain damage and its potential reversibility. Alcohol Clin Exp Res 10:226–232, 1986

Carlen PL, McAndrews MP, Weiss RT, et al: Alcohol-related dementia in the institutionalized elderly. Alcohol Clin Exp Res 18:1330–1334, 1994

Carota A, Schnider A: Dramatic recovery from prolonged Wernicke-Korsakoff disease. Eur Neurol 53:45–46, 2005

Chang MM, Kwon J, Hamada RS, et al: Effect of combined substance use on laboratory markers of alcoholism. J Stud Alcohol 51:361–365, 1990

Chen J, Conigrave KM, Macaskill P, et al: Combining carbohydrate-deficient transferrin and gamma-glutamyltransferase to increase diagnostic accuracy for problem drinking. Alcohol Alcohol 38:574–582, 2003

Ciraulo DA, Shader RI, Ciraulo AM: Alcoholism and its treatment, in Manual of Psychiatric Therapeutics, 3rd Edition. Edited by Shader RI. Philadelphia, PA, Lippincott Williams & Wilkins, 2003, pp 127–142

Ciraulo DA, Ciraulo JA, Sands BF, et al: Sedative-hypnotics, in Clinical Manual of Addiction Psychopharmacology. Edited by Kranzler HR, Ciraulo DA. Washington, DC, American Psychiatric Publishing, 2005, pp 111–162

Cullen KM, Halliday GM, Caine D, et al: The nucleus basalis (Ch4) in the alcoholic Wernicke-Korsakoff syndrome: reduced cell number in both amnesic and non-amnesic patients. J Neurol Neurosurg Psychiatry 63:315–320, 1997

Cushman P: Delirium tremens: update on an old disorder. Postgrad Med 82:117–122, 1987

Daeppen J-B, Gache P, Landry U, et al: Symptom-triggered vs. fixed-schedule doses of benzodiazepine for alcohol withdrawal. Arch Intern Med 162:1117–1121, 2002

De Witte P, Littleton J, Parot P, et al: Neuroprotective and abstinence-promoting effects of acamprosate. CNS Drugs 19:517–537, 2005

D'Onofrio G, Rathlev NK, Ulrich AS, et al: Lorazepam for the prevention of recurrent seizures related to alcohol. N Engl J Med 340:915–919, 1999

Epstein S, Renner JA, Ciraulo DA, et al: Opioids, in Clinical Manual of Addiction Psychopharmacology. Edited by Kranzler HR, Ciraulo DA. Washington, DC, American Psychiatric Publishing, 2005, pp 55–110

Feuerlein W, Reiser E: Parameters affecting the course and results of delirium tremens treatment. Acta Psychiatr Scand 73:120–123, 1986

Fiellin DA, O'Connor PG, Holmboe ES, et al: Risk for delirium tremens in patients with alcohol withdrawal syndrome. Subst Abuse 23:83–94, 2002

Fink A, Tsai MC, Hays RD, et al: Comparing the Alcohol-Related Problems Survey (ARPS) to traditional alcohol screening measures in elderly outpatients. Arch Gerontol Geriatr 34:55–78, 2002

Fleming MF, Manwell LB, Barry KL, et al: Brief physician advice for alcohol problems in older adults: a randomized community-based trial. J Fam Pract 48:378–384, 1999

Forsberg L, Halldin J, Ekman S, et al: Screening of binge drinking among patients on an emergency surgical ward. Alcohol 27:77–82, 2002

Fuller RK, Neiderhiser DH: Evaluation and application of a urinary diethylamine method to measure compliance with disulfiram therapy. J Stud Alcohol 42:202–207, 1980

Giordano J, Beckman K: Alcohol use and abuse in old age: an examination of type II alcoholism. J Gerontol Soc Work 9:65–83, 1985

Glass IB: Alcoholic hallucinosis: a psychiatric enigma—1T the development of an idea. Br J Addict 84:29–41, 1989

Goldman D, Oroszi G, O'Malley S, et al: COMBINE genetics study: the pharmacogenetics of alcoholism treatment response: genes and mechanisms. J Stud Alcohol Suppl 15:56–64, 2005

Gomberg ESL: Ethnic minorities and the elderly, in The American Psychiatric Publishing Textbook of Substance Abuse Treatment, 3rd Edition. Edited by Galanter M, Kleber HD. Washington, DC, American Psychiatric Publishing, 2004, pp 519–527

Gomez A, Conde A, Aguiar A, et al: Diagnostic usefulness of carbohydrate-deficient transferrin for detecting alcohol-related problems in hospitalized patients. Alcohol Alcohol 36:266–270, 2001

Gonzales D, Rennard SI, Nides M, et al: Varenicline, an $\alpha4\beta2$ nicotinic acetylcholine receptor partial agonist, vs sustained-release bupropion and placebo for smoking cessation. JAMA 296:47–55, 2006

Gorelick DA: Pharmacological treatment, in Recent Developments in Alcoholism. Edited by Galanter M. New York, Plenum Press, 1993, pp 413–427

Gorelick DA, Paredes A: Effect of fluoxetine on alcohol consumption in male alcoholics. Alcohol Clin Exp Res 16:261–265, 1992

Grant BF, Dawson DA, Stinson FS, et al: The 12-month prevalence and trends in DSM-IV alcohol abuse and dependence: United States, 1991–1992 and 2001–2002. Drug Alcohol Depend 74:223–234, 2004a

Grant BF, Stinson FS, Dawson DA, et al: Prevalence and co-occurrence of substance use disorders and independent mood and anxiety disorders. Arch Gen Psychiatry 61:807–816, 2004b

Grant I, Adams KM, Reed R: Aging, abstinence, and medical risk factors in the prediction of neuropsychologic deficit among long-term alcoholics. Arch Gen Psychiatry 41:710–718, 1984

Hajak G, Muller WE, Wittchen HU, et al: Abuse and dependence potential for the non-benzodiazepine hypnotics zolpidem and zopiclone: a review of case reports and epidemiological data. Addiction 98:1371–1378, 2003

Hammett-Stabler CA, Pesce AJ, Cannon DJ: Urine drug screening in the medical setting. Clin Chim Acta 315:125–135, 2002

Harding A, Halliday G, Caine D, et al: Degeneration of anterior thalamic nuclei differentiates alcoholics with amnesia. Brain 123:141–154, 2000

Heap LC, Pratt OE, Ward RJ, et al: Individual susceptibility to Wernicke-Korsakoff syndrome and alcoholism-induced cognitive deficit: impaired thiamine utilization found in alcoholics and alcohol abusers. Psychiatr Genet 12:217–224, 2002

Holroyd S, Duryee JJ: Substance use disorders in a geriatric psychiatry outpatient clinic: prevalence and epidemiologic characteristics. J Nerv Ment Dis 185:627–632, 1997

Horwitz RI, Gottlieb LD, Kraus ML: The efficacy of atenolol in the outpatient management of the alcohol withdrawal syndrome. Results of a randomized clinical trial. Arch Intern Med 149:1089–1093, 1989

Hughes JR, Stead LF, Lancaster T: Antidepressants for smoking cessation. The Cochrane Database of Systematic Reviews, Issue 4, Article No: CD000031. DOI: 10.1002/14651858.CD000031, 2004

Hurt RD, Dale LC, Offord KP, et al: Inpatient treatment of severe nicotine dependence. Mayo Clin Proc 67:823–828, 1992

Jernigan TL, Schafer K, Butters N, et al: Magnetic resonance imaging of alcoholic Korsakoff patients. Neuropsychopharmacology 4:175–186, 1991

Johnson BA, Roache JD, Javors MA, et al: Ondansetron for reduction of drinking among biologically predisposed alcoholic patients: a randomized controlled trial. JAMA 284:963–971, 2000

Johnson BA, Ait-Daoud N, Bowden CL, et al: Oral topiramate for treatment of alcohol dependence: a randomised controlled trial. Lancet 361:1677–1685, 2003

Johnson BA, Ait-Daoud N, Akhtar FZ, et al: Oral topiramate reduces the consequences of drinking and improves the quality of life of alcohol-dependent individuals. Arch Gen Psychiatry 61:905–912, 2004

Jorenby DE, Leischow SJ, Nides MA, et al: A controlled trial of sustained-release bupropion, a nicotine patch, or both for smoking cessation. N Engl J Med 340:685–691, 1999

Jorenby DE, Hayes JT, Rigotti NA, et al: Efficacy of varenicline, an a4b2 nicotinic acetylcholine receptor partial agonist, vs placebo or sustained-release bupropion for smoking cessation. JAMA 296:56–63, 2006

Kim KY, Ke V, Adkins LM: Donepezil for alcohol-related dementia: a case report. Pharmacotherapy 24:419–421, 2004

Koob GF, Le Moal M: Drug addiction, dysregulation of reward, and allostasis. Neuropsychopharmacology 24:97–129, 2001

Kopelman MD: The Korsakoff syndrome. Br J Psychiatry 166:154–173, 1995

Kraemer KL, Mayo-Smith MF, Calkins DR: Impact of age on the severity, course, and complications of alcohol withdrawal. Arch Intern Med 157:2234–2241, 1997

Kranzler HR, Ciraulo DA: Alcohol, in Clinical Manual of Addiction Psychopharmacology. Edited by Kranzler HR, Ciraulo DA. Washington, DC, American Psychiatric Publishing, 2005, pp 1–54

Kraus ML, Gottlieb LD, Horwitz RI, et al: Randomized clinical trial of atenolol in patients with alcohol withdrawal. N Engl J Med 313:905–909, 1985

LaCroix AZ, Lang J, Scherr P, et al: Smoking and mortality among older men and women in three communities. N Engl J Med 324:1619–1625, 1991

Lesch OM, Walter H, Freitag H, et al: Carbohydrate-deficient transferrin as a screening marker for drinking in a general hospital population. Alcohol Alcohol 31:249–256, 1996

Limosin F, Loze J-Y, Boni C, et al: The A9 allele of the dopamine transporter gene increases the risk of visual hallucinations during alcohol withdrawal in alcohol-dependent women. Neurosci Lett 362:91–94, 2004

Mahowald ML, Singh JA, Majeski P: Opioid use by patients in an orthopedics spine clinic. Arthritis Rheum 52:312–321, 2005

Malcolm R, Ballenger JC, Sturgis ET, et al: Double-blind controlled trial comparing carbamazepine to oxazepam treatment of alcohol withdrawal. Am J Psychiatry 146:617–621, 1989

Mant A, Duncan-Jones P, Saltman D, et al: Development of long-term use of psychotropic drugs by general practice patients. Br Med J (Clin Red Ed) 296:251–254, 1988

Mayo-Smith MF, Cushman P, Hill AJ, et al: Pharmacological management of alcohol withdrawal: a meta-analysis and evidence-based practice guideline. JAMA 278:144–151, 1997

Mayo-Smith MF, Beecher LH, Fischer TL, et al: Management of alcohol withdrawal delirium. Arch Intern Med 164:1405–1412, 2004

McEvoy GK, Snow EK, Kester L, et al: AHFS Drug Information. Bethesda, MD, American Society of Health-System Pharmacists, 2006

Meine TJ, Patel MR, Washam JB, et al: Safety and effectiveness of transdermal nicotine patch in smokers admitted with acute coronary syndromes. Am J Cardiol 95:976–978, 2005

Mellinger GD, Balter MB, Uhlenhuth EH: Prevalence and correlates of the long-term regular use of anxiolytics. JAMA 251:375–379, 1984

Moore RD, Bone LR, Geller G, et al: Prevalence, detection, and treatment of alcoholism in hospitalized patients. JAMA 261:403–407, 1989

Mowe M, Bohmer T: Increased levels of alcohol markers (GGT, MCV, ASAT, ALAT) in older patients are not related to high alcohol intake. J Am Geriatr Soc 44:1136–1137, 1996

Mueller TI, Stout RL, Rudden S, et al: A double-blind, placebo-controlled pilot study of carbamazepine for the treatment of alcohol dependence. Alcohol Clin Exp Res 21:86–92, 1997

Nakada T, Knight RT: Alcohol and the central nervous system. Med Clin North Am 68:121–131, 1984

Naranjo CA, Bremner KE, Lanctot KL: Effects of citalopram and a brief psychosocial intervention on alcohol intake, dependence and problems. Addiction 90:87–99, 1995

Nyblom H, Berggren U, Balldin J, et al: High AST/ALT ratio may indicate advanced alcoholic liver disease rather than heavy drinking. Alcohol Alcohol 39:336–339, 2004

O'Malley SS, Jaffe AJ, Chang G, et al: Six-month follow-up of naltrexone and psychotherapy for alcohol dependence. Arch Gen Psychiatry 53:217–224, 1996

Oncken CA, George TP: Tobacco, in Clinical Manual of Addiction Psychopharmacology. Edited by Kranzler HR, Ciraulo DA. Washington, DC, American Psychiatric Publishing, 2005, pp 315–338

Onen S-H, Onen F, Mangeon J-P, et al: Alcohol abuse and dependence in elderly emergency department patients. Arch Gerontol Geriatr 41:191–200, 2005

Oscar-Berman M, Kirkley SM, Gansler DA, et al: Comparisons of Korsakoff and non-Korsakoff alcoholics on neuropsychological tests of prefrontal brain functioning. Alcohol Clin Exp Res 28:667–675, 2004

Oslin DW: Alcohol use in late life: disability and comorbidity. J Geriatr Psychiatry Neurol 13:134–140, 2000

Oslin DW: Treatment of late-life depression complicated by alcohol dependence. Am J Geriatr Psychiatry 13:491–500, 2005

Oslin D, Liberto JG, O'Brien J, et al: Naltrexone as an adjunctive treatment for older patients with alcohol dependence. Am J Geriatr Psychiatry 5:324–332, 1997a

Oslin DW, Streim JE, Parmelee P, et al: Alcohol abuse: a source of reversible functional disability among residents of a VA nursing home. Int J Geriatr Psychiatry 12:825–832, 1997b

Oslin D, Atkinson RM, Smith DM, et al: Alcohol related dementia: proposed clinical criteria. Int J Geriatr Psychiatry 13:203–212, 1998

Oslin DW, O'Brien CP, Katz IR: The disabling nature of comorbid depression among older DUI recipients. Am J Addict 8:128–135, 1999

Oslin DW, Katz IR, Edell WS, et al: Effects of alcohol consumption on the treatment of depression among elderly patients. Am J Geriatr Psychiatry 8:215–220, 2000

Oslin DW, Berrettini W, Kranzler HR, et al: A functional polymorphism of the mu-opioid receptor gene is assocated with naltrexone response in alcohol-dependent patients. Neuropsychopharmacology 28:1546–1552, 2003

Page RD, Linden JD: "Reversible" organic brain syndrome in alcoholics. Q J Stud Alcohol 35:98–107, 1974

Paille FM, Guelfi JD, Perkins AC, et al: Double-blind randomized multicentre trial of acamprosate in maintaining abstinence from alcohol. Alcohol Alcohol 30:239–247, 1995

Pbert L, Ockene JK, Reiff-Hekking S: Tobacco, in The American Psychiatric Publishing Textbook of Substance Abuse Treatment, 3rd Edition. Edited by Galanter M, Kleber HD. Washington, DC, American Psychiatric Publishing, 2004, pp 217–234

Petrovic M, Vandierendonck A, Mariman A, et al: Personality traits and socio-epidemiological status of hospitalised elderly benzodiazepine users. Int J Geriatr Psychiatry 17:733–738, 2002

Pfefferbaum A, Rosenbloom M, Crusan K, et al: Brain CT changes in alcoholics: effects of age and alcohol consumption. Alcohol Clin Exp Res 12:81–87, 1988

Pfefferbaum A, Sullivan EV, Rosenbloom MJ, et al: Increase in brain cerebrospinal fluid volume is greater in older than in younger alcoholic patients: a replication study and CT/MRI comparison. Psychiatry Res 50:257–274, 1993

Reoux JP, Saxon AJ, Malte CA, et al: Divalproex sodium in alcohol withdrawal: a randomized double-blind placebo-controlled clinical trial. Alcohol Clin Exp Res 25:1324–1329, 2001

Rodrigo EK, King MB, Williams P: Health of long-term benzodiazepine users. Br Med J (Clin Res Ed) 296:603–606, 1988

Ron MA: The alcoholic brain: CT scan and psychological findings. Psychol Med (Monogr Suppl) 3:1–33, 1983

Rosse RB, Riggs RL, Dietrich AM, et al: Frontal cortical atrophy and negative symptoms in patients with chronic alcohol dependence. J Neuropsychiatry Clin Neurosci 9:280–282, 1997

Rubino FA: Neurologic complications of alcoholism. Psychiatr Clin N Am 15:359–372, 1992

Russell RM: Vitamin and trace mineral deficiency and excess, in Harrison's Principles of Internal Medicine, 16th Edition. Edited by Kasper DL, Fauci AS, Longo DL, et al. New York, McGraw-Hill, 2005, pp 403–411

Salive ME, Cornoni-Huntley J, LaCroix AZ, et al: Predictors of smoking cessation and relapse in older adults. Am J Public Health 82:1268–1271, 1992

Salmon DP, Butters N: The etiology and neuropathology of alcoholic Korsakoff's syndrome: some evidence for the role of the basal forebrain. J Clin Exp Neuropsychol 7:181–210, 1985

Schuckit MA, Segal DS: Opioid drug abuse and dependence, in Harrison's Principles of Internal Medicine, 16th Edition. Edited by Kasper DL, Fauci AS, Longo DL, et al. New York, McGraw-Hill, 2005, pp 2567–2570

Schuckit MA, Tapert S: Alcohol, in The American Psychiatric Publishing Textbook of Substance Abuse Treatment, 3rd Edition. Edited by Galanter M, Kleber HD. Washington, DC, American Psychiatric Publishing, 2004, pp 151–166

Sellers EM, Higgins GA, Sobell MB: 5-HT and alcohol abuse. Trends Pharmacol Sci 13:69–75, 1992

Semla TP, Beizer JL, Higbee MD: Geriatric Dosage Handbook, 11th Edition. Hudson, OH, Lexi-Comp Inc, 2006

Sofuoglu M, Kosten TR: Pharmacologic management of relapse prevention in addictive disorders. Psychiatr Clin North Am 27:627–648, 2004

Soyka M, Bottlender R, Moller H-J: Epidemiological evidence for a low abuse potential of zolpidem. Pharmacopsychiatry 33:138–141, 2000

Spies CD, Neuner B, Neumann T, et al: Intercurrent complications in chronic alcoholic men admitted to the intensive care unit following trauma. Intensive Care Med 22:286–293, 1996

Stranges S, Freudenheim JL, Muti P, et al: Differential effects of alcohol drinking pattern on liver enzymes in men and women. Alcohol Clin Exp Res 28:949–956, 2004

Stuppaeck CH, Pycha R, Miller C, et al: Carbamazepine versus oxazepam in the treatment of alcohol withdrawal: a double-blind study. Alcohol Alcohol 27:153–158, 1992

Sullivan EV: Compromised pontocerebellar and cerebellothalamocortical systems: speculations on their contributions to cognitive and motor impairment in nonamnesic alcoholism. Alcohol Clin Exp Res 27:1409–1419, 2003a

Sullivan EV: Hippocampal volume deficits in alcoholic Korsakoff's syndrome. Neurology 61:1716–1719, 2003b

Sullivan JT, Sykora K, Schneiderman J, et al: Assessment of alcohol withdrawal: the revised Clinical Institute Withdrawal Assessment for Alcohol Scale (CIWA-Ar). Br J Addict 84:1353–1357, 1989

Swift RM: Pharmacologic treatments for drug and alcohol dependence: experimental and standard therapies. Psychiatr Ann 23:697–702, 1998

Tonstad S, Tonnesen P, Hajek P, et al: Effect of maintenance therapy with varenicline on smoking cessation. JAMA 296:64–71, 2006

Verheul R, Lehert P, Geerlings PJ, et al: Predictors of acamprosate efficacy: results from a pooled analysis of seven European trials including 1,485 alcohol-dependent patients. Psychopharmacology (Berl) 178:167–173, 2005

Vocci FJ, Acri J, Elkashef A: Medication development for addictive disorders: the state of the science. Am J Psychiatry 162:1432–1440, 2005

Weintraub D, Linder MW: Amphetamine positive toxicology screen secondary to bupropion. Depress Anxiety 12:53–54, 2000

Whitworth AB, Fischer F, Lesch OM, et al: Comparison of acamprosate and placebo in long-term treatment of alcohol dependence. Lancet 347:1438–1442, 1996

Willenbring ML: Organic mental disorders associated with heavy drinking and alcohol dependence. Clin Geriatr Med 4:869–887, 1988

Wojnar M, Bizon Z, Wasilewski D: The role of somatic disorders and physical injury in the development and course of alcohol withdrawal delirium. Alcohol Clin Exp Res 23:209–213, 1999

Generic name	acamprosate
Trade name	Campral
Class	GABA agonist/glutamate antagonist
Half-life	20–33 hours
Mechanism of action	Not fully elucidated; appears to attenuate glutamatergic transmission via glutamate receptor antagonism and allosteric modulation at NMDA receptor
Available preparations	Tablets (enteric-coated, delayed-release): 333 mg
Starting dose	333 mg tid
Titration	Increase after 7 days to 666 mg tid
Typical daily dose	666 mg tid
Dose range	333–666 mg tid
Therapeutic serum level	Not established

Comments: A treatment for alcohol dependence but not for alcohol withdrawal syndrome. Understudied in the elderly population. Treatment is initiated as soon as possible after abstinence has been achieved and maintained for 12 months or longer, even through relapses. High first-pass metabolism, with bioavailability of 11%. Negligible protein binding. Not metabolized. Excreted in urine as unchanged drug. Lower dose should be used in renal impairment. *Drug interactions:* No significant interactions identified. Formulation may contain sulfites. *Adverse effects:* Diarrhea, suicidal ideation and suicide attempts, syncope, palpitations, edema, insomnia, anxiety, depression, weakness, nausea, vomiting, and constipation. *Uncommon but serious adverse effects:* Renal failure, seizures, angina, myocardial infarction, and pancreatitis.

Generic name	buprenorphine
Trade name	Suboxone (with naloxone), Subutex
Class	μ opioid partial agonist
Half-life	2.2–3 hours
Mechanism of action	As a partial agonist at the μ opioid receptor, buprenorphine has effects similar to abused opioids, but maximal effects are less; also blocks effects of full agonists
Available preparations	Tablets (Suboxone): 2, 8 mg
Starting dose	See text and information provided/required for certification.
Titration	
Typical daily dose	
Dose range	
Therapeutic serum level	

Comments: Used for treatment of opioid dependence, although understudied in the elderly population. As a Schedule III drug with a relatively wide margin of safety, can be dispensed from an office by a certified clinician. Recommended inpatient Suboxone detoxification regimens include a flexible (4- to 6-day) program and several fixed (3-, 7-, or 10-day) programs. Recommended outpatient regimens include a flexible (5- to 8-day) and fixed (20- to 36-day) programs. Doses are not well worked out for elders; these patients are likely to require doses at the lower end of recommended ranges. Extensive first-pass metabolism (low oral bioavailability). Sublingual form (Suboxone) dissolves in 3–10 minutes. It is dosed one time a day and has a duration of 96 hours, so dosing three times a week is possible. Metabolized mainly in the liver via CYP3A4, and excreted mainly in feces but also in urine. Addition of naloxone to Suboxone formulation intended to prevent diversion to intravenous use by heroin-dependent individuals; would not necessarily prevent diversion by buprenorphine-dependent or nonopioid-dependent patients. *Drug interactions:* CYP3A4 inducers and inhibitors (see Table 2–2), additive respiratory and CNS depression with other CNS depressants (may be significant). *Common adverse effects (>10%) for Suboxone:* Headache, pain, insomnia, anxiety, depression, nausea, abdominal pain, constipation, back pain, weakness, rhinitis, and withdrawal syndrome. *Less common adverse effects (1%–10%):* Chills, nervousness, vomiting, and flu-like syndrome. Patients with hepatitis who are treated with buprenorphine must have liver function tests monitored closely.

Generic name	bupropion
Trade name	Zyban, Wellbutrin SR
Class	Atypical antidepressant
Half-life	Parent compound approximately 20 hours; metabolites > 30 hours (unclear whether longer in elderly)
Mechanism of action	Probably noradrenergic; inhibition of dopamine reuptake at doses greater than usual antidepressant doses
Available preparations	SR tablets: 100, 150 mg (Zyban is 150-mg SR tablet)
Starting dose	100 mg/day or 150 mg/day SR while patient is still smoking
Titration	Increase after 4–7 days to 100 mg SR bid or 150 mg SR bid
Typical daily dose	100–150 mg SR bid (SR doses should be separated by 8 hours)
Dose range	As above
Therapeutic serum level	Not established, although levels > 40 ng/mL may be poorly tolerated

Comments: A first-line drug in elderly patients for treatment of tobacco dependence; approximately doubles quit rate. When used for this indication, the drug is continued for 7–12 weeks and then stopped. Well absorbed orally. In healthy adults, peak levels in 3 hours for extended release. Metabolized in the liver by CYP2B6. Two active metabolites: hydroxy-bupropion and threo-hydro-bupropion; metabolite levels may be much higher than parent drug. High metabolite levels are associated with poor response and psychotic symptoms. Clearance decreased in elderly and in those with renal or hepatic insufficiency, so lower doses are generally used. Dosage adjustment not needed for dialysis patients. *Important drug interactions:* Levodopa, potentially monoamine oxidase inhibitors (MAOIs); use therapeutic nicotine with caution. *Common adverse effects (>10%):* Agitation, dry mouth, insomnia, headache, nausea, constipation, weight loss or gain, and tremor. Hypertension may occur. As noted in text, bupropion may be associated with false-positive urine tests for amphetamines. *Serious but uncommon effect:* Seizures.

Generic name	clonidine
Trade name	Catapres
Class	α_2 adrenergic agonist
Half-life	6–20 hours
Mechanism of action	Stimulates α_2 adrenoceptors in the brain stem, resulting in reduced sympathetic outflow from the CNS
Available preparations	Tablets: 0.1, 0.2, 0.3 mg
Starting dose	After test dose: 0.1 mg po tid on withdrawal day 1
Titration	0.2 mg po tid on withdrawal day 2 if tolerated 0.3 mg po tid on withdrawal day 3 if tolerated Decrease dose by 0.2 mg/day on withdrawal days 4–10 until discontinued
Typical daily dose	N/A
Dose range	As above
Therapeutic serum level	Not established

Comments: Used for the treatment of opioid withdrawal, although not necessarily recommended in elderly patients. Treats autonomic symptoms of withdrawal, but not restlessness, insomnia, or drug craving. Test dose is given before use to determine effects on pulse and blood pressure (see text). Onset of action in 30–60 minutes, with peak effects within 2–4 hours and duration of 6–10 hours. Oral bioavailability 75%–95%. Metabolized in the liver to inactive metabolites. Half-life prolonged in renal impairment to 18–41 hours. Sixty-five percent excreted in urine. *Drug interactions:* Additive hypotensive effect with antipsychotics (especially low-potency) and opioid analgesics; bradycardia with β-blockers; rebound hypertension on clonidine discontinuation with β-blockers, mirtazapine, and tricyclic antidepressants; additive sedative effects with other CNS depressants; decreased sensitivity to hypoglycemia with oral antidiabetic drugs; mirtazapine and TCAs may antagonize antihypertensive effects of clonidine; and increased cyclosporine (and possibly tacrolimus) levels. Clonidine should not be discontinued abruptly, or rapid increases in blood pressure and pulse can occur, along with other signs of autonomic hyperactivity. *Common adverse effects (>10%):* Drowsiness, dizziness, and dry mouth. *Less common adverse effects (1%–10%):* Orthostasis, fatigue, constipation, nausea, and vomiting.

Generic name	disulfiram
Trade name	Antabuse
Class	Aldehyde dehydrogenase inhibitor
Half-life	20% of drug remains in the body 6 days after a single 2-g dose
Mechanism of action	Inhibits the enzyme involved in conversion of toxic intermediate acetaldehyde to acetic acid; when alcohol is coingested, symptoms of flushing, nausea, palpitations, and hypotension occur
Available preparations	Tablets: 250 mg
Starting dose	250 mg/day
Titration	Dose is continued for 1–2 weeks, then maintenance therapy is started
Typical daily dose	Maintenance therapy: 125 mg/day
Dose range	125–500 mg/day
Therapeutic serum level	Not established

Comments: Not a preferred drug in elderly patients because of potential adverse effects and drug interactions. Patient must be abstinent from alcohol for a minimum of 12 hours before use. Full effect takes 12 hours from time of ingestion. Duration of effect from 1–2 weeks after last dose. Rapidly absorbed. Metabolized in liver via CYP1A2, 2A6, 2B6, 2D6, 2E1, and 3A4. Potent inhibitor of CYP2E1; also inhibits CYP1A2, 2A6, 2B6, 2C8/9, 2D6, and 3A4. *Drug interactions:* Increased concentrations of benzodiazepines that are oxidatively metabolized; increased cocaine concentrations; disulfiram reaction (flushing, nausea, palpitations, and hypotension) with alcohol-containing drugs such as Bactrim, metronidazole, tolbutamide, or diphenhydramine syrup; increased levels of CYP2E1 substrates such as theophylline; adverse CNS effects with isoniazid, TCAs, MAOIs, and metronidazole; increased phenytoin levels; and inhibition of warfarin metabolism with increased international normalization ratio. *Adverse effects:* Drowsiness, headache, fatigue, psychosis, rash, dermatitis, metallic aftertaste, impotence, hepatitis, polyneuritis, peripheral neuropathy, and optic neuritis.

Generic name	methadone
Trade name	Dolophine, Methadose, Methadone Intensol
Class	Opioid
Half-life	>36 hours
Mechanism of action	μ receptor agonist
Available preparations	Tablets: 5, 10 mg Oral solution: 5 mg/5mL, 10 mg/5 mL Oral concentrate: 10 mg/mL
Starting dose	10 mg po
Titration	Dose can be repeated after several hours if needed
Typical daily dose	10 mg bid; when stable for several days, taper begun (see text)
Dose range	5–20 mg bid
Therapeutic serum level	Variable

Comments: Used for the treatment of opioid dependence, but not necessarily a recommended drug in elderly patients because of complex and changing pharmacokinetics. Well absorbed orally, with peak concentrations in 4 hours, minimizing euphoric effects. Large extravascular reservoir because of high lipophilicity; plasma half-life of 1–2 days avoids withdrawal between doses. Duration of action increases substantially with repeated dosing. Wide variability among individuals in serum levels at a given dose. Extensively metabolized, primarily via CYP3A4. Renal excretion is dose dependent, and renal reabsorption is dependent on urinary pH. *Drug interactions:* Drugs such as phenobarbital, phenytoin, carbamazepine, isoniazid, rifampin, nevirapine, and high-dose vitamin C may significantly reduce methadone levels. Drugs such as ketoconazole, fluconazole, sertraline, amitriptyline, paroxetine, fluvoxamine, fluoxetine, diazepam, alprazolam, and zidovudine are associated with increased methadone levels (other metabolic routes involved). *Adverse effects:* Tolerance develops to sedative effect, but may not develop to constipation, increased sweating, decreased libido, and sexual dysfunction. EEG sleep abnormalities resolve with time, but insomnia may persist. Same toxic effects as other opioids, except methadone also has the potential to prolong QTc.

Generic name	naltrexone
Trade name	ReVia, Depade, Vivitrol (long-acting injectable)
Class	Opioid antagonist
Half-life	4 hours; 6-β-naltrexol metabolite: 13 hours
Mechanism of action	Blocks opioid effects by competitive antagonism
Available preparations	Tablets: 25, 50, 100 mg
Starting dose	25 mg/day
Titration	As needed and tolerated
Typical daily dose	25 mg
Dose range	25–50 mg/day
Therapeutic serum level	Not established

Comments: Understudied in the geriatric population; not a preferred drug in elderly patients because of the risk of hepatotoxicity, which is dose-related. This is particularly true for the injectable form, which results in a three- to fourfold higher concentration compared to a 50-mg oral dose. Contraindicated in patients with acute hepatitis or hepatic failure. Patient must be opioid-free for 7 days with heroin or other short-acting drug or 10 days with methadone or other long-acting drug before naltrexone is initiated. Give with food or antacids after meals. Almost completely absorbed; about 60 minutes to peak level with oral dosing. With injection, initial peak level is in 2 hours, with second peak 2–3 days later. Levels of injected drug begin to decline 14 days after injection; measureable levels detected for more than 30 days. Extensive first-pass metabolism to 6-β-naltrexol with oral dosing. Also glucuronidated; no CYP450 involvement. Excreted in urine. Drug interactions: Decreased effects of opioid analgesics, may precipitate withdrawal; lethargy and somnolence with thioridazine. Common adverse effects (>10%): Insomnia, nervousness, headache, low energy, abdominal cramping, nausea, vomiting, and arthralgia. Less common adverse effects (1%–10%): Feeling down, irritability, dizziness, anxiety, somnolence, polydipsia, diarrhea, constipation, and impotence; injection site reactions occurred in patients administered Vivitrol. Uncommon but serious adverse effects: Depression, suicide attempts, disorientation, hallucinations, and paranoia.

Generic name	nicotine replacements
Trade name	Chewing gum: Nicorette, generic brands Lozenge: Commit Transdermal patch: NicoDerm, Nicotrol, generic brands
Class	Nicotine replacement therapy
Half-life	About 4 hours
Mechanism of action	Nicotine replaces smoking
Available preparations	See Table 7–5
Starting dose	
Titration	
Typical daily dose	
Dose range	
Therapeutic serum level	

Comments: Although understudied in the elderly population, nicotine replacement therapy is a first-line treatment for tobacco dependence. For elders, the transdermal patch may be the preferred vehicle because of slow absorption. Although these products generally provide lower peak nicotine levels and slower onset compared with smoking, caution is advised in using them in patients with coronary artery disease, severe or worsening angina, recent myocardial infarction, uncontrolled hypertension, or serious cardiac dysrhythmia. When nicotine replacement therapy is initiated, the patient should stop smoking to avoid toxic nicotine levels. The intended duration of replacement therapy is 8–12 weeks. These products are most effective when used on a fixed schedule rather than at varying intervals. Details regarding preparations and instructions for use of selected products are shown in Table 7–5. Absorption is slow for transdermal preparation and relatively rapid for gum and lozenge preparations. Nicotine is metabolized in the liver, primarily to cotinine (one-fifth as active; can be assayed in saliva). Eliminated via kidneys, with rate dependent on pH. *Drug interactions:* Hypertension with bupropion, increased nicotine concentrations with cimetidine, increased hemodynamic and atrioventricular blocking effects of adenosine. Lozenge contains phenylalanine; manufacturer recommends caution in its use in frail elders with anxiety, hypertension, or diabetes. *Common adverse effects (>10%) with gum/lozenge:* Tachycardia, headache, nausea, vomiting, indigestion, excessive salivation, belching, increased appetite, mouth/throat soreness, jaw muscle ache, and hiccups. *Less common adverse effects (1%–10%) with gum/lozenge:* Insomnia, dizziness, nervousness, GI distress, muscle pain, and hoarseness. *Uncommon but serious adverse effects with gum/lozenge:* Atrial fibrillation, hypersensitivity reactions. *Common adverse effects (>10%) with transdermal patch:* Insomnia, abnormal dreams, pruritis, cough, and pharyngitis. *Less common adverse effects with transdermal patch:* Chest pain, dysphoria, anxiety, somnolence, dizziness, difficulty concentrating, diarrhea, dyspepsia, nausea, dry mouth, constipation, anorexia, abdominal pain, arthralgia, and myalgia. *Uncommon but serious adverse effects with transdermal patch:* Atrial fibrillation, hypersensitivity reactions, nervousness, taste perversion, thirst, and tremor.

Generic name	varenicline
Trade name	Chantix
Class	Nicotinic receptor partial agonist
Half-life	17–24 hours
Mechanism of action	Partial agonist at α4β2 nicotinic acetylcholine receptor; binds with greater affinity than nicotine; blocks nicotine from binding; receptor stimulation leads to release of dopamine
Available preparations	Tablets: 0.5, 1 mg
Starting dose	0.5 mg/day
Titration	0.5 mg/day for 3 days, then 0.5 mg bid for 4 days, then 1 mg bid for 12 weeks. Patients who quit smoking may continue for another 12 weeks
Typical daily dose	1 mg bid
Dose range	1–2 mg/day divided bid
Therapeutic serum level	Not established

Comments: A potentially useful agent in treating tobacco dependence, although understudied in elderly patients. This drug is started 1 week before the target date to quit smoking. Rapidly absorbed through the gastric mucosa and reaches peak plasma concentration in about 4 hours. It is minimally metabolized; excreted unchanged through the kidneys. Dosage should be reduced in patients with severe renal impairment. *Drug interactions:* Cimetidine decreases renal clearance of varenicline, increasing level by 29%. *Adverse effects:* Nausea, vomiting, constipation, flatulence, insomnia, abnormal dreams, headache, xerostomia, and weight gain. Coadministration with nicotine replacement therapies may worsen adverse effects. Physical dependence may occur.

8

Treatment of
Movement Disorders

Introduction

This chapter focuses on clinically relevant information about diagnosis, differential diagnosis, and basic treatment of selected movement disorders in the geriatric patient. It is intended to assist geriatric psychiatrists and geriatricians in the detection of movement abnormalities, in decisions about neurological or neuropsychiatric referral, and in evaluation of care provided by consultants. Medications effective for various movement-related disorders are identified in the text and described more fully in the Specific Drug summaries at the end of this chapter.

Aging is associated with motor changes, including variable decline in vestibular, visual, and proprioceptive functions, increases in postural sway, and motor and psychomotor slowing (Rajput and Rajput 2004). In addition, certain movement disorders not only are more prevalent in old age but have a much higher incidence after 65 years of age. These include parkinsonism, essential tremor (ET), stroke-related movement abnormalities (hemiballismus, dystonia, parkinsonism), orofacial dyskinesias, and neuroleptic-induced dyskinesias (Rajput and Rajput 2004). The differentiation of normal from abnormal motor findings in the elderly patient requires attention to specific features of the clinical examination.

The first step in diagnosis of a movement disorder is careful observation and description of the movement abnormality itself. The abnormality is then labeled, using one of the terms defined in the following section, and a differential diagnosis of etiology is formulated. Most movement abnormalities represent either idiopathic or secondary disorders.

Abnormalities of Movement

Akinesia, Bradykinesia, and Hypokinesia

Akinesia is slowness in the initiation of movement, *bradykinesia* is decreased velocity of movement, and *hypokinesia* is reduced amplitude of movement. In practice, the term *bradykinesia* is often used as an overarching term, to include all three abnormalities. Bradykinesia is among the most disabling of movement abnormalities and significantly affects the patient's ability to perform activities of daily living. It is a core deficit from which other signs are derived, including masklike facies (decreased blinking), drooling (decreased swallowing), hypophonia, and micrographia. Bradykinesia that is a consequence of aging is generalized and symmetric, whereas bradykinesia due to pathology is often asymmetric. Severe bradykinesia is usually pathological.

Athetosis

Athetosis is a type of dystonia seen as continuous, slow, twisting movements (sometimes described as wormlike), usually in the fingers and hands. Athetosis may occur in combination with chorea as choreoathetosis, as seen in Huntington's disease (HD). Athetosis is not commonly seen in elderly patients.

Chorea

Chorea refers to arrhythmic, jerky, purposeless, involuntary movements occurring in a random sequence. The movements can be brisk or slow and involve limbs, face, or trunk. Etiologies of chorea in elderly patients are listed in Table 8–1. Movement disorders in which chorea is prominent include tardive dyskinesia (TD), HD, and edentulous dyskinesia.

Dystonia

Involuntary, sustained muscle contraction that results in twisting, unusual postures, or repetitive movements is termed *dystonia*. Dystonia is classified as *focal* (e.g., blepharospasm, torticollis, writer's cramp), *segmental* or *hemidystonia* (e.g., secondary to stroke or tumor), *multifocal*, or *generalized* (Kishore and Calne 1997). Causes of dystonia are listed in Table 8–2. Dystonia at rest is usually a more severe symptom than action dystonia, such as writer's cramp. Dystonia is relieved by rest and sleep and worsened by stress, fatigue, and emotional upset (Kumar and Calne 2004). Patients can sometimes suppress dystonias with sensory tricks such as touching the skin around a blepharospastic eye (Kumar and Calne 2004). Along with other dystonias, writer's cramp can be effectively treated with periodic injections of botulinum toxin into forearm muscles (Jankovic and Schwartz 1993). Acute and tardive dystonias secondary to neuroleptic drug exposure are discussed later in this chapter.

Gait and Postural Instability

Increased postural sway and loss of postural reflexes are seen with usual aging, and thus the gait of the elderly individual may be slightly wide-based, with short, slow strides (Rajput and Rajput 2004). Heel strike and armswing are normal and symmetric. Gait that is excessively slow or that deviates significantly from this description is abnormal. Abnormal gait in elderly patients may be due to any one of a number of conditions particularly afflicting elders, including arthritis, weakness, gait apraxia from frontal lobe disease, and parkinsonism, among others, or may have no identifiable cause (Rajput and Rajput 2004).

Hemiballismus

Hemiballismus is a flinging, rotatory movement of the limbs on one side of the body usually resulting from ischemia of the subthalamic nucleus and/or other areas of the striatum (Rajput and Rajput 2004). Onset is usually sudden, and the movements either resolve or are transformed into choreiform movements over several weeks. Symptoms can often be managed, at least over the short term, using haloperidol or other neuroleptics (Rajput and Rajput 2004).

Table 8–1. Etiologies of chorea in elderly patients

Hereditary diseases
Huntington's disease
Neuroacanthocytosis
Benign hereditary chorea
Central nervous system degenerations
Olivopontocerebellar atrophy
Machado-Joseph disease
Kufs' disease
Dentatorubropallidoluysian atrophy
Aging-related
Spontaneous orofacial dyskinesia
Edentulous orodyskinesia
"Senile chorea"
Drug-induced
Neuroleptics, antiparkinsonian drugs, lithium, benzodiazepines, tricyclic
antidepressants, monoamine oxidase inhibitors, carbamazepine,
amphetamines, methylphenidate, methadone, steroids, estrogens
(including vaginal cream), antihistamines, digoxin, and other drugs
Metabolic
Hyperthyroidism
Hypoparathyroidism
Hypo- and hypernatremia, hypomagnesemia, hypocalcemia
Hypo- and hyperglycemia
Acquired hepatocerebral degeneration, Wilson's disease
Infectious
Encephalitis
Subacute bacterial endocarditis
Creutzfeldt-Jakob disease
Toxins
Alcohol intoxication/withdrawal, anoxia, carbon monoxide, manganese,
mercury, toluene, thallium

Table 8–1.   Etiologies of chorea in elderly patients *(continued)*

Immunological

    Systemic lupus erythematosus

    Sydenham's chorea (recurrence)

    Primary anticardiolipin antibody syndrome

Vascular

    Infarction (usually striatum, subthalamic nucleus)

    Hemorrhage

    Arteriovenous malformation

    Polycythemia rubra vera

    Migraine

Tumors

Trauma: subdural hematoma

Miscellaneous: paroxysmal choreoathetosis

Source.   Reprinted from Jackson GR, Lang AE: "Hyperkinetic Movement Disorders," in *The American Psychiatric Press Textbook of Geriatric Neuropsychiatry,* 2nd Edition. Edited by Coffey CE, Cummings JL. Washington, DC, American Psychiatric Press, 2000, p. 535. Used with permission.

Myoclonus

Myclonic movements are sudden, brief, shock-like, and usually irregular (Kumar and Calne 2004). They can be physiologic, as in the case of hiccups or "sleep starts," idiopathic (essential), or secondary. Myoclonus can be triggered by stimuli such as noise, light, touch, or muscle stretch (as with asterixis). Myoclonic movements can be distinguished from tremor by distinct pauses between jerks, and distinguished from tics by suppressibility of the latter. Myoclonus in the geriatric population is usually seen in the context of degenerative diseases such as Alzheimer's disease or Parkinson's disease (PD), but it is also seen in toxic-metabolic encephalopathies (often as asterixis). New-onset myoclonus can be the harbinger of seizures, as has been noted in patients taking clozapine (Sajatovic and Meltzer 1996). Etiologies of myoclonus are shown in Table 8–3.

Table 8–2. Etiologies of late-onset dystonia

Idiopathic dystonia

Focal dystonias

    Spasmodic torticollis

    Cranial dystonia: blepharospasm, oromandibular dystonia, spasmodic dysphonia

    Writer's cramp

Segmental/Multifocal dystonia

Generalized dystonia (rare)

Secondary dystonia

Drugs: neuroleptics (including metoclopramide), dopamine agonists, anticonvulsants, antimalarial drugs

Stroke: hemorrhage or infarction

Other focal lesions: vascular malformation, tumor, abscess, demyelination

Trauma: head injury or peripheral injury and subdural hematoma

Encephalitis

Toxins: manganese, carbon monoxide poisoning, methanol, carbon disulfide

Paraneoplastic

Hypoparathyroidism

Central pontine myelinolysis

Degenerative diseases

    Parkinson's disease

    Progressive supranuclear palsy

    Cortical-basal ganglionic degeneration

    Multiple system atrophy

Disorders simulating dystonia

    Psychogenic dystonia

    Atlantoaxial subluxation

    Seizures

    Posterior fossa tumor

    Oculomotor disturbance

Source. Adapted from Jackson GR, Lang AE: "Hyperkinetic Movement Disorders," in *The American Psychiatric Press Textbook of Geriatric Neuropsychiatry,* 2nd Edition. Edited by Coffey CE, Cummings JL. Washington, DC, American Psychiatric Press, 2000, p. 545. Used with permission.

Rigidity

Rigidity is an increase in muscle tone during passive movement through flexion and extension (e.g., bending the arm at the elbow) and is usually more evident around distal joints such as the wrist. *Lead-pipe rigidity* is smooth, whereas *cogwheeling* is a ratchet-like movement thought to arise from the incorporation of a tremor. Lead-pipe rigidity can be seen in the patient with neuroleptic malignant syndrome (NMS), as discussed later in this chapter and in Chapter 3 of this volume, "Antipsychotics." To be examined for rigidity, the patient must be capable of relaxing the tested limb. Rigidity secondary to medications or other causes is often (but not always) symmetric; asymmetric rigidity may suggest the presence of PD (Kumar and Calne 2004). Spasticity is a velocity-dependent catch followed by release without further resistance to movement ("clasp-knife" phenomenon) characteristic of corticospinal tract disease (Rajput and Rajput 2004).

Tics

Tics are involuntary, rapid, repetitive, stereotyped vocalizations or movements. They can be simple (e.g., blinking, shrugging, throat clearing, sniffing) or complex (e.g., touching, obscene gestures, echolalia, coprolalia). They are worsened by stress, anxiety, and fatigue and may be relieved by concentration on another task (Kumar and Calne 2004). Tics usually are multifocal but commonly involve the upper body. The subjective experience is one of a buildup of tension, followed by relief when the movement occurs. Patients may be able to suppress tics temporarily, but this can lead to rebound exacerbation. In elderly patients, tics can be seen after a head injury, after a stroke, with certain medications, or in developmentally disabled individuals. Tics can also occur as a tardive syndrome after chronic neuroleptic exposure (Kumar and Calne 2004). A list of etiologies of tics is shown in Table 8–4.

Tremor

Tremor is a rhythmic oscillation of a body part that may involve the upper or lower limbs, lips, tongue, neck, or voice (Kumar and Calne 2004). It can be coarse or fine and can vary in frequency. Types of tremor include resting, postural, and kinetic (present with action). A *resting tremor* sub-

Table 8–3.   Etiologies of myoclonus in elderly patients

Physiological myoclonus

Hiccups, "starts" while falling asleep or wakening, exercise-induced, anxiety-induced

Essential myoclonus

Secondary myoclonus

Metabolic causes

    Hepatic failure, renal failure, dialysis syndrome, hyponatremia, hypoglycemia, nonketotic hyperglycemia

Viral encephalopathies

    Herpes simplex encephalitis, arbovirus encephalitis, encephalitis lethargica, postinfectious encephalomyelitis

Drugs: tricyclic antidepressants, levodopa, monoamine oxidase inhibitors, antibiotics, lithium, selective serotonin reuptake inhibitors

Toxins: bismuth, heavy metal poisons, methyl bromide, dichlorodiphenyltrichloroethane (DDT)

Physical encephalopathies

    Postanoxic (Lance-Adams syndrome)

    Posttraumatic

    Heat stroke

    Electric shock

    Decompression injury

Dementing and degenerative diseases

    Creutzfeldt-Jakob disease

    Alzheimer's disease

    Cortical-basal ganglionic degeneration

    Parkinson's disease

    Huntington's disease

    Multiple-system atrophy

    Pallidal degenerations

Focal central nervous system damage

    Poststroke

    Olivodentate lesions (palatal myoclonus)

Table 8–3. Etiologies of myoclonus in elderly patients *(continued)*

Spinal cord lesions (segmental/spinal myoclonus)
Tumor
Trauma
Postthalamotomy (often unilateral asterixis)

Source. Adapted from Jackson GR, Lang AE: "Hyperkinetic Movement Disorders," in *The American Psychiatric Press Textbook of Geriatric Neuropsychiatry,* 2nd Edition. Edited by Coffey CE, Cummings JL. Washington, DC, American Psychiatric Press, 2000, p. 549. Used with permission.

sides with action and with assumption of a posture (Kumar and Calne 2004). In some classifications, *kinetic tremor* is further subdivided into *simple kinetic* and *intentional,* the latter being worse during the completion of target-directed movements (Deuschl et al. 1998). Tremor is tested first by observation of the patient sitting, with hands on thighs (*resting*); then arms are extended away from the body (*kinetic*) and held out parallel to the floor (*postural*). The patient is then asked to touch a target, such as the examiner's finger (*intentional*). Latent resting and postural tremors may be elicited by asking the patient to perform a distracting activity such as drawing the figure *8* in the air while the examiner observes the opposite hand. The presence of tremor, particularly resting tremor, is one of the signs that best distinguishes normal aging from a movement disorder (Rajput and Rajput 2004). Etiologies of tremor in elderly patients are listed in Table 8–5. Important tremor syndromes discussed below include PD, drug-induced tremor, and ET. Movement abnormalities seen in the context of serotonin syndrome and NMS are discussed later in this chapter and in relevant chapters throughout this volume.

Treatment of Selected Movement Disorders and Syndromes

Degenerative and Other Movement Disorders

Corticobasal Degeneration

Corticobasal degeneration (CBD) is an insidiously developing, progressive disease of late life involving motor signs, higher cortical dysfunction,

Table 8–4.   Etiologies of tics in elderly patients

Idiopathic

Persistent childhood-onset tic disorder

Simple tic

Multiple motor tics

Tourette's syndrome (multiple motor and vocal tics)

Adult-onset tic disorder

Secondary

Postencephalitic

Head injury

Carbon monoxide poisoning

Poststroke

Drugs: stimulants, levodopa, neuroleptics, carbamazepine, phenytoin, and
   phenobarbital

Mental retardation syndromes (including chromosomal abnormalities)

Source.   Adapted from Jackson GR, Lang AE: "Hyperkinetic Movement Disorders," in
The American Psychiatric Press Textbook of Geriatric Neuropsychiatry, 2nd Edition. Edited by
Coffey CE, Cummings JL. Washington, DC, American Psychiatric Press, 2000, p. 551.
Used with permission.

and neuropsychiatric abnormalities (Stover et al. 2004). It is more common in women than men and appears not to be familial. It is classified
pathologically as a tauopathy, along with several other diseases (progressive supranuclear palsy [PSP], Pick's disease, and frontotemporal dementia) involving defective processing of the microtubule-associated protein
tau (Stover et al. 2004). Distinguishing features of CBD include asymmetric onset of motor findings and absence of gait abnormality.

Although either motor dysfunction or cognitive impairment may
occur first, CBD most often presents with asymmetric limb clumsiness
or asymmetric progressive parkinsonism of the akinetic-rigid type. The
clinical triad that develops in most cases is that of akinesia, rigidity, and
apraxia (Stover et al. 2004). Many other motor signs may also be seen,
however, including kinetic and postural tremor, dystonia, and myoclo-

Table 8–5. Etiologies of tremor in elderly patients

Resting tremor

Parkinson's disease

Secondary parkinsonian syndromes

Rubral (midbrain) tremor

Postural tremor

Physiological tremor

Exaggerated physiological tremor

Endocrine

> Hypoglycemia, thyrotoxicosis, pheochromocytoma, steroids

Drugs/Toxins

> β-Agonists, dopamine agonists, lithium, tricyclic antidepressants, neuroleptics, serotonergic drugs (serotonin syndrome), theophylline, caffeine, valproate, amphetamines, alcohol withdrawal, mercury, lead, arsenic, etc.

Essential tremor

Primary writing tremor

Parkinson's disease

Akinetic-rigid syndromes

Idiopathic dystonia (including focal dystonia)

Tremor with peripheral neuropathy

Cerebellar tremor

Kinetic tremor (simple or intentional)

Vascular

Tumor

Acquired hepatocerebral degeneration

Drugs/Toxins (e.g., mercury)

Multiple sclerosis

Miscellaneous tremor syndromes

Psychogenic tremor

Orthostatic tremor

Rhythmical myoclonus (e.g., palatal, spinal)

Asterixis

Clonus

Epilepsia partialis continua

Source. Adapted from Jackson GR, Lang AE: "Hyperkinetic Movement Disorders," in *The American Psychiatric Press Textbook of Geriatric Neuropsychiatry,* 2nd Edition. Edited by Coffey CE and Cummings JL. Washington, DC, American Psychiatric Press, 2000, p. 532. Used with permission.

nus. When tremor is seen, it is more irregular and of a higher frequency (6–8 Hz) than is usually seen with PD (Stover et al. 2004). Higher cortical impairments can include limb apraxia and alien limb phenomenon. Although different kinds of apraxia can be seen, the most common is probably ideomotor apraxia, which is characterized by impairment in timing, sequencing, spatial organization, and mimicking of movements (Stover et al. 2004). Alien limb phenomenon, the failure to recognize an extremity as one's own in the absence of visual cues, develops in half of patients with CBD. Neuropsychiatric symptoms can include depression, apathy, irritability, anxiety, disinhibition, delusions, and agitation (Stover et al. 2004). As with lesions from stroke, depression is more common with left hemisphere involvement.

Structural and functional neuroimaging findings often are asymmetric, as described in Table 8–6, and consulting radiologists should be asked to look specifically for asymmetries. In later disease stages, magnetic resonance imaging or computed tomography may show asymmetric frontoparietal cortical atrophy (contralateral to affected limbs) and an electroencephalogram may show slowing over the involved hemisphere (Stover et al. 2004).

Treatment of CBD is symptomatic. Poor response is seen to levodopa or dopamine agonists. Kinetic tremor and myoclonus may respond to clonazepam, and rigidity to baclofen (Stover et al. 2004). Botulinum toxin injections may provide relief for painful focal dystonias or blepharospasm (Stover et al. 2004).

Dementia With Lewy Bodies

As discussed in Chapter 3 of this volume, "Antipsychotics," dementia with Lewy bodies (DLB) is a degenerative dementia associated with α-synuclein accumulation. Characteristic features of DLB include parkinsonian symptoms (with or without tremor), fluctuating cognitive impairment, and psychosis (particularly visual hallucinations). Falls are common, and episodic loss of consciousness may occur, as may delusions and depression. A neuroleptic sensitivity reaction can be seen in response to antipsychotic treatment, with sudden onset of rigidity, immobility, increased confusion, and sedation (Aarsland et al. 2005).

Cholinesterase inhibitors are a mainstay of treatment for DLB, with improvement often noted in motor signs in addition to cognition. Motor

Table 8–6.   Neuroimaging in selected movement disorders

Movement disorder	Structural findings (MRI)	Functional findings (PET)
Huntington's disease	Caudate atrophy	Hypometabolism in caudate and frontal lobes
Wilson's disease	Hypo- or hyperintensities in basal ganglia, thalamus, midbrain, and frontal lobes	Hypometabolism in striatum, frontoparietal cortices, and white matter Reduced fluorodopa uptake
Parkinson's disease	Normal	Reduced fluorodopa uptake in striatum, especially putamen Hypermetabolism in pallidum by fluorodeoxyglucose scan
Progressive supranuclear palsy	Midbrain atrophy	Reduced fluorodopa uptake in striatum
Multi-system atrophy (Shy-Drager syndrome)	Cerebellar and brain stem atrophy Hyperintensity in dorsolateral putamen	Reduced fluorodopa uptake in caudate and putamen Frontal and striatal hypometabolism by fluorodeoxyglucose scan
Corticobasal degeneration	Contralateral and later bilateral frontoparietal atrophy	Asymmetric parietal and frontal hypometabolism by fluorodeoxyglucose scan Asymmetric reduction of striatal fluorodopa uptake

Note.   MRI=magnetic resonance imaging; PET=positron emission tomography.
Source.   Adapted from Kumar A, Calne DB: "Approach to the Patient With a Movement Disorder and Overview of Movement Disorders," in *Movement Disorders: Neurologic Principles and Practice,* 2nd Edition. Edited by Watts RL, Koller WC. New York, McGraw-Hill Health Professions Division, 2004, p. 13. Used with permission.

signs are usually poorly responsive to levodopa or respond only partially at extremely low dosages (e.g., Sinemet at 10–100 mg/day). As discussed in Chapter 3, antipsychotic medications must be used carefully (if at all) and at low doses because of neuroleptic sensitivity. If antipsychotic drugs must be used in the treatment of patients with DLB, preferred drugs include quetiapine and clozapine.

Essential Tremor

ET is a common syndrome that may have onset at any age, but both incidence and prevalence increase markedly in older age (Rajput and Rajput 2004). It is often familial. ET is a coarse, postural tremor that usually first involves the hands. The tremor frequency varies from 4 to 12 cycles/second and is inversely related to amplitude. With aging, tremor amplitude increases and frequency decreases, and tremor may extend to other parts of the body (Rajput and Rajput 2004) such as the tongue, head, voice, or trunk. Because disability relates to tremor amplitude, the oldest old are most affected. Functional disability involves handwriting, eating with utensils, drinking from a cup, and use of objects such as hand tools or knitting needles. Some of those afflicted report that ingestion of alcohol markedly reduces this tremor, but over time this effect is lost (Rajput and Rajput 2004).

First-line therapies for ET include propranolol and primidone. Propranolol is more effective than selective β-blockers and should be used at a dosage of at least 120 mg/day. The usual therapeutic dosage for this indication is 160–320 mg/day (Louis 2001). The long-acting formulation of propranolol may improve compliance. Primidone is poorly tolerated by elderly patients, partly because one of its metabolites is a barbiturate. Initial nausea, vomiting, and ataxia can be seen even at low starting doses. Over the long-term, however, primidone may be better tolerated than propranolol (Louis 2001). The usual therapeutic dosage of primidone for treatment of ET is 62.5–1,000 mg/day (Louis 2001). Second-line therapies for ET include gabapentin at a dosage of 1,200–3,600 mg/day and alprazolam at dosages up to 2.75 mg/day, the latter not necessarily recommended for the treatment of elderly patients (Louis 2001). Up to 55% of patients may not respond to pharmacologic treatment for ET. In refractory cases, deep brain stimulation to the ventral intermediate nucleus of the thalamus has been used successfully to treat ET (Louis 2001).

Huntington's Disease

HD usually has onset before 65 years of age, with peaks before 20 years of age and in the fifth and sixth decades. It can, however, become symptomatic for the first time in later life, and when it does, it often progresses more slowly and involves less severe cognitive impairment than early-onset forms (Myers et al. 1985). HD is a complex disorder involving progressive abnormalities in motor function, cognition, behavior, and functional ability. In many cases, the presenting symptom is depression or suicidal behavior. Motor dysfunctions include prominent chorea, eye movement abnormalities, and later-appearing parkinsonism, dystonia, dysarthria, and dysphagia (Marshall 2004). The dementia of HD is a frontal/subcortical type. Behavioral disorders include mood disorders (particularly depression), apathy, risk of suicide, psychosis, compulsive and ritualistic behaviors (e.g., hand washing), early personality changes, and sleep disorders (Marshall 2004). HD is diagnosed on the basis of clinical signs. Genetic testing for polymorphic trinucleotide (CAG) repeat expansion shows high sensitivity (98.8%) and specificity (100%) (Kremer et al. 1994).

The motor symptoms of HD in some ways resemble those of TD, but the two syndromes can be distinguished by clinical signs. Compared with TD, in HD there is often a prominent appearance of forehead chorea (e.g., eyebrow movements), flowing or athetoid movements, dysarthria, facial apraxia, impersistence of tongue protrusion, oculomotor defects, gait disorder, postural instability, and swallowing difficulties. Compared with HD, there is often a more prominent appearance of mouth movements and stereotyped movements in TD (Wojcieszek and Lang 1994). As shown in Table 8–6, neuroimaging abnormalities in HD include caudate atrophy and hypometabolism in caudate and frontal lobes.

The movement abnormalities of HD suggest overactivity of the dopaminergic system. In the early stages of the disease, dopamine D_2 receptor antagonists active in the dorsal striatum (e.g., haloperidol) may be helpful as palliative treatment for motor symptoms; usual antipsychotic doses for geriatric patients are employed. Atypical antipsychotics are expected to be less useful for this indication, although several cases were reported in which risperidone at 3–6 mg/day was helpful in treating motor and psychiatric disturbances in patients with HD (Dallocchio et al.

1999). Antiglutamatergic agents (e.g., riluzole) and cellular energy-enhancing drugs (e.g., coenzyme Q_{10}) are currently under study for HD, as are other neuroprotective strategies (Marshall 2004).

Parkinson's Disease

Degeneration of dopaminergic neurons in the basal ganglia (substantia nigra) underlies idiopathic PD. Risk of developing PD increases with advancing age and is higher in males. All ethnic groups are affected. The classic triad of clinical symptoms in PD consists of tremor, bradykinesia, and rigidity. The presence of a resting tremor is highly suggestive of PD, although tremor is not present in all cases (Nutt and Wooten 2005). In idiopathic PD, tremor and bradykinesia are usually asymmetric on initial presentation. Bradykinesia involves fine movements, especially on repetition, so the patient might report inability to fasten buttons or to brush teeth (Nutt and Wooten 2005). Rigidity might be reported as stiffness and aching in a limb. Even in early PD, gait may be slowed, with foot dragging and decreased armswing on the affected side (Nutt and Wooten 2005). With further development of postural instability and the development of festination (accelerating, shuffling gait) and en bloc turning, the risk of falls is greatly increased. PD also may be associated with dementia, depression, and generalized anxiety, syndromes that are discussed in other chapters. Idiopathic PD can be distinguished from secondary parkinsonism (e.g., neuroleptic-induced) by the prominence of resting tremor, asymmetry of signs and symptoms, and better response to levodopa therapy (Lang and Lozano 1998a). PD can be distinguished from other neurodegenerative disorders by clinical examination findings; there are no laboratory tests to confirm the diagnosis. Neuroimaging may be of use in ruling out other diseases (see Table 8–6). In addition, there is some evidence that dopamine transporter imaging using single photon emission computed tomography (SPECT) scanning may be helpful in diagnosis when PD findings are equivocal (Nutt and Wooten 2005), and that positron emission tomography (PET) and SPECT imaging may help distinguish PD from DLB (Colloby and O'Brien 2004). At present, however, these technologies are available only in research settings in the United States.

Patients newly diagnosed with PD need education and reassurance that the disease varies considerably among individuals, that it may be only gradually progressive over decades, and that many treatments are now available to control symptoms (Nutt and Wooten 2005). A number of Web sites are available that provide helpful information to patients, including http://www.apdaparkinson.org, http://www.michaeljfox.org, and http://www.parkinson.org (Nutt and Wooten 2005). Patients are counseled about fitness maintenance, including exercise and balance training.

Treatment for PD is initiated when symptoms become disabling or excessively bothersome to the patient. Although a number of agents are available for treatment of PD, levodopa and dopamine agonists are recommended as first-line agents and are the mainstays of treatment. Anticholinergic medications are not recommended for treatment of PD in elderly patients because the risk of adverse anticholinergic effects outweighs the small benefit (Lang and Lozano 1998b). Amantadine and the selective monoamine oxidase B inhibitor (MAO B) selegiline are used, but provide at best moderate benefit (Lang and Lozano 1998b). When selegiline is prescribed, pyridoxine (vitamin B_6) at 100 mg/day should be coprescribed to prevent development of peripheral neuropathy.

Levodopa is the most effective antiparkinsonian agent in current use. It is combined with carbidopa to prevent peripheral decarboxylation before the drug reaches the brain. Carbidopa-levodopa (Sinemet) should be initiated in elderly patients at a dose of one-half of a 25/100 tablet (25 mg of carbidopa and 100 mg of levodopa) two times a day and titrated to clinical effect, with the goal of alleviating disability rather than eliminating all symptoms (Scharre and Mahler 1994). The usual dose is one to two tablets three times a day. Food affects levodopa absorption significantly, so this medication should be given consistently with respect to meals—preferably before meals on an empty stomach. Further information about levodopa-carbidopa pharmacology appears in the Specific Drug summary at the end of this chapter.

Nonresponse to levodopa in idiopathic PD is not common but can be seen with an inadequate trial of levodopa, with concomitant use of neuroleptics (including antiemetics and metoclopramide), with an inaccurate diagnosis, or with the use of tremor as an indicator of response (Nutt and Wooten 2005). Rigidity and bradykinesia are generally more responsive than tremor to levodopa treatment. An adequate trial of levodopa is at least 3 months in duration, with slow titration to a daily dose not exceeding

1,000 mg (Nutt and Wooten 2005) or the maximum tolerated dose.

After a variable number of years on levodopa, motor complications often occur (Scharre and Mahler 1994). These include dyskinesias (chorea, dystonia, myoclonus), earlier wearing off of the drug with time after a dose, and unpredictable periods in which parkinsonian symptoms acutely and transiently recur (known as *on-off phenomena*). Levodopa-induced dyskinesias may respond to a gradual lowering of levodopa dosage. In a small, open-label study, clozapine at a mean dosage of 30 mg/day added to the treatment regimen resulted in significant improvement in dyskinesias as early as 1 week and lasting for the 4-month study duration (Pierelli et al. 1998). Controlled-release Sinemet does not alleviate dyskinesias or on-off phenomena but does reduce wearing off. When it is necessary to discontinue levodopa or any of the other dopamine agonists, the drugs should be tapered because of the risk of inducing NMS with abrupt discontinuation.

Catechol *O*-methyltransferase (COMT) inhibitors such as tolcapone and entacapone prolong the action of levodopa and increase brain concentrations of dopamine, thus reducing wearing-off effects (Gottwald et al. 1997). These agents lack antiparkinsonian activity themselves, so they should not be administered without levodopa. When they are used in combination with levodopa, adverse effects such as hallucinations or increased dyskinesias may necessitate a reduction in levodopa dose (Lang and Lozano 1998b).

Dopamine agonists may be used as initial treatment for PD or may be added when levodopa proves ineffective (Scharre and Mahler 1994). These agents are less likely to introduce dyskinesias and motor fluctuations in the first years of therapy but may not be as effective as levodopa (Nutt and Wooten 2005). Dopamine agonists should be used judiciously in patients with dementia or psychiatric diagnoses because of the risk of inducing hallucinations. Dopamine agonists currently marketed for PD include the ergot derivatives bromocriptine (Parlodel) and pergolide (Permax) and the newer non-ergoline agents, pramipexole (Mirapex) and ropinirole (Requip). Of the dopamine agonists, the non-ergoline drugs pramipexole and ropinirole are often preferred for treatment of PD because they appear to have a better adverse-effect profile than the ergot derivatives. Bromocriptine and pergolide have been associated with fibrosis (retroperitoneal, pleural, and pericardial), and pergolide has been associated with restrictive valvular disease (Nutt and Wooten 2005). All dopaminergic drugs have side effects, however, and considering that some are shared with levodopa, these medications are best dosed apart in time when used in combination.

Pramipexole should be given initially at 0.125 mg, three times a day, and titrated slowly to a dose of 0.5–1.5 mg, three times a day. Ropinirole should be given initially at 0.25 mg, three times a day, and titrated slowly to 3–8 mg three times a day. Other details regarding use of these medications are included in the Specific Drug summaries at the end of this chapter.

In later stages of PD, surgical options may be considered. Deep brain stimulation (pallidal or subthalamic) or pallidotomy can improve motor symptoms in patients who have responded to medications but suffer from severe dyskinesias and/or motor fluctuations (Nutt and Wooten 2005). Thalamic stimulation using implanted electrodes or thalamotomy may be helpful for disabling tremor that is unresponsive to medication (Nutt and Wooten 2005).

Progressive Supranuclear Palsy

PSP is a nonfamilial disorder characterized by the unusual constellation of impaired vertical gaze, prominent axial rigidity, extensor posturing of the neck, bradykinesia, early dysarthria, frequent falls, frontal/subcortical dementia, behavioral decline, and poor response to levodopa (Kumar and Calne 2004; Scully et al. 1997). Neuroimaging findings in PSP are shown in Table 8–6.

In general, pharmacotherapy for PSP is relatively ineffective. High doses of levodopa-carbidopa (twice the dose used for PD) may be effective in alleviating symptoms in some cases (Golbe 2004). Alternatively, a trial of amantadine starting at 100 mg/day and increasing to 100 mg two times a day may be helpful (Golbe 2004). If no improvement is seen after 1 month, amantadine should be tapered and discontinued. A preliminary study found that zolpidem at 5 mg was associated with improvement in motor function in PSP, with effects seen in 40–60 minutes and lasting about 2 hours (Daniele et al. 1999). Botulinum toxin injection may be helpful for certain dystonic symptoms of PSP. Electroconvulsive therapy (ECT) has been reported to make motor and cognitive symptoms worse (Golbe 2004).

Restless Legs Syndrome

The essential feature of restless legs syndrome (RLS), also known as *Ekbom syndrome,* is an unpleasant sensation in the legs with an urge to move that worsens during periods of rest or inactivity and is relieved by movement and symptoms most marked or occurring only during the evening or nighttime hours (Trenkwalder et al. 2005). Both subjective and objective features resemble those of akathisia, but nighttime predominance of symptoms results in significant sleep disruption. Periodic limb movements of sleep are often associated with RLS, but these are distinct clinical phenomena. Periodic limb movements are discussed in the section on sleep disorders in Chapter 6 of this volume, "Anxiolytic and Sedative-Hypnotic Medications."

RLS is seen in up to 15% of the general population and 24% of primary care populations (Thorpy 2005). Given that the syndrome has a strong correlation with panic disorder, generalized anxiety disorder, and major depression (Winkelmann et al. 2005), it is likely to be even more prevalent among psychiatric patients. It is more common in women than men, and most patients seen clinically are middle-aged or older (Trenkwalder et al. 2005).

In the idiopathic form of RLS, a positive family history is often elicited. Secondary forms are most commonly due to iron deficiency in conditions such as end-stage renal disease (Thorpy 2005). In the elderly population, other associated conditions include diabetes, chronic obstructive pulmonary disease, and PD (Hornyak and Trenkwalder 2004). With increasing age, iron deficiency as a cause becomes more prevalent, and idiopathic RLS becomes less common (O'Keeffe 2005).

Abnormalities of dopaminergic neurotransmission have been implicated in RLS, and attempts to localize pathology have focused on the A11 dopaminergic neurons in the midbrain as well as spinal pathways (Trenkwalder et al. 2005). Symptoms may be caused or worsened by neuroleptics, antidepressants, or exogenous antihistamines (Thorpy 2005).

The patient who presents with symptoms consistent with RLS should have serum ferritin concentration and chemistries checked (particularly glucose, blood urea nitrogen, and creatinine). The current list of medications should be reviewed, including over-the-counter antihistamines. Changing or stopping offending medications may result in improvement of symptoms (Thorpy 2005).

Sensible sleep hygiene measures should be recommended to the patient, as should limitation of nicotine, caffeine, and alcohol, all of which contribute to symptoms. Moderate but not overly strenuous daily exercise is helpful (Thorpy 2005). If symptoms continue despite conservative treatment, pharmacologic therapy should be considered.

The following medications are recommended in the treatment of RLS, but suggested dosages are not specifically directed toward the geriatric population, so lower maxima may be appropriate in some instances (Thorpy 2005):

- Gabapentin: initially 300 mg at bedtime, titrated to 2,400 mg/day (divided three times a day); the dose for patients receiving hemodialysis is 200–300 mg after each dialysis session.
- Clonazepam: initially 0.25 mg at bedtime, increased to 0.5 mg at bedtime.
- Pramipexole: initially 0.125 mg at bedtime, titrated slowly to clinical effect; maximum 1.5 mg/day, at bedtime.
- Ropinirole: initially 0.25 mg at bedtime, titrated slowly to clinical effect; maximum 4 mg/day, at bedtime.
- Oxycodone: initially 5 mg at bedtime, titrated to 20–30 mg/day, divided two to three times a day.

Some specialists recommend starting with gabapentin or clonazepam and then moving on to trials of dopamine agonists or oxycodone only if these drugs are unsuccessful in controlling symptoms. If dopamine agonists are used, the patient should be monitored for symptom augmentation and rebound (Trenkwalder et al. 2005). *Augmentation* refers to onset of symptoms earlier in the day (or more severe symptoms, or more anatomic involvement) (Trenkwalder et al. 2005). Severe augmentation is treated by withdrawal of the medication. Milder augmentation can be managed by adding another dose of medication earlier in the day. *Rebound* refers to the reappearance of symptoms between doses when a dose of drug has been sufficiently eliminated from the body (Trenkwalder et al. 2005). Troublesome rebound could be treated by dosing medication more than one time a day.

Tic Disorders

Tourette's syndrome is not often highly symptomatic in elderly patients because most patients with the syndrome improve as they age, and residual symptoms of Tourette's in late life are mild (Bruun 1988; Burd et al. 1986). In the geriatric population, tics secondary to cerebral insults such as traumatic brain injury or stroke are more often seen than Tourette's syndrome (Table 8–4). Treatment aims to suppress tics sufficiently that the patient's function is reasonably restored (e.g., social interaction is resumed). Drugs of choice for this indication include the α-agonists guanfacine and clonidine and the atypical antipsychotics risperidone, olanzapine, and ziprasidone (Kurlan 2004). For painful dystonic tics, botulinum toxin injection may be helpful.

Vascular Parkinsonism

Parkinsonism secondary to cerebrovascular disease is believed to account for 4.4%–12% of cases of parkinsonism (Thanvi et al. 2005). With the exception of resting tremor, most features of PD are seen in the classic form of vascular parkinsonism. In addition, legs are involved more than arms, involvement may be symmetric, and the course of disease is more rapid than PD (Thanvi et al. 2005). Patients typically exhibit prominent gait difficulty, postural instability, hyperactive reflexes, incontinence, dementia, and pseudobulbar affect (Winikates and Jankovic 1999). Neuroimaging findings usually consist of lacunar infarcts and/or white matter lesions (Thanvi et al. 2005). Definitive diagnosis requires a clinical diagnosis of parkinsonism along with pathological confirmation of the presence of vascular lesions in the absence of Lewy bodies (Thanvi et al. 2005). Treatment of vascular parkinsonism should be directed toward control of risk factors for cerebrovascular disease such as hypertension, hyperlipidemia, sedentary lifestyle, and smoking. It has been thought that vascular parkinsonism is unresponsive to levodopa. However, some investigators have recently begun to question this belief. A retrospective study involving 17 patients with pathologically confirmed vascular parkinsonism found that 12 had experienced a good to excellent response to levodopa, and of those 12, 10 had vascular lesions in the basal ganglia or substantia nigra (Zijlmans et al. 2004). It may be, as has been speculated elsewhere, that patients with lesions in the nigrostriatal pathway selectively respond to dopaminergic medication such as levodopa (Thanvi et al. 2005).

Drug-Induced Syndromes

Akathisia

Akathisia is a subjective feeling of restlessness, with an irresistible urge to move; observed behaviors include pacing, stomping, tapping, running, and crossing and uncrossing of legs. Akathisia is often mislabeled as agitation in elderly patients. The excessive motor activity of akathisia particularly involves the lower extremities. Akathisia is the most common neurological adverse effect of conventional antipsychotics and can occur as an acute or tardive syndrome. It can also be seen with the use of atypical antipsychotics, selective serotonin reuptake inhibitor (SSRI) antidepressants, and calcium channel blockers (Sachdev 2005).

The acute syndrome of akathisia usually develops within a few days of initiation or incremental increase in dose of an antipsychotic or a change to a high-potency agent; almost all cases occur within 2 weeks (Sachdev 2005). The risk is greater in patients who have developed drug-induced parkinsonism (Sachdev 2005).

The preferred treatment for akathisia is a switch to an atypical antipsychotic at a lower dose (if possible), although lowering the dose of a conventional antipsychotic also can be effective. Propranolol at 20–80 mg/day or a benzodiazepine such as lorazepam can lessen symptom severity. Anecdotal evidence exists for the efficacy of gabapentin in nonelderly patients (Pfeffer et al. 2005). Anticholinergic medication is generally not helpful for akathisia unless parkinsonism is also present.

Dystonia (Acute)

Dystonia is sustained muscle contraction often affecting the neck and face musculature. It can occur within minutes to hours of neuroleptic exposure or with abrupt discontinuation of anticholinergic medication. The neck is seen to twist and to pull back (retrocollis), the jaw muscles may lock, and blepharospasm may occur. Other manifestations include oculogyric crisis or opisthotonos. Less commonly, laryngeal musculature is affected, with respiratory compromise. Acute dystonia occurs less frequently in elderly patients than younger patients but can be seen in geriatric populations. Risk of dystonia is greatest with use of conventional antipsychotics (particularly high-potency agents) and with parenteral use of antipsychotics and is increased in the presence of hyperthyroidism, hyperparathyroidism, and hypocalcemia (Sachdev 2005). Acute dystonia can be treated with benztropine (Cogentin), 0.5–1 mg intramuscularly or intravenously, or diphenhydramine (Benadryl), 25 mg intramuscularly or intravenously. This can be followed up with an oral anticholinergic, given for a temporary period while the dose of neuroleptic is lowered or a switch is made to an atypical antipsychotic. Indefinite continuation of the anticholinergic is often associated with adverse events such as delirium, constipation, or urinary retention in elderly patients. Patients maintained chronically on anticholinergic drugs can often be successfully tapered off these medications.

Pisa syndrome is a rare truncal dystonia in which the patient presents with lateral flexion of the spine and backward axial rotation, a posture reminiscent of the Leaning Tower of Pisa (Villarejo et al. 2003). In its acute form, the syndrome may respond to withdrawal of a neuroleptic. In one reported case, the syndrome resolved with discontinuation of a cholinesterase inhibitor (donepezil) (Villarejo et al. 2003).

Neuroleptic Malignant Syndrome

NMS is a potentially fatal derangement of dopaminergic neurotransmission usually resulting from neuroleptic exposure but also seen in patients who have been abruptly withdrawn from dopamine agonists. Symptoms come on acutely and are fully developed within 24–48 hours (Sachdev 2005). Central features of NMS include fever, muscle rigidity, fluctuating consciousness, and autonomic instability. Rigidity may be of the lead-pipe or cogwheel variety and may be severe enough to cause rhabdomyolysis (Sachdev 2005). Catatonia or delirium may be seen. Autonomic features may include diaphoresis, pallor or flushing, tachycardia, hypertension, hypotension, labile blood pressure, cardiac dysrhythmia, tachypnea, dyspnea, and urinary incontinence (Sachdev 2005). Movement abnormalities may include bradykinesia, tremor, dystonia, and myoclonus. Dystonia may manifest as blepharospasm, opisthotonos, oculogyric crisis, trismus, chorea, or oral-buccal dyskinesia resembling TD (Sachdev 2005). NMS is often confounded by a comorbid medical illness or by complications of the syndrome itself. These complications include pneumonia, pulmonary embolism, cardiac arrest or dysrhythmia, and renal failure (Sachdev 2005). In addition, the presentation of NMS is quite variable, and even the central features are not present in all cases or are not present simultaneously. NMS is also discussed in Chapter 3.

Laboratory abnormalities in NMS typically include elevation in creatine phosphokinase (ranging from 200 IU/L to > 100,000 IU/L), elevation in white blood cell count (often with left shift), and elevation in liver function test values. Acute renal failure can occur as a consequence of myoglobinuria. In the experience of the authors, *formes frustes* of NMS may be seen in elderly patients, with less extreme muscle rigidity and temperature elevation. These patients respond to usual treatments for NMS. For this reason, the possibility of NMS should be considered for any elderly patient with unexplained fever and drug exposure. Cases of atypical NMS with the absence of muscle rigidity have been described with atypical antipsychotics (Ananth et al. 2004).

Risk factors for NMS include dehydration and infection. The question of why some patients develop NMS on antipsychotic drugs and others do not—given equal medical debility—remains unanswered. Investigation of genetic factors underlying NMS as a failure of dopaminergic neurotransmission may hold promise. In a recent case report, a patient suffering from NMS was found to carry the A1 allele of the DRD2 gene, which is associated with reduced dopamine activity (Del Tacca et al. 2005).

NMS represents a medical emergency best managed in a monitored setting, in which neuroleptic medication is discontinued, aggressive hydration and cooling are initiated, and comorbid medical illnesses are treated. These are the mainstays of management; as yet there are no specific rescue medications that have been well validated in the treatment of NMS. Nevertheless, when creatine kinase levels are very high or increasing or when there is persistent rigidity or fever, use of bromocriptine and sodium dantrolene should be considered. Bromocriptine is a dopamine agonist. Dantrolene reduces muscle rigidity by blocking release of calcium from the sarcoplasmic reticulum. Suggested dosing of these medications is as follows:

- Bromocriptine: 2.5 mg orally or via nasogastric tube three times a day, titrated up to 5 mg three times a day as tolerated.
- Dantrolene: 1 mg/kg, repeated up to a cumulative dose of 10 mg/kg. When the patient has been stabilized, intravenous dantrolene may be switched to oral dantrolene at 4–8 mg/kg/day in four divided doses.

Patients with NMS secondary to abrupt withdrawal of levodopa also should be restarted on levodopa. One randomized study of patients with PD and NMS looked at usual care (including bromocriptine and dantrolene) versus usual care plus methylprednisolone (1 g/day intravenously for 3 days) and found that the patients given the steroid recovered more quickly and had less severe symptoms (Sato et al. 2003). These medications, although possibly helpful in NMS, are not necessarily benign in terms of adverse effects. In severe cases of NMS, an alternative that should be considered early is ECT, which is very effective in facilitating a rapid resolution of NMS. In the experience of the authors, significant improvement can be seen within the first few ECT treatments. When ECT is used, it may be advisable to avoid succinylcholine as a muscle relaxant because of the risk of cardiac dysrhythmias in patients with hyperkalemia secondary to rhabdomyolysis.

Other medications may have a role in NMS treatment. Benzodiazepines may be used, although it remains controversial whether these drugs treat NMS per se (as a form of catatonia) or only serve to alleviate agitation or anxiety. Amantadine may be used at a dose of 100 mg orally or via nasogastric tube two times a day, titrated up to 200 mg two times a day as tolerated. For patients who have been administered decanoate formulations of neuroleptics, very slow clearance is highly problematic when NMS develops; plasmapheresis has been used successfully in these cases (Gaitini et al. 1997).

About one-third of patients will have recrudescence of symptoms when neuroleptics are reintroduced (Kipps et al. 2005). A minimum of 2 weeks should elapse before any neuroleptic is used. Most patients treated with conventional neuroleptics should be switched to an atypical agent, even though there is still no conclusive evidence that rates of NMS are substantially lower with use of atypical drugs. Patients with PD or other preexisting central nervous system (CNS) diseases may have persistent sequelae after an episode of NMS (Adityanjee et al. 2005).

Parkinsonism

Secondary parkinsonism is most commonly due to cerebrovascular disease or medications (Scharre and Mahler 1994). Neuroleptics are the most common cause, although lithium, SSRI antidepressants, metoclopramide

(Bateman et al. 1985), and other drugs can be implicated, as shown in Table 8–7. In contrast to idiopathic parkinsonism, drug-induced parkinsonism is more often characterized by the absence of prominent tremor and the presence of bilateral rigidity and akinesia/bradykinesia. Rigidity is often of the cogwheeling type (suggesting that tremor is present, although subtle). Drug-induced parkinsonism is not seen as early as either dystonia or akathisia in the course of treatment, but most cases develop within the first week (Sachdev 2005). Risk factors include old age, female gender, high dose of drug, high potency of drug, and rapid rate of dose escalation (Sachdev 2005).

Treatment of drug-induced parkinsonism in elderly patients involves switching to an atypical antipsychotic, lowering the dose of antipsychotic, switching to a lower-potency agent, or discontinuation of antipsychotic. In most cases, drug-induced parkinsonism is slowly reversible with these treatments, but parkinsonism persists in some cases for months to years. For these patients, careful consideration should be given to the use of anticholinergic medications such as benztropine or trihexyphenidyl. For many elderly patients, the risk introduced by anticholinergic drugs used to treat drug-induced parkinsonism outweighs the benefit of reduced symptoms of parkinsonism. When anticholinergic agents are used, the patient should be followed closely for adverse effects such as constipation and urinary retention, and duration of therapy should be limited. Suggested doses of several anticholinergic drugs are shown in Table 8–8. Amantadine (50–200 mg two times a day) is an alternative when the decision is made against the use of anticholinergic drugs, although this agent carries some risk of exacerbation of psychosis (Wilcox and Tsuang 1990–1991).

Serotonin Syndrome

Serotonin syndrome is characterized by mental status changes, neuromuscular signs, and autonomic hyperactivity—all thought to be caused by overstimulation of postsynaptic serotonin receptors (Boyer and Shannon 2005). Serotonin syndrome has a more rapid onset than NMS and is marked by prominent neuromuscular findings, including clonus, tremor, rigidity, and hyperreflexia, with lower extremities more involved than upper extremities (Boyer and Shannon 2005). Other motor signs

Table 8–7. Causes of secondary parkinsonism

Cerebrovascular disease*
Degeneration
    Basal ganglia calcification (Fahr's disease)
    Dementia with Lewy bodies
    Olivopontocerebellar atrophy
    Parkinsonism-dementia complex of Guam
    Progressive supranuclear palsy
    Shy-Drager syndrome
    Striatonigral degeneration
    Wilson's disease
Drug-induced*
    Amiodarone
    Antiemetics
    Antipsychotics (conventional and atypical)*
    Lithium
    Methyldopa
    Metoclopramide
    Reserpine
    Valproate
Endocrine
    Hypoparathyroidism
    Hypothyroidism
Hydrocephalus, normal-pressure
Infection
    AIDS
    Jakob-Creutzfeldt disease
    Postencephalitic (Von Economo's) encephalitis
Intoxication
    Carbon monoxide
    Manganese
    1-methyl-4-phenyl-1,2,5,6-tetrahydropyridine (MPTP)
Traumatic encephalopathy
Tumors, basal ganglia
    Arteriovenous malformations
    Neoplasms

*Major cause.

Table 8–8.   Selected anticholinergic drugs

Generic name	Trade name	Dosage
benztropine	Cogentin	0.5–2 mg/day
biperiden	Akineton	2–4 mg/day
diphenhydramine	Benadryl	50–75 mg/day
procyclidine	Kemadrin	5–10 mg/day
trihexyphenidyl	Artane	6–10 mg/day

include akathisia, increased tone (greater in lower extremities), and a stereotypy involving repetitive head rotation with neck in extension (Boyer and Shannon 2005). In contrast to NMS, motor signs in serotonin syndrome are primarily hyperkinetic rather than hypokinetic. In addition, shivering, diarrhea, and hypomania are more commonly observed in serotonin syndrome than NMS (Sternbach 1991). Serotonin syndrome is discussed further in Chapter 4 of this volume, "Antidepressants."

Laboratory abnormalities in serotonin syndrome include metabolic acidosis, elevated creatinine, and elevated liver transaminases (aspartate transaminase [AST] and alanine transaminase [ALT]). The syndrome may have a rapid progression; delirium, seizures, shock, rhabdomyolysis, renal failure, and disseminated intravascular coagulation may ensue, with a fatal outcome. Implicated drugs are listed in Chapter 4. Treatment of serotonin syndrome involves discontinuation of the offending drugs, supportive care, control of agitation, use of 5-HT$_{2A}$ antagonists, control of autonomic instability, and treatment of hyperthermia (Boyer and Shannon 2005). Details of these treatments are discussed in Chapter 4. Benzodiazepines can help reduce the autonomic component, eliminate excessive muscle activity in mild to moderate cases, and improve survival (Boyer and Shannon 2005). As noted in Chapter 4, physical restraints must be avoided in the management of serotonin syndrome.

In severe cases, where fever is very high (>41.1°C or 106°F), the patient should be sedated, paralyzed, and intubated, with the goal of eliminating excessive muscle activity that is the source of the hyperthermia (Boyer and Shannon 2005). Antipyretics are avoided early in treatment as the fever is followed diagnostically. In severe cases, super high-flux hemofiltration may be used, as noted in Chapter 4.

Tardive Dyskinesia

As discussed in Chapter 3, TD is a syndrome of abnormal involuntary movements associated with chronic antipsychotic medication treatment. The clinical appearance is characteristic, involving mouthing, chewing, puckering, smacking, sucking, licking, and other orolingual movements, also known as *buccolinguomasticatory* movements. Choreic movements of fingers, hands, arms, and feet are also seen, and truncal TD is occasionally reported. Associated speech abnormalities include impaired phonation and intelligibility and slowed rate of speech production (Khan et al. 1994).

TD occurs more frequently in women, patients with conditions other than schizophrenia (Wirshing 2001), patients with diabetes (Caligiuri and Jeste 2004), and elderly patients, particularly those who are institutionalized (Byne et al. 1998). Other risk factors for the development of TD include long duration of antipsychotic use, coadministration of anticholinergic drugs, the presence of an affective disorder, alcohol abuse or dependence, degenerative brain disease, diabetes (Casey 1997; Jeste et al. 1995), history of interruption of neuroleptic treatment (van Harten et al. 1998), extrapyramidal symptoms (EPS) early in treatment (Woerner et al. 1998), presence of negative symptoms (Liddle et al. 1993), and high serum ferritin levels (Wirshing et al. 1998).

Most importantly, the cumulative incidence of TD is related to duration of antipsychotic use. Among older patients, TD is identified in 3.4% after 1 month of neuroleptic treatment, in 5.9% after 3 months of treatment (Jeste et al. 1999), and in 60% after 3 years of treatment (Jeste et al. 1995). A variety of candidate genes have been studied as possible contributors to TD susceptibility among neuroleptic-treated patients, with positive results suggested for a *DRD3* Ser9Gly polymorphism (Lerer et al. 2002), certain cytochrome P450 (CYP) 2D6 mutations (Nikoloff et al. 2002), and the C/C genotype of 5-HT$_{2A}$ (Lattuada et al. 2004).

TD has been reported in association with all conventional and all atypical antipsychotics. It is widely believed that atypical drugs carry substantially less risk than conventional drugs, but in fact this has not been conclusively demonstrated. A recent population-based retrospective cohort study performed in Canada found that the risk for developing TD in the year after initiation of atypical antipsychotics (5.19/100 person-years) was not significantly different from the risk for conventional antipsychotics (5.24/100 person-years) (Lee et al. 2005). The European Schizophrenia Outpatient Health Outcomes (SOHO) Study, on the other hand, found a lower incidence and less persistence of TD among patients treated with atypical agents over a 6-month period (Tenback et al. 2005). Findings from the Clinical Antipsychotic Trials in Intervention Effectiveness (CAT-IE) study also support a lower incidence of TD with atypical agents, although the study was performed in nonelders over a relatively short period of time (18 months) (Lieberman et al. 2005). As noted in Chapter 3, it has been observed that patients with preexisting TD who go on to treatment with atypical agents (including clozapine, olanzapine, risperidone, quetiapine, aripiprazole, and ziprasidone) may exhibit improvement in dyskinetic movements.

The increased risk of developing TD among elderly patients necessitates frequent reassessment for dyskinetic movements for those treated with antipsychotics. For this purpose, a standardized instrument such as the Abnormal Involuntary Movement Scale (AIMS) is recommended (Figure 8–1). For elderly patients, these assessments are recommended at baseline, 4 weeks, 8 weeks, and at least every 6 months thereafter, as shown in Table 3–7 in Chapter 3.

The risk of TD can be reduced by minimizing the dose of neuroleptic used (Morgenstern and Glazer 1993) and possibly by avoiding routine use of adjunctive anticholinergic medications (Bergen et al. 1992). In addition, current evidence suggests that risk is reduced with use of atypical agents, as noted above. These same measures can be used when symptoms of TD occur; progression of TD may be halted by reducing neuroleptic doses, avoiding anticholinergic drugs, and switching to atypical agents. Taper and discontinuation of a typical neuroleptic will result in remission of TD in up to one-half of cases. If the taper is too rapid, however, a syndrome of withdrawal dyskinesia may occur, possibly related to activation of hypersensitive D_2 receptors that are now exposed (Glazer et al. 1989).

Three Cochrane Reviews of treatments for TD found insufficient evidence for efficacy of any of the following treatments: γ-aminobutyric acid (GABA) agonists (baclofen, γ-vinyl GABA, γ-acetylenic GABA, progabide, muscimol, sodium valproate, and tetrahydroisoxazolopyridine (Soares et al. 2004), cholinergic drugs (arecoline, choline, deanol, lecithin, meclofenoxate, physostigmine, RS-86, tacrine, methoxytacrine, galantamine, ipidacrine, donepezil, rivastigmine, eptastigmine, metrifonate, xanomeline, and cevimeline) (Tammenmaa et al. 2002), or miscellaneous drugs or treatments (botulinum toxin, endorphin, essential fatty acids, EX11582A, ganglioside, insulin, lithium, naloxone, estrogen, cyproheptadine, phenylalanine, piracetam, stepholidine, tryptophan, neurosurgery, or ECT) (Soares-Weiser and Joy 2003).

At present, there is no well-validated pharmacologic treatment for TD. Various drugs and treatment strategies have been tried, and several have been reported anecdotally to be effective. Atypical antipsychotics at usual therapeutic doses may be associated with symptomatic improvement in TD (Chouinard 1995). Propranolol at dosages up to 30 mg three times a day may be effective. Of the calcium channel blockers, nifedipine was found to be most effective, and diltiazem was found to be least effective (Cates et al. 1993; Loonen et al. 1992). With nifedipine, better response was seen in cases of severe TD, among elderly patients, and with high nifedipine doses (e.g., 80 mg) (Cates et al. 1993; Kushnir and Ratner 1989). Clonazepam improved TD symptoms (especially tardive dystonia) in nongeriatric patients (Thaker et al. 1990). For reasons discussed in Chapter 9 of this volume, "Medications to Treat Dementia and Other Cognitive Disorders," vitamin E is no longer recommended for treatment or for prevention of TD.

The prognosis for patients with TD may not be as grim as once thought, although incidence and prevalence data appear to conflict in this regard. For example, it was reported that among older, institutionalized patients with TD, 30% improved over time and 28% recovered completely (Cavallaro et al. 1993). In population studies, prevalence was reported to be stable over 10 years of treatment, even when conventional neuroleptics were continued (Gardos et al. 1994). These data are difficult to reconcile with the incidence data reported above. This issue aside, the real problem is that it is impossible to predict which patients will suffer the (possibly rare) outcome of relentless disease progression. For this

Abnormal Involuntary Movement Scale (ECDEU version)

Instructions

Movement ratings: Rate highest severity observed. Rate movements that occur upon activation one *less* than those observed spontaneously.

Code: 0 = None
1 = Minimal, may be extreme normal
2 = Mild
3 = Moderate
4 = Severe

		Circle one				
Facial and oral movements	1. Muscles of facial expression (e.g., movements of forehead, eyebrows, periorbital area, cheeks; include frowning, blinking, smiling, grimacing)	0	1	2	3	4
	2. Lips and periorbital area (e.g., puckering, pouting, smacking)	0	1	2	3	4
	3. Jaw (e.g., biting, clenching, chewing, mouth opening, lateral movement)	0	1	2	3	4
	4. Tongue Rate only increase in movement both in and out of mouth, not inability to sustain movement	0	1	2	3	4
Extremity movements	5. Upper (arms, wrists, hands, fingers) Include choreic movements, (i.e., rapid, objectively purposeless, irregular, spontaneous), athetoid movements (i.e., slow, irregular, complex, serpentine) Do not include tremor (i.e., repetitive, regular, rhythmic)	0	1	2	3	4
	6. Lower (legs, knees, ankles, toes) (e.g., lateral knee movement, foot tapping, heel dropping, foot squirming, inversion and eversion of foot)	0	1	2	3	4
Trunk movements	7. Neck, shoulders, hips (e.g., rocking, twisting, squirming, pelvic gyrations)	0	1	2	3	4

Figure 8–1. Abnormal Involuntary Movement Scale.

Global judgments	8. Severity of abnormal movements	None, normal	0
		Minimal	1
		Mild	2
		Moderate	3
		Severe	4
	9. Incapacitation due to abnormal movements	None, normal	0
		Minimal	1
		Mild	2
		Moderate	3
		Severe	4
	10. Patient's awareness of abnormal movements Rate only patient's report	No awareness	0
		Aware, no distress	1
		Aware, mild distress	2
		Aware, moderate distress	3
		Aware, severe distress	4
Dental status	11. Current problems with teeth and/or dentures	No	0
		Yes	1
	12. Does patient usually wear dentures?	No	0
		Yes	1

Figure 8–1.   Abnormal Involuntary Movement Scale. *(Continued)*

reason, it has been recommended that long-term use of conventional antipsychotics in elderly patients be minimized.

Aside from the classic syndrome of TD, a variety of other tardive syndromes have been described, including tardive dystonia, tardive akathisia, tardive tremor, and tardive myoclonus. Tardive dystonia is discussed in the section that follows. Tardive akathisia carries a poor prognosis in that it is often persistent and treatment resistant. A less common manifestation of tardive dyskinesia is respiratory dyskinesia, which is characterized by irregular respiratory movements, dyspnea, grunting, and gasping (Kruk et al. 1995). Complications of this syndrome include respiratory alkalosis and aspiration pneumonia. Both reserpine and olanzapine have been reported to treat respiratory dyskinesia (Gotto 1999). TD has also been reported to present as severe dysphagia as an isolated movement abnormality (Gregory et al. 1992).

Tardive Dystonia

Tardive dystonia can occur as a consequence of neuroleptic exposure. Like acute dystonia, this is not common as a new diagnosis in elderly patients but has been reported (Kiriakakis et al. 1998). It is usually focal initially, involving the craniocervical region, but it can progress in many cases to involve other areas of the body. The dystonia known as *Pisa syndrome* (described above) can be seen as a tardive as well as acute syndrome. Dystonia rarely remits completely (Gironell et al. 1999) and can cause significant pain and disability (Wojcik et al. 1991). Treatment involves discontinuation of the neuroleptic. A switch to clozapine (or possibly to other atypical agents) may be helpful. In addition, this is the one tardive syndrome for which anticholinergic agents (e.g., benztropine) may be useful (Goetz and Horn 2004). Finally, botulinum toxin injection may be helpful, as it is for other dystonias (Jankovic and Brin 1991).

Tremor

As noted earlier, tremor is a less prominent manifestation of drug-induced parkinsonism than of idiopathic PD. When it occurs with neuroleptic use, it is characteristically a resting tremor of large amplitude with a frequency of 4–5 cycles/second and symmetric at onset. One tremor variant is rabbit syndrome, which involves muscles of the perinasal and oral region. Drug-induced tremors usually abate when the neuroleptic is discontinued. If ongoing therapy is required, a switch to an atypical antipsychotic or to a less potent neuroleptic is indicated. Use of anticholinergic medication to treat drug-induced parkinsonism (including tremor) is discussed in an earlier section.

Many psychotropics have the potential to cause an exaggeration of physiologic tremor that is different from the classic neuroleptic-induced tremor. The exaggerated physiologic tremor is of relatively small amplitude, prominent more distally (at the fingertips), and best seen when the patient is holding a posture (e.g., arms outstretched with fingers slightly spread). Some of the medications that can cause this tremor are listed in Table 8–5. These tremors may require little intervention other than reassurance. When the tremors are persistent and disabling, usual management involves withdrawal of the offending drug. It has been observed clinically that fine drug-induced tremors may become coarser with the development of drug-induced toxicity, as is the case with lithium. When such a progression is seen, toxicity should be suspected and the medication dose reduced or withheld until the tremor improves.

Chapter Summary

- The first step in the diagnosis of a movement disorder is careful observation and description of the movement abnormality itself.
- The presence of tremor, particularly resting tremor, is one of the signs that best distinguishes the effects of normal aging from a movement disorder.
- The classic triad of clinical symptoms in Parkinson's disease (PD) consists of tremor, bradykinesia, and rigidity. The presence of a resting tremor is highly suggestive of PD, although tremor is not present in all cases.
- First-line agents for treatment of PD include levodopa and the dopamine agonists pramipexole and ropinirole.
- Essential features of restless legs syndrome include an unpleasant sensation in the legs with an urge to move that worsens during periods of rest or inactivity, is relieved by movement, and has symptoms that are most marked or occur only during the evening or nighttime hours.
- Restless legs syndrome can be treated with gabapentin, clonazepam, dopamine agonists, or oxycodone.
- In the geriatric population, tics secondary to cerebral insults such as traumatic brain injury or stroke are more often seen than Tourette's syndrome.
- With the exception of resting tremor, most features of PD are seen in the classic form of vascular parkinsonism. In addition, legs are usually involved more than arms, involvement may be symmetrical, and the course of disease may be more rapid than PD.
- Akathisia is often mislabeled as agitation in elderly patients.
- The preferred treatment for akathisia is a switch to an atypical antipsychotic at a lower dose (if possible), although lowering the dose of a typical neuroleptic can be effective.
- For many elderly patients, the risk introduced by anticholinergic drugs used to treat drug-induced parkinsonism outweighs the benefit of reduced symptoms of parkinsonism.
- It has been observed clinically that fine drug-induced tremors may become coarser with the development of drug-induced toxicity, as is the case with lithium.

References

Aarsland D, Perry R, Larsen JP, et al: Neuroleptic sensitivity in Parkinson's disease and parkinsonian dementias. J Clin Psychiatry 66:633–637, 2005

Adityanjee, Sajatovic M, Munshi KR: Neuropsychiatric sequelae of neuroleptic malignant syndrome. Clin Neuropharmacol 28:197–204, 2005

Ananth J, Parameswaran S, Burgoyne K, et al: Neuroleptic malignant syndrome and atypical antipsychotic drugs. J Clin Psychiatry 65:464–470, 2004

Bateman DN, Rawlings MD, Simpson JM: Extrapyramidal reactions with metoclopramide. Br Med J (Clin Res Ed) 291:930–932, 1985

Bergen J, Kitchin R, Berry G: Predictors of the course of tardive dyskinesia in patients receiving neuroleptics. Biol Psychiatry 32:580–594, 1992

Boyer EW, Shannon M: The serotonin syndrome. N Engl J Med 352:1112–1120, 2005

Bruun RD: The natural history of Tourette's syndrome, in Tourette's Syndrome and Tic Disorders. Edited by Cohen DJ, Bruun RD, Leckman JF. New York, Wiley, 1988, pp 21–40

Burd L, Kerbeshian J, Wilkenheiser M, et al: Prevalence of Gilles de la Tourette's syndrome in North Dakota adults. Am J Psychiatry 143:787–788, 1986

Byne W, White L, Parella M, et al: Tardive dyskinesia in a chronically institutionalized population of elderly schizophrenic patients: prevalence and association with cognitive impairment. Int J Geriatr Psychiatry 13:473–479, 1998

Caligiuri MP, Jeste DV: Association of diabetes with dyskinesia in older psychosis patients. Psychopharmacology (Berl) 176:281–286, 2004

Casey DE: The relationship of pharmacology to side effects. J Clin Psychiatry 58 (suppl 10):55–62, 1997

Cates M, Lusk K, Wells BG: Are calcium-channel blockers effective in the treatment of tardive dyskinesia? Ann Pharmacother 27:191–196, 1993

Cavallaro R, Regazzetti MG, Mundo E, et al: Tardive dyskinesia outcomes: clinical and pharmacologic correlates of remission and persistence. Neuropsychopharmacology 8:233–239, 1993

Chouinard G: Effects of risperidone in tardive dyskinesia: an analysis of the Canadian Multicenter Risperidone Study. J Clin Psychopharmacol 15 (suppl 1):36S–44S, 1995

Colloby S, O'Brien J: Functional imaging in Parkinson's disease and dementia with Lewy bodies. J Geriatr Psychiatry Neurol 17:158–163, 2004

Dallocchio C, Buffa C, Tinelli C, et al: Effectiveness of risperidone in Huntington chorea patients. J Clin Psychopharmacol 19:101–103, 1999

Daniele A, Moro E, Bentivoglio AR: Zolpidem in progressive supranuclear palsy. N Engl J Med 341:543–544, 1999

Del Tacca M, Lattanzi L, Lastella M, et al: Genotype A1/A2 associated with neuroleptic malignant syndrome. Bipolar Disord 7:390–391, 2005

Deuschl G, Bain P, Brin M: Consensus statement of the Movement Disorder Society on Tremor. Ad Hoc Scientific Committee. Mov Disord 13 (suppl 3):2–23, 1998

Gaitini L, Fradis M, Vaida S, et al: Plasmapheresis in neuroleptic malignant syndrome. Anaesthesia 52:165–168, 1997

Gardos G, Casey DE, Cole JO, et al: Ten-year outcome of tardive dyskinesia. Am J Psychiatry 151:836–841, 1994

Gironell A, Kulisevsky J, Barbanoj M, et al: A randomized placebo-controlled comparative trial of gabapentin and propranolol in essential tremor. Arch Neurol 56:475–480, 1999

Glazer WM, Bowers MBJ, Charney DS, et al: The effect of neuroleptic discontinuation on psychopathology, involuntary movements, and biochemical measures in patients with persistent tardive dyskinesia. Biol Psychiatry 26:224–233, 1989

Goetz CG, Horn S: Tardive dyskinesia, in Movement Disorders: Neurologic Principles and Practice, 2nd Edition. Edited by Watts RL, Koller WC. New York, McGraw-Hill, Health Professionals Division, 2004, pp 629–637

Golbe LI: Progressive supranuclear palsy, in Movement Disorders: Neurologic Principles and Practice, 2nd Edition. Edited by Watts RL, Koller WC. New York, McGraw-Hill Medical Publishing, 2004, pp 339–358

Gotto J: Treatment of respiratory dyskinesia with olanzapine. Psychosomatics 40:257–259, 1999

Gottwald MD, Bainbridge JL, Dowling GA, et al: New pharmacotherapy for Parkinson's disease. Ann Pharmacother 31:1205–1217, 1997

Gregory RP, Smith PT, Rudge P: Tardive dyskinesia presenting as severe dysphagia. J Neurol Neurosurg Psychiatry 55:1203–1204, 1992

Hornyak M, Trenkwalder C: Restless legs syndrome and periodic limb movement disorder in the elderly. J Psychosom Res 56:543–548, 2004

Jankovic J, Brin MF: Therapeutic uses of botulinum toxin. N Engl J Med 324:1186–1194, 1991

Jankovic J, Schwartz KS: Use of botulinum toxin in the treatment of hand dystonia. J Hand Surg [Am] 18:883–887, 1993

Jeste DV, Caligiuri MP, Paulsen JS, et al: Risk of tardive dyskinesia in older patients: a prospective longitudinal study of 266 outpatients. Arch Gen Psychiatry 52:756–765, 1995

Jeste DV, Lacro JP, Palmer B, et al: Incidence of tardive dyskinesia in early stages of low-dose treatment with typical neuroleptics in older patients. Am J Psychiatry 156:309–311, 1999

Khan R, Jampala VC, Dong K, et al: Speech abnormalities in tardive dyskinesia. Am J Psychiatry 151:760–762, 1994

Kipps CM, Fung VSC, Grattan-Smith P, et al: Movement disorder emergencies. Mov Disord 20:322–334, 2005

Kiriakakis V, Bhatia KP, Quinn NP, et al: The natural history of tardive dystonia. A long-term follow-up study of 107 cases. Brain 121:2053–2066, 1998

Kishore A, Calne DB: Approach to the patient with a movement disorder and overview of movement disorders, in Movement Disorders: Neurologic Principles and Practice. Edited by Watts RL, Koller WC. New York, McGraw-Hill, 1997, pp 3–14

Kremer B, Goldberg P, Andrew SE, et al: A worldwide study of the Huntington's disease mutation: the sensitivity and specificity of measuring CAG repeats. N Engl J Med 330:1401–1406, 1994

Kruk J, Sachdev P, Singh S: Neuroleptic-induced respiratory dyskinesia. J Neuropsychiatry Clin Neurosci 7:223–229, 1995

Kumar A, Calne DB: Approach to the patient with a movement disorder and overview of movement disorders, in Movement Disorders: Neurologic Principles and Practice, 2nd Edition. Edited by Watts RL, Koller WC. New York, McGraw-Hill Medical Publishing, 2004, pp 3–15

Kurlan R: Tourette's syndrome, in Movement Disorders: Neurologic Principles and Practice, 2nd Edition. Edited by Watts RL, Koller WC. New York, McGraw-Hill Medical Publishing, 2004, pp 569–575

Kushnir SL, Ratner JT: Calcium channel blockers for tardive dyskinesia in geriatric psychiatric patients. Am J Psychiatry 146:1218–1219, 1989

Lang AE, Lozano AM: Parkinson's disease: first of two parts. N Engl J Med 339:1044–1053, 1998a

Lang AE, Lozano AM: Parkinson's disease: second of two parts. N Engl J Med 339:1130–1143, 1998b

Lattuada E, Cavallaro R, Serretti A, et al: Tardive dyskinesia and DRD2, DRD3, DRD4, 5-HT2A variants in schizophrenia: an association study with repeated assessment. Int J Neuropsychopharmacol 7:489–493, 2004

Lee PE, Sykora K, Gill SS, et al: Antipsychotic medications and drug-induced movement disorders other than parkinsonism: a population-based cohort study in older adults. J Am Geriatr Soc 53:1374–1379, 2005

Lerer B, Segman RH, Fangerau H, et al: Pharmacogenetics of tardive dyskinesia: combined analysis of 780 patients supports association with dopamine D3 receptor gene Ser9Gly polymorphism. Neuropsychopharmacology 27:105–119, 2002

Liddle PF, Barnes TRE, Speller J, et al: Negative symptoms as a risk factor for tardive dyskinesia in schizophrenia. Br J Psychiatry 163:776–780, 1993

Lieberman JA, Stroup TS, McEvoy JP, et al: Effectiveness of antipsychotic drugs in patients with chronic schizophrenia. N Engl J Med 353:1209–1223, 2005

Loonen AJM, Verwey HA, Roels PR, et al: Is diltiazem effective in treating the symptoms of (tardive) dyskinesia in chronic psychiatric inpatients? A negative, double-blind, placebo-controlled trial. J Clin Psychopharmacol 12:39–42, 1992

Louis ED: Essential tremor. N Engl J Med 345:887–891, 2001

Marshall FJ: Clinical features and treatment of Huntington's disease, in Movement Disorders: Neurologic Principles and Practice, 2nd Edition. Edited by Watts RL, Koller WC. New York, McGraw-Hill Medical Publishing, 2004, pp 589–601

Morgenstern H, Glazer WM: Identifying risk factors for tardive dyskinesia among long-term outpatients maintained with neuroleptic medications. Arch Gen Psychiatry 50:723–733, 1993

Myers RH, Sax DS, Schoenfeld M, et al: Late onset of Huntington's disease. J Neurol Neurosurg Psychiatry 48:530–534, 1985

Nikoloff D, Shim J-C, Fairchild M, et al: Association between CYP2D6 genotype and tardive dyskinesia in Korean schizophrenics. Pharmacogenomics J 2:400–407, 2002

Nutt JG, Wooten GF: Diagnosis and initial management of Parkinson's disease. N Engl J Med 353:1021–1027, 2005

O'Keeffe ST: Secondary causes of restless legs syndrome in older people. Age Ageing 34:349–352, 2005

Pfeffer G, Chouinard G, Margolese HC: Gabapentin in the treatment of antipsychotic-induced akathisia in schizophrenia. Int Clin Psychopharmacol 20:179–181, 2005

Pierelli F, Adipietro A, Soldati G, et al: Low dosage clozapine effects on L-dopa induced dyskinesias in parkinsonian patients. Acta Neurol Scand 97:295–299, 1998

Rajput AH, Rajput A: Movement disorders and aging, in Movement Disorders: Neurologic Principles and Practice, 2nd Edition. Edited by Watts RL, Koller WC. New York, McGraw-Hill Medical Publishing, 2004, pp 837–853

Sachdev PS: Neuroleptic-induced movement disorders: an overview. Psychiatr Clin North Am 28:255–274, 2005

Sajatovic M, Meltzer HY: Clozapine-induced myoclonus and generalized seizures. Biol Psychiatry 39:367–370, 1996

Sato Y, Asoh T, Metoki N, et al: Efficacy of methylprednisolone pulse therapy on neuroleptic malignant syndrome in Parkinson's disease. J Neurol Neurosurg Psychiatry 74:574–576, 2003

Scharre DW, Mahler ME: Parkinson's disease: making the diagnosis, selecting drug therapies. Geriatrics 49:14–23, 1994

Scully RE, Mark EJ, McNeely WF, et al: Case records of the Massachusetts General Hospital (Case 26–1997). N Engl J Med 337:549–556, 1997

Soares KVS, Rathbone J, Deeks JJ: Gamma-aminobutyric acid agonists for neuroleptic-induced tardive dyskinesia. The Cochrane Database of Systematic Reviews, Issue 4, Article No: CD000203. DOI: 10.1002/14651858.CD000203, 2004

Soares-Weiser KVS, Joy C: Miscellaneous treatments for neuroleptic-induced tardive dyskinesia. The Cochrane Database of Systematic Reviews, Issue 2, Article No: CD000208. DOI: 10.1002/14651858.CD000208, 2003

Sternbach H: The serotonin syndrome. Am J Psychiatry 148:705–713, 1991

Stover NP, Wainer BH, Watts RL: Corticobasal degeneration, in Movement Disorders: Neurologic Principles and Practice, 2nd Edition. Edited by Watts RL, Koller WC. New York, McGraw-Hill Medical Publishing, 2004, pp 764–778

Tammenmaa IA, McGrath JJ, Sailas E, et al: Cholinergic medication for neuroleptic-induced tardive dyskinesia. The Cochrane Database of Systematic Reviews, Issue 3, Article No: CD000207. DOI: 10.1002/14651858.CD000207, 2002

Tenback DE, van Harten PN, Slooff CJ, et al: Effects of antipsychotic treatment on tardive dyskinesia: a 6-month evaluation of patients from the European Schizophrenia Outpatient Health Outcomes (SO43HO) Study. J Clin Psychiatry 66:1130–1133, 2005

Thaker GK, Nguyen JA, Strauss ME, et al: Clonazepam treatment of tardive dyskinesia: a practical GABAmimetic strategy. Am J Psychiatry 147:445–451, 1990

Thanvi B, Lo N, Robinson T: Vascular parkinsonism—an important cause of parkinsonism in older people. Age Aging 34:114–119, 2005

Thorpy MJ: New paradigms in the treatment of restless legs syndrome. Neurology 64 (supp 3):S28–S33, 2005

Trenkwalder C, Paulus W, Walters AS: The restless legs syndrome. Lancet Neurol 4:465–475, 2005 van Harten PN, Hoek HW, Matroos GE, et al: Intermittent neuroleptic treatment and risk for tardive dyskinesia: Curacao Extrapyramidal Syndromes Study III. Am J Psychiatry 155:565–567, 1998

Villarejo A, Camacho A, Garcia-Ramos R, et al: Cholinergic-dopaminergic imbalance in Pisa syndrome. Clin Neuropharmacol 26:119–121, 2003

Wilcox JA, Tsuang J: Psychological effects of amantadine on psychotic subjects. Neuropsychobiology 23:144–146, 1990–1991

Winikates J, Jankovic J: Clinical correlates of vascular parkinsonism. Arch Neurol 56:98–102, 1999

Winkelmann J, Prager M, Pfister H, et al: "Anxietas tibiarum": depression and anxiety disorders in patients with restless legs syndrome. J Neurol 252:67–71, 2005

Wirshing DA, Bartzokis G, Pierre JM, et al: Tardive dyskinesia and serum iron indices. Biol Psychiatry 44:493–498, 1998

Wirshing WC: Movement disorders associated with neuroleptic treatment. J Clin Psychiatry 62 (suppl 21):15–18, 2001

Woerner MG, Alvir JMJ, Saltz BL, et al: Prospective study of tardive dyskinesia in the elderly: rates and risk factors. Am J Psychiatry 155:1521–1528, 1998

Wojcieszek JM, Lang AE: Hyperkinetic movement disorders, in The American Psychiatric Press Textbook of Geriatric Neuropsychiatry. Edited by Coffey CE, Cummings JL. Washington, DC, American Psychiatric Press, 1994, pp 405–431

Wojcik JD, Falk WE, Fink JS, et al: A review of 32 cases of tardive dystonia. Am J Psychiatry 148:1055–1059, 1991

Zijlmans JCM, Katzenschlager R, Daniel SE, et al: The L-dopa response in vascular parkinsonism. J Neurol Neurosurg Psychiatry 75:545–547, 2004

Generic name	amantadine
Trade name	Symmetrel (generic available)
Class	Dopamine agonist
Half-life	24–29 hours
Mechanism of action	Blocks reuptake of dopamine, increases dopamine release from presynaptic neuron
Available preparations	Tablets: 100 mg Capsules: 100 mg Syrup: 50 mg/5 mL
Starting dose	100 mg/day (or 100 mg bid)
Titration	Increase to 100 mg bid after 1–2 weeks.
Typical daily dose	50–100 mg bid
Dose range	50–200 mg/day (latter divided bid)
Therapeutic serum level	Not established

Comments: Used in some cases of drug-induced parkinsonism and NMS. Duration of therapeutic benefit may be limited to a few months. Onset of action usually within 48 hours. Well absorbed orally. About 67% protein bound. Not appreciably metabolized. Excreted unchanged in urine by glomerular filtration and tubular secretion. Use with caution in patients with congestive heart failure, peripheral edema, orthostatic hypotension, untreated psychosis, seizures, hepatic disease, or renal disease. Special dosing required for patients with renal impairment. No appreciable anticholinergic effect. *Drug interactions:* Thiazide diuretics, triamterene, and trimethoprim, all of which increase potential for toxicity with amantadine. *Adverse effects (1%–10%):* Orthostasis, peripheral edema, insomnia, depression, anxiety, dizziness, hallucinations, ataxia, somnolence, agitation, confusion, nausea, anorexia, constipation, diarrhea, dry mouth, and dermatologic changes (*livedo reticularis*). *Uncommon but severe adverse effects:* Amnesia, congestive heart failure, seizures, dyspnea, hypertension, blood dyscrasias, psychosis, dysarthria, and urinary retention. Abrupt discontinuation associated with NMS, delirium, and psychosis.

Generic name	benztropine
Trade name	Cogentin (generic available)
Class	Anticholinergic agent
Half-life	Unknown (duration of activity 6–48 hours)
Mechanism of action	Anticholinergic, antihistaminergic; may also inhibit dopamine reuptake
Available preparations	Tablets: 0.5, 1, 2 mg Injection: 1 mg/mL
Starting dose	0.5 mg/day to bid (acute dystonia: 1–2 mg im/iv)
Titration	Increase by 0.5 mg every 5–6 days as needed and tolerated
Typical daily dose	0.5–2 mg
Dose range	0.25–4 mg/day
Therapeutic serum level	Not established

Comments: Not a preferred drug for elderly patients because of adverse-effect profile. May be indicated for secondary parkinsonism, rabbit syndrome, or acute dystonia. Not used prophylactically for EPS in elderly patients. Time to peak serum concentration 60–90 minutes. Half-life not found in published sources. Effects of oral drug are cumulative and may not be apparent until several days after drug initiation. Eliminated primarily in urine. Contraindicated in patients with narrow-angle glaucoma, pyloric or duodenal obstruction, stenosing peptic ulcer, bladder neck obstruction, achalasia, or myasthenia gravis. Patients are warned regarding use in hot weather or during exercise and use with cardiovascular disease, liver or kidney disorders, or prostatic hyperplasia. *Many adverse effects:* Tachycardia, confusion, disorientation, memory impairment, toxic psychosis, visual hallucinations, rash, heat stroke, hyperthermia, dry mouth, nausea, vomiting, constipation, ileus, urinary retention, dysuria, blurred vision, mydriasis, fever, and exacerbation of tardive dyskinesia. *Drug interactions:* Additive effects with other anticholinergic drugs, opposes the effects of cholinergic drugs (e.g., cholinesterase inhibitors), increased bioavailability of atenolol, increased amount of digoxin absorbed, decreased amount of levodopa absorbed, antagonism of some therapeutic effects of neuroleptic drugs.

Generic name	biperiden
Trade name	Akineton
Class	Anticholinergic agent
Half-life	18.4–24.3 hours
Mechanism of action	Inhibition of striatal cholinergic receptors
Available preparations	Tablets: 2 mg
Starting dose	2 mg/day
Titration	As needed and tolerated
Typical daily dose	2 mg bid
Dose range	2–4 mg/day
Therapeutic serum level	Not established

Comments: Not a preferred drug for elderly patients because of adverse-effect profile. May be indicated for secondary parkinsonism, rabbit syndrome, or acute dystonia. Not used prophylactically for EPS in elderly patients. Given that this drug mainly affects tremor, may be less useful for secondary parkinsonism than other agents. (See text for discussion of symptoms of drug-induced parkinsonism.) Time to peak serum concentration is 1–1.5 hours. Contraindicated in patients with ileus, gastrointestinal (GI) obstruction, genitourinary obstruction or urinary retention, heart failure, edema, achalasia, narrow-angle glaucoma, or myasthenia gravis. Patients are warned regarding use in hot weather or during exercise, and use with cardiovascular disease, liver or kidney disorders, or prostatic hyperplasia. *Many adverse effects:* Orthostasis, bradycardia, drowsiness, euphoria, disorientation, agitation, sleep disorder, constipation, dry mouth, urinary retention, choreic movements, blurred vision, and exacerbation of tardive dyskinesia. *Drug interactions:* Additive effects with other anticholinergic drugs, opposes the effects of cholinergic drugs (e.g., cholinesterase inhibitors), increased bioavailability of atenolol, increased amount of digoxin absorbed, decreased amount of levodopa absorbed, antagonism of some therapeutic effects of neuroleptic drugs.

Generic name	bromocriptine
Trade name	Parlodel (generic available)
Class	Dopamine agonist
Half-life	Biphasic: 6–8 hours/50 hours
Mechanism of action	Activates postsynaptic dopamine receptors
Available preparations	Tablets: 2.5 mg Capsules: 5 mg
Starting dose	2.5 mg orally or via nasogastric tube tid
Titration	As tolerated
Typical daily dose	5 mg tid
Dose range	2.5–5 mg tid
Therapeutic serum level	Not established

Comments: Used in some cases of NMS. 90%–96% protein bound. Peak serum concentration in 1–2 hours. Metabolized in the liver. Major substrate of CYP3A4. Eliminated mainly in bile. Ergot alkaloids are contraindicated in patients with uncontrolled hypertension, severe ischemic heart disease, or peripheral vascular disease. Use with caution in patients with impaired renal or hepatic function, history of cardiovascular disease or psychosis, peptic ulcer disease, or dementia. *Drug interactions:* Do not give bromocriptine with potent CYP3A4 inhibitors. (See Table 2–2.) Use caution in combination with antihypertensive drugs. May cause serotonin syndrome in combination with monoamine oxidase inihibitors (MAOIs), sibutramine, and other serotonergic drugs. Diminished bromocriptine effects in combination with dopamine blockers (neuroleptics). *Common adverse effects (>10%):* Headache, dizziness, and nausea. *Less common adverse effects (1%–10%):* Orthostasis, fatigue, light-headedness, drowsiness, anorexia, vomiting, abdominal cramps, constipation, and nasal congestion. *Less common but serious adverse effects:* Arrhythmias, hair loss, insomnia, paranoia, and visual hallucinations.

Generic name	clonazepam
Trade name	Klonopin (generic available)
Class	Benzodiazepine
Half-life	19–50 hours
Mechanism of action	Potentiates effects of GABA by binding to GABA$_A$-benzodiazepine receptor complex
Available preparations	Tablets: 0.5, 1, 2 mg Orally disintegrating wafer: 0.125, 0.25, 0.5, 1, 2 mg
Starting dose	0.25–0.5 mg/day (evening or at bedtime)
Titration	Increase by 0.25–0.5 mg every 4–5 days
Typical daily dose	1–2 mg/day (evening or at bedtime)
Dose range	0.5 mg every other day to 4 mg/day (evening or before bedtime)
Therapeutic serum level	Not established for movement abnormalities

Comments: A drug of choice for RLS; also used in some cases of myoclonus and tremor (e.g., in CBD). Some reported efficacy for TD. Rapidly and well absorbed orally. 85% protein bound . Onset of action in 20–60 minutes, duration of action 12 hours. Extensively metabolized in the liver to inactive metabolites. Major substrate of CYP3A4. Metabolites excreted as glucuronide or sulfate conjugates. Contraindicated in patients with significant hepatic impairment. Use with caution in elderly patients and in those with renal impairment, respiratory disease, or impaired gag reflex. Additive effects with alcohol and other CNS depressants; increased risk of falls. *Drug interactions:* CYP3A4 inducers and inhibitors (see Table 2–2), increased clonazepam level with disulfiram, clonazepam possibly diminishes effect of levodopa, theophylline diminishes effect of clonazepam, absence seizures when clonazepam and valproate combined. *Adverse effects:* Amnesia, ataxia, dysarthria, sedation, incoordination, dizziness, depression with suicidality, confusion, hallucinations, emotional lability, paradoxical aggression, insomnia, behavioral problems, anorexia, constipation, dehydration, diarrhea, nausea, dry mouth, dysuria, change in frequency of urination, nocturia, urinary retention, encopresis, blood dyscrasias, abnormal liver function test values, weakness, myalgia, blurred vision, and increased respiratory secretions.

Generic name	dantrolene
Trade name	Dantrium
Class	Skeletal muscle relaxant
Half-life	8.7 hours
Mechanism of action	Interferes with release of calcium ion from sarcoplasmic reticulum; by reducing rigidity, reduces or prevents catabolic processes associated with NMS
Available preparations	Capsules: 25, 50, 100 mg Injection (powder for reconstitution): 20 mg (contains mannitol)
Starting dose	1 mg/kg iv When the patient has been stabilized, iv dantrolene may be switched to po dantrolene 4–8 mg/kg/day in four divided doses
Titration	Repeat dose until patient is stabilized (up to a cumulative dose of 10 mg/kg), then make switch to po/nasogastric tube (NGT) dosing
Typical daily dose	6 mg/kg (in four divided doses) po/NGT
Dose range	4–8 mg/kg/day (in four divided doses) po/NGT
Therapeutic serum level	Not established

Comments: Used with bromocriptine in severe cases of NMS. Slow and incomplete absorption when taken orally. Slowly metabolized in the liver. Major substrate of CYP3A4. Eliminated mainly in feces via bile; 25% eliminated in urine. Use with caution in patients with cardiac or pulmonary dysfunction. *Drug interactions:* Expected interactions with CYP3A4 inhibitors and inducers (see Table 2–2); increased toxicity with warfarin, clofibrate, tolbutamide; hepatotoxicity with estrogens; sedation with CNS depressants; increased neuromuscular blockade with MAOIs, phenothiazines, clindamycin; hyperkalemia and cardiac depression with verapamil. Potential hepatotoxicity. *Common adverse effects (> 10%):* Drowsiness, dizziness, light-headedness, fatigue, rash, diarrhea, vomiting, and muscle weakness. *Less common adverse effects (1%–10%):* Pleural effusion with pericarditis, chills, fever, headache, insomnia, nervousness, depression, diarrhea, constipation, anorexia, stomach cramps, blurred vision, and respiratory depression. *Less common but serious effects:* Confusion, hepatic necrosis, hepatitis, and seizures.

Generic name	diphenhydramine
Trade name	Benadryl and others (generic available)
Class	Antihistamine (with anticholinergic side effects)
Half-life	13.5 hours
Mechanism of action	Antiparkinsonian effects mediated by anticholinergic activity
Available preparations	Tablets: 25, 50 mg Capsules: 25, 50 mg Oral solution: 12.5 mg/5mL Oral suspension: 25 mg/5mL Injection: 50 mg/mL
Starting dose	25 mg bid
Titration	Increase as needed and tolerated
Typical daily dose	25–50 mg bid
Dose range	25 mg/day (qhs) to 100 mg bid
Therapeutic serum level	Not established (toxic >0.1 µg/mL)

Comments: Not a preferred drug for elderly patients because of adverse-effect profile. May be indicated for secondary parkinsonism, rabbit syndrome, or acute dystonia. Not used prophylactically for EPS in elderly patients. About 65% is absorbed orally. Extensively metabolized in the liver (less in lung and kidney). Moderate inhibitor of CYP2D6. Peak concentration in 2–4 hours. Peak levels significantly elevated in elderly. Clearance significantly reduced in elderly. Elderly patients should be warned that antihistamines are more likely to cause dizziness, excessive sedation, syncope, hypotension, and confusional states. Use with caution in patients with narrow-angle glaucoma, peptic ulcer disease, urinary tract obstruction, or hypothyroidism. *Adverse reactions:* Hypotension, palpitations, tachycardia, sedation, dizziness, incoordination, fatigue, nervousness, insomnia, confusion, nausea, vomiting, diarrhea, dry mouth, anorexia or increased appetite, urinary retention or increased frequency, thrombocytopenia, agranulocytosis, tremor, blurred vision, and thickening of bronchial secretions. *Drug interactions:* Increased levels of CYP2D6 substrates, decreased effect of CYP2D6 prodrug substrates, additive effects with other anticholinergic drugs, opposes effects of cholinergic drugs (e.g., cholinesterase inhibitors), increased bioavailability of atenolol, increased amount of digoxin absorbed, decreased amount of levodopa absorbed, antagonism of some therapeutic effects of neuroleptic drugs, additive effects with other CNS depressants, Antabuse reactions with syrup form (contains alcohol) in patients on disulfiram.

Generic name	gabapentin
Trade name	Neurontin (generic available)
Class	Anticonvulsant structurally related to GABA
Half-life	5–7 hours
Mechanism of action	Structurally related to GABA, but mechanism has not been elucidated
Available preparations	Capsules: 100, 300, 400 mg Tablets: 100, 300, 400, 600, 800 mg Oral solution: 250 mg/5 mL
Starting dose	Essential tremor (ET): 100 mg tid Restless legs syndrome (RLS): 300 mg qhs
Titration	ET: increase by 100 mg tid every 1–2 days RLS: increase to 300 mg bid in 1–2 days, then 300 mg tid in 1–2 days, then continue increasing by 300 mg as tolerated to target dose
Typical daily dose	ET: 1,200–3,600 mg RLS: 2,400 mg (divided tid)
Dose range	900–3,600 mg/day (divided tid)
Therapeutic serum level	Obtainable, but not used clinically

Comments: A first-line drug for RLS and a second-line drug for ET; anecdotal evidence for efficacy in treating akathisia. 50%–60% absorbed from proximal small intestine via L-amino transport system. Less than 3% protein bound. Bioavailability inversely proportional to dose (60% at 900 mg/day, 33% at 3,600 mg/day). Not appreciably metabolized. Excreted in urine as unchanged drug; clearance proportional to renal function. Half-life greatly prolonged in anuria (132 hours), shortened during dialysis (3.8 hours). For hemodialysis patients, dose is 200–300 mg after each dialysis session. Generally well tolerated, with adverse effects that are mild to moderate in severity and self-limiting. *Drug interactions:* Additive sedation from other CNS depressants. *Common adverse effects (>10%):* Somnolence, dizziness, ataxia, and fatigue. *Less common adverse effects (1%–10%):* Peripheral edema, diarrhea, nausea, vomiting, dry mouth, constipation, tremor, weakness, nystagmus, diplopia, and blurred vision. *Uncommon but serious adverse effects:* Acute renal failure, asterixis, encephalopathy, induction of rapid cycling, and others.

Generic name	levodopa/carbidopa
Trade name	Sinemet, Sinemet CR, Parcopa
Class	Dopamine agonist
Half-life	1–2 hours
Mechanism of action	Increases striatal dopamine concentration
Available preparations	Immediate-release (IR) tablets: 10/100 (10 mg carbidopa/100 mg levodopa), 25/100, 25/250 IR orally disintegrating tablets (contain phenylalanine): 10/100 (10 mg carbidopa/100 mg levodopa), 25/100, 25/250 Sustained-release (SR) tablets: 25/100, 50/200
Starting dose	Half of 25/100 mg tablet bid (12.5/50 mg bid)
Titration	Increase by one-half to 1 tablet every week
Typical daily dose	25/100 mg, 1–2 tablets tid
Dose range	Levodopa up to 1,000 mg/day
Therapeutic serum level	Not established

Comments: First-line drug for treatment of Parkinson's disease. Contraindicated in patients with narrow-angle glaucoma, patients taking MAOIs, and patients with history of melanoma or undiagnosed skin lesions. Used with caution in patients with history of myocardial infarction, arrhythmias, asthma, wide-angle glaucoma, or peptic ulcer disease. Food (particularly high-protein meals) reduces absorption, so medication should be given consistently with respect to meals, preferably before meals on an empty stomach. If GI upset occurs, can be given with food. Effects of IR drug peak in 1 hour and last 3–8 hours. Eliminated primarily in urine as dopamine, norepinephrine, and homovanillic acid. *Drug interactions:* These are numerous; among psychotropics, antipsychotics and benzodiazepines inhibit the antiparkinsonian effects of levodopa, and anticholinergics and tricyclic antidepressants reduce levodopa absorption. *Adverse effects:* These are numerous and include orthostasis, hypertension, arrhythmias, syncope, confusion, hallucinations, insomnia, memory impairment, peripheral neuropathy, increased libido, nausea, vomiting, diarrhea, constipation, GI bleeding, sialorrhea, change in urinary frequency, blood dyscrasias, abnormalities in liver function test values, and dyskinetic movements. Abrupt discontinuation of levodopa may be associated with NMS or exacerbation of parkinsonism.

Generic name	pramipexole
Trade name	Mirapex
Class	Dopamine agonist
Half-life	12 hours
Mechanism of action	Activates postsynaptic dopamine receptors in the striatum and substantia nigra
Available preparations	Tablets: 0.125, 0.25, 0.5, 1, 1.5 mg
Starting dose	0.125 mg bid
Titration	Increase by 0.125 mg bid every 7 days
Typical daily dose	1 mg bid
Dose range	1–3 mg/day (divided bid to tid)
Therapeutic serum level	Not established

Comments: A drug of choice in treating Parkinson's disease and RLS. Absorption is rapid but delayed by food. Bioavailability >90%. Minimally metabolized. 90% eliminated unchanged in urine. Clearance reduced in direct proportion to reduced glomerular filtration rate. *Drug interactions:* Neuroleptics decrease pramipexole's efficacy due to dopamine antagonism, cimetidine increases serum concentrations and half-life of pramipexole, and drugs secreted by the cationic transport system (e.g., diltiazem, ranitidine) reduce pramipexole clearance by about 20%. *Common adverse effects (>10%):* Orthostasis, asthenia, dizziness, somnolence, insomnia, hallucinations, abnormal dreams, constipation, weakness, dyskinesia, and EPS. *Less common adverse effects (1%–10%):* Edema, syncope, tachycardia, chest pain, confusion, amnesia, dystonias, akathisia, myoclonus, paranoia, fever, decreased libido, anorexia, dry mouth, dysphagia, urinary frequency or incontinence, visual abnormalities, and dyspnea. *Uncommon but serious adverse effects:* Rhabdomyolysis and increased liver transaminases. Also causes daytime somnolence that is dose-related.

Generic name	primidone
Trade name	Mysoline (generic available)
Class	Anticonvulsant
Half-life	Primidone: 10–12 hours Phenylethylmalonamide (PEMA): 16 hours Phenobarbital: up to 118 hours
Mechanism of action	Decreases neuronal excitability
Available preparations	Tablets: 50, 250 mg
Starting dose	125 mg tid
Titration	Increase by 125 mg every 3–7 days
Typical daily dose	250 mg tid
Dose range	125–250 mg tid
Therapeutic serum level	Not established for tremor

Comments: In spite of being a first-line agent for treatment of essential tremor, this is not a preferred drug in elderly patients because one of its metabolites is a barbiturate with a long half-life (phenobarbital). Bioavailability 60%–80%. Peak serum concentration within 4 hours. 99% protein bound. Metabolized in the liver to phenobarbital and PEMA. Phenobarbital metabolite strongly induces CYP1A2, 2B6, 2C8/9, and 3A4. Excreted in urine. Dose adjustment needed in renal and hepatic impairment. Drug interactions are numerous, in part because of CYP450 induction. *Adverse effects:* Drowsiness, vertigo, ataxia, lethargy, behavior change, fatigue, hyperirritability, nausea, vomiting, anorexia, impotence, agranulocytosis, anemia, diplopia, and nystagmus.

Generic name	procyclidine
Trade name	Kemadrin
Class	Anticholinergic agent
Half-life	12 hours
Mechanism of action	Blocks acetylcholine at cerebral synapses
Available preparations	Tablets: 5 mg
Starting dose	2.5 mg/day
Titration	As tolerated by 2.5 mg
Typical daily dose	5 mg
Dose range	5–10 mg/day
Therapeutic serum level	Not established

Comments: Not a preferred drug for elderly patients because of adverse-effect profile. May be indicated for secondary parkinsonism, rabbit syndrome, or acute dystonia. Not used prophylactically for EPS in elderly patients. Onset of action in 30–40 minutes; duration 4–6 hours with residual effects at 12 hours. Metabolized in the liver and eliminated in urine. Contraindicated in patients with narrow-angle glaucoma or myasthenia gravis. Carries warnings regarding use in hot weather or during exercise and for patients with cardiovascular disease, liver or kidney disorders, or prostatic hyperplasia. *Adverse effects:* Tachycardia, confusion, drowsiness, headache, loss of memory, fatigue, ataxia, light-headedness, constipation, dry mouth, nausea, vomiting, epigastric discomfort, difficulty with urination, weakness, blurred vision, mydriasis, decreased diaphoresis, and exacerbation of tardive dyskinesia. *Drug interactions:* Additive effects with other anticholinergic drugs, opposes the effects of cholinergic drugs (e.g., cholinesterase inhibitors), increased bioavailability of atenolol, increased amount of digoxin absorbed, decreased amount of levodopa absorbed, and antagonism of some therapeutic effects of neuroleptic drugs.

Generic name	propranolol
Trade name	Inderal, Inderal LA, InnoPran XL (generic available)
Class	β-Adrenergic receptor antagonist (nonselective)
Half-life	4–6 hours
Mechanism of action	Competitive blockade of β_1 and β_2 adrenergic receptors
Available preparations	Tablets: 10, 20, 40, 60, 80 mg Capsule (SR): 60, 80, 120, 160 mg Capsule (XL): 80, 120 mg Oral solution: 4 mg/mL, 8 mg/mL
Starting dose	10 mg bid
Titration	Increase dose every 3–7 days
Typical daily dose	80 mg bid
Dose range	40–120 mg bid
Therapeutic serum level	Not established

Comments: First-line agent for treatment of essential tremor. Reduced hemodynamic response may be seen in elderly compared with younger patients because of age-related changes in the β-adrenergic system. Serum levels and clearance affected by food, especially changes in dietary protein intake. β–Blockade occurs within 1–2 hours of ingestion, lasts about 6 hours. Extensive first-pass metabolism (bioavailability 30%–40%). 93% protein bound. Metabolized in the liver to active and inactive metabolites. Major substrate of CYP1A2 and 2D6; weakly inhibits same isoenzymes. Eliminated primarily in urine. Numerous drug interactions among psychotropics, with diazepam, fluoxetine, and haloperidol. Important interactions with antiarrhythmics and warfarin. *Adverse effects:* Bradycardia, congestive heart failure, hypotension, syncope, depression, amnesia, hyperglycemia, hyperlipidemia, hyperkalemia, constipation, vomiting, diarrhea, and thrombocytopenia, among others.

Generic name	ropinirole
Trade name	Requip
Class	Dopamine agonist
Half-life	6 hours
Mechanism of action	Activates postsynaptic dopamine receptors in the striatum
Available preparations	Tablets: 0.25, 0.5, 1, 2, 3, 4, 5 mg
Starting dose	Parkinson's disease (PD): 0.25 mg tid Restless legs syndrome (RLS): 0.25 mg 1–3 hours before bedtime
Titration	PD: increase by 0.25 mg tid every 7 days RLS: increase to 0.5 mg before bedtime after 2 days, then to 1 mg after 7 days; further dose increases made at weekly intervals
Typical daily dose	PD: 1 mg tid RLS: 3 mg, 1–3 hours before bedtime
Dose range	PD: 0.75–6 mg/day (divided tid) RLS: up to 4 mg before bedtime
Therapeutic serum level	Not established

Comments: A drug of choice in the treatment of Parkinson's disease and restless legs syndrome. Peak concentration in 1–2 hours. Absorption delayed by food. Bioavailability about 55%. Extensively metabolized in the liver to inactive metabolites. Major substrate of CYP1A2; strong inhibitor of CYP2D6. Clearance reduced by 30% in elderly. Expected drug interactions with CYP1A2 and 2D6 substrates, inhibitors, and inducers. Neuroleptics oppose pharmacodynamic effects of ropinirole. Quinolone antibiotics (e.g., ciprofloxacin) and estrogen increase levels of ropinirole. Rate of adverse effects influenced by coadministration of levodopa. *Common adverse effects when used without levodopa (>10%):* Syncope, somnolence, dizziness, fatigue, nausea, and vomiting. *Less common adverse effects (1%–10%):* Edema, orthostasis, hypertension, pain, confusion, hallucinations, constipation, dyspepsia, abdominal pain, dry mouth, diarrhea, weakness, abnormal vision, and diaphoresis. Numerous uncommon but serious adverse effects.

Generic name	trihexyphenidyl
Trade name	Artane (generic available)
Class	Anticholinergic
Half-life	5.6–10.2 hours
Mechanism of action	Anticholinergic
Available preparations	Tablets: 2, 5 mg Elixir: 2 mg/5 mL
Starting dose	1 mg/day
Titration	Increase by 2 mg every 3–5 days as needed and tolerated
Typical daily dose	2 mg tid
Dose range	6–10 mg/day (divided tid to qid)
Therapeutic serum level	Not established

Comments: Not a preferred drug for elderly patients because of adverse-effect profile. May be indicated for secondary parkinsonism, rabbit syndrome, or acute dystonia. Not used prophylactically for EPS in elderly patients. Peak effects within 60 minutes; peak serum concentrations within 60–90 minutes. Eliminated primarily in urine. Contraindicated in patients with narrow-angle glaucoma, pyloric or duodenal obstruction, stenosing peptic ulcer, bladder neck obstruction, achalasia, or myasthenia gravis. Carries warnings regarding use in hot weather or during exercise and use in patients with cardiovascular disease, liver or kidney disorders, or prostatic hyperplasia. *Adverse effects:* Tachycardia, confusion, drowsiness, agitation, euphoria, headache, dizziness, nervousness, delusions, hallucinations, paranoia, constipation, dry mouth, ileus, nausea, vomiting, parotitis, urinary retention, weakness, blurred vision, mydriasis, increased intraocular pressure, glaucoma, blindness, decreased diaphoresis, and exacerbation of tardive dyskinesia. *Drug interactions:* Additive effects with other anticholinergic drugs, opposes the effects of cholinergic drugs (e.g., cholinesterase inhibitors), increased bioavailability of atenolol, increased amount of digoxin absorbed, decreased amount of levodopa absorbed, and antagonism of some therapeutic effects of neuroleptic drugs.

9

Medications to Treat Dementia and Other Cognitive Disorders

Introduction

The relative proportions of various dementing diseases among patients in developed countries of the world have been estimated at 35% for Alzheimer's disease (AD), 15% for dementia with Lewy bodies (DLB), 15% for mixed vascular dementia/AD, 10% for vascular dementia, and 5% for frontotemporal dementia, with the remainder a mix of movement disorder–related dementia and others (Mendez and Cummings 2003). In spite of the fact that environmental and pharmacologic treatments for these diseases differ in important ways, it is still relatively common to encounter elderly patients in the clinical setting who carry only the syndromic diagnosis of dementia.

As detailed in the following sections, explicit diagnostic criteria have been formulated for AD (McKhann et al. 1984), vascular dementia (Chui et al. 1992; Roman et al. 1993), and DLB (McKeith et al. 1996), and proposed for frontotemporal dementia (FTD) (Lund and Manchester Groups 1994) and alcohol-related dementia (ARD) (Oslin et al. 1998). In general, the application of disease criteria to individual patients is straightforward, and documentation of signs and symptoms with reference to criteria establishes a foundation for later consideration of existing and emerging pharmacologic and environmental treatments.

A certain amount of complexity is introduced to the diagnostic evaluation by the existence of other medical conditions that can give rise to secondary dementia syndromes, as listed in Table 9–1. For many of these conditions, other disease-specific treatments are indicated, and the role of antidementia drugs, such as cholinesterase inhibitors or N-methyl-D-aspartate (NMDA) receptor antagonists, is not fully understood.

The database regarding pharmacologic options for dementia treatment is rapidly evolving, largely because of the explosion of research into pathogenesis and prevention of AD. As new drugs are added, drugs once thought to be promising are called into question, such as vitamin E and estrogen therapies. These issues are discussed further later in this chapter.

Neuropsychiatric disturbances in dementia may reflect degeneration of brain areas involving emotion and behavioral control or may be a consequence of a mismatch between vulnerable patients and the demands placed on them in particular environments. These complex phenomena are in fact likely to be multifactorial in origin. There is evidence from positron emission tomography (PET) studies that certain clinical-pathologic correlates are regionally specific, with agitation and disinhibition associated with frontotemporal hypometabolism, anxiety and depression with parietal hypometabolism, and psychosis with frontal hypometabolism (Sultzer et al. 1995). In addition, behavioral symptoms in AD such as agitation/aggression and psychosis may be linked to specific neurotransmitters such as serotonin (Assal et al. 2004). Even so, initial interventions in most cases should center on behavioral, interpersonal, or environmental approaches.

Evaluation of the Cognitively Impaired Elder

The initial evaluation of the elderly patient presenting with evidence of cognitive dysfunction includes a history, physical and neurologic examinations, mental status examination, and laboratory evaluation. The history of interest relates to cognitive decline, linked temporally to holidays or important personal dates such as birthdays or anniversaries. Deficits can be inferred from problems that have developed with activities of daily living (e.g., missed appointments, misplaced keys, mistakes in keeping a check-

Table 9–1.   Causes of dementia in the elderly population

Degenerative disorders	Organ failure
Alzheimer's disease	Hepatic encephalopathy
Mixed dementia (Alzheimer's plus vascular dementia)	Uremic encephalopathy
	Pulmonary insufficiency
Dementia with Lewy bodies	**Vitamin deficiencies**
Parkinson's disease with dementia	B_{12} cyanocobalamin
Frontotemporal dementia	B_1 thiamine
Progressive supranuclear palsy	Others (e.g., folate, niacin, ?B_6)
Corticobasal degeneration	**Toxicities**
Multisystem atrophy	Prescribed medications
Amyotrophic lateral sclerosis	Heavy metals (arsenic, mercury, lead)
Huntington's disease	Poisons (pesticides, fertilizers)
Hereditary ataxia	**Chronic infections**
Multiple sclerosis	Neurosyphilis
Cerebrovascular diseases	HIV/AIDS
Multi-infarct dementia	Creutzfeldt-Jakob disease
Strategic single-infarct dementia	Gerstmann-Sträussler-Scheinker syndrome
Small-vessel disease	
Watershed area hypoperfusion	Progressive multifocal leukoencephalopathy
Endocrine diseases	
Hypothyroidism	Tuberculosis
Cushing's syndrome	Fungal or protozoal infection
Adrenal insufficiency	Sarcoidosis
Hypoparathyroidism	Whipple's disease
Hyperparathyroidism	**Other causes**
Brain injuries	Vasculitis
Postanoxic	Normal-pressure hydrocephalus
Postencephalitic	Nonconvulsive status epilepticus
Chronic subdural hematoma	Acute intermittent porphyria

Source.   Adapted from Bird TD, Miller BL: "Alzheimer's Disease and Other Dementias," in *Harrison's Principles of Internal Medicine,* 16th Edition. Edited by Kasper DL, Fauci AS, Longo DL, et al. New York, McGraw-Hill, 2005, pp. 2393–2406. Used with permission.

book, mishaps in the kitchen, getting lost on familiar routes, motor vehicle accidents, or problems recognizing family members). Neurologic symptoms of trouble walking, urinary incontinence, slurred speech, swallowing problems, stiffness, tremor, slowing, falling, loss of consciousness, weakness, incoordination, seizures, and headache should be elicited. Psychiatric symptoms of disinhibition, neglect of personal hygiene, aggression, apathy, depression, irritability, delusions, suicidal ideation, misidentifications, hallucinations, and personality changes should also be elicited. A complete list of medical problems and current medications should be obtained.

At a minimum, physical evaluation should include cardiac, pulmonary, and neurologic examinations. Some dementia specialists perform these evaluations themselves, while others work in tandem with colleagues in general medicine. The neurologic screening examination should particularly address cranial nerve dysfunction, weakness, tremor, rigidity, akinesia, myoclonus, asymmetry of reflexes, abnormal reflexes (Babinski, grasp), dysmetria, clumsiness, and ambulation difficulties.

Components of the mental status examination especially relevant to a dementia evaluation include the level of conscious awareness and attention, presence of psychotic symptoms (delusions, hallucinations), abnormalities of mood, and cognition. Assessment of cognition should include tests of verbal and nonverbal memory, language, praxis, visuospatial performance, and executive system function. Several valid and reliable screening instruments for cognitive impairment are published. The most widely used is the Mini-Mental State Examination (MMSE; Folstein et al. 1975), which uncovers mainly cortical deficits. The MMSE can be supplemented with tests such as the Trail Making Test (Parts A and B), timed naming (e.g., types of animals), clock drawing, and Luria hand sequences to identify frontal-subcortical dysfunction (Cummings and Benson 1992). Cognitive screening may be inadequate for certain individuals undergoing evaluation (e.g., a patient with superior premorbid intelligence and clear decline who achieves perfect scores on screens, or a patient with a low level of education who scores in the impaired ranges at baseline). One approach to this problem is to evaluate patients on functional measures in tandem with cognitive measures. When the two measures are discrepant (e.g., test scores in the normal range with function clearly impaired), further investigation is indicated. Such patients can be referred for neuropsychologic testing, using a more extensive battery with a more fully developed normative database.

Dementia is a syndrome of acquired intellectual impairment characterized in DSM-IV-TR by persistent deficits in memory (amnesia) and at least one other domain: language (aphasia), motor function (apraxia), recognition (agnosia), or executive function. Some definitions require three domains of impairment for the diagnosis and include personality change as one of the domains. Patients with FTD such as Pick's disease may be quite severely affected before memory impairment is evident. For this reason, not all definitions require the presence of memory impairment for a dementia diagnosis to be made. In general, the order in which symptoms become apparent, and their relative severity, depends on the etiology of dementia.

In the first stage of the evaluation, a syndromic diagnosis is made (e.g., mild cognitive impairment [MCI], delirium, or dementia). In patients with MCI, memory impairment compared with age-matched peers is found, with normal cognitive function in other domains and no functional evidence of dementia. In delirium, the acute onset of impairment and waxing and waning of symptoms (even when subtle) are important clues to diagnosis. Cognitive dysfunction can be compounded when disorders coexist; for example, delirium may be identified in a patient with preexisting dementia. In the discussion to follow, the disorders are considered separately for the sake of clarity, but it is recognized that cases encountered clinically may be more ambiguous.

In the next stage of the evaluation, a differential diagnosis of etiology is formulated. Although a detailed history and careful examination provide the most significant information about etiology, laboratory investigation is required to rule out causes of dementia that require specific treatment. In at least some of these conditions (e.g., early B_{12} deficiency), the cognitive impairment will improve or even remit with treatment.

As shown in Table 9–2, the standard laboratory workup for the diagnosis of dementia etiology includes a complete blood count, chemistries, liver function tests, thyroid function tests, vitamin B_{12} and folate levels, and syphilis serology. Since negative rapid plasma reagin (RPR) and Venereal Disease Research Laboratory (VDRL) results can be reported in a substantial minority of patients with tertiary syphilis, fluorescent trep-

Table 9–2.   Laboratory workup for dementia

Routine tests

Complete blood count	White blood cell count with differential; red blood cell count with indices, hemoglobin, hematocrit, and platelet count
Chemistries	Glucose, blood urea nitrogen, creatinine, sodium, potassium, chloride, CO_2, anion gap, calcium, magnesium, phosphorus, AST, ALT, LDH, alkaline phosphatase, bilirubin, thyroid-stimulating hormone, free T_4 index, vitamin B_{12}, and syphilis serology (RPR or VDRL)
Structural neuroimaging study	MRI or CT

Ancillary tests

Lumbar puncture	Cerebrospinal fluid studies: protein, glucose, cell count with differential; other tests depend on clinical presentation
Electroencephalogram	Wakefulness, drowsiness, and sleep with hyperventilation and photic stimulation; patient may need stimulation to ensure that a sample of awake state is obtained
HIV serology	CD4 cell count, HIV RNA (viral load)
Lyme disease titers	ELISA, Western blot for antibodies; polymerase chain reaction for spirochete DNA
Heavy metal screening	Lead, mercury, manganese, arsenic, copper, and aluminum
Functional neuroimaging	SPECT, PET, fMRI

Note.   ALT = alanine transaminase; AST = aspartate transaminase; CT = computed tomography; ELISA = enzyme-linked immunosorbent assay; LDH = lactate dehydrogenase; fMRI = functional MRI; MRI = magnetic resonance imaging; PET = positron emission tomography; RPR = rapid plasma reagin; SPECT = single photon emission computed tomography; T_4 = thyroxine; VDRL = Venereal Disease Research Laboratory.

onemal antibody absorption (FTA-ABS) testing may be necessary. A structural neuroimaging study is required for the differential diagnosis of vascular dementia and to diagnose other conditions associated with dementia such as tumor or hydrocephalus. Although a head computed tomography (CT) scan may be sufficient, magnetic resonance imaging (MRI) is superior in detecting white matter lesions and is therefore the procedure of choice. MRI may be contraindicated in patients with any metal in the body (prostheses, heart valves, or foreign bodies such as metal slivers in the globe of the eye from a prior industrial accidents), so screening for metal is necessary. If MRI is obtained, it is important to avoid overinterpretation of white matter changes seen only on T2-weighted studies (Small et al. 1997).

Lumbar puncture should be performed in cases where symptoms have been of short duration, especially in the presence of fever, nuchal rigidity, or elevated erythrocyte sedimentation rate; where symptoms are rapidly progressive; where metastatic cancer is suspected; or where the FTA-ABS test confirming syphilis is positive. An electroencephalogram should be performed in patients with a seizure history, with rapid progression of dementia, or in a prolonged confusional (delirious) state. HIV testing, Lyme disease titers, or heavy metal screening should be done in patients with a possible history of exposure. Functional neuroimaging (PET, single photon emission computed tomography, or functional MRI) can be helpful if the etiology of dementia remains unclear at this point in the workup.

APOE genotyping can help to increase the specificity of diagnosis in the patient who meets clinical diagnostic criteria for AD (Mayeux et al. 1998), but is not useful in predicting whether the disease will develop in an asymptomatic individual. This test is not a recommended part of the routine dementia evaluation. Also not routinely recommended is a urine test for neural thread protein, a putative biomarker for AD. The test kit was judged nonapprovable by the U.S. Food and Drug Administration (FDA) in mid-2005 because of concerns about its validity, specificity, and utility in dementia diagnosis. Its use is presently considered investigational by most health insurance plans.

Medications Used to Treat Dementia

Cholinesterase Inhibitors

At present, cholinesterase inhibitors constitute the mainstay of dementia treatment, particularly for AD and DLB, even though these medications lack FDA labeling for the latter indication. Other potential uses for these drugs are discussed in later sections. For AD, cholinesterase inhibitors confer a modest benefit: up to half of patients with mild to moderate disease show cognitive improvement, stabilization of daily function, and some delay of disease progression (Mendez and Cummings 2003). The magnitude of the cognitive and functional benefit in AD is relatively small, and is best detected by scales such as the Alzheimer's Disease Assessment Scale–Cognitive Subscale (ADAS-Cog) and the Clinician's Interview-Based Impression of Change (CIBIC+) rather than by screening instruments such as the MMSE (Mendez and Cummings 2003). There is some suggestion that these drugs may also exert neuroprotective effects as measured by N-acetylaspartate concentrations and hippocampal volumes (Krishnan et al. 2003).

There are four drugs labeled for AD in the class of cholinesterase inhibitors (Table 9–3). One of the drugs, tacrine, is largely outmoded because of hepatotoxic effects. As shown in Figure 9–1, all the drugs in this class share the mechanism of acetylcholinesterase inhibition. Rivastigmine also inhibits butyrylcholinesterase, and galantamine binds allosterically to the nicotinic acetylcholine receptor and may thereby potentiate the action of agonists such as acetylcholine. In fact, the clinical significance of these other mechanisms is not clear; to date, there is no convincing evidence that any one of these drugs is superior to the others at any stage of disease. Extended-release oral physostigmine has also been studied for AD but has been found to have an unacceptably high rate of gastrointestinal (GI) side effects (van Dyck et al. 2000).

Drug interactions involving cholinesterase inhibitors are both pharmacodynamic and pharmacokinetic, with the former potentially more significant. Pharmacodynamic interactions include potentiation of the response to succinylcholine-type muscle relaxants used in anesthesia (including anesthesia for electroconvulsive therapy), additive effects with other agents that reduce heart rate, and antagonistic effects with anticho-

Table 9–3. Cholinesterase inhibitors

Generic name	Trade name	Mechanism	Chemical class	Half-life (hours)	Metabolism
donepezil	Aricept	AChEI (reversible)	Piperidine derivative	70	CYP2D6, CYP3A4, glucuronidation
galantamine	Razadyne (changed from Reminyl)	AChEI (reversible, competitive), nicotinic receptor modulator	Phenanthrene alkaloid	6–8	CYP2D6, CYP3A4, demethylation, glucuronidation
rivastigmine	Exelon	AChEI, BuChEI	Carbamate derivative	1.5	Hydrolysis
tacrine	Cognex	AChEI (reversible)	Monoamine acridine	Serum: 2–4 Steady-state: 24–36	Extensively metabolized, mostly by CYP1A2

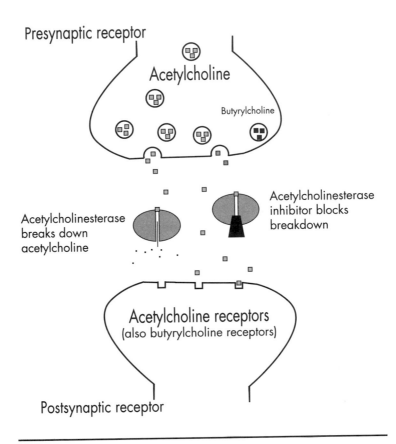

Figure 9–1.   Mechanism of action of acetylcholinesterase inhibitors.

Note.   Butyrylcholinesterase inhibition works by the same mechanism.

linergic medications. Known pharmacokinetic effects relate mainly to coadministration of cytochrome P450 (CYP) inhibitors or inducers with donepezil, galantamine, and tacrine. Rivastigmine is unique in being metabolized by local cholinesterases and is devoid of pharmacokinetic interactions. Both donepezil and galantamine also are metabolized by uridine 5'-diphosphate glucuronosyltransferases (UGTs). This information is summarized in Table 9–4.

Table 9–4.   Dementia drugs: known metabolic pathways

Drug	Metabolic pathways	Enzyme(s) inhibited	Enzyme(s) induced
Cholinesterase inhibitors			
Donepezil	CYP2D6, **3A4**, UGTs	None known	None known
Galantamine	CYP2D6, 3A4, UGTs; 50% excreted in urine unchanged	None known	None known
Rivastigmine	Local cholinesterases	None known	None known
Tacrine	**CYP1A2**, 2D6	CYP1A2	None known
Other drugs			
Clopidogrel	CYP1A2, 3A4	CYP2C8/9	None known
Memantine	Insignificant P450 metabolism	None known	None known
Selegiline	?CYP2D6, ?3A4, ?2B6, ?2C19	2C19	None known

Note.   CYP = cytochrome P450; UGT = uridine 5′-diphosphate glucuronosyltransferases. Bold type indicates major pathway.
Source.   Adapted from Cozza et al. 2003.

The issue of when to start and when to stop a cholinesterase inhibitor in probable AD remains controversial. In the ideal case, the drug would be started as early as possible, some degree of cognitive benefit would be noted, and the drug would be continued throughout disease progression. In the later stages of the disease, these drugs are believed to exert a meaningful effect in preventing behavioral disturbances but not in treating problematic behaviors that have already developed. In cases where cognitive benefit is not clear or where adverse effects are noted, a risk-benefit assessment should be made to determine whether the patient should remain on the medication. Drug cost is one of the factors to be taken into account.

Prescribing information for individual cholinesterase inhibitors is included in the Specific Drug summaries at the end of this chapter. Treated patients should be monitored for bradycardia and GI bleeding. Once a cholinesterase inhibitor is titrated to effect and tolerability, it should not be stopped abruptly in the absence of serious adverse effects. There is evidence that abrupt discontinuation may be associated with rapid cognitive and functional decline (Minett et al. 2003). It is not clear whether this represents a withdrawal phenomenon or whether underlying cognitive impairment is unmasked by abrupt discontinuation. Clinical experience suggests that in certain patients, baseline function is not achieved again, even with reinstitution of therapy. In addition, if therapy has been stopped for more than a day or two, it is necessary to reinitiate and retitrate the medication.

NMDA Receptor Antagonists

Several older drugs, including amantadine and dextromethorphan, are believed to act as antagonists at the NMDA receptor. However, it was not until 2003, when memantine was introduced, that an NMDA antagonist was specifically labeled for treatment of dementia (in this case, moderate to severe AD). Memantine blocks the action of glutamate at the NMDA receptor, as shown in Figure 9–2. Glutamate is an excitatory neurotransmitter that plays a number of important physiologic roles in learning and memory. In pathologic conditions such as Alzheimer's disease, persistent activation of the NMDA receptor can cause nerve cells to degenerate. When memantine is used, physiologic functions of glutamate are theoretically spared because memantine has only a low to moderate affinity for the receptor and can be dis-

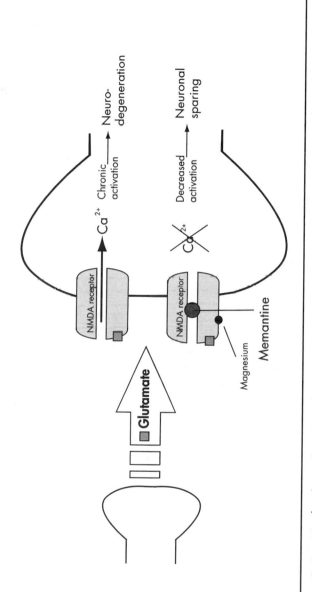

Figure 9–2.   Mechanism of action of memantine.

Note.   NMDA = *N*-methyl-D-aspartate. Under pathological conditions of NMDA receptor overactivation by glutamate, memantine acts by blocking the NMDA receptor. Under physiological conditions, glutamate binds to the receptor as usual.

placed under normal conditions by glutamate itself. Memantine also has low to moderate affinity as an antagonist at the serotonin 5-HT$_3$ receptor, and very low affinity as an antagonist at the nicotinic acetylcholine receptor.

Since memantine's putative mechanism involves a process basic to neurodegeneration in general, it may prove useful at earlier stages of AD as well as for a range of other dementing diseases. A review concluded that it also has a beneficial effect on cognitive function in vascular dementia (Areosa Sastre et al. 2005). Results from a randomized controlled trial in which memantine was added to a stable dose of the cholinesterase inhibitor donepezil in patients with moderate to severe AD suggest that the combination was well tolerated, and the treated group scored significantly better than the placebo group on measures of cognition, activities of daily living, global outcome, and behavior (Tariot et al. 2004). Based in part on these findings, many clinicians now consider optimal pharmacologic care for patients with AD to include a combination of a cholinesterase inhibitor with memantine.

Vitamin E (α-Tocopherol)

A 1997 study by Sano and colleagues reported the results of a 2-year controlled study of vitamin E and/or selegiline in patients with moderately severe AD. They found that 10 mg/day of selegiline and 2,000 IU/day of vitamin E were both effective in delaying the progression of disease. At the time, it was thought that vitamin E therapy was harmless, even at high doses, so it became standard practice to administer vitamin E (along with a cholinesterase inhibitor) for AD, despite the fact that the Sano study was never replicated. More recently, there has been some interest in determining whether these AD treatments could be extended to patients with MCI (discussed below). A study of vitamin E and donepezil in patients with MCI found no benefit for those treated with vitamin E (Petersen et al. 2005).

Recent investigations have called into question the safety of vitamin E supplementation. The results of the longitudinal Heart Outcomes Prevention Evaluation (HOPE) and The Ongoing Outcomes (HOPE-TOO) studies of daily vitamin E (400 IU) indicate that supplemented patients had higher rates of heart failure compared to control patients (Lonn et al. 2005). In addition, a meta-analysis of 19 clinical trials concluded that high-dose vitamin E (≥400 IU/day) was associated with an increase in all-cause mortality (E.R. Miller et al. 2005). Although controversial, these findings have raised legitimate questions about the routine use of vitamin E in AD and related disorders. At this point, the recommendation to clinicians and their patients is to taper vitamin E to discontinuation. No safe dose has yet been established.

Selegiline

Selegiline is a selective monoamine oxidase type B (MAO B) inhibitor used to treat Parkinson's disease (PD) with or without dementia. It is presumed to act by potentiating dopamine in degenerating nigrostriatal neurons, and possibly also by inhibiting neuronal injury from reactive products of oxidative metabolism. In studies of selegiline as a treatment for AD, effects have been modest overall. A Cochrane Review published in 2003 concluded that although there was no evidence of significant adverse events with this drug, there was also no evidence of a clinically meaningful benefit (Birks and Flicker 2003). It is important to note that selegiline loses its selectivity for MAO B at dosages higher than those recommended (>10 mg/day). MAO-type drug and food interactions are minimized by keeping the dose low, and dietary restrictions are not needed at the lower doses. This holds true for the transdermal form of selegiline as well as the oral form. Further pharmacologic and prescribing information for this drug is included in the Specific Drug summary at the end of this chapter.

Secretase Inhibitors

Evidence has accumulated to support the hypothesis advanced by Selkoe and others that accumulation, aggregation, and deposition of the β-amyloid peptide, $A\beta_{42}$, are central to the pathogenesis of AD (Zhou et al. 2003). Levels of $A\beta_{42}$ have been found to be reduced in the presence of certain nonsteroidal anti-inflammatory drugs (NSAIDs; e.g., indomethacin, sulindac, or ibuprofen) but not others (e.g., naproxen, meloxicam, or piroxicam), suggesting a possible mediation by inhibition of the small G protein ρ (Zhou et al. 2003) or other mechanisms (Morihara et al. 2005). Cleavage of amyloid precursor protein gives rise to either soluble products or the insoluble $A\beta_{42}$, depending on the site of cleavage. With α-secretase, soluble products are formed. With β- and γ-secretases, the insoluble $A\beta_{42}$ is formed, as shown in Figure 9–3. As the figure illustrates, inhibition of β-

and/or γ-secretase has the potential to reduce the deposition of Aβ_{42}, which forms the core of the plaque characteristic of AD and possibly other neurodegenerative conditions.

There has been intense competition to develop the first viable secretase inhibitor for clinical use, one that crosses the blood-brain barrier, is highly selective for the targeted enzyme, is readily taken up by neurons, and does not interfere with other signaling pathways or the function of other proteases (Maiorini et al. 2002). Although information in the public domain is limited, it appears that a number of pharmaceutical companies are working actively in this area. Secretase inhibitors may offer an important new clinical strategy for AD treatment and prevention in the near future.

Alzheimer's Vaccine

A vaccine designed to stimulate the body's immune response to β-amyloid in the brain was developed by Elan Corporation and brought through Phase I trials in the United States and United Kingdom in collaboration with Wyeth-Ayerst Pharmaceuticals. Initially, the vaccine appeared to be safe and well tolerated. When Phase IIA trials began, however, a number of cases of cerebritis (inflammation of the brain and spinal cord) were noted among vaccine recipients, so the trials were halted in the United States. Among subjects who continued the trial in Europe, findings were promising not only in slowing progression of cognitive decline but also in apparently improving cognitive function (by implication, through removal of plaques already formed). In addition, autopsy results from one of the vaccinated subjects suggested that plaque reduction in the brain was apparent but that β-amyloid deposits in blood vessels were unaffected, as were neurofibrillary tangles (Nicoll et al. 2003). At present, although the details are not available publicly, it appears that efforts are under way to refine the vaccine.

Ginkgo Biloba

In a review of the use of *Ginkgo biloba* for cognitive impairment and dementia, Birks and Grimley Evans (2002) noted poor methodology of early trials, and inconsistent results of later trials, but nonetheless concluded that the ginkgo extract appears to hold promise as far as effects on cognition and function. It has been noted elsewhere, however, that the effects of this extract are not as robust as those of cholinesterase inhibitors and

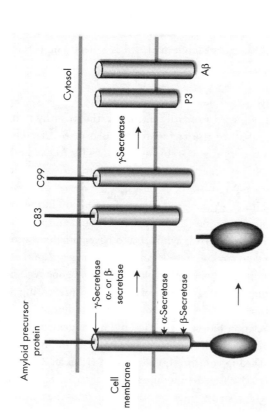

Figure 9–3. Amyloid precursor protein processing.

Note. Amyloid precursor protein is processed by α- or β-secretase to products C83 or C99, respectively. γ-Secretase processes C83 and C99 to P3 and Aβ, respectively. β-Amyloid then can polymerize to form oligomers $(A\beta)_n$ in the amyloid plaque.

Source. Reprinted from Rosenberg RN: "Translational Research on the Way to Effective Therapy for Alzheimer Disease." *Archives of General Psychiatry* 62:1186–1192, 2005. Used with permission.

that the extract is less convenient because of the need for dosing three times a day (Flint and Van Reekum 1998). In addition, rare case reports have associated ginkgo with episodes of serious bleeding, including subdural hematoma (L.G. Miller and Freeman 2002; Rowin and Lewis 1996) and bleeding into the anterior chamber of the eye (Rosenblatt and Mindel 1997), and this concern cannot be dismissed using meta-analytic methods on primary studies that may not have been designed to detect bleeding events. Finally, concerns persist about product purity and potency, as ginkgo is not FDA regulated, but marketed as a dietary supplement.

Statin Drugs

Statin drugs, or 3-hydroxy-3-methylglutaryl coenzyme A (HMG-CoA) reductase inhibitors, are used primarily in the treatment of hyperlipidemia, one of the established risk factors for vascular dementia. These drugs have been under scrutiny as possible risk reducers for AD and other dementing illnesses. It has been shown that cholesterol drives amyloid precursor protein processing to favor β cleavage (see earlier discussion about secretase inhibitors), so that lowering cholesterol would theoretically reduce β-amyloid deposition (Zandi et al. 2005). In addition, statin drugs reportedly inhibit nitric oxide synthase and have antiatherothrombotic actions on platelets, smooth muscle, and macrophages (Zandi et al. 2005). From the standpoint of pathophysiology, there was good reason to think that statin drugs could have beneficial effects in preventing and slowing the progression of AD. Early cross-sectional studies did in fact confirm an inverse relationship between AD (and other dementias) and statin drug use. More recently, however, several large, community-based, prospective studies failed to confirm this association (Li et al. 2004; Rea et al. 2005; Zandi et al. 2005). Randomized, clinical trials are currently under way, but at present, statin drugs are not indicated for the treatment of AD or any other type of dementia, including vascular dementia.

Estrogen

Findings from the Women's Health Initiative (WHI) Memory Study, a large, randomized, double-blind, placebo-controlled trial of estrogen (0.625 mg) and estrogen plus progestin (0.625 mg/2.5 mg) in postmenopausal women have had a major impact on estrogen prescribing practices

(Espeland et al. 2004; Shumaker et al. 2004). This study found that not only was the incidence of dementia and MCI not reduced in treated patients, but the risk for these events was actually increased. When these results are coupled with the findings from the WHI study itself related to increased risk of cardiovascular events with estrogen use, a convincing argument against the use of standard estrogen therapy for dementia treatment and prevention can be made, in spite of earlier positive reports from smaller, uncontrolled studies. Other estrogenic drugs are currently under investigation. Findings from the Multiple Outcomes of Raloxifene Evaluation (MORE) study, for example, suggested that the selective estrogen receptor modulator raloxifene might reduce the risk of developing cognitive impairment in postmenopausal women at particular doses (Yaffe et al. 2005).

Nonsteroidal Anti-Inflammatory Drugs

Evidence of inflammatory mechanisms contributing to neurodegeneration in AD has stimulated interest in the use of various anti-inflammatory drugs as possible treatments (Aisen and Davis 1997). Findings have been conflicting (Hanlon et al. 1997; in t' Veld et al. 2001). The most recent randomized controlled trial found that neither rofecoxib (a COX-2-selective inhibitor) nor naproxen was associated with slowed cognitive decline over 1 year in patients with mild to moderate AD (Aisen et al. 2003). The particular choice of NSAID may be significant, since only some of these drugs are known to be associated with reduced levels of $A\beta_{42}$ peptide, as discussed above in the section on secretase inhibitors. It may be that NSAIDs will have a role in AD prevention or even treatment in the future, when mechanisms are more fully elucidated. At present, however, routine use of NSAIDs in the treatment of dementia, including AD, is not recommended because they are known to have adverse effects that are sometimes serious in the elderly (including nephrotoxicity and GI bleeding).

Treatment of Specific Dementing Diseases and Other Cognitive Syndromes

Alcohol-Related Dementia

Proposed clinical criteria for probable and possible ARD are shown in Table 9–5. Characteristic radiologic findings in ARD include cerebellar

Table 9–5.   Alcohol-related dementia: proposed
criteria

Dementia

Dementia is defined as a significant deterioration of cognitive function sufficient
to interfere in social or occupational functioning. As defined by DSM-IV-TR,
this requires a deterioration in memory and at least one other area of intellectual
functioning. Moreover, the cognitive changes are not attributable to the presence
of delirium or substance-induced intoxication or withdrawal.

Definite alcohol-related dementia

At the current time there are no acceptable criteria to definitively define alcohol-
related dementia.

Probable alcohol-related dementia

A.   The criteria for the clinical diagnosis of probable alcohol-related dementia
include the following:

1.   A clinical diagnosis of dementia at least 60 days after the last exposure
to alcohol.

2.   Significant alcohol use as defined by a minimum average of 35 standard
drinks per week for men (28 for women) for greater than a period of
5 years. The period of significant alcohol use must occur within 3 years
of the initial onset of dementia.

B.   The diagnosis of alcohol-related dementia is supported by the presence of
any of the following:

1.   Alcohol-related hepatic, pancreatic, gastrointestinal, cardiovascular, or
renal disease (i.e., other end-organ damage).

2.   Ataxia or peripheral sensory polyneuropathy (not attributable to other
specific causes).

3.   Beyond 60 days of abstinence, cognitive impairment stabilizes or improves.

4.   After 60 days of abstinence, any neuroimaging evidence of ventricular
or sulcal dilatation improves.

5.   Neuroimaging evidence of cerebellar atrophy, especially of the vermis.

C.   The following clinical features cast doubt on the diagnosis of alcohol-related
dementia:

1.   The presence of language impairment, especially dysnomia or anomia.

2.   The presence of focal neurologic signs or symptoms (except ataxia or
peripheral sensory polyneuropathy).

Table 9–5. Alcohol-related dementia: proposed criteria *(continued)*

Probable alcohol-related dementia *(continued)*

    3. Neuroimaging evidence for cortical or subcortical infarction, subdural hematoma, or other focal brain pathology.

    4. Elevated Hachinski Ischemia Scale score.

D. Clinical features that neither are supportive nor cast doubt on the diagnosis of alcohol-related dementia include:

    1. Neuroimaging evidence of cortical atrophy.

    2. The presence of periventricular or deep white matter lesions on neuroimaging in the absence of focal infarct(s).

    3. The presence of the apolipoprotein ε4 allele.

E. The diagnosis of *possible* alcohol-related dementia may be made when there is:

    1. A clinical diagnosis of dementia at least 60 days after the last exposure to alcohol.

    2. Either significant alcohol use as defined by a minimum average of 35 standard drinks per week for men (28 for women) for 5 years or more, and the period of significant alcohol use occurred more than 3 years but less than 10 years prior to the initial onset of cognitive deficits; or possibly significant alcohol use as defined by a minimum average of 21 standard drinks per week for men (14 for women) but no more than 34 drinks per week for men (27 for women) for 5 years; the period of significant alcohol use must have occurred within 3 years of the onset of cognitive deficits.

Mixed dementia

A diagnosis of mixed dementia is reserved for clinical cases that appear to have more than one cause for dementia. The classification of probable or possible should continue to be used to convey the certainty of the diagnosis of alcohol-related dementia. The classification of mixed dementia should not be used to convey uncertainty of the diagnosis or to imply a differential diagnosis.

Table 9–5.   Alcohol-related dementia: proposed criteria *(continued)*

Alcohol as a contributing factor in the development or course of dementia

The designation of alcohol as a contributing factor is used for the situation in which alcohol is used but not to the degree required or within the time required to meet the classification of probable or possible alcohol-related dementia. This designation should not preclude the use of probable vascular dementia or probable dementia of the Alzheimer type.

Source.   Reprinted from Oslin D, Atkinson RM, Smith DM, et al: "Alcohol-Related Dementia: Proposed Clinical Criteria." *International Journal of Geriatric Psychiatry* 13:203–212, 1998. Used with permission.

atrophy, especially of the vermis, and in later disease stages, generalized atrophy, possibly more prominent in frontal areas.

Treatment of ARD requires abstinence from alcohol, and any treatment that helps to maintain abstinence—pharmacologic and nonpharmacologic—may be of use. As discussed more fully in Chapter 7, "Treatment of Substance-Related Disorders," medications used in the geriatric population for this purpose include acamprosate, naltrexone, disulfiram, and possibly serotonergic antidepressants and mood stabilizers. In addition, there is limited anecdotal evidence that cholinesterase inhibitor therapy may be of benefit in ARD (Kim et al. 2004; Levy et al. 1999). As discussed in a later section in this chapter on vascular dementia, this would presuppose that cholinergic pathways are affected in ARD. Since glutamatergic mechanisms are also likely to be implicated in the pathogenesis of ARD, memantine may also prove useful.

Alzheimer's Disease

National Institute of Neurological and Communicative Disorders and Stroke–Alzheimer's Disease and Related Disorders Association (NINCDS-ADRDA) criteria for the diagnosis of AD are shown in Table 9–6 (Roman et al. 1993). For patients who meet criteria for probable or possible AD, currently recommended treatments include cholinesterase inhibitors and memantine. As discussed earlier, treatments recommended in the past but now considered possibly harmful include high-dose vitamin E and estrogen. Treatments for which there is conflicting evidence regarding benefit or risk/benefit in AD include statin drugs, selegiline, NSAIDs, and *Ginkgo biloba*.

Although there is evidence of efficacy in AD for donepezil (Feldman et al. 2001; Rogers et al. 1998), rivastigmine (Rosler et al. 1999), and galantamine (Raskind et al. 2000; Tariot et al. 2000; Wilcock et al. 2000), the benefit from these drugs is generally modest. Positive effects may be seen in cognitive function, general function, and behavior. It appears that patients in all stages of disease may benefit (Kurz et al. 2004) and that those who initiate therapy early in the course of disease may benefit the most (Doraiswamy et al. 2002). As noted above, in later disease stages, these medications may help prevent behavioral disturbances, but they are not as helpful in treating behavioral disturbances that have already developed. There is no convincing evidence of any difference in efficacy among the agents currently marketed.

As noted above, there is no uniform practice with regard to when cholinesterase inhibitors are started and when they are stopped in the course of AD progression. Many clinicians initiate therapy with one of these drugs early and continue the drug as long as possible throughout disease progression. Others initiate therapy when the diagnosis is made, and then reevaluate risk and benefit of the drug after several months. In either case, doses should be titrated slowly (Tariot et al. 2000) to the highest tolerable dose, as there is evidence that benefit is dose dependent. It is preferable not to interrupt treatment; when these medications are stopped abruptly, patients typically have a rapid decline in cognitive and behavioral function (Minett et al. 2003).

As discussed earlier, memantine is a drug in a new class of antidementia treatment, and evidence to date suggests that it is associated with beneficial effects on cognitive function, functional decline, and behavior in moderate to severe AD (Areosa Sastre et al. 2005; Reisberg et al. 2003). Because the putative mechanism of this drug involves prevention of neurotoxicity through dampening of glutamatergic effects, it might be that therapy should be initiated earlier; this question awaits further study, as does combining therapy with cholinesterase inhibitors. Although there are data regarding tolerability of the combination of memantine and donepezil in the first 6 months of treatment, long-term data are not yet available (Tariot et al. 2004).

Table 9–6. Alzheimer's disease: NINCDS-ADRDA criteria

I. The criteria for the clinical diagnosis of *probable* Alzheimer's disease include:

   A. Dementia established by clinical examination and documented by the Mini-Mental State Examination, the Blessed Dementia Scale, or some similar examination, and confirmed by neuropsychologic tests

   B. Deficits in two or more areas of cognition

   C. Progressive worsening of memory and other cognitive functions

   D. No disturbance of consciousness

   E. Onset between ages 40 and 90 years, most often after age 65 years

   F. Absence of systemic disorders or other brain diseases that themselves could account for the progressive deficits in memory and cognition

II. The diagnosis of *probable* Alzheimer's disease is supported by:

   A. Progressive deterioration of specific cognitive functions such as language (aphasia), motor skills (apraxia), and perceptions (agnosia)

   B. Impaired activities of daily living and altered patterns of behavior

   C. Family history of similar disorders, particularly if confirmed neuropathologically

   D. Laboratory results of:

      1. Normal lumbar puncture as evaluated by standard techniques

      2. Normal pattern or nonspecific changes in electroencephalogram, such as increased slow-wave activity

      3. Evidence of cerebral atrophy on computed tomography, with progression documented by serial observation

III. Other clinical features consistent with the diagnosis of *probable* Alzheimer's disease, after exclusion of causes of dementia other than Alzheimer's disease, include:

   A. Plateaus in the course of progression of the illness

   B. Associated symptoms of depression; insomnia; incontinence; delusions; illusions; hallucinations; catastrophic verbal, emotional, or physical outbursts; sexual disorders; and weight loss

Table 9–6. Alzheimer's disease: NINCDS-ADRDA criteria *(continued)*

   C. Other neurologic abnormalities in some patients, especially in those with more advanced disease and exhibiting motor signs such as increased muscle tone, myoclonus, or gait disorder

   D. Seizures in advanced disease

   E. Computed tomography normal for age

IV. Features that make the diagnosis of *probable* Alzheimer's disease uncertain or unlikely include:

   A. Sudden, apoplectic onset

   B. Focal neurologic findings such as hemiparesis, sensory loss, visual field deficits, and incoordination early in the course of the illness

   C. Seizures or gait disturbances at the onset or very early in the course of the illness

V. Clinical diagnosis of *possible* Alzheimer's disease:

   A. May be made on the basis of the dementia syndrome, in the absence of other neurologic, psychiatric, or systemic disorders sufficient to cause dementia, and in the presence of variations in the onset, presentation, or clinical course

   B. May be made in the presence of a second systemic or brain disorder sufficient to produce dementia, which is not considered to be the cause of the dementia

   C. Should be used in research studies when a single, gradually progressive severe cognitive deficit is identified in the absence of other identifiable causes

VI. Criteria for diagnosis of *definite* Alzheimer's disease are:

   A. The clinical criteria for probable Alzheimer's disease

   B. Histopathologic evidence obtained from a biopsy or autopsy

Note. NINCDS-ADRDA = National Institute of Neurological and Communicative Disorders and Stroke–Alzheimer's Disease and Related Disorders Association.
Source. Reprinted from McKhann G, Drachman D, Folstein M, et al: "Clinical Diagnosis of Alzheimer's Disease: Report of the NINCDS-ADRDA Work Group Under the Auspices of Department of Health and Human Services Task Force on Alzheimer's Disease." *Neurology* 34:939–944, 1984. Used with permission.

Amnestic Disorder

Isolated memory impairment can be found in association with head trauma, thiamine and other vitamin deficiency states, infections such as herpes encephalitis, cerebrovascular insufficiency, and other medical conditions afflicting the elderly. The primary intervention for an amnestic disorder is timely treatment of the underlying medical condition. For example, aggressive thiamine replacement in Wernicke's encephalopathy or intravenous antiviral therapy in herpes encephalitis can be associated with relatively rapid resolution of amnesia. With cerebrovascular insufficiency, one pattern that can be seen is that of transient global amnesia, in which memory impairment occurs in spells lasting minutes to hours. When this pattern is recognized and the underlying cerebrovascular disease is managed effectively, the spells can resolve, and stroke can be prevented.

With head trauma, amnesia can resolve gradually, over several years following injury. With any serious cerebral insult, however, persistent amnesia can be seen. There is some evidence that pathology of the cholinergic system may represent a final common pathway in these amnestic conditions (Siegfried 2000). Although this area has been little researched, there have been case reports of galantamine efficacy in Wernicke-Korsakoff syndrome, a persistent amnesia attributed to thiamine deficiency that is most commonly found in association with alcoholism (Phillips et al. 2004).

Delirium

The use of antipsychotic medication for symptomatic treatment of delirium is discussed in Chapter 3 of this volume, "Antipsychotics." The discussion here focuses on delirium as a cognitive disorder, as it is classified in DSM-IV-TR. Delirium is believed to be a hypocholinergic state, despite lack of direct evidence in cases other than anticholinergic toxicity. The only medication ever labeled for delirium treatment is physostigmine (Antilirium). With the availability of less toxic cholinesterase inhibitors (discussed earlier), a number of case reports have appeared reporting efficacy of these drugs in delirium of differing etiologies (Fischer 2001; Gleason 2003; Hori et al. 2003). Only one randomized, double-blind, placebo-controlled trial of a cholinesterase inhibitor (donepezil) in delirium has been reported (Liptzin et al. 2005). In that study, 80 patients received donepezil or placebo for 14 days before and 14 days after elective orthopedic surgery, and no difference was found between the donepezil-treated and placebo groups in frequency or duration of delirium (Liptzin et al. 2005). Of note in that study was an unusually low prevalence of delirium.

In the experience of the authors, when cholinesterase inhibitors are used for delirium, effects on confusion and memory impairment are generally modest, unlike the robust effects seen with antipsychotic medications in treating the psychotic symptoms of delirium. In addition, the effects are not as rapidly achieved as the effects of antipsychotics, often taking several days before any benefit is noted. The drugs are usually maintained at the initial dose (e.g., donepezil at 5 mg) unless the duration of delirium is very prolonged, as could be seen with stroke affecting the right parietal area.

Dementia Syndrome of Depression

In late life, the syndromes of dementia and depression can be interrelated in several ways: depression can represent a prodrome to dementia, occur in the context of an established dementia, or be associated with reversible cognitive impairment in the "dementia of depression" (Alexopoulos et al. 1993). In the latter case, depression is associated with a slowing of information processing, a fundamental impairment that influences all aspects of frontal/subcortical function (Butters et al. 2004). Effective treatment of depression in elderly patients does result in cognitive improvement, but many affected patients do not return to their premorbid cognitive baseline (Butters et al. 2000). Improvement is seen in domains such as initiation, perseveration, and conceptualization but not necessarily in memory or executive function (Butters et al. 2000). In a sizable subset of the elderly population with depression and cognitive impairment, it appears that the depression heralds the onset of a dementia. In fact, in about half of elderly patients who present with major depression and cognitive impairment, irreversible cognitive impairment is seen within 5 years (Alexopoulos et al. 1993; Copeland et al. 1992).

Cognitive impairment in executive systems appears to be associated with slow or poor antidepressant response (Kalayam and Alexopoulos 1999), residual depressive symptoms, and relapse and recurrence of major depression (Alexopoulos et al. 2000). The association of late-life depression with subcortical cerebrovascular disease is of note here, possibly providing an explanation for treatment resistance. Patients with vascular depression and vascular cognitive impairment merit aggressive antidepressant treatment, along with treatment for vascular dementia, as discussed below. By convention, treatment for vascular depression is started with selective serotonin reuptake inhibitor (SSRI) antidepressants, but clinical experience suggests that these patients often require adjunctive agents or treatment with dual-acting drugs such as venlafaxine or duloxetine. Treatment of vascular depression is discussed more fully in Chapter 4 of this volume, "Antidepressants."

Frontal Lobe and Frontotemporal Dementia

FTD is the third most common cause of cortical dementia, after AD and DLB (Neary et al. 1998). Consensus diagnostic criteria for FTD are shown in Table 9–7. The age at onset of FTD varies but is usually before 65 years of age (Mendez and Cummings 2003), so when these patients are encountered in the geriatric clinic, they may have been symptomatic for some time. Personality changes in the form of disinhibition and social inappropriateness are the hallmark of FTD, with frontotemporal atrophy seen by MRI or CT that corresponds to the severity of symptoms. Memory impairment may not manifest until late in the disease process.

There is no specific treatment for FTD. Certain symptoms, such as perseverative behaviors and disinhibition, may respond to treatment with SSRI antidepressants (Mendez and Cummings 2003). In some patients with hyperorality, anticonvulsants such as valproate or carbamazepine may be useful (Mendez and Cummings 2003). Although unstudied for this indication, memantine might prove useful by virtue of neuroprotective effects. There is anecdotal evidence that amantadine may be of benefit, but this is based on experience with traumatic brain injury to anterior brain regions, mostly in nongeriatric populations (Kraus and Maki 1997). Amantadine shares with memantine the mechanism of NMDA receptor antagonism, so could theoretically also have neuroprotective effects. There is currently no evidence that cholinesterase inhibitors are of any benefit in FTD.

Table 9–7. Consensus criteria for frontotemporal dementia

I. Core diagnostic features
  A. Insidious onset and gradual progression
  B. Early decline in social interpersonal conduct
  C. Early impairment in regulation of personal conduct
  D. Early emotional blunting
  E. Early loss of insight

II. Supportive diagnostic features
  A. Behavioral disorder
    1. Decline in personal hygiene and grooming
    2. Mental rigidity and inflexibility
    3. Distractibility and impersistence
    4. Hyperorality and dietary changes
    5. Perseverative and stereotyped behavior
    6. Utilization behavior
  B. Speech and language
    1. Altered speech output
       a. Aspontaneity and economy of speech
       b. Press of speech
    2. Stereotypy of speech
    3. Echolalia
    4. Perseveration
    5. Mutism
  C. Physical signs
    1. Primitive reflexes
    2. Incontinence
    3. Akinesia, rigidity, and tremor
    4. Low and labile blood pressure
  D. Investigations
    1. Neuropsychology: significant impairment on frontal lobe tests in the absence of severe amnesia, aphasia, or perceptuospatial disorder
    2. Electroencephalography: normal on conventional electroencephalogram despite clinically evident dementia
    3. Brain imaging (structural and/or functional): predominant frontal and/or anterior temporal abnormality

Source. Reprinted from Neary D, Snowden JS, Gustafson L, et al: "Frontotemporal Lobar Degeneration: A Consensus on Clinical Diagnostic Criteria." *Neurology* 51:1546–1554, 1998. Used with permission.

Dementia With Lewy Bodies

DLB is a progressive dementia that presents with cognitive symptoms and parkinsonism and has genetic relationships to both AD and PD (Saitoh and Katzman 1996). Psychiatric symptoms are prominent and include vivid visual hallucinations, delusions, and depression (Papka et al. 1998). Unusual features include dramatic fluctuation in symptoms, repeated falls, and frequent, transient episodes of loss of consciousness (McKeith et al. 1996).

Consensus criteria for the diagnosis of DLB are shown in Table 9–8. These criteria were validated in a prospective study of 50 cases that went to autopsy, and the consensus criteria for DLB performed as well as the NINCDS-ADRDA criteria for AD and the National Institute of Neurological Disorders and Stroke and Association Internationale pour la Recherché et l'Enseignement en Neurosciences (NINDS-AIREN) criteria for vascular dementia (McKeith et al. 2000a). In the validation study, it was noted that DLB can occur in the absence of extrapyramidal features and in the presence of comorbid vascular disease, and that fluctuation of symptoms is a particularly important diagnostic indicator (McKeith et al. 2000a).

Like AD, DLB is associated with markedly reduced levels of choline acetyltransferase, the enzyme that catalyzes synthesis of acetylcholine, particularly in the temporal and parietal cortices (Papka et al. 1998). These reductions may be quite severe for patients with visual hallucinations (Papka et al. 1998). Patients with DLB may benefit from cholinesterase inhibitors, in some cases with marked improvement in cognitive, behavioral, and functional realms (McKeith et al. 2000c; Samuel et al. 2000). Although most studies of these drugs in DLB have been faulted on methodological grounds (Simard and van Reekum 2004), there is at least one randomized controlled trial showing efficacy (McKeith et al. 2000b). In that study, treated patients exhibited less apathy and anxiety, had fewer delusions and hallucinations, and showed improved attention and faster performance on cognitive tasks (McKeith et al. 2000b).

Although not studied, memantine might prove useful in the treatment of DLB, since DLB is understood to be a neurodegenerative disease. Treatment of motor symptoms in DLB is discussed in Chapter 8 of this volume, "Treatment of Movement Disorders." It is worth reiterating

Table 9–8. Dementia with Lewy bodies: consensus criteria for clinical diagnosis

I.   Progressive cognitive decline of sufficient magnitude to interfere with normal social or occupational function.

II. Two of the following are essential for a *probable* diagnosis; one is consistent with a *possible* diagnosis:

    A. Fluctuating cognition

    B. Recurrent visual hallucinations

    C. Spontaneous parkinsonism

III. Features supportive of the diagnosis

    A. Repeated falls

    B. Syncope

    C. Transient losses of consciousness

    D. Neuroleptic sensitivity

    E. Systematized delusions

    F. Hallucinations in other modalities

IV. Diagnosis is less likely in the presence of

    A. Stroke confirmed by clinical focal findings and/or brain imaging

    B. Evidence of other physical illness or brain disorder that may account for the clinical findings

Source. Reprinted from McKeith IG, Galasko D, Kosaka K, et al: "Consensus Guidelines for the Clinical and Pathologic Diagnosis of Dementia With Lewy Bodies (DLB): Report of the Consortium on DLB International Workshop." *Neurology* 47:1113–1124, 1996. Used with permission.

that patients with DLB are exquisitely sensitive to extrapyramidal effects of neuroleptic medication, and conventional and atypical antipsychotics should be avoided in this population. This issue is discussed further in Chapter 3 of this volume. Future research on treatment of DLB will likely focus on the pathogenetic role of α-synuclein accumulation, a model analogous to that of β-amyloid accumulation in AD. Research is under way to develop gene transfer technology for genes that block α-synuclein accumulation (Hashimoto et al. 2004).

Mild Cognitive Impairment

MCI is characterized by a mild deficit in memory or other aspects of cognitive function in the absence of dementia. To date, most attention has focused on the amnestic form of MCI, but in fact not all patients have memory impairment. Some have impairment in a single domain other than memory, and others have mild impairment in multiple domains (Petersen et al. 2001). Criteria for the diagnosis of the amnestic form of MCI are as follows (Petersen et al. 2001):

- Memory complaint, preferably corroborated by an informant
- Impaired memory function for age and education
- Preserved general cognitive function
- Intact activities of daily living
- Not demented

Amnestic MCI is increasingly understood as a transitional state in many patients from the cognitive changes of normal aging to those of early AD (Petersen et al. 2005). Although the same agents useful in treating AD could theoretically also be useful for MCI, there is little evidence that this is the case. One randomized controlled trial of donepezil over 24 weeks did not find significant treatment effects (Salloway et al. 2004). Another randomized controlled trial over 3 years found no effect of vitamin E at 2,000 IU/day, and an effect of donepezil only during the first year, with reduced rates of progression to AD among treated patients (Petersen et al. 2005). Another randomized controlled trial showed no effect of *Ginkgo biloba* (van Dongen et al. 2000). In the future, it is likely that the focus of treatment efforts in MCI will turn to drugs that actually influence disease progression at cellular and molecular levels, such as the class of secretase inhibitors.

Parkinson's Disease With Dementia

A substantial minority of PD patients (40% or more) develops dementia (Hobson and Meara 1999; Mayeux et al. 1992). In general, dementia is more common in patients with early gait and balance difficulties than in those with tremor-dominant disease (Cummings 1995). The dementia of PD is characterized by attention deficit, executive system dysfunction, and secondary effects on memory (Emre 2004). There is some evidence that the dementia is associated with a cholinergic deficit (Levy et al. 1999), but use of cholinergic agents is complicated by the underlying dopaminergic deficit central to PD; in theory, increasing central cholinergic neurotransmission could shift the dopamine-to-acetylcholine ratio in favor of increased extrapyramidal symptoms. Nonetheless, numerous open-label studies; several small placebo-controlled trials; and one large, randomized controlled trial have found positive effects of cholinesterase inhibitors on cognition, neuropsychiatric symptoms, and global function in patients with PD-associated dementia (Aarsland et al. 2004; Emre 2004). As could be expected, dropout rates in these studies were high (>20%), mostly secondary to worsening motor symptoms (tremor) and cholinergic excess (nausea and vomiting).

As discussed above, memantine may have utility in the treatment of neurodegenerative disorders other than AD, and its use in PD is under study. The selective MAO B inhibitor selegiline, useful for its antioxidant as well as possible neuroprotective effects, has been used for a number of years in PD with dementia. Finally, it should be noted that conventional treatment for the motor symptoms of PD is often associated with perceived cognitive improvement, probably mediated by better performance on timed tasks.

Schizophrenia-Related Cognitive Dysfunction

Elderly patients with schizophrenia may present with a marked degree of cognitive impairment, a consequence of slow decline over the years that in many cases appears to accelerate in old age (Harvey 2001). A low level of education and increased age represent risk factors (Harvey et al. 1999). Domains of cognition affected in schizophrenia include serial learning, executive function, vigilance, and attentional ability/distractibility (Friedman et al. 1999). Drugs that may be useful in treatment of cognitive dysfunction in schizophrenia include atypical antipsychotics, α_2 adrenergic agonists, cholinesterase inhibitors, and possibly memantine. Atypical antipsychotics can be associated with improvement in prefrontal functions, such as working memory and executive function (Friedman et al. 1999). In addition, treatment of negative symptoms such as apathy could be expected to exert a positive effect on cognition. α_2 Adrenergic agonists, such as guanfacine and clonidine, can be associated with improvements in serial learning, working memory, and attention (Friedman et al. 1999); guanfacine may be preferred to clonidine for this indication (Friedman et al. 1999). In general, however, use of α_2 agonists is affected by problems with hypotension and rebound hypertension and angina on abrupt discontinuation in elderly patients. Cholinergic drugs can be associated with improvement in memory, language, and praxis (Friedman et al. 1999). Finally, because the mechanism underlying cognitive deterioration in schizophrenia could be glutamatergic, memantine may prove to be useful for this indication by virtue of its antiglutamatergic activity. This is an area of current National Institute of Mental Health–sponsored research.

Vascular Dementia

Diagnostic evaluation of the patient with suspected vascular dementia should include the following elements: a standardized, quantitative assessment of cognitive deficits; determination of risk factors for stroke; localization of cerebrovascular lesions (by history, examination, and neuroimaging); establishment of a temporal relationship between cognitive deficits and cerebrovascular lesions; exclusion of other etiologies of dementia; and establishment of the diagnosis of possible or probable vascular dementia using accepted criteria (Konno et al. 1997). NINDS-AIREN criteria for the diagnosis of vascular dementia are listed in Table 9–9.

Types of vascular dementia include the following (Konno et al. 1997):

- Multi-infarct dementia: multiple large infarctions, usually resulting from cardiac emboli or emboli from atherosclerotic plaques.
- Strategically placed infarct(s) in thalamus, frontal white matter, basal ganglia, or angular gyrus.
- Lacunar infarctions: multiple, cumulative, subcortical lesions usually associated with hypertension and/or diabetes; this is the most common type of vascular dementia.
- Binswanger's disease, hemorrhagic infarcts, familial syndromes, and combinations of disease patterns, including vascular dementia with AD.

Treatment of vascular dementia first involves the control of vascular risk factors to reduce the incidence of recurrent infarction. Well-documented risk factors for stroke include hypertension, smoking, diabetes, carotid stenosis, atrial fibrillation, and hyperlipidemia (Goldstein et al. 2001). Risk reduction is effected by control of hypertension, cessation of smoking, carotid angioplasty or endarterectomy, control of atrial fibrillation, and decrease of cholesterol levels through diet and exercise or lipid-lowering drugs (mainly HMG-CoA reductase inhibitors [statins]). As discussed in an earlier section, the evidence for statin use has recently been called into question (Rea et al. 2005; Suribhatla et al. 2005). Except for patients with recurrent hemorrhagic strokes, antithrombotic/antiplatelet agents such as aspirin or clopidogrel are also a mainstay of treatment for vascular dementia.

A meta-analysis of randomized controlled trials of antiplatelet therapies to prevent death, myocardial infarction, and stroke in patients at high risk for these events (including those with ischemic brain disease) showed that aspirin is effective at a dosage of 75–150 mg/day (Antithrombotic Trialists' Collaboration 2002). Several studies have shown clopidogrel to be more effective than aspirin in high-risk populations (Hirsh and Bhatt 2004), but the cost of clopidogrel is significantly greater than aspirin; so this medication often is reserved for patients intolerant of aspirin or for whom aspirin is ineffective. The combination of extended-release dipyridamole and aspirin (Aggrenox) is now prescribed less often, in part because of a nonsignificant reduction of risk found with this drug versus aspirin in the Aggrenox versus Aspirin Therapy Evaluation (AGATE) trial (Serebruany et al. 2004).

Studies of cholinesterase inhibitors in vascular dementia have generally been plagued by the application of AD methodologies to a heterogeneous group of patients whose diseases do not have the same course or the same neuropathologic progression as AD. The fundamental methodological problem is that patients with vascular dementia who are receiving appropriate antithrombotic and risk reduction therapies should not suffer disease progression over short (e.g., 6-month) study intervals, as would patients with AD. In addition, measures of cortical impairment designed for AD studies will not adequately capture deficits that characterize subcortical vascular cognitive impairment. In spite of these concerns, controlled and open-label studies have generally reported positive results with all

Table 9–9.   Vascular dementia: NINDS-AIREN criteria

I.   The criteria for the clinical diagnosis of *probable* vascular dementia include all of the following:

    A.   *Dementia* is defined by cognitive decline from a previously higher level of functioning and manifested by impairment of memory and of two or more cognitive domains (orientation, attention, language, visuospatial functions, executive functions, motor control, and praxis), preferably established by clinical examination and documented by neuropsychological testing; deficits should be severe enough to interfere with activities of daily living and not due to physical effects of stroke alone.

        1.   *Exclusion criteria:* cases with disturbance of consciousness, delirium, psychosis, severe aphasia, or major sensorimotor impairment precluding neuropsychological testing. Also excluded are systemic disorders or other brain diseases (such as Alzheimer's disease) that themselves could account for deficits in memory and cognition.

    B.   *Cerebrovascular disease* is defined by the presence of focal signs on neurological examination, such as hemiparesis, lower facial weakness, Babinski sign, sensory deficit, hemianopia, and dysarthria consistent with stroke (with or without history of stroke), and evidence of relevant CVD by brain imaging (CT or MRI), including multiple large-vessel infarcts or a single strategically placed infarct (angular gyrus, thalamus, basal forebrain, or PCA or ACA territories), as well as multiple basal ganglia and white matter lacunes or extensive periventricular white matter lesions, or combinations thereof.

    C.   A *relationship between the above two disorders* is manifested or inferred by the presence of one or more of the following: 1) onset of dementia within 3 months following a recognized stroke, 2) abrupt deterioration in cognitive functions or fluctuating, stepwise progression of cognitive deficits.

II.   Clinical features consistent with the diagnosis of *probable* vascular dementia include

    A.   Early presence of a gait disturbance (small-step gait or marche à petits pas, or magnetic, apraxic-ataxic or parkinsonian gait)

    B.   History of unsteadiness and frequent, unprovoked falls

Table 9–9.   Vascular dementia: NINDS-AIREN
criteria *(continued)*

    C. Early urinary frequency, urgency, and other urinary symptoms not explained by urologic disease

    D. Pseudobulbar palsy

    E. Personality and mood changes, abulia, depression, emotional incontinence, or other subcortical deficits, including psychomotor retardation and abnormal executive function

III. Features that make the diagnosis of vascular dementia uncertain or unlikely include

    A. Early onset of memory deficit and progressive worsening of memory and other cognitive functions such as language (transcortical sensory aphasia), motor skills (apraxia), and perception (agnosia), in the absence of corresponding focal lesions on brain imaging

    B. Absence of focal neurological signs, other than cognitive disturbance

    C. Absence of cerebrovascular lesions on brain CT or MRI

IV. Clinical diagnosis of possible vascular dementia may be made in the presence of dementia (section I-A) with focal neurological signs in patients in whom brain imaging studies to confirm definite CVD are missing; or in the absence of clear temporal relationship between dementia and stroke; or in patients with subtle onset and variable course (plateau or improvement) of cognitive deficits and evidence of relevant CVD.

V. Criteria for diagnosis of *definite* vascular dementia are

    A. Clinical criteria for probable vascular dementia

    B. Histopathologic evidence of CVD obtained from biopsy or autopsy

    C. Absence of neurofibrillary tangles and neuritic plaques exceeding those expected for age

    D. Absence of other clinical or pathological disorder capable of producing dementia

---

Note.   ACA = anterior cerebral artery; CT = computed tomography; CVD = cerebrovascular disease; MRI = magnetic resonance imaging; PCA = posterior cerebral artery.
Source.   Reprinted from Roman GC, Tatemichi TK, Erkinjuntti T, et al: "Vascular Dementia: Diagnostic Criteria for Research Studies. Report of the NINDS-AIREN International Workshop." *Neurology* 43:250–260, 1993. Used with permission.

three cholinesterase inhibitors in vascular dementia (Erkinjuntti et al. 2002; Moretti et al. 2003; Wilkinson et al. 2003). However, one study looked at vascular dementia, AD, and mixed dementia and found significant positive results only for the AD and mixed groups (Erkinjuntti et al. 2002). Another study had an unacceptably high dropout rate in the high-dose donepezil group (Wilkinson et al. 2003). A review of rivastigmine for vascular cognitive impairment that identified no randomized controlled trials to analyze nonetheless concluded that there was some evidence of benefit (Craig and Birks 2004).

It is in fact likely that some patients with vascular dementia do have significant cholinergic system dysfunction (Erkinjuntti et al. 2004; Roman 2005), whereas others do not (Perry et al. 2005), depending on brain regions affected. It would be helpful to have a means of determining the degree of cholinergic involvement in individual cases. The issue of drug efficacy is confounded by the fact that cholinergic stimulation generally increases cortical blood flow (Roman 2005) and could exert nonspecific effects.

As a relatively new drug to the market, memantine has been little studied in application to vascular dementia, but because of its more fundamental mechanism involving putative protection from neural degeneration through dampening of glutamatergic activity, it might be expected to have positive effects. One memantine-versus-placebo study conducted over 7 months in patients with mild to moderate vascular dementia found that memantine was associated with a small degree of cognitive improvement, whereas placebo was associated with cognitive decline, and that neither global function nor behavior deteriorated in the memantine-treated group (Orgogozo et al. 2002). (See discussion above for methodological difficulties in studying vascular dementia.)

Treatment of Selected Behavioral Disturbances in Dementia

Various neuropsychiatric syndromes associated with dementia may also be associated with behaviors that are disturbing to others or problematic for the affected individual. Certain syndromes—depression, anxiety, and psychosis—have already been discussed in earlier chapters. This section will focus on two areas of behavioral disturbance commonly seen in patients with dementia that do not fit neatly into the earlier chapters because their treatment crosses boundaries of pharmacologic class: agitation/aggression and sundowning. These disturbances may be seen in dementia of very diverse etiologies, and they are generally more prevalent in later disease stages.

Agitation and Aggression

Among patients with dementia, behaviors on the spectrum of agitation and aggression may be the most disruptive and potentially dangerous. Since *agitation* ranges broadly, from repetitive vocalization through non-aggressive physical behavior (e.g., pacing) to aggressive physical behavior, a critical first step in treating agitation or aggression in the patient with dementia is to list and describe target behaviors. For this purpose, a scale such as the Neuropsychiatric Inventory (NPI) can be used (Cummings et al. 1994).

Consensus Guidelines have been formulated for the management of agitation in dementia (Alexopoulos et al. 1998). The following discussion is based on those guidelines as well as the experience of the authors. For all types of agitation, reversible precipitants should be identified and corrected. Pain, nicotine withdrawal, covert medical or neurologic illness, and environments that are either overly demanding or understimulating are examples of precipitants indicating specific interventions. Careful attention should be paid to the pattern of behavioral disturbance, such as occurrence during shift changes or mealtimes, because stimulation may exacerbate agitation or elicit aggression. Environmental interventions should be used liberally. For example, bathing is often the precipitant for impulsive aggressive acts; environmental interventions (e.g., keeping the shower room and bathwater warm, avoiding water spray to the face) are strongly recommended for patients who resist bathing (Kovach and Meyer-Arnold 1997; Sloane et al. 1995). Environmental interventions are also often appropriate for pacing, which is sometimes managed simply by creating a hazard-free path, and for repetitive vocalization (Bourgeois et al. 1997).

A complete evaluation of the patient facilitates the subtyping of agitation into one of several categories, each with a specific algorithm for intervention:

- If the *patient is delirious:* the underlying medical cause should be treated; environmental interventions should be instituted (Inouye et al. 1999); antipsychotics should be used for symptomatic treatment only if needed, and only acutely. (See Chapter 3.)
- If the *patient is in pain:* the cause of the pain should be treated directly, if possible; both pharmacologic and nonpharmacologic treatments should be used. (See Chapter 10 of this volume, "Analgesic Medications.")
- If the *patient has akathisia* from use of an antipsychotic (including drugs such as metoclopramide or prochlorperazine): the antipsychotic dose should be lowered or the drug discontinued, if possible. If not possible, pharmacologic treatment for akathisia should be added. (See Chapter 8.)
- If the *patient is medically ill:* the illness should be treated; environmental interventions may also help reduce discomfort.
- If the *patient has signs or symptoms to suggest any of the following medication-responsive syndromes* (whether or not all DSM-IV-TR criteria are met), then syndrome-specific medications should be used:

  a. Antidepressants for depression (oppositional behavior, negativism, irritability, dysphoria, anxiety)
  b. Antipsychotics for psychosis (suspiciousness, paranoia, hallucinations, delusions)
  c. Atypical antipsychotics or mood stabilizers for mania or hypomania (pressured speech, overactivity, decreased sleep, extreme irritability, persistent agitation)

Safety concerns regarding the use of antipsychotic medications in elderly patients with dementia are discussed in Chapter 3. Use of any of the above medications in this population should be undertaken with caution.

When an algorithm such as the the one provided in the bulleted list is followed, many cases of agitation will be adequately treated. In a subset of patients, however, agitation will persist. Reconsideration of dementia etiology (e.g., AD versus FTD) at this point might guide a productive change in treatment of the hypothesized core neurotransmitter deficit. There is evidence that treatment of AD with cholinesterase inhibitors such as donepezil (Cummings et al. 2000; Weiner et al. 2000) and galantamine (Cummings et al. 2004) can be associated with reduced levels of agitation (pacing, attempting to leave) and aggression (threatening behavior). As noted in an earlier section, benefit applies more to prevention of behavioral disturbance than treatment of existing disturbance. Patients with FTD may be more likely to benefit from treatment with serotonergic medications (SSRIs) than cholinesterase inhibitors.

A number of medications have been recommended for nonspecific treatment of agitation and aggression in dementia. First-line treatment includes serotonergic antidepressants, which may be supplanting atypical antipsychotics in view of new concerns about cerebrovascular adverse effects and increased mortality associated with the latter drugs (discussed in Chapter 3). Other possible treatments include β-blockers, gabapentin, and selegiline. Estrogen was once considered for certain patients with dementia-associated agitation but is no longer recommended because of adverse effects, as discussed earlier in this chapter.

The SSRI antidepressant citalopram at dosages of 10–30 mg/day has been associated with improvement in irritability, hostility, anxiety, agitation, and disruptive vocalization in patients with dementia (Nyth and Gottfries 1990; Pollock et al. 1997). Citalopram's effect on disruptive vocalization deserves further study because this behavior is generally not responsive to pharmacologic intervention (Bourgeois et al. 1997). Fluoxetine, paroxetine, sertraline, and escitalopram are also commonly used for this indication. Although trazodone has been reported anecdotally to be effective in some patients at a standing dosage ranging from 12.5 mg two times a day to 100 mg three times a day (or used as needed), a randomized controlled trial of trazodone found no significant behavioral effect (Teri et al. 2000). In addition, as noted in Chapter 4, trazodone can be associated with significant orthostatic hypotension and falls and so should be used with caution in the elderly dementia population.

Other medications have been reported anecdotally to be effective for certain patients with dementia-associated agitation and aggression:

propranolol at dosages of 10–80 mg/day (Shankle et al. 1995), gabapentin at dosages of 300–2,400 mg/day, divided three times a day (Hawkins et al. 2000; Herrmann et al. 2000; Roane et al. 2000), and selegiline at 10 mg/day (Goad et al. 1991). Recommendations regarding the use of these agents await controlled study. Valproate has been found in several randomized controlled trials to be ineffective in controlling problematic behaviors in dementia (Lonergan and Luxenberg 2006).

Certain patients may still require treatment with atypical antipsychotics. Risperidone at a dosage of 1 mg/day has been shown effective for treating agitation and aggression in AD, vascular dementia, and mixed dementia (Bhana and Spencer 2000; Rabinowitz et al. 2004; Sink et al. 2005). The dosage of risperidone is critical: 1 mg/day is associated with a reduced rate of falls, but 2 mg/day is associated with an increased rate of falls (Katz et al. 2004). Olanzapine at a dosage of 5–10 mg/day has also been shown effective in treating agitation and aggression in AD patients (Sink et al. 2005; Street et al. 2000), although not without adverse effects, including somnolence and gait disturbance (Street et al. 2000). The risks of using antipsychotic medications are discussed in Chapter 3.

Sundowning

Sundowning refers to a specific pattern of agitation in which symptoms worsen acutely at a regular time each day, often in the evening hours (although it can occur at other times). Sundowning is associated with both delirium and dementia; in patients with dementia, the new onset of sundowning may signal the presence of a superimposed delirium. This pattern of agitation may be related to light exposure, sleep cycles, or the timing of medication use (Martin et al. 2000), among other factors.

Chronobiologic treatments that may be useful in treating sundowning include exogenous administration of the sleep-inducing hormone *melatonin* (Cohen-Mansfield et al. 2000), bright light therapy, and natural sun exposure during the morning hours. Decreased melatonin levels are found in a subset of elderly patients, possibly more often in those with AD (Liu et al. 1999).

Given the risks of using antipsychotic medications (discussed in Chapter 3), these agents should be reserved for patients with the most severe sundowning symptoms. In the past, atypical antipsychotics were the agents of choice in the treatment of sundowning, and it is not yet clear that other drugs will be effective for this indication. When an antipsychotic is used, it should be given on a standing rather than as-needed basis about 1–2 hours before the time of usual behavioral disturbance. For example, if agitation regularly occurs around 5:00 P.M., 0.5 mg of risperidone could be given orally at 3:00 P.M., and another 0.5 mg could be administered orally at bedtime. Alternatively, 25 mg of quetiapine could be given at 3:00 P.M. and at bedtime. Olanzapine and aripiprazole may also be effective when used on this split-dose schedule.

Chapter Summary

- At present, cholinesterase inhibitors constitute the mainstay of treatment for Alzheimer's disease (AD).
- Since memantine's putative mechanism involves a process basic to neurodegeneration in general, it may prove useful at earlier stages of AD as well as for a range of other dementing diseases.
- β- and γ-secretase inhibitors may offer an important new clinical strategy for AD treatment and prevention in the near future.
- Memantine is a drug in a new class of antidementia treatment, and evidence to date suggests that it is associated with modest beneficial effects on cognitive function, functional decline, and behavior in moderate to severe AD.
- Patients with dementia with Lewy bodies (DLB) may benefit from cholinesterase inhibitors, in some cases with marked improvement in cognitive, behavioral, and functional realms.
- Conventional and atypical antipsychotics should be avoided in patients with DLB.
- Treatment of vascular dementia first involves the control of vascular risk factors to reduce the incidence of recurrent infarction.
- Except for patients with recurrent hemorrhagic strokes, antithrombotic/antiplatelet agents such as aspirin (75–150 mg/day) or clopidogrel are a mainstay of treatment for vascular dementia.
- Wherever possible, specific causes of agitation and aggression in patients with dementia should be identified and treated.
- For nonspecific treatment of agitation and aggression, first-line pharmacologic treatment includes serotonergic antidepressants, which may be supplanting atypical antipsychotics because of safety concerns with the latter drugs.

588   Clinical Manual of Geriatric Psychopharmacology

References

Aarsland D, Mosimann UP, McKeith IG: Role of cholinesterase inhibitors in Parkinson's disease and dementia with Lewy bodies. J Geriatr Psychiatry Neurol 17:164–171, 2004

Aisen PS, Davis KL: Anti-inflammatory therapy for Alzheimer's disease: a status report. International Journal of Geriatric Psychopharmacology 1:2–5, 1997

Aisen PS, Schafer KA, Grundman M, et al: Effects of rofecoxib or naproxen vs placebo on Alzheimer disease progression: a randomized, controlled trial. JAMA 289:2819–2826, 2003

Alexopoulos GS, Meyers BS, Young RC, et al: The course of geriatric depression with "reversible dementia": a controlled study. Am J Psychiatry 150:1693–1699, 1993

Alexopoulos GS, Silver JM, Kahn DA, et al: The expert consensus guideline series: treatment of agitation in older persons with dementia. Postgrad Med (Special No):1–88, 1998

Alexopoulos GS, Meyers BS, Young RC, et al: Executive dysfunction and long-term outcomes of geriatric depression. Arch Gen Psychiatry 57:285–290, 2000

Antithrombotic Trialists' Collaboration: Collaborative meta-analysis of randomised trials of antiplatelet therapy for prevention of death, myocardial infarction, and stroke in high risk patients. BMJ 324:71–86, 2002

Assal F, Alarcon M, Solomon EC, et al: Association of the serotonin transporter and receptor gene polymorphisms in neuropsychiatric symptoms in Alzheimer disease. Arch Neurol 61:1249–1253, 2004

Bhana N, Spencer CM: Risperidone: a review of its use in the management of the behavioural and psychological symptoms of dementia. Drugs Aging 16:451–471, 2000

Birks J, Grimley Evans J: Ginkgo biloba for cognitive impairment and dementia. The Cochrane Database of Systematic Reviews, Issue 4, Article No: CD003120. DOI: 003110.001002/14651858.CD14003120, 2002

Birks J, Flicker L: Selegiline for Alzheimer's disease. The Cochrane Database of Systematic Reviews, Issue 1, Article No: CD000442. DOI: 10.1002/14651858.CD000442, 2003

Bourgeois MS, Burgio LD, Schulz R, et al: Modifying repetitive verbalizations of community-dwelling patients with AD. Gerontologist 37:30–39, 1997

Butters MA, Becker JT, Nebes RD, et al: Changes in cognitive functioning following treatment of late-life depression. Am J Psychiatry 157:1949–1954, 2000

Butters MA, Whyte EM, Nebes RD, et al: The nature and determinants of neuropsychological functioning in late-life depression. Arch Gen Psychiatry 61:587–595, 2004

Chui HC, Victoroff JI, Margolin D, et al: Criteria for the diagnosis of ischemic vascular dementia proposed by the State of California Alzheimer's Disease Diagnostic and Treatment Centers. Neurology 42:473–480, 1992

Cohen-Mansfield J, Garfinkel D, Lipson S: Melatonin for treatment of sundowning in elderly persons with dementia—a preliminary study. Arch Gerontol Geriatr 31:65–76, 2000

Copeland JR, Davidson IA, Dewey ME, et al: Alzheimer's disease, other dementias, depression and pseudodementia: prevalence, incidence and three-year outcome in Liverpool. Br J Psychiatry 161:230–239, 1992

Cozza KL, Armstrong SC, Oesterheld JR: Concise Guide to Drug Interaction Principles for Medical Practice, 2nd Edition. Washington, DC, American Psychiatric Publishing, 2003

Craig D, Birks J: Rivastigmine for vascular cognitive impairment. Cochrane Database of Systematic Reviews, Issue 2, Article No: CD004744. DOI: 10.1002/14651858.CD004744, 2004

Cummings JL: Dementia: the failing brain. Lancet 345:1481–1484, 1995

Cummings JL, Benson DF: Dementia: A Clinical Approach, 2nd Edition. Boston, MA, Butterworth-Heinemann, 1992

Cummings JL, Mega MS, Gray K, et al: The Neuropsychiatric Inventory: comprehensive assessment of psychopathology in dementia. Neurology 44:2308–2314, 1994

Cummings JL, Donohue JA, Brooks RL: The relationship between donepezil and behavioral disturbances in patients with Alzheimer's disease. Am J Geriatr Psychiatry 8:134–140, 2000

Cummings JL, Schneider L, Tariot PN, et al: Reduction of behavioral disturbances and caregiver distress by galantamine in patients with Alzheimer's disease. Am J Psychiatry 161:532–538, 2004

Doraiswamy PM, Krishnan KRR, Anand R, et al: Long-term effects of rivastigmine in moderately severe Alzheimer's disease: does early initiation of therapy offer sustained benefits? Prog Neuropsychopharmacol Biol Psychiatry 26:705–712, 2002

Emre M: Dementia in Parkinson's disease: cause and treatment. Curr Opin Neurol 17:399–404, 2004

Erkinjuntti T, Kurz A, Gauthier S, et al: Efficacy of galantamine in probable vascular dementia and Alzheimer's disease combined with cerebrovascular disease: a randomised trial. Lancet 359:1283–1290, 2002

Erkinjuntti T, Roman G, Gauthier S: Treatment of vascular dementia—evidence from clinical trials with cholinesterase inhibitors. J Neurol Sci 226:63–66, 2004

Espeland MA, Rapp SR, Shumaker SA, et al: Conjugated equine estrogens and global cognitive function in postmenopausal women: Women's Health Initiative Memory Study. JAMA 291:2959–2968, 2004

Feldman H, Gauthier S, Hecker J, et al: A 24-week, randomized, double-blind study of donepezil in moderate to severe Alzheimer's disease. Neurology 57:613–620, 2001

Fischer P: Successful treatment of nonanticholinergic delirium with a cholinesterase inhibitor (letter). J Clin Psychopharmacol 21:118, 2001

Flint AJ, Van Reekum R: The pharmacologic treatment of Alzheimer's disease: a guide for the general psychiatrist. Can J Psychiatry 43:689–697, 1998

Folstein MF, Folstein SE, McHugh PR: "Mini-mental state": a practical method for grading the cognitive state of patients for the clinician. J Psychiatr Res 12:189–198, 1975

Friedman JI, Temporini H, Davis KL: Pharmacologic strategies for augmenting cognitive performance in schizophrenia. Biol Psychiatry 45:1–16, 1999

Gleason OC: Donepezil for postoperative delirium. Psychosomatics 44:437–438, 2003

Goad DL, Davis CM, Liem P, et al: The use of selegiline in Alzheimer's patients with behavior problems. J Clin Psychiatry 52:342–345, 1991

Goldstein LB, Adams R, Becker K, et al: Primary prevention of ischemic stroke: a statement for healthcare professionals from the Stroke Council of the American Heart Association. Circulation 103:163–182, 2001

Hanlon JT, Schmader KE, Landerman LR, et al: Relation of prescription nonsteroidal antiinflammatory drug use to cognitive function among community-dwelling elderly. Ann Epidemiol 7:87–94, 1997

Harvey PD: Cognitive and functional impairments in elderly patients with schizophrenia: a review of the recent literature. Harv Rev Psychiatry 9:59–68, 2001

Harvey PD, Silver JM, Mohs RC, et al: Cognitive decline in late-life schizophrenia: a longitudinal study of geriatric chronically hospitalized patients. Biol Psychiatry 45:32–40, 1999

Hashimoto M, Rockenstein E, Mante M, et al: An antiaggregation gene therapy strategy for Lewy body disease utilizing beta-synuclein lentivirus in a transgenic model. Gene Ther 11:1713–1723, 2004

Hawkins JW, Tinklenberg JR, Sheikh JI, et al: A retrospective chart review of gabapentin for the treatment of aggressive and agitated behavior in patients with dementias. Am J Geriatr Psychiatry 8:221–225, 2000

Herrmann N, Lanctot K, Myszak M: Effectiveness of gabapentin for the treatment of behavioral disorders in dementia. J Clin Psychopharmacol 20:90–93, 2000

Hirsh J, Bhatt DL: Comparative benefits of clopidogrel and aspirin in high-risk patient populations: lessons from the CAPRIE and CURE studies. Arch Intern Med 164:2106–2110, 2004

Hobson P, Meara J: The detection of dementia and cognitive impairment in a community population of elderly people with Parkinson's disease by use of the CAMCOG neuropsychological test. Age Ageing 28:39–43, 1999

Hori K, Tominaga I, Inada T, et al: Donepezil-responsive alcohol-related prolonged delirium. Psychiatry Clin Neurosci 57:603–604, 2003

Inouye SK, Bogardus ST, Charpentier PA, et al: A multicomponent intervention to prevent delirium in hospitalized older patients. N Engl J Med 340:669–676, 1999

in t' Veld BA, Ruitenberg A, Hofman A, et al: Nonsteroidal antiinflammatory drugs and the risk of Alzheimer's disease. N Engl J Med 345:1515–1521, 2001

Kalayam B, Alexopoulos GS: Prefrontal dysfunction and treatment response in geriatric depression. Arch Gen Psychiatry 56:713–718, 1999

Katz IR, Rupnow M, Kozma C, et al: Risperidone and falls in ambulatory nursing home residents with dementia and psychosis or agitation: secondary analysis of a double-blind, placebo-controlled trial. Am J Geriatr Psychiatry 12:499–508, 2004

Kim KY, Ke V, Adkins LM: Donepezil for alcohol-related dementia: a case report. Pharmacotherapy 24:419–421, 2004

Konno S, Meyer JS, Terayama Y, et al: Classification, diagnosis and treatment of vascular dementia. Drugs Aging 11:361–373, 1997

Kovach CR, Meyer-Arnold EA: Preventing agitated behaviors during bath time. Geriatr Nurs 18:112–114, 1997

Kraus MF, Maki PM: Effect of amantadine hydrochloride on symptoms of frontal lobe dysfunction in brain injury: case studies and review. J Neuropsychiatry Clin Neurosci 9:222–230, 1997

Krishnan KR, Charles HC, Doraiswamy PM, et al: Randomized, placebo-controlled trial of the effects of donepezil on neuronal markers and hippocampal volumes in Alzheimer's disease. Am J Psychiatry 160:2003–2011, 2003

Kurz A, Farlow M, Quarg P, et al: Disease stage in Alzheimer disease and treatment effects of rivastigmine. Alzheimer Dis Assoc Disord 18:123–128, 2004

Levy ML, Cummings JL, Kahn-Rose R: Neuropsychiatric symptoms and cholinergic therapy for Alzheimer's disease. Gerontology 45 (suppl 1):15–22, 1999

Li G, Higdon R, Kukull WA, et al: Statin therapy and risk of dementia in the elderly. Neurology 63:1624–1628, 2004

Liptzin B, Laki A, Garb JL, et al: Donepezil in the prevention and treatment of post-surgical delirium. Am J Geriatr Psychiatry 13:1100–1106, 2005

Liu RY, Zhou JN, van Heerikhuize J, et al: Decreased melatonin levels in post-mortem cerebrospinal fluid in relation to aging, Alzheimer's disease, and apo-lipoprotein E-epsilon 4/4 genotype. J Clin Endocrinol Metab 84:323–327, 1999

Lonergan ET, Luxenberg J: Valproate preparations for agitation in dementia. The Cochrane Database of Systematic Reviews, Issue 2, Article No: CD003945. DOI: 003910.001002/14651858.CD14003945.pub14651852, 2006

Lonn E, Bosch J, Yusuf S, et al: Effects of long-term vitamin E supplementation on cardiovascular events and cancer: a randomized controlled trial. JAMA 293:1338–1347, 2005

Lund and Manchester Groups: Clinical and neuropathological criteria for fron-totemporal dementia. J Neurol Neurosurg Psychiatry 57:416–418, 1994

Maiorini AF, Gaunt MJ, Jacobsen TM, et al: Potential novel targets for Alzheimer pharmacotherapy, I: secretases. J Clin Pharm Ther 27:169–183, 2002

Martin J, Marler M, Shochat T, et al: Circadian rhythms of agitation in institu-tionalized patients with Alzheimer's disease. Chronobiol Int 17:405–418, 2000

Mayeux R, Denaro J, Hemenegildo N, et al: A population-based investigation of Parkinson's disease with and without dementia. Relationship to age and gen-der. Arch Neurol 49:492–497, 1992

Mayeux R, Saunders AM, Shea S, et al: Utility of the apolipoprotein E genotype in the diagnosis of Alzheimer's disease. N Engl J Med 338:506–511, 1998

McKeith IG, Galasko D, Kosaka K, et al: Consensus guidelines for the clinical and pathologic diagnosis of dementia with Lewy bodies (DLB): report of the Consortium on DLB International Workshop. Neurology 47:1113–1124, 1996

McKeith IG, Ballard CG, Perry RH, et al: Prospective validation of consensus criteria for the diagnosis of dementia with Lewy bodies. Neurology 54:1050–1058, 2000a

McKeith IG, Del Ser T, Spano PF, et al: Efficacy of rivastigmine in dementia with Lewy bodies: a randomised, double-blind, placebo-controlled international study. Lancet 356:2031–2036, 2000b

McKeith IG, Grace JB, Walker Z, et al: Rivastigmine in the treatment of dementia with Lewy bodies: preliminary findings from an open trial. Int J Geriatr Psychiatry 15:387–392, 2000c

McKhann G, Drachman D, Folstein M, et al: Clinical diagnosis of Alzheimer's disease: report of the NINCDS-ADRDA Work Group under the auspices of Department of Health and Human Services Task Force on Alzheimer's Disease. Neurology 34:939–944, 1984

McShane R, Areosa Sastre A, Minakaran N: Memantine for dementia. The Cochrane Database of Systematic Reviews, Issue 2, Article No: CD003154. DOI: 10.1002/14651858.CD003154, 2006

Mendez MF, Cummings JL: Dementia: A Clinical Approach, 3rd Edition. Philadelphia, PA, Butterworth-Heinemann, 2003

Miller ER, Pastor-Barriuso R, Dalal D, et al: Meta-analysis: high-dosage vitamin E supplementation may increase all-cause mortality. Ann Intern Med 142:37–46, 2005

Miller LG, Freeman B: Possible subdural hematoma associated with Ginkgo biloba. J Herb Pharmacother 2:57–63, 2002

Minett TSC, Thomas A, Wilkinson LM, et al: What happens when donepezil is suddenly withdrawn? an open label trial in dementia with Lewy bodies and Parkinson's disease with dementia. Int J Geriatr Psychiatry 18:988–993, 2003

Moretti R, Torre P, Antonello RM, et al: Rivastigmine in subcortical vascular dementia: a randomized, controlled, open 12-month study in 208 patients. Am J Alzheimers Dis Other Demen 18:265–272, 2003

Morihara T, Teter B, Yang F, et al: Ibuprofen suppresses interleukin-1β induction of pro-amyloidogenic α1-antichymotrypsin to ameliorate β-amyloid (Aβ) pathology in Alzheimer's models. Neuropsychopharmacology 30:1111–1120, 2005

Neary D, Snowden JS, Gustafson L, et al: Frontotemporal lobar degeneration: a consensus on clinical diagnostic criteria. Neurology 51:1546–1554, 1998

Nicoll JA, Wilkinson D, Holmes C, et al: Neuropathology of human Alzheimer disease after immunization with amyloid-beta peptide: a case report. Nat Med 9:448–452, 2003

Nyth AL, Gottfries CG: The clinical efficacy of citalopram in treatment of emotional disturbances in dementia disorders. Br J Psychiatry 157:894–901, 1990

Orgogozo JM, Rigaud AS, Stoffler A, et al: Efficacy and safety of memantine in patients with mild to moderate vascular dementia. Stroke 33:1834–1839, 2002

Oslin D, Atkinson RM, Smith DM, et al: Alcohol-related dementia: proposed clinical criteria. Int J Geriatr Psychiatry 13:203–212, 1998

Papka M, Rubio A, Schiffer RB: A review of Lewy body disease, an emerging concept of cortical dementia. J Neuropsychiatry Clin Neurosci 10:267–279, 1998

Perry EK, Ziabreva I, Perry R, et al: Absence of cholinergic deficits in "pure" vascular dementia. Neurology 64:132–133, 2005

Petersen RC, Doody R, Kurz A, et al: Current concepts in mild cognitive impairment. Arch Neurol 58:1985–1992, 2001

Petersen RC, Thomas RG, Grundman M, et al: Vitamin E and donepezil for the treatment of mild cognitive impairment. N Engl J Med 352:2379–2388, 2005

Phillips BK, Ingram MV, Grammer GG: Wernicke-Korsakoff syndrome and galantamine. Psychosomatics 45:366–368, 2004

Pollock BG, Mulsant BH, Sweet R, et al: An open pilot study of citalopram for behavioral disturbances of dementia: plasma levels and real-time observations. Am J Geriatr Psychiatry 5:70–78, 1997

Rabinowitz J, Katz IR, De Deyn PP, et al: Behavioral and psychological symptoms in patients with dementia as a target for pharmacotherapy with risperidone. J Clin Psychiatry 65:1329–1334, 2004

Raskind MA, Peskind ER, Wessel T, et al: Galantamine in AD: a 6-month randomized, placebo-controlled trial with a 6-month extension. Neurology 54:2261–2268, 2000

Rea TD, Breitner JC, Psaty BM, et al: Statin use and the risk of incident dementia: the Cardiovascular Health Study. Arch Neurol 62:1047–1051, 2005

Reisberg B, Doody R, Stoffler A, et al: Memantine in moderate-to-severe Alzheimer's disease. N Engl J Med 348:1333–1341, 2003

Roane DM, Feinberg TE, Meckler L, et al: Treatment of dementia-associated agitation with gabapentin. J Neuropsychiatry Clin Neurosci 12:40–43, 2000

Rogers SL, Farlow MR, Doody RS, et al: A 24-week, double-blind, placebo-controlled trial of donepezil in patients with Alzheimer's disease. Neurology 50:136–145, 1998

Roman GC: Cholinergic dysfunction in vascular dementia. Curr Psychiatry Rep 7:18–26, 2005

Roman GC, Tatemichi TK, Erkinjuntti T, et al: Vascular dementia: diagnostic criteria for research studies. Report of the NINDS-AIREN International Workshop. Neurology 43:250–260, 1993

Rosenblatt M, Mindel J: Spontaneous hyphema associated with ingestion of Ginkgo biloba extract (letter). N Engl J Med 336:1108, 1997

Rosler M, Anand R, Cicin-Sain A, et al: Efficacy and safety of rivastigmine in patients with Alzheimer's disease: international randomised controlled trial. BMJ 318:633–640, 1999

Rowin J, Lewis SL: Spontaneous bilateral subdural hematomas associated with chronic Ginkgo biloba ingestion. Neurology 46:1775–1776, 1996

Saitoh T, Katzman R: Genetic correlations in Lewy body disease, in Dementia With Lewy Bodies. Edited by Perry R, McKeith I, Perry E. Cambridge, UK, Cambridge University Press, 1996, pp 336–349

Salloway S, Ferris S, Kluger A, et al: Efficacy of donepezil in mild cognitive impairment: a randomized, placebo-controlled trial. Neurology 63:651–657, 2004

Samuel W, Caligiuri M, Galasko D, et al: Better cognitive and psychopathologic response to donepezil in patients prospectively diagnosed as dementia with Lewy bodies: a preliminary study. Int J Geriatr Psychiatry 15:794–802, 2000

Sano M, Ernesto C, Thomas RG, et al: A controlled trial of selegiline, alpha-tocopherol, or both as treatment for Alzheimer's disease. N Engl J Med 336:1216–1222, 1997

Serebruany VL, Malinin AI, Sane DC, et al: Magnitude and time course of platelet inhibition with Aggrenox and aspirin in patients after ischemic stroke: the Aggrenox versus Aspirin Therapy Evaluation (AGATE) trial. Eur J Pharm 499:315–324, 2004

Shankle WR, Nielson KA, Cotman CW: Low-dose propranolol reduces aggression and agitation resembling that associated with orbitofrontal dysfunction in elderly demented patients. Alzheimer Dis Assoc Disord 9:233–237, 1995

Shumaker SA, Legault C, Kuller L, et al: Conjugated equine estrogens and incidence of probable dementia and mild cognitive impairment in postmenopausal women. JAMA 291:2947–2958, 2004

Siegfried KR: Cholinergic approaches to cognition and dementia, in Pharmacotherapy for Mood, Anxiety, and Cognitive Disorders. Edited by Halbreich U, Montgomery SA. Washington, DC, American Psychiatric Press, 2000, pp 519–533

Simard M, van Reekum R: The acetylcholinesterase inhibitors for treatment of cognitive and behavioral symptoms in dementia with Lewy bodies. J Neuropsychiatry Clin Neurosci 16:409–425, 2004

Sink KM, Holden KF, Yaffe K: Pharmacological treatment of neuropsychiatric symptoms of dementia. JAMA 293:596–608, 2005

Sloane PD, Rader J, Barrick AL, et al: Bathing persons with dementia. Gerontologist 35:672–678, 1995

Small GW, Rabins PV, Barry PP, et al: Diagnosis and treatment of Alzheimer disease and related disorders. JAMA 278:1363–1371, 1997

Street JS, Clark WS, Gannon KS, et al: Olanzapine treatment of psychotic and behavioral symptoms in patients with Alzheimer disease in nursing care facilities: a double-blind, randomized, placebo-controlled trial. Arch Gen Psychiatry 57:968–976, 2000

Sultzer DL, Mahler ME, Mandelkern MA, et al: The relationship between psychiatric symptoms and regional cortical metabolism in Alzheimer's disease. J Neuropsychiatry Clin Neurosci 7:476–484, 1995

Suribhatla S, Dennis MS, Potter JF: A study of statin use in the prevention of cognitive impairment of vascular origin in the UK. J Neurol Sci 229–230:147–150, 2005

Tariot PN, Solomon PR, Morris JC, et al: A 5-month, randomized, placebo-controlled trial of galantamine in AD. The Galantamine USA-10 Study Group. Neurology 54:2269–2276, 2000

Tariot PN, Farlow MR, Grossberg GT, et al: Memantine treatment in patients with moderate to severe Alzheimer disease already receiving donepezil. JAMA 291:317–324, 2004

Teri L, Logsdon RG, Peskind E, et al: Treatment of agitation in AD: a randomized, placebo-controlled trial. Neurology 55:1271–1278, 2000

van Dongen MC, van Rossum E, Kessels AG, et al: The efficacy of ginkgo for elderly people with dementia and age-associated memory impairment: new results of a randomized clinical trial. J Am Geriatr Soc 48:1183–1194, 2000

van Dyck CH, Newhouse P, Falk WE, et al: Extended-release physostigmine in Alzheimer disease: a multicenter, double-blind, 12-week study with dose enrichment. Arch Gen Psychiatry 57:157–164, 2000

Weiner MF, Martin-Cook K, Foster BM, et al: Effects of donepezil on emotional/behavioral symptoms in Alzheimer's disease patients. J Clin Psychiatry 61:487–492, 2000

Wilcock GK, Lilienfeld S, Gaens E: Efficacy and safety of galantamine in patients with mild to moderate Alzheimer's disease: multicentre randomised controlled trial. BMJ 321:1445–1449, 2000

Wilkinson D, Doody R, Helme R, et al: Donepezil in vascular dementia: a randomized, placebo-controlled study. Neurology 61:479–486, 2003

Yaffe K, Krueger K, Cummings SR, et al: Effect of raloxifene on prevention of dementia and cognitive impairment in older women: the Multiple Outcomes of Raloxifene Evaluation (MORE) randomized trial. Am J Psychiatry 162:683–690, 2005

Zandi PP, Sparks L, Khachaturian AS, et al: Do statins reduce risk of incident dementia and Alzheimer's disease? Arch Gen Psychiatry 62:217–224, 2005

Zhou Y, Su Y, Li B, et al: Nonsteroidal anti-inflammatory drugs can lower amyloidogenic Aβ42 by inhibiting Rho. Science 302:1215–1217, 2003

Generic name	clopidogrel
Trade name	Plavix
Class	Antiplatelet agent
Half-life	7–8 hours
Mechanism of action	Blocks adenosine diphosphate receptor and prevents binding of fibrinogen, which reduces platelet adhesion/aggregation
Available preparations	Tablet: 75 mg
Starting dose	75 mg/day
Titration	None
Typical daily dose	75 mg
Dose range	N/A
Therapeutic serum level	Not established

Comments: Second-line antiplatelet agent for patients intolerant of aspirin because of GI bleeding/distress or who have evidence of continued ischemic events despite aspirin therapy. Slightly more effective than aspirin. Well absorbed; metabolized in the liver to an active metabolite. Minor substrate of CYP1A2 and 3A4; weakly inhibits CYP2C8/9. *Drug interactions:* Additive effects with other antiplatelet and anticoagulant drugs, increased risk of GI bleeding with NSAIDs, attenuated clopidogrel effects with atorvastatin and macrolide antibiotics, increased effects of clopidogrel with rifampin. *Common adverse effects (>10%):* Abdominal pain, vomiting, dyspepsia, gastritis, and constipation. *Less common adverse effects (1%–10%):* Chest pain, hypertension, edema, headache, dizziness, arthralgia, back pain, and flu-like syndrome. *Uncommon but serious adverse effects:* Agranulocytosis and other blood dyscrasias, bronchospasm, hepatitis, abnormal liver function test values, and intracranial hemorrhage.

599

Generic name	donepezil
Trade name	Aricept
Class	Central acetylcholinesterase inhibitor
Half-life	70 hours
Mechanism of action	Reversibly and noncompetitively inhibits acetylcholinesterase, which breaks down acetylcholine
Available preparations	Tablets: 5, 10 mg Orally disintegrating tablets: 5, 10 mg
Starting dose	5 mg/day po
Titration	Increase to 10 mg/day po after 4–6 weeks as tolerated
Typical daily dose	10 mg po
Dose range	5–10 mg/day po
Therapeutic serum level	Not established

Comments: A first-line drug for cognition and prevention of behavioral disturbance in AD and in DLB. Well absorbed orally. Time to peak plasma concentration is 3–4 hours. Extensively protein bound. Metabolized in liver via glucuronidation; minor substrate of CYP2D6 and CYP3A4. Eliminated mainly in urine. Use with caution in patients with sick sinus syndrome or other supraventricular conduction problems, peptic ulcer disease, bladder outflow obstruction, seizures, or chronic obstructive pulmonary disease or asthma. *Drug interactions:* Synergistic effects with other cholinergic agents, antagonistic effects with anticholinergic drugs, potential for increased extrapyramidal symptoms with antipsychotics. *Common adverse effects (>10%):* Insomnia, nausea, and diarrhea. *Less common adverse effects (1%–10%):* Syncope, hypotension, hypertension, dizziness, fatigue, headache, anorexia, vomiting, and muscle cramps. In certain AD patients at some stages of disease, may be associated with worsening of agitation, which is often transient.

Generic name	galantamine
Trade name	Razadyne, Razadyne ER (trade name changed from Reminyl)
Class	Central acetylcholinesterase inhibitor
Half-life	7 hours
Mechanism of action	Reversible, competitive cholinesterase inhibitor (decreases acetylcholine breakdown) and nicotinic receptor modulator (increases acetylcholine release)
Available preparations	Extended-release (ER) capsules: 8, 16, 24 mg Immediate-release (IR) tablets: 4, 8, 12 mg Oral solution (IR): 4 mg/mL
Starting dose	IR: 4 mg bid with meals ER: 8 mg/day with meal
Titration	IR: increase after 4 weeks to 8 mg bid; if tolerated, increase again after 4 weeks to 12 mg bid. ER: increase after 4 weeks to 16 mg/day; if tolerated, increase again after 4 weeks to 24 mg/day
Typical daily dose	IR: 8 mg bid with meals ER: 16 mg/day with meal
Dose range	IR: 16–24 mg/day in two divided doses ER: 16–24 mg/day
Therapeutic serum level	Not established

Comments: A first-line drug for cognition and prevention of behavioral disturbance in AD and in DLB. Rapidly and completely absorbed, with bioavailability over 80%. Linear pharmacokinetics. 18% protein bound. Dose in patients with moderate renal or hepatic dysfunction should be ≤16 mg/day; use is not recommended in severe renal or hepatic disease. Several metabolic pathways, including oxidation (minor substrate of CYP2D6 and 3A4), demethylation, and glucuronidation. Use with caution in patients with sick sinus syndrome or other supraventricular conduction problems, peptic ulcer disease, bladder outflow obstruction, seizures, or chronic obstructive pulmonary disease or asthma. *Drug interactions:* Synergistic effects with other cholinergic agents; antagonistic effects with anticholinergic drugs; potential for increased extrapyramidal symptoms with antipsychotics; bradycardia with amiodarone, β-blockers, diltiazem, and verapamil; atrioventricular block with digoxin; GI bleeding with NSAIDs; enhanced neuromuscular blockade with succinylcholine. *Common adverse effects (>10%):* Nausea, vomiting, and diarrhea. *Less common adverse effects (1%–10%):* Bradycardia, syncope, chest pain, dizziness, headache, depression, anorexia, and weight loss.

Generic name	memantine
Trade name	Namenda
Class	NMDA receptor antagonist
Half-life	60–80 hours
Mechanism of action	Blocks excessive stimulation of the NMDA receptor by glutamate
Available preparations	Tablets: 5, 10 mg Oral solution: 2 mg/mL
Starting dose	5 mg at bedtime
Titration	Increase by 5 mg at weekly intervals, as tolerated: Week 2: 5 mg morning/5 mg bedtime Week 3: 5 mg morning/10 mg bedtime Week 4: 10 mg morning/10 mg bedtime
Typical daily dose	10 mg bid
Dose range	5–10 mg bid
Therapeutic serum level	Not established

Comments: First NMDA receptor antagonist to be labeled for treatment of dementia, approved first for moderate to severe AD. May prove useful in early AD and for a range of other diseases. Well absorbed orally; taken without regard to meals. 45% protein bound. Peak plasma concentrations in 3–7 hours. Three metabolites with minimal NMDA-blocking activity. Insignificant CYP450 metabolism. Eliminated in urine; 57%–82% of drug excreted unchanged. Dose reduction recommended in moderate renal impairment; use not recommended in severe renal impairment. No pharmacokinetic data with hepatic impairment, but clearance expected to be little affected. Potential interactions with other drugs secreted by renal tubular cationic transport, including cimetidine, ranitidine, hydrochlorothiazide, nicotine, quinidine, and triamterene. Competition could alter plasma concentrations of these drugs as well as memantine, although available data suggest effect is insignificant. Potential for significantly reduced clearance of memantine with alkalinizing drugs such as sodium bicarbonate and carbonic anhydrase inhibitors; memantine clearance reduced by 80% with alkaline urine (pH = 8). *Less common adverse effects (1%–10%):* Hypertension, cardiac failure, syncope, stroke, transient ischemic attack, dizziness, confusion, headache, and constipation.

Generic name	rivastigmine
Trade name	Exelon
Class	Central acetylcholinesterase inhibitor
Half-life	1.5 hours
Mechanism of action	Noncompetitive, reversible acetylcholinesterase and butyrylcholinesterase inhibitor
Available preparations	Capsules: 1.5, 3, 4.5, 6 mg Oral solution: 2 mg/mL
Starting dose	1.5 mg bid
Titration	Increase by 1.5 mg bid every 2–4 weeks
Typical daily dose	6 mg bid
Dose range	4.5–6 mg bid
Therapeutic serum level	Not established

Comments: A first-line drug for cognition and prevention of behavioral disturbance in AD and in DLB. Rapidly absorbed, with peak concentrations in 1 hour; absorption delayed by food. Duration of cholinesterase inhibition is about 10 hours after a single dose. 40% protein bound. Extensively metabolized in the brain, with metabolite undergoing N-demethylation and/ or sulfate conjugation in the liver. Minimal role of CYP450 enzymes in metabolism. Nonlinear kinetics at doses >6 mg/day. Eliminated primarily in urine. Clearance 30% lower in elderly. *Drug interactions:* Synergistic effects with other cholinergic agents; antagonistic effects with anticholinergic drugs; potential for increased extrapyramidal symptoms with antipsychotics; bradycardia with β-blockers, calcium channel blockers, and digoxin; decreased clearance with smoking; increased neuromuscular blockade with depolarizing blockers. *Common adverse effects (>10%):* Dizziness, headache, nausea, vomiting, diarrhea, anorexia, and abdominal pain. *Less common adverse effects (1%–10%):* Fatigue, insomnia, confusion, depression, syncope, hypertension, dyspepsia, and weakness. Adverse effects are more likely with faster titration (every 2 weeks rather than every 4 weeks).

Generic name	selegiline
Trade name	Eldepryl (generic available), EMSAM
Class	MAO B inhibitor
Half-life	10 hours
Mechanism of action	Selective MAO B inhibitor (at doses < 10 mg/ day) that increases dopaminergic activity; psychostimulant
Available preparations	Capsules: 5 mg Tablets: 5 mg Transdermal patch: 6, 9, 12 mg every 24 hours
Starting dose	5 mg with breakfast
Titration	Increase in 1–3 days by 5 mg, as tolerated
Typical daily dose	5 mg bid, with breakfast and lunch
Dose range	5–10 mg/day
Therapeutic serum level	Not established

Comments: May be useful by virtue of its antioxidant and neuroprotective effects for patients with AD as well as PD with cognitive impairment (both off-label uses). Onset of effect for oral preparation within 1 hour; duration 24–72 hours. Little is known about pharmacokinetics of the transdermal patch in elders. Metabolized in liver to amphetamine and methamphetamine. *Drug interactions (at recommended low dose):* Amphetamines, fluoxetine and other SSRIs, serotonergic antidepressants such as nefazodone and venlafaxine, meperidine and other opioids, nonselective monoamine oxidase inhibitors, possibly linezolid. Major metabolism via CYP2B6 and 2C8/9, so levels can be increased with concomitant administration of inhibitors listed in Table 2–2. Foods with high tyramine content are problematic only at higher doses (or higher levels, through drug interactions). *Adverse effects:* Orthostasis, arrhythmias, hypertension, angina, edema, syncope, hallucinations, confusion, depression, insomnia, agitation, nausea, vomiting, dry mouth, constipation, anorexia, weight loss, tremor, loss of balance, and bradykinesia.

10

Analgesic Medications

Introduction

The prevalence of pain increases significantly with age. Pain-related problems are identified in up to 50% of elders living in the community (Chodosh et al. 2004), and pain-related functional impairment is identified in up to 80% of nursing home residents (Davis and Srivastava 2003). Pain is commonly reported among hospitalized elders, and many patients—particularly the oldest old—are dissatisfied with pain control (Desbiens et al. 1997). The older the patient, the less likely it is that pain will be adequately treated, and this is particularly true among minority group members (Bernabei et al. 1998). Even in home hospice care, breakthrough pain may be underestimated and undertreated (Fine and Busch 1998). Poor recognition and control of pain in elders has unfortunate consequences, including depression, anxiety, insomnia, poor nutrition, curtailment of activities, functional dependence, and subtle attentional and memory problems (Davis and Srivastava 2003). Pain also may be a contributing factor to delirium. The presence of dementia is associated with reduced ability to communicate effectively about pain symptoms, even though perception of pain remains intact (Davis and Srivastava 2003).

For all of these reasons, pain management has become the purview of many practicing psychiatrists, particularly consultants working with elderly patients in general medical/surgical settings. Moreover, there is an important interplay between depression and pain that places the psychiatrist in a unique position to provide effective treatment. As discussed below, the use of antidepressant medication not only is critical to the success of treatment in the presence of comorbid depression, but also can be helpful adjunctive therapy when depression is not present.

A distinction is made between acute pain and chronic pain because these are different phenomena. *Acute pain* reflects the extent of tissue injury and subsides with healing. With acute pain, there is an immediate need to identify and treat the cause, such that the medical model of management serves the patient well. *Chronic pain* is not simply a continuation of acute pain; it is best understood as a disease unto itself, with its own neurobiology and with important psychological and social ramifications. Chronic pain is better managed using a multidisciplinary model in which the psychiatrist may have a central role in assessment as well as ongoing treatment. The goal of chronic pain management in the elderly patient is to treat pain so that function is satisfactory; the complete elimination of the pain is not always a realistic goal (Davis and Srivastava 2003).

Pain and the Mechanisms of Analgesia

Pain is the unpleasant sensory and emotional experience associated with tissue injury. One component of pain is *nociception*, which is neural activity set in motion by a physical stimulus that may be injurious to tissue. Nociception serves the adaptive function of setting reflexes and other behaviors into action to remove the individual from the painful stimulus. The pain pathway begins with pain receptors (*nociceptors*) in the periphery, which activate dorsal horn neurons in the spinal cord, which project via the spinothalamic tract to the thalamus and then to other areas of the brain, including the limbic system and frontal cortex.

In practice, two subtypes of *nociceptive pain* are described: somatic pain, which emanates from skin, bone, muscle, or ligaments and is characterized as constant, aching, gnawing, sharp, stabbing, or throbbing; and visceral pain, characterized as paroxysmal, deep, dull, crampy, or squeezing. Somatic pain is well localized, while visceral pain is usually poorly localized. In most cases, nociceptive pain is time-limited (e.g., postoperative or posttraumatic); however, arthritic pain is an important exception.

Neuropathic pain results from malfunctioning nerves, either peripheral or central, and occurs in the absence of ongoing tissue injury. It may be triggered initially by tissue injury, but then is persistent, apparently sustained by abnormal somatosensory processing in the peripheral or central nervous system (CNS) (Cheville et al. 2000). Abnormal peripheral processing gives rise to conditions such as stump pain after amputation or pain from shingles. Abnormal central processing gives rise to deafferentation syndromes, involving pain due to loss of sensory input to the CNS, such as phantom limb pain. Neuropathic pain is described as burning, lancinating, tingling, shooting, or electric shock–like. *Hyperalgesia* (exquisite sensitivity) and *allodynia* (pain from nonpainful stimuli, such as a light touch) may be features of neuropathic pain, and these sensations may lie outside the distribution of the affected nerve (Likar and Sittl 2005).

The term *idiopathic pain* is used to describe pain without evidence of an organic cause or pain that is out of proportion to the severity of organic pathology. In DSM-IV-TR, this type of pain is coded as 307.89, "pain disorder associated with both psychological factors and a general medical condition" or 307.8, "pain disorder associated with psychological factors." In such cases, the patient's pain experience is present and the nociceptive component is absent. The important task with these disorders, as with any pain disorder, is to identify nociceptive and non-nociceptive factors that may be contributing to or sustaining pain so that a meaningful treatment plan can be devised (Cheville et al. 2000).

There is no evidence that elderly patients have different physiological responses to pain compared with younger individuals. Just as in younger patients, the physiological overflow of pain in elders is associated with autonomic signs, including hypertension, tachycardia, facial flushing or blanching, and changes in gastrointestinal (GI) motility. For cultural or other reasons, however, elders might complain less about the pain they experience.

Indications for Analgesics

Analgesia is defined as relief of pain without loss of consciousness. Mechanisms of analgesia can be peripheral or central. Peripheral mechanisms involve reduction or inhibition of synthesis or release of endogenous pain-producing substances, such that pain sensation is decreased; non-steroidal anti-inflammatory drugs (NSAIDs) and nerve blocks work by this mechanism. Central mechanisms involve actions on the brain's limbic system, such that concern about pain is decreased and tolerability of pain is increased; opioids work by these mechanisms. Traditionally, it has been taught that nociceptive pain responds to opioids, NSAIDs, salicylates, acetaminophen, and surgical interventions, whereas neuropathic pain may respond less well to opioids and has a variable but better response to antidepressants, anticonvulsants, and sympatholytics. Nonspecific factors, such as the patient's expectations regarding pain relief, also influence analgesia (Amanzio et al. 2001).

Elderly patients may be affected by a variety of painful conditions, both acute and chronic. An important principle of pain management for these individuals is that a variety of strategies for pain prevention and control should be used, both pharmacologic and nonpharmacologic. For the treatment of chronic pain in particular, benign interventions such as heat/cold packs, exercise or physical therapy, and therapeutic massage should be tried first. (Other nonpharmacologic therapies are listed in a later section of this chapter.) Patients who have no response to these initial strategies may then move on to the analgesic medication ladder, with or without adjuvant medications.

A list of painful conditions affecting elderly patients is shown in Table 10–1. Specific recommendations for treatment of selected conditions from this list are covered in a later section of this chapter.

Pharmacology of Major Analgesic Medications

The two major classes of analgesic medications discussed in this chapter are opioids and nonopioids (acetaminophen, salicylates, and NSAIDs). Selected opioid preparations are listed in Table 10–2, and nonopioid preparations are listed in Table 10–3. Adjuvant medications used in the treatment of neuropathic pain (e.g., anticonvulsants, antidepressants) are discussed in a later section. Both pharmacokinetics and pharmacodynamics for opioids and NSAIDs are altered with aging (Davis and Srivastava 2003). In general, opioids have a narrower therapeutic index in the elderly

Table 10–1.   Painful conditions affecting elderly patients

Nociceptive pain syndromes

    Postoperative pain

    Cancer

    Fall with fracture

    Osteoporosis with compression fracture

    Phantom limb pain

    Osteoarthritis

    Gout

    Rheumatoid arthritis

    Cardiac pain

    Paget's disease

    Polymyalgia rheumatica

Neuropathic pain syndromes

    Postherpetic neuralgia

    Diabetic peripheral neuropathy

    Nutritional neuropathy

    Poststroke syndrome

population, so these patients require closer monitoring of drug effects. NSAIDs have renal, cardiovascular, and GI effects that may be highly problematic for elders. For all analgesics, there is a greater risk of drug interaction in the elderly because of polypharmacy, and there is an increased risk of inducing adverse effects, such as constipation and delirium.

Opioid medications fall into three families:

- Lipophilic agents: methadone, fentanyl
- Codeine family: hydrocodone, oxycodone, codeine, tramadol
- Morphine-related family (hydrophilic): morphine, hydromorphone

The lipophilic agents are metabolized primarily by cytochrome P450 (CYP) 3A4, the codeine family agents by CYP2D6, and the morphine-

Table 10–2. Selected opioids: available preparations

Codeine	Tablets: 15, 30, 60 mg
	Oral solution: 15 mg/5 mL
	Injection: 15 mg/mL, 30 mg/mL
Codeine and acetaminophen	Tablets:
	TC#3: 300 mg acetaminophen/30 mg codeine
	TC#4: 300 mg acetaminophen/60 mg codeine
	Oral solution: 120 mg acetaminophen/12 mg codeine per 5 mL
Fentanyl	Lozenges: 200, 400, 600, 800, 1,200, 1,600 μg
	Transdermal: 12.5, 25, 50, 75, 100 μg/hr
	Injection: 0.05 mg/mL. Infusion also available.
Hydrocodone and acetaminophen	Tablets: 2.5/500, 5/325, 5/400, 5/500, 7.5/325, 7.5/400, 7.5/500, 7.5/650, 7.5/750, 10/325, 10/400, 10/500, 10/650, 10/660, 10/750 mg
	Capsules: 5/500 mg
	Oral solution: 7.5/325 mg per 15 mL, 7.5/500 mg per 15 mL
Hydromorphone	Tablets: 2, 4, 8 mg
	Suppository: 3 mg
	Oral liquid: 1 mg/mL
	Injection: 1, 2, 4, 10 mg/mL
Methadone	Tablets: 5, 10 mg
	Dispersible tablets: 40 mg
	Oral solution: 5 mg/5 mL, 10 mg/5 mL
	Oral concentrate: 10 mg/mL
	Injection: 10 mg/mL
Morphine	Tablets: 15, 30 mg
	Controlled-release tablets: 15, 30, 60, 100, 200 mg
	Extended-release tablets: 15, 30, 60, 100, 200 mg
	Sustained-release tablets: 20, 30, 50, 60, 100 mg

Table 10–2. Selected opioids: available preparations *(continued)*

Morphine *(continued)*	Capsules: 15, 30, 60, 90, 120 mg
	Extended-release capsules: 30, 60, 90, 120 mg
	Sustained-release capsules: 20, 30, 50, 60, 100 mg
	Oral solution: 10 mg/5 mL, 20 mg/5 mL, 20 mg/mL, 100 mg/5 mL
	Injection: 0.5 mg/mL, 1 mg/mL, 2 mg/mL, 4 mg/mL, 5 mg/mL, 8 mg/mL, 10 mg/mL, 15 mg/mL, 25 mg/mL, 50 mg/mL. Infusion also available.
	Rectal suppositories: 5, 10, 20, 30 mg
Oxycodone	Tablets: 5, 10, 15, 20, 30 mg
	Capsules: 5 mg
	Controlled-release tablets: 10, 20, 40, 80, 160 mg
	Extended-release tablets: 10, 20, 40, 80 mg
	Oral solution: 5 mg/5 mL
	Oral concentrate: 20 mg/mL
Oxycodone and acetaminophen	Tablets: 2.5/325, 5/325, 7.5/325, 7.5/500, 10/325, 10/650 mg
	Capsules: 5/500 mg
	Caplets: 5/500 mg
	Oral solution: 5/325 mg per 5 mL
Oxycodone and aspirin	Tablets: 4.5 oxycodone HCl + 0.38 oxycodone terephthalate/325 mg aspirin
Oxymorphone	Suppository: 5 mg
	Injection: 1 mg in 1 mL, 1.5 mg/mL (10 mL)
Tramadol	Tablets: 50 mg
	Extended-release tablets: 100, 200, 300 mg
Tramadol and acetaminophen	Tablets: 37.5 mg tramadol/325 mg acetaminophen

Note. TC = tylenol with codeine.
Source. Adapted from McEvoy et al. 2006; Semla et al. 2006.

Table 10–3.   Selected nonopioids: available preparations

Acetaminophen	Tablets: 325, 500 mg
	Capsules: 500 mg
	Extended-release caplets/geltabs: 650 mg
	Oral solution: 160 mg/5 mL, 500 mg/15 mL
	Suppositories: 80, 120, 125, 325, 650 mg
Aspirin	Tablets: 325, 500 mg
	Buffered tablets: 325, 500 mg
	Enteric-coated tablets: 81, 325, 500, 650, 975 mg
	Controlled-release tablets: 800 mg
	Suppositories: 300, 600 mg
Celecoxib	Capsules: 100, 200, 400 mg
Ibuprofen	Tablets: 200, 400, 600, 800 mg
	Capsules: 200 mg
	Oral suspension: 100 mg/5 mL
Ketorolac	Tablets: 10 mg
	Injection: 15 mg/mL (1 mL), 30 mg/mL (1 mL, 2 mL, 10 mL)
Naproxen	Tablets: 250, 375, 500 mg
	Tablets as sodium: 220 mg (200 mg naproxen), 275 mg (250 mg), 550 mg (500 mg)
	Caplets/Gelcaps: 220 mg (200 mg naproxen)
	Controlled-release tablets as sodium: 550 mg (500 mg naproxen), 421.5 mg (375 mg)
	Delayed-release tablets: 375, 500 mg
	Oral suspension: 125 mg/5 mL

Source.   Adapted from McEvoy et al. 2006; Semla et al. 2006.

related agents by glucuronidation. Pharmacodynamic effects of opioids occur through binding to μ, κ, and δ opioid receptors in the CNS. Methadone's analgesic effects also are mediated by *N*-methyl-D-aspartate (NMDA) and monoamine receptors (Davis and Srivastava 2003). Tramadol is an opioid, but it binds to the μ receptor with relatively low affinity and so theoretically has less abuse potential than other opioids.

The nonopioids (aspirin, acetaminophen, and NSAIDs) are rapidly absorbed with oral administration. Aspirin, buffered aspirin, and the related salicylate choline magnesium trisalicylate (Trilisate) are absorbed in the stomach, whereas enteric-coated aspirin is absorbed mostly from the small intestine. Opioids are well absorbed orally, but substantial first-pass effects make it necessary to give larger doses orally rather than parenterally. Distribution of opioids is greatest for the lipophilic agents methadone and fentanyl and smallest for the hydrophilic agents morphine and hydromorphone. Significant accumulation of the more lipophilic agents can occur with continued administration of these drugs. Pharmacokinetic data for opioid and nonopioid analgesics are discussed in the Specific Drug summaries at the end of this chapter.

Metabolic pathways for opioid medications are listed in Table 10–4. As noted above, several opioids are metabolized mainly via oxidation by CYP3A4 or 2D6 isoenzymes. Many also undergo glucuronidation. With morphine, glucuronidation forms the active metabolite M6G, which is 50 times more potent than the parent compound (Armstrong and Cozza 2003). Codeine, hydrocodone, propoxyphene, and tramadol are prodrugs that are metabolized to active analgesics. In the case of tramadol, the active analgesic metabolite (M_1) is formed by the CYP2D6 oxidative pathway, and in poor metabolizers, barely detectable levels of active drug are found at 2D6 (Poulsen et al. 1996). Codeine presents a more complex case. Although this medication is a prodrug metabolized in part by CYP2D6, it is believed that neither poor metabolism at 2D6 nor coadministration of 2D6 inhibitors affects analgesia (Cozza et al. 2003). Other factors may underlie poor analgesic response to codeine (Poulsen et al. 1998).

Acetaminophen is metabolized primarily by glucuronidation, with only 5%–9% undergoing oxidation, mostly by CYP2E1 (McEvoy et al. 2006). The latter reaction forms a toxic intermediate known as NAPQI, which is further conjugated with glutathione to form nontoxic products. There has been concern that patients with liver disease might form the toxic intermediate without being able to complete the processing to nontoxic products. In part because of the small proportion of drug that undergoes oxidation, the effect may not be clinically significant. Contrary

Table 10–4. Opioids: known metabolic pathways

Drug	Metabolic pathways	Enzyme(s) inhibited
Alfentanil	CYP3A4	None
Buprenorphine	CYP3A4, ?2D6, UGT2B7	None
Codeine	CYP3A4, 2D6, UGT2B7	UGT2B7
Diphenoxylate	Unknown	None
Fentanyl	CYP3A4	?CYP3A4
Hydrocodone	CYP2D6, 3A4, reduction by unknown enzymes	None
Hydromorphone	UGT1A3, UGT2B7, others	None
Loperamide	Unknown	None
Meperidine	?CYP3A4, ?other P450 enzymes, ?UGT1A4, ?other UGTs	Unknown
Methadone	CYP3A4, ?2D6	CYP3A4, ?UGT2B7
Morphine	CYP2D6, 3A4, UGT2B7, UGT1A3	UGT2B7
Nalbuphine	?Unspecified P450 enzymes, reduction by unknown enzymes, conjugation by UGT2B7	None
Oxycodone	CYP2D6, ?3A4, UGT2B7	None
Oxymorphone	UGT2B7, others	None

Table 10–4. Opioids: known metabolic pathways *(continued)*

Drug	Metabolic pathways	Enzyme(s) inhibited
Propoxyphene	CYP3A4	CYP3A4
Remifentanil	Esterases	None
Sufentanil	CYP3A4, 2D6	None
Tramadol	CYP2D6, 3A4, 2B6, unspecified UGTs	None

Note. CYP = cytochrome P450; UGT = uridine 5'-diphosphate glucuronosyltransferase.
Source. Adapted from Cozza KL, Armstrong SC, Oesterheld JR: *Concise Guide to Drug Interaction Principles for Medical Practice,* 2nd Edition. Washington, DC, American Psychiatric Publishing, 2003. Used with permission.

to popular medical belief, not only do patients with liver disease tolerate usual doses of acetaminophen but this medication can be used for pain and fever in patients with acute viral hepatitis or interferon-related side effects in hepatitis C (Benson et al. 2005).

Many of the nonopioid analgesics are metabolized by CYP2C9, which has a known poor metabolizer phenotype and is inhibited by medications such as fluvoxamine and fluconazole. When CYP2C9 inhibition occurs, the drugs are eliminated instead through conjugation, so inhibition is probably rarely encountered as a clinical problem. Several nonselective NSAIDs and salicylates inhibit uridine 5′-diphosphate glucuronosyltransferase (UGT) 2B7, which has valproate and lorazepam as substrates, along with many other analgesics and a number of important nonpsychotropics, such as cyclosporine and tacrolimus. Metabolic pathways for nonopioid analgesics are listed in Table 10–5.

Salicylates are excreted almost exclusively in urine. Other opioid and nonopioid analgesics are excreted primarily in urine, and to a lesser extent in feces. Pharmacokinetics of most analgesics may be significantly affected by renal dysfunction. Patients with renal failure who are given morphine, for example, may accumulate the active metabolite morphine-6-glucuronide to extremely high levels. Toxicity may be reduced in a subset of the population by a mutation in the μ opioid receptor gene (Lotsch et al. 2002).

Drug Interactions

Both opioid and nonopioid analgesics are subject to drug interactions that may be significant. The potential nephrotoxicity of NSAIDs makes these drugs unsuitable for coadministration with other drugs affecting renal function, including acetaminophen. Selective COX-2 inhibitors should not be given with aspirin (and possibly warfarin) because of loss of gastroprotective effect (Borer and Simon 2005). The fentanyl patch should not be used with CYP3A4 inhibitors such as ciprofloxacin, erythromycin, nefazodone, or grapefruit juice because of inhibition of metabolism. Other analgesic drug interactions are listed in Table 10–6.

Efficacy of Analgesics and Adjuvants

When analgesic medications are used for intermittent pain such as headache, they can be used on an as-needed basis; when they are used for ongoing pain, they should be prescribed on a scheduled basis. This is because it is easier to prevent pain than to control it and easier to control mild pain than severe pain. This applies to acute pain as well as chronic pain and to noncancer as well as cancer pain.

NSAIDs have an important role in treating acute and chronic pain, especially of the nociceptive type. NSAIDs have anti-inflammatory as well as analgesic effects while acetaminophen has only analgesic effects. Ibuprofen at 200 mg has analgesic efficacy equal to 650 mg of aspirin or 650 mg of acetaminophen. Ibuprofen at 400 mg is superior to these standard doses of aspirin and acetaminophen.

Partial opioid agonists, mixed agonist-antagonists, and weak opioids (e.g., codeine and tramadol) are ultimately limited in analgesic efficacy by ceiling effects. In contrast, high-potency, direct agonist opioids (e.g., morphine) have no ceiling effect. These drugs are efficacious in even the most severe nociceptive pain (e.g., cancer pain), given adequate doses. In neuropathic pain, opioids are generally less efficacious, although it may be that individual drugs differ from one another in efficacy. There is some evidence that buprenorphine may provide better control of neuropathic pain compared with other agents (McCormack 1999), although further research is needed in this area.

Adjuvants can be used to improve pain control and/or to mitigate adverse effects of opioids. Noradrenergic antidepressants and anxiolytics are effective adjuvants because of direct neurotransmitter effects and because treatment of depression and anxiety can substantially reduce the burden of pain. Anticonvulsants are mostly used in the treatment of neuropathic pain syndromes. Psychostimulants, including methylphenidate, dextroamphetamine, and modafinil, can be used in patients with advanced cancer to reverse opioid-induced sedation and to increase energy, hedonic tone, and motivation for end-of-life work. Some evidence suggests that cholinesterase inhibitors such as donepezil can also be useful in reversing opioid-induced sedation (Bruera et al. 2003; Slatkin et al. 2001). Corticosteroids are potent analgesics with appetite-stimulating

Table 10–5. Metabolic pathways: nonopioid analgesics

Drug	Metabolic pathways	Enzyme(s) inhibited
Acetaminophen	CYP2E1, other P450 enzymes, UGT1A1, UGT1A6, UGT1A9, sulfation (SULT1A1)	None
Aspirin	Metabolized to salicylic acid by carboxylesterases	None
Salicylic acid	UGT2B7, other UGTs, glycine conjugation	UGT2B7, ?other UGTs, SULTs
Salsalate	UGT2B7, other UGTs, split by esterases into two salicylates	UGT2B7, ?other UGTs, SULTs
Celecoxib	CYP2C9, unspecified UGTs	CYP2D6
Rofecoxib	Non-P450 reduction	None
Valdecoxib	CYP3A4, 2C9, unspecified UGTs	CYP2C19
Diclofenac	CYP2C9, 2C8, 2C18, 2C19, 3A4, UGT2B7, other UGTs, sulfation	UGT2B7, ?SULTs
Etodolac	Unspecified P450 enzymes and UGTs	None
Meloxicam	CYP2C9, 3A4	None
Nabumetone	Unspecified phase I enzyme and UGTs	None
Diflunisal	UGT1A3, UGT1A9	UGT1A9, SULTs
Fenoprofen	UGT1A3, UGT2B7	UGT2B7

Table 10–5. Metabolic pathways: nonopioid analgesics *(continued)*

Drug	Metabolic pathways	Enzyme(s) inhibited
Flurbiprofen	CYP2C9, unspecified UGTs	None
Ibuprofen	CYP2C9, UGT1A3, UGT2B7	UGT2B7
Indomethacin	CYP2C9, 2C19, unspecified UGTs	UGT2B7
Ketoprofen	?CYP2C9, UGT1A3, UGT1A6, UGT2B7	?CYP2C9, UGT2B7
Ketorolac	Unspecified P450 enzyme and UGT	None
Mefenamic acid	CYP2C9, UGT1A9, other UGTs	SULTs
Naproxen	CYP2C9, 2C8, 1A2, UGT1A3, UGT1A6, UGT1A9, UGT2B7	UGT2B7
Oxaprozin	Unspecified P450 enzymes, UGTs	None
Piroxicam	CYP2C9, ?other P450 enzymes	None
Sulindac	Unspecified UGTs; activation by FMO_3	None
Tolmetin	Unspecified P450 enzymes and UGTs	None

Note. CYP = cytochrome P450; FMO_3 = flavin-containing monooxygenase 3; SULT = sulfotransferase; UGT = uridine 5'-diphosphate glucuronosyltransferase.
Source. Adapted from Cozza KL, Armstrong SC, Oesterheld JR: *Concise Guide to Drug Interaction Principles for Medical Practice,* 2nd Edition. Washington, DC, American Psychiatric Publishing, 2003. Used with permission.

Table 10–6. Analgesic drug interactions

Analgesic	Interacting agent	Potential interaction
Acetaminophen	Alcohol	Potential hepatotoxicity (reduced glutathione stores)
	Barbiturates, carbamazepine, hydantoins, isoniazid, rifampin, sulfinpyrazone	Decreased analgesia, increased hepatotoxic potential of acetaminophen
	Cholestyramine	Decreased acetaminophen absorption
	Warfarin	Enhanced anticoagulant effect
Aspirin	ACE inhibitors	Effects of ACE inhibitors blunted
	Carbonic anhydrase inhibitors, steroids	Altered salicylate concentration
	Heparin, low-molecular-weight heparin, warfarin, platelet inhibitors	Increased risk of bleeding
	Methotrexate	Increased methotrexate levels
	NSAIDs	Increased risk of GI bleeding, reduced cardioprotective effect of aspirin, reduced concentration of NSAID
	Probenecid	Effects antagonized by aspirin
	Valproate	Valproate β-oxidation impaired; may lead to valproate toxicity
	Verapamil	Potentiates prolongation of bleeding time with aspirin

Table 10–6. Analgesic drug interactions *(continued)*

Analgesic	Interacting agent	Potential interaction
Celecoxib	ACE inhibitors, β-blockers, hydralazine, loop diuretics (furosemide), thiazide diuretics (hydrochlorothiazide)	Decreased effect of interacting drugs
	Aminoglycosides	Increased aminoglycoside levels
	Aspirin	GI toxicity
	Bile acid sequestrants	Decreased NSAID absorption
	Cyclosporine	Increased cyclosporine level and potential nephrotoxicity
	Fluconazole	Doubled celecoxib concentration
	Lithium	Increased lithium levels (about 17%)
	Methotrexate	Bone marrow suppression, aplastic anemia, GI toxicity
	Vancomycin	Increased vancomycin levels
	Warfarin	Bleeding events
Codeine	CYP2D6 inhibitors, cigarette smoking	Decreased analgesic effect
	CNS depressants, TCAs, MAOIs, phenothiazines, guanabenz, neuromuscular blockers, other opioids	Increased toxicity

Table 10–6.   Analgesic drug interactions *(continued)*

Analgesic	Interacting agent	Potential interaction
Fentanyl	CYP3A4 inhibitors	Increased levels and effect of fentanyl; can be fatal with potent inhibitors (see Table 2–2)
	MAOIs	Potentiation of opioid (serious)
	CNS depressants, phenothiazines	Increased sedation
Hydrocodone	CYP2D6 inhibitors	Decreased analgesic effect
	CNS depressants	Additive effects
	MAOIs, TCAs	Increased effects of hydrocodone and coadministered drug
Hydromorphone	CNS depressants	Additive effects
	Pegvisomant	Decreased effect of pegvisomant
	Phenothiazines	Enhanced hypotension and CNS depression
	SSRIs	Serotonin syndrome
Ibuprofen	ACE inhibitors, angiotensin II antagonists, hydralazine	Decreased antihypertensive effect
	Anticoagulants, antiplatelet agents	Increased bleeding
	Aspirin	Reduced cardioprotective effect of aspirin

Table 10–6. Analgesic drug interactions *(continued)*

Analgesic	Interacting agent	Potential interaction
Ibuprofen *(continued)*	Corticosteroids	Increased risk GI ulceration
	Cyclosporine	Increased cyclosporine level
	Lithium	Increased lithium level
	Loop diuretics	Reduced diuretic efficacy
	Methotrexate	Bone marrow suppression, aplastic anemia, GI toxicity
	Warfarin	Increased international normalized ratio
Meperidine	MAOIs, chlorpromazine, thioridazine	Potential for serious toxicity; do not coadminister meperidine with MAOIs
Morphine	Diuretics	Decreased effect of diuretics due to release of antidiuretic hormone
	CNS depressants, dextroamphetamine, TCAs, MAOIs	Increased toxicity
Opioids (all)	SSRIs	Serotonin syndrome
Oxycodone	CNS depressants, general anesthetics, MAOIs, TCAs, dextroamphetamine	Potentiate effects of opioid
	CYP2D6 inhibitors	Decreased oxycodone levels

Table 10–6. Analgesic drug interactions *(continued)*

Analgesic	Interacting agent	Potential interaction
Oxymorphone	Phenothiazines	Decreased opioid effect
	CNS depressants, TCAs, dextroamphetamine	Potentiated opioid effects; possible toxicity
Tramadol	Amphetamines	Increased seizure risk
	Carbamazepine	Decreased tramadol half-life
	CYP2D6 inhibitors	Decreased tramadol level/effects
	Linezolid, MAOIs, selegiline, TCAs, SSRIs, neuroleptics, other opioids	Increased risk of seizures
	SSRIs	Serotonin syndrome
	Digoxin	Digoxin toxicity
	Quinidine	Increased tramadol concentration
	Warfarin	Potentiated anticoagulant effect

Note. ACE=angiotensin-converting enzyme; CNS=central nervous system; CYP=cytochrome P450; GI=gastrointestinal; MAOI=monoamine oxidase inhibitor; NSAID=nonsteroidal anti-inflammatory drug; SSRI=selective serotonin reuptake inhibitor; TCA=tricyclic antidepressant.
Source. Adapted from McEvoy et al. 2006; Semla et al. 2006.

effects, but they can precipitate psychosis and mood changes and also may have serious long-term effects. Other adjuvants used include calcitonin, which can relieve pain from bone resorption in conditions such as metastatic cancer and osteoporosis, and pamidronic acid, which can be effective in relieving pain from bony metastases (e.g., from breast cancer or myeloma) (Davis and Srivastava 2003).

Clinical Use of Analgesics and Adjuvants

Pain Assessment

Whether pain is treated in a multidisciplinary clinic, hospital, or private office, a clinical evaluation is needed before analgesics are prescribed. This evaluation should include the following elements:

- Pain history: Where is the pain? What is it like (stabbing, burning, throbbing, aching, dull, crampy)? Is it constant or intermittent? What makes it better? What makes it worse? How bad is it right now? How bad is it at its worst? What effect has it had on your ability to do activities of daily living, such as work, drive, walk, etc.? Have you changed your social or recreational activities because of the pain?
- Examination: Look for objective indicators of pain, including signs of sympathetic overactivity (hypertension, tachycardia, facial flushing or blanching, or diaphoresis), antalgic (painful) gait, writhing, moaning, grimacing, guarding, splinting, or crying. Assess for depression, suicidal ideation, anxiety, delirium, and cognitive dysfunction using a standardized instrument such as the Mini-Mental State Examination.

The location of the pain provides important clues as to etiology, in some cases helping to identify the anatomic source directly. In other cases, the pain is referred along predictable neural pathways. Pain of hepatic or gallbladder origin may be referred to the scapula on the right side; pain of cardiac origin may be referred to the left arm, shoulder, or jaw; pain of diaphragmatic origin may be referred to the cap of the shoulder on the same side; and pain from the pancreas may be referred to the mid back (Cheville et al. 2000; Massie 2000). The description of the pain can be helpful in determining whether it is primarily neuropathic or primarily nociceptive in nature. Because pain by nature waxes and wanes in intensity, it is not uncommon to see patients appear more mobile and less distressed at times, and this should not be taken as evidence that the patient's report of pain is exaggerated.

Any one of several scales can be used to rate pain severity. As shown in Figure 10–1, these include a 0–10 rating, a verbal description, the Wong-Baker FACES Pain Rating Scale, and a functional limitation scale. The same scale(s) can be used serially to determine response to treatment.

Sympathetic signs and other objective signs of pain are not always present. When pain becomes chronic, signs of sympathetic overactivity may be absent. In addition, medications such as β-blockers and other antihypertensives may mask these signs. A patient with delirium, advanced dementia, or severe depression may not exhibit antalgic behaviors when in pain but may withdraw from interaction or cooperation with caregivers.

Choice of Drug

Except in the immediate postoperative period or after trauma, it is recommended that analgesics be started at a low dose and titrated slowly to the effective dose for elderly patients. After surgery or trauma, opioids may be used as sole agents for a limited period, starting with effective doses and tapering off as the wound or injury heals. For chronic or subacute nociceptive pain, the three steps of the World Health Organization (WHO) analgesic ladder should guide treatment:

1. Nonopioid with or without adjuvants
2. Weak opioid plus nonopioid with or without adjuvants
3. Strong opioid with or without nonopioid with or without adjuvants

Nonopioids include acetaminophen, aspirin and other salicylates, and NSAIDs. Weak opioids include codeine, hydrocodone, and tramadol. Strong opioids include morphine, hydromorphone, methadone, and fentanyl. Oxycodone is an opioid of intermediate potency.

Among nonopioids, acetaminophen is preferable to NSAIDs as initial analgesic treatment for elders because of low propensity to cause GI and cardiovascular adverse effects. Although acetaminophen can have

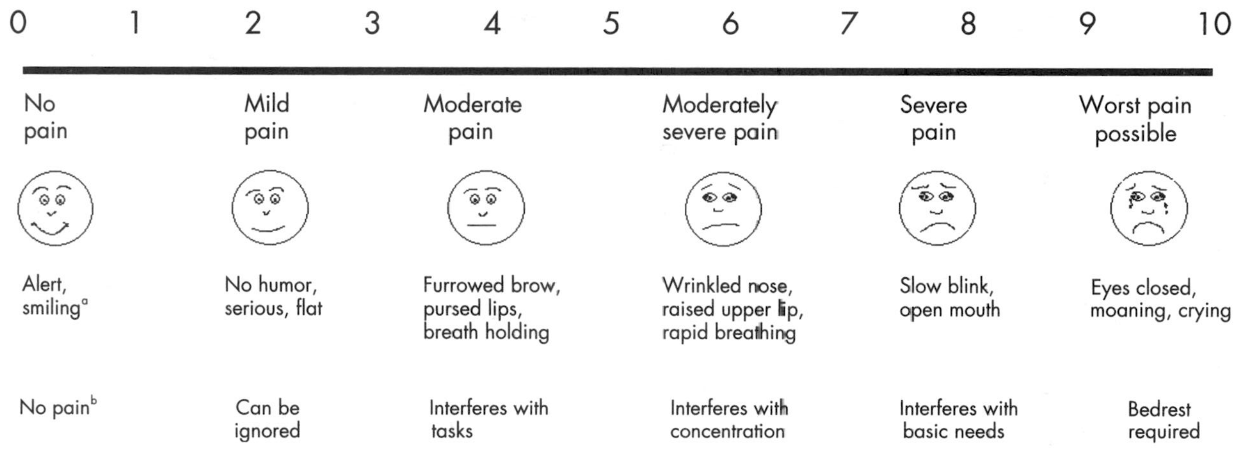

0   1   2   3   4   5   6   7   8   9   10

No pain — Mild pain — Moderate pain — Moderately severe pain — Severe pain — Worst pain possible

Alert, smiling[a] — No humor, serious, flat — Furrowed brow, pursed lips, breath holding — Wrinkled nose, raised upper lip, rapid breathing — Slow blink, open mouth — Eyes closed, moaning, crying

No pain[b] — Can be ignored — Interferes with tasks — Interferes with concentration — Interferes with basic needs — Bedrest required

Figure 10–1. Pain assessment scales.

[a] Wong-Baker FACES Pain Rating Scale.
[b] Activity Tolerance Scale.

Source. Reprinted from Hockenberry MJ, Wilson D, Winkelstein ML: *Wong's Essentials of Pediatric Nursing,* 7th Edition. St. Louis, MO, Mosby, 2005, p. 1259. Copyright, Mosby. Used with permission.

adverse renal effects with prolonged use, the risk of renal toxicity is much lower than with NSAIDs. However, acetaminophen is a centrally acting analgesic without anti-inflammatory effects, so it generally has weaker analgesic activity than NSAIDs. NSAIDs should be used one at a time when prescribed and should not be combined with steroids or even acetaminophen because of the potential for GI and renal toxicity (Davis and Srivastava 2003). For Step 2 treatment, a commercially available combination drug (opioid plus nonopioid) could be used. This has the potential to improve compliance but also has the disadvantage of imposing a ceiling dose by virtue of the presence of the nonopioid.

Drugs that should be avoided in elders because of potential adverse effects include meperidine, propoxyphene, indomethacin, mefenamic acid, and pentazocine and other mixed agonist-antagonist drugs (except possibly buprenorphine). Drugs that should be avoided for long-term use in the elderly include ketorolac, naproxen, oxaprozin, and piroxicam, as noted in Table 1–3 in Chapter 1 of this volume, "The Practice of Geriatric Psychopharmacology" (Davis and Srivastava 2003; Fick et al. 2003). Fentanyl is commonly used in the geriatric population despite its complex kinetics. This drug is among the most lipophilic of the opioids and can accumulate in fat, muscle, lung, and GI tract with continuous administration. At some threshold of drug accumulation, mental status changes (confusion and delirium) may be seen. In addition, drug effects can be erratic when the drug redistributes from storage sites, resulting in problems such as delayed ventilatory depression (Davis and Srivastava 2003).

As the safety of NSAIDs (whether COX-2-selective or not) is called into question, the balance is shifting toward the use of acetaminophen monotherapy, opioid monotherapy, or opioids in combination with acetaminophen for treatment, particularly of elderly patients. The WHO ladder has not yet been revised in light of new findings regarding cardiovascular adverse effects of NSAIDs.

Opioid medications of choice in elderly patients include codeine, hydrocodone, hydromorphone, morphine, oxycodone, oxymorphone, and tramadol. Nonopioids of choice include acetaminophen, salicylates, ibuprofen, and (for short-term use) naproxen. Other NSAIDs with a short half-life also may be useful. Elimination of oxycodone is unaffected by age but is affected by gender; the drug is eliminated 25% more slowly in women (Davis and Srivastava 2003). Adverse effects of oxycodone are no more common in elders than in younger patients. Hydromorphone has the advantage of few drug interactions because it is metabolized solely by conjugation and does not inhibit any P450 isoenzymes. It may be less likely than morphine to produce hallucinations. A sustained-release form of hydromorphone (Palladone) has been withdrawn from the market because of the risk of serious interaction with alcohol. Tramadol is a weak opioid (it has one-tenth the potency of morphine) given as a prodrug that has to be metabolized via CYP2D6 for analgesic effects. Tramadol may be ineffective when administered to patients who are poor metabolizers at CYP2D6 or who are coadministered 2D6 inhibitors.

Opioids: Alternative Formulations and Routes of Administration

Ideally, opioid medications are given orally or through a feeding tube. A variety of alternative routes exist for patients who are unable to take medications enterally, including intravenous, subcutaneous, intrathecal, transmucosal, sublingual, rectal, and transdermal administrations. In general, intravenous administration of opioids results in a faster effect and shorter duration of action compared with oral dosing and a faster development of tolerance to analgesic effects at a given dose. The subcutaneous route can be used to administer opioids at home, with family members or other caregivers trained to monitor the infusion site. Spinal analgesia begun operatively can be continued for pain control during the immediate postoperative period. For all elderly patients, intramuscular dosing should be avoided because it is painful and discourages patients from accepting analgesia, and absorption by this route is erratic. Rectal administration is also erratic and should be used as a last resort.

Dosing and Dose Titration

As with other drug classes, analgesic medications should be started at low doses and titrated as tolerated for elders, either to clinical effect or limiting side effects. Nonopioids have ceiling doses that should not be exceeded. In elderly patients, the duration of effect from a single dose can be prolonged because of decreased clearance, so frail elders may require longer dosing intervals or smaller doses initially. Final doses required to achieve analgesia, however, do not correlate well with body weight or even initial pain severity (Davis and Srivastava 2003). Elders may be more sensitive to adverse effects of opioids such as respiratory depression.

Analgesic doses for ongoing pain should be scheduled around the clock and should be given at times tailored to the pain pattern of the patient. Often, patients experience greater pain at night; therefore, nighttime doses may be larger than daytime doses. Patients already beset with severe pain may require high doses of analgesics to get the pain under control initially; they then continue to experience adequate analgesia as the dose is tapered and maintained at a lower level. Breakthrough pain in patients with cancer (particularly those with metastases to bone) is a very significant problem that is often underestimated by caregivers (Fine and Busch 1998). For these patients, fast-onset, short-acting drugs such as oxycodone, fentanyl, or hydromorphone should be prescribed as needed at short intervals. When baseline pain is controlled but breakthrough pain occurs intermittently, the scheduled dose should not be increased; supplementation with adequate as-needed (prn) doses can be used indefinitely.

Dosing recommendations for individual drugs are given in the Specific Drug summaries at the end of this chapter. Initially, each as-needed dose for breakthrough pain should be the same as each standing dose except for extended- (XR) or sustained-release preparations. Careful attention should then be paid to the pattern of as-needed use, so that adjustments can be made to standing as well as as-needed doses and schedules. Equianalgesic doses of opioids are provided in the Specific Drug summaries so that conversions can be made from one opioid to another. Note that in converting intramuscular (or intravenous) hydromorphone or morphine to oral medication, the number of milligrams increases considerably because the oral bioavailability of these drugs is poor. Intravenous, intramuscular, and subcutaneous doses are approximately equivalent. Doses administered orally and rectally are approximately equivalent.

Monitoring Treatment

A patient who is receiving intravenous dosing of opioids should be observed for oversedation and respiratory depression. With chronic opioid use, concerns include constipation and risk of falls. At each visit, pain severity should be assessed using one of the pain scales discussed in an earlier section of this chapter. Little is needed in the way of laboratory monitoring for patients prescribed opioids. For patients receiving NSAIDs, follow-up evaluation is recommended to look for GI bleeding (hematocrit, stool Hemoccult) and renal effects (electrolytes, creatinine, and calculation or measurement of creatinine clearance). Although cardiovascular adverse effects of NSAIDs (particularly COX-2 inhibitors) are now known, guidelines for follow-up assessment have not been established.

Management of Inadequate Response

When a patient prescribed an opioid reports pain escalating before a dose, the pain can be treated either by shortening the dosing interval or increasing the dose. A dose increase is indicated for pain that is inadequately controlled during the whole dosing interval. When adverse effects limit dosing or dose increases appear to have no effect, progression to the next WHO step is indicated. It is very common for patients with neuropathic pain to report inadequate pain control on the WHO ladder. For these patients, anticonvulsant or antidepressant medications should be considered. Treatment of neuropathic pain is discussed separately in a later section of this chapter.

Stopping Opioid Treatment

When an opioid is to be discontinued, it is best to taper the medication to avoid withdrawal symptoms. The recommended rate of taper is slow: 10% every 24–72 hours (Gershwin and Hamilton 1998), the exact rate depending upon the clinical situation.

Switching Analgesics

A patient who has become tolerant to the effects of one opioid may not be as tolerant to the effects of a second opioid. When a switch is made, the equianalgesic dose of the second opioid should be calculated, and the patient should initially be prescribed 50%–75% of that dose to avoid overdose. When switching from tramadol to another opioid, the dose should be lowered substantially because of the possibility that the patient may be a poor metabolizer at CYP2D6 and little conversion to active drug may have taken place, such that the patient is in essence opioid-naive. When switching from normal-release to sustained-release morphine or oxycodone or from parenteral drug to sustained-release morphine, a 2-hour overlap may be needed to maintain analgesia. When switching from a normal-release opioid to a fentanyl patch, a 12- to 18-hour overlap of the two is required (both standing and as-needed doses). When switching from a continuous intravenous infusion of fentanyl to a patch of equivalent dose, a graded dose reduction over 12–18 hours has been found effective (Davis and Srivastava 2003).

Acute Analgesic Overdose

Acute salicylate overdose is a serious condition marked by fever, dyspnea, confusion, ataxia, asterixis, seizures, oliguria, prolonged bleeding, metabolic acidosis with respiratory alkalosis, and elevated blood urea nitrogen. The syndrome is potentially fatal. Treatment includes forced diuresis with urinary alkalinization to increase drug clearance, emesis, and administration of vitamin K to restore coagulation.

Acetaminophen overdose should be treated with acetylcysteine (oral Mucomyst or intravenous Acetadote). For the oral solution, a loading dose of 140 mg/kg should be given, followed by 17 doses of 70 mg/kg every 4 hours. For the intravenous infusion, a loading dose of 150 mg/kg should be given over 15 minutes, and then 50 mg/kg should be infused over 4 hours, then 100 mg/kg over 16 hours. The entire dosing regimen should be completed even when acetaminophen levels return to normal (Fuller and Sajatovic 2005).

Acute and subacute opioid overdose has been reported with all agents and all routes of administration. Signs of opioid overdose include decreased respiratory rate (2–4 breaths/minute) or Cheyne-Stokes respiration, cyanosis from decreased oxygen saturation, hypothermia, miosis (except with meperidine), sedation, coma, pyramidal signs (e.g., extensor plantar response), and loss of skeletal muscle tone. Acute overdose should be treated with parenteral opioid antagonists such as naloxone (Narcan) or nalmefene (Revex). Naloxone has onset in 2–5 minutes and a duration of effect of 20–60 minutes, and nalmefene has onset in 5–15 minutes and a duration of effect of several hours (Fuller and Sajatovic 2005). Either of these medications can precipitate acute withdrawal in opioid-dependent patients. Naltrexone is an oral medication with a prolonged latency to effect that is sometimes used in cases of overdose with long-acting medications such as methadone.

Issues of Tolerance, Abuse, and Dependence

Tolerance is an intrinsic change in receptor sensitivity that occurs as a consequence of continued exposure to a drug, necessitating a higher dose. With opioids, tolerance develops over time to analgesic and euphoric effects, but less or not at all to other effects. Tolerance develops more rapidly with intravenous or spinal administration of opioids than with oral or rectal administration. In the cancer patient, both tolerance to opioids and tumor progression can contribute to the need for dose escalation. Tolerance per se often first becomes manifest as a decrease in duration of effect at a particular opioid dose. When this trend appears, either a dose increase or a switch to a different opioid is indicated. Alternatively, nonopioids, adjuvants, or nondrug therapies could be added.

In patients without a history of prior substance abuse, even chronic opioid treatment for pain control is rarely associated with psychological dependence or addiction. On the other hand, the syndrome of *pseudoaddiction* is often seen in the clinical setting. This is drug-seeking behavior that occurs as a consequence of inadequate dosing of prescribed medication. It can be seen with as-needed use of medication in the patient with continuous pain, with dosing intervals that are too long, or with drugs that are too low-potency for the severity of pain being treated. Pseudoaddiction can be mistaken for real addiction, but when adequate scheduled doses of analgesia are prescribed, this variant of drug-seeking behavior usually subsides.

All patients who take opioids for a sufficient length of time will become physically dependent, meaning that they will experience exacerbation of pain upon withdrawal of the medication, and some will experience withdrawal symptoms (hypertension, tachycardia, nausea, diarrhea, anxiety/agitation). As noted earlier, few will exhibit signs or symptoms of psychological dependence or drug craving.

Adverse Effects of Analgesics by Class

Acetaminophen

Chronic, high-dose acetaminophen use is associated with nephrotoxicity, and doses >4 g/day are associated with hepatotoxicity. The latter may be exacerbated by alcohol use or fasting, both factors known to deplete liver stores of glutathione, the enzyme responsible for metabolism of acetaminophen's hepatotoxic intermediate NAPQI. Laboratory abnormalities that may be associated with acetaminophen use include increased chloride, uric acid, glucose, ammonia, bilirubin, and alkaline phosphatase; decreased sodium, bicarbonate, and calcium; and anemia and blood dyscrasias, including pancytopenia (Semla et al. 2006).

Aspirin and Other Salicylates

Chronic use of aspirin may be associated with prolonged bleeding time, GI irritation, and renal insufficiency. Aspirin irreversibly inhibits platelet function and for this reason is best discontinued in advance of certain surgical procedures. Choline magnesium trisalicylate (Trilisate) reportedly does not have the same effect on platelet function. Salicylates also inhibit synthesis of certain clotting factors in the liver and can cause hemolysis in patients with G6PD deficiency. Aspirin sensitivity may manifest as symptoms of rhinitis, bronchospasm, and/or urticaria.

Nonsteroidal Anti-Inflammatory Drugs

NSAIDs cause GI irritation and bleeding as well as renal toxicity. Gastric irritation may permit invasion by *Helicobacter pylori,* leading to ulceration. Bleeding is caused by reversible inhibition of platelet function (unlike the case with aspirin); platelet function returns when most of the drug has been eliminated. The Beers criteria specifically mention longer half-life, non–COX-2-selective NSAIDs (naproxen, oxaprozin, and piroxicam) as problematic with long-term use in elders (Fick et al. 2003). COX-2-selective inhibitors do not alter hemostasis or increase the risk of GI bleeding but are as renally toxic as other NSAIDs. More importantly, it is increasingly recognized that these drugs may increase the risk of significant cardiovascular events. It is not yet clear whether the risk applies to all NSAIDs or only to the COX-2-selective drugs. Less frequent adverse effects of NSAIDs include anxiety, dizziness, tinnitus, drowsiness, confusion, bronchospasm in aspirin-sensitive individuals, urticaria, pruritus, and photophobia (Semla et al. 2006).

Opioids

Opioids can cause significant respiratory depression, hypotension, orthostasis, bradycardia, cognitive impairment, confusion, delirium, sedation, nausea and vomiting, constipation, and urinary retention. Individual agents differ in relative severity of each of these effects. Table 10–7 summarizes major adverse effects of opioids.

System-Specific Adverse Effects

Cardiovascular Effects

The COX-2-selective drugs rofecoxib and valdecoxib have been withdrawn from the market because of a reported association with serious cardiovascular adverse effects, including myocardial infarction and stroke. The risk may extend to nonselective NSAIDs. Although the mechanism of increased risk is not yet known, it has been suggested that it could be a consequence of sodium and water retention associated with the drugs (Borer and Simon 2005). This could in turn cause an increase in blood pressure (and in some patients, worsened congestive heart failure). Celecoxib (the only COX-2-selective drug still on the market) now carries a boxed warning regarding cardiovascular risks.

Gastrointestinal Effects

Bleeding

The risk of upper GI bleeding with NSAIDs is greater for elderly patients, women, those with a history of peptic ulcer disease or previous GI bleeding, those on high-dose therapy, and those on concomitant selective serotonin reuptake inhibitor antidepressants. GI symptoms are reported by about a quarter of elderly NSAID users (slightly more by chronic users and slightly less by acute users) (Pilotto et al. 2003), and 40% of patients stop NSAIDs because of GI intolerance. The worst offenders are

Table 10–7.   Summary of adverse effects of opioids

Drug	Analgesic	Antitussive	Constipation	Respiratory depression	Sedation	Emesis
Phenanthrenes						
Codeine	+	+++	+	+	+	+
Hydrocodone	+	+++		+		
Hydromorphone	++	+++	+	++	+	+
Levorphanol	++	++	++	++	++	+
Morphine	++	+++	++	++	++	++
Oxycodone	++	+++	++	++	++	++
Oxymorphone	++	+	++	+++		+++
Phenylpiperidines						
Alfentanil	++					
Fentanyl	++			+	+	+
Meperidine	++	+	+	++		
Remifentanil	++			++	+++	++
Sufentanil	+++					

Table 10–7. Summary of adverse effects of opioids *(continued)*

Drug	Analgesic	Antitussive	Constipation	Respiratory depression	Sedation	Emesis
Diphenylheptanes						
Methadone	++	++	++	++	+	+
Propoxyphene	+			+	+	+
Agonist-Antagonists						
Buprenorphine	++	N/A	+++	+++	++	++
Butorphanol	++	N/A	+++	+++	++	+
Dezocine	++		+	++	+	++
Nalbuphine	++	N/A	+++	+++	++	++
Pentazocine	++	N/A	+	++	++ or stimulation	++

Source. Adapted from Semla TP, Beizer JL, Higbee MD: *Geriatric Dosage Handbook*, 11th Edition. Hudson, OH, Lexi Comp, 2006. Used with permission, p. 1495.

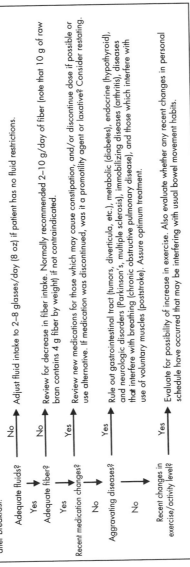

Define constipation as no more than two bowel movements per week or straining upon defecation 25% of the time or more. If possible, educate resident about this definition to develop cooperation.

Verify constipation with digital exam and/or X ray (radiography) if impaction is suspected. Establish baseline and toilet daily, 30 minutes after breakfast.

Adequate fluids? — No → Adjust fluid intake to 2–8 glasses/day (8 oz) if patient has no fluid restrictions.

Yes ↓

Adequate fiber? — No → Review for decrease in fiber intake. Normally recommended 2–10 g/day of fiber (note that 10 g of raw bran contains 4 g fiber by weight) if not contraindicated.

Yes ↓

Recent medication changes? — Yes → Review new medications for those which may cause constipation, and/or discontinue dose if possible or use alternative. If medication was discontinued, was it a promotility agent or laxative? Consider restarting.

No ↓

Aggravating diseases? — Yes → Rule out gastrointestinal tract (tumors, diverticula, etc.), metabolic (diabetes), endocrine (hypothyroid), and neurologic disorders (Parkinson's, multiple sclerosis), immobilizing diseases (arthritis), diseases that interfere with breathing (chronic obstructive pulmonary disease), and those which interfere with use of voluntary muscles (poststroke). Assure optimum treatment.

No ↓

Recent changes in exercise/activity level? — Yes → Evaluate for possibility of increase in exercise. Also evaluate whether any recent changes in personal schedule have occurred that may be interfering with usual bowel movement habits.

Once constipation is identified and contributing factors are ruled out, determine if any signs or symptoms of fecal impaction are exhibited (distended abdomen, fever, vomiting, confusion).

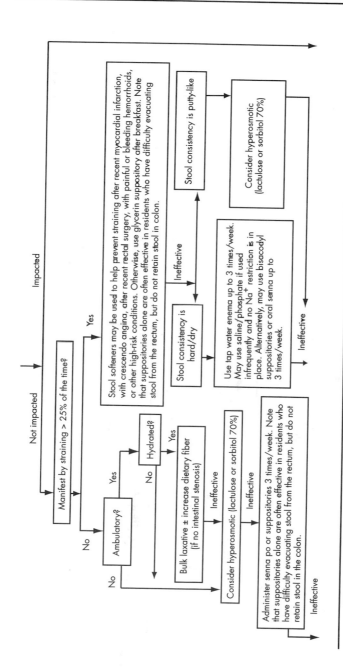

Figure 10–2.   Algorithm for treatment of constipation.

Note.   MOM=Milk of Magnesia; po=orally; prn=as needed.

Source.   Reprinted from Semla TP, Beizer JL, Higbee MD: *Geriatric Dosage Handbook*, 11th Edition. Hudson, OH, Lexi Comp, 2006, p. 1518. Used with permission.

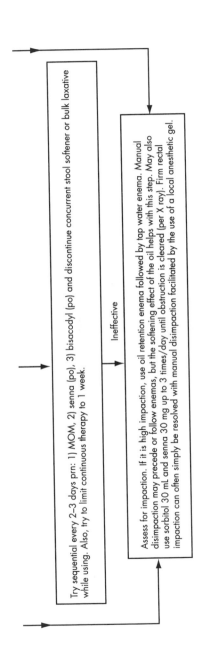

Try sequential every 2–3 days prn: 1) MOM, 2) senna (po), 3) bisacodyl (po) and discontinue concurrent stool softener or bulk laxative while using. Also, try to limit continuous therapy to 1 week.

Ineffective

Assess for impaction. If it is high impaction, use oil retention enema followed by tap water enema. Manual disimpaction may precede or follow enemas, but the softening effect of the oil helps with this step. May also use sorbitol 30 mL and senna 30 mg up to 3 times/day until obstruction is cleared (per X ray). Firm rectal impaction can often simply be resolved with manual disimpaction facilitated by the use of a local anesthetic gel.

Figure 10–2.   Algorithm for treatment of constipation. (*Continued*)

indomethacin, ketorolac, piroxicam, and mefenamic acid (Davis and Srivastava 2003). The NSAIDs that offend least are etodolac, ibuprofen, nabumetone, and meloxicam (Davis and Srivastava 2003). Use of H_2 antagonists and proton pump inhibitors only partially alleviates the problem. Alternative medications in high-risk patients include low-dose opioids, nonacetylated salicylates, low-dose steroids, and the COX-2-selective drug celecoxib. COX-2-selective drugs lose gastroprotective effects when aspirin is coadministered, even at low doses (e.g., baby aspirin).

Constipation

Constipation is a common adverse effect of opioids that should be prevented by ensuring that the patient is adequately hydrated, maintains mobility, and is started on a bowel regimen at the time the opioid is initiated (e.g., 100 mg of docusate sodium [Colace] two times a day and two tablets of bisacodyl [Dulcolax] at bedtime). When used alone, bulk laxatives such as psyllium are not adequate for this purpose and should be avoided. Figure 10–2 shows a more complete algorithm for prevention and treatment of constipation in the elderly patient.

Nausea

Elders started on treatment with opioids also commonly experience nausea, which often dissipates as tolerance develops, usually within several days. Although drugs such as metoclopramide or prochlorperazine could theoretically be used, these drugs are best avoided in elders because of adverse effects. When nausea persists, the dose of opioid should be reduced, the medication should be given by another route, or a different opioid should be used.

Hepatotoxicity

Acetaminophen is hepatotoxic at dosages above 4 g/day. This threshold for liver injury may be lower for those with preexisting liver disease, in alcoholic patients (with drinking), or in those who are fasting, as discussed in an earlier section.

Neuropsychiatric Effects

Delirium

Delirium can be a consequence of the disease for which the opioid is prescribed or a complication of opioid treatment. In addition, constipation is a common side effect of opioid use and contributes significantly to the risk of developing delirium. When delirium occurs, the dose of opioid should be reduced, the medication should be given by another route, or a switch to another drug should be made. In end-of-life care, the opioid could be continued based on the preference of the patient and family, and the delirium could be treated with a cholinesterase inhibitor (e.g., donepezil, 5 mg/day) (Slatkin and Rhiner 2004). If symptoms of delirium persist, the dose of the opioid could be lowered. If hallucinations or delusions develop, the option of adding an antipsychotic medication could then be discussed with the patient and family.

Myoclonus

Myoclonus is a common, although benign, adverse effect of opioids. Myoclonus in this case comes from the spinal cord and is not a harbinger of seizure. It may be necessary to decrease the dose of opioid or switch to another opioid. If a switch is not possible, a benzodiazepine (lorazepam or clonazepam), valproate, or gabapentin could be used for treatment (Davis and Srivastava 2003).

Sedation

Sedation is a common effect of opioids in the early stages of therapy. Tolerance usually develops to this effect within the first week, so reassurance may be all that is needed. In end-of-life care, sedation can be reduced in some cases with the use of donepezil (Bruera et al. 2003; Slatkin et al. 2001) or a psychostimulant such as modafinil (Webster et al. 2003).

Renal Effects

NSAIDs affect renal function by decreasing prostaglandin and renin secretion. Their use may be associated with the development of renal insufficiency, hyperkalemia, sodium and water retention, interstitial nephritis, and acute renal failure. The risk of adverse renal effects is increased with advanced age, female gender, preexisting renal disease, cirrhosis, diabetes, infection, congestive heart failure, volume depletion, use of an extended-release NSAID, or coadministration of diuretics or angiotensin-converting enzyme (ACE) inhibitors. The progression of renal insufficiency can be reversed if the condition is recognized early and treated effectively. Offending medications should be discontinued.

Respiratory Effects

Respiratory depression can occur with rapid escalation of opioid dosing, particularly with intravenous use or with acute renal failure and consequent opioid accumulation. In addition, respiratory depression can be seen in patients treated with opioids who experience sudden relief of pain (and thus removal of respiratory stimulation) through successful nerve block if the usual opioid dose is continued.

Treatment of Selected Pain Syndromes Affecting Elderly Patients

Whether pain is acute versus chronic or nociceptive versus neuropathic determines appropriate treatment. Acute, single-episode, nociceptive pain such as muscle strain or postoperative state is an indication for rest, graded physical therapy, and analgesic medication adequate to the severity of tissue injury. Recurrent acute pain such as headache or gout should be treated using the acute pain model, applied again with each episode.

For chronic nociceptive pain such as that due to arthritis, treatment is more complex; the element of time is introduced, with the need for follow-up, and the more important need for analgesics that do no harm when used long-term. In general, the treatment algorithm should follow the WHO ladder discussed earlier.

Many chronic pain syndromes, including cancer pain, involve a combination of nociceptive and neuropathic pain components. For these conditions, a combination of the treatments for nociceptive pain and the treatments listed in the sections that follow for neuropathic pain should be used. In addition, surgical approaches (e.g., tumor debulking) and nerve blocks may be effective.

Neuropathic pain can be difficult to treat. Of the numerous medications studied for treatment of neuropathic pain, the most effective appear to be gabapentin, pregabalin, carbamazepine, venlafaxine, and possibly duloxetine (Goldstein et al. 2005; Mendell and Sahenk 2003; Wiffen et al. 2005). High doses are needed when opioids are used for neuropathic pain relief, and for many patients analgesia is never achieved or adverse effects are intolerable (Rowbotham et al. 2003).

Back Pain

In elderly patients, back pain may be associated with osteoarthritis (discussed further below), vertebral compression fractures, disk disease, spinal stenosis, multiple myeloma, or primary or metastatic cancer, among other conditions. Vertebral compression fractures in the patient with osteoporosis can at times occur with minor trauma, such as coughing or sneezing. Pain ranges from mild to severe, depending in part on the severity of the fracture. Pain is well localized over the vertebral body and is exacerbated by percussion. In general, the pain subsides over 4–6 weeks as the fracture heals. Short-term therapy should target the pain (using the WHO ladder), while long-term therapy should aim to restore bone mass. Thoracic epidural block may be very effective for patients who do not respond to systemic analgesics (Waldman 2002).

Pathology affecting lumbar spine disks, facets, and/or ligaments that worsens with age may culminate in spinal stenosis, a narrowing of the spinal canal. The patient usually presents reporting pain and weakness in the legs and calves when walking (*neurogenic claudication*) accompanied by lower-extremity pain (Waldman 2002). Numbness, weakness, and loss of reflexes may be found on examination. The appearance of bowel or bladder dysfunction is an indication for urgent neurosurgical consultation. Lumbar spine magnetic resonance imaging (MRI) is the diagnostic test of choice, with computed tomography or myelography used where MRI is contraindicated. Electromyogram and nerve conduction testing provide information about the integrity of individual nerve roots and the nerve plexus. Spinal stenosis can be treated with surgery, physical therapy (heat, deep massage), NSAIDs, skeletal muscle relaxants, epidural nerve blocks with a local anesthetic and steroid, and a hypnotic to ensure sleep (Waldman 2002).

Cancer Pain

Pain may occur at any stage of cancer and can be acute (e.g., postoperative) or chronic. As noted in an earlier section, pain among older cancer patients is often underappreciated by clinicians and thus undertreated, particularly among minority patients residing in nursing home settings. Undertreated or untreated pain can result in depression, anxiety, undernutrition, and poor sleep quality, with further debilitation. Pain in the cancer patient may be related to the cancer itself, to treatment, to deconditioning arising from immobility, or to unrelated pathology. Most pain syndromes are a consequence of direct tumor involvement, with the primary mass or metastatic lesions impinging upon bones, nerves, or organs. Elderly cancer patients also are more susceptible to neuropathic pain syndromes resulting from chemotherapy or radiation. A multi-modal approach to treatment should be used to treat cancer pain in elders.

- If pain is severe on presentation, the most potent opioid analgesics (e.g., morphine, hydromorphone) should be used as a first step to get control of the pain.
- If pain is mild to moderate, the WHO ladder should be used: acetaminophen, NSAIDs, or weak opioids should be initial treatments. NSAIDs may be particularly effective in treating bone pain.
- Neuropathic pain should be treated with antidepressants and anticonvulsants.
- To supplement pharmacologic approaches, a range of nonpharmacologic treatment options should be used, including heat/cold packs, massage, ultrasound, transcutaneous electrical nerve stimulation (TENS), physical therapy, occupational therapy, cognitive-behavioral therapy, and distracting activities (e.g., listening to music).
- Frequent reassessments of pain may be necessary, since medications should generally be started at a low dose and titrated slowly.
- Exact dosing of pain medication will have to be determined empirically. For example, larger doses may be needed at night because of more severe pain.
- If the patient experiences persistent sedation at an opioid dose providing adequate pain control, consideration should be given to use of a cholinesterase inhibitor such as donepezil or a psychostimulant such as modafinil.

Diabetic Neuropathy

Diabetic neuropathy, the most prevalent of the peripheral neuropathies, is more frequently recognized when it involves the lower extremities than when it involves the trunk. In the lower extremities, symptoms include numbness, tingling, burning, sharp pains, cramps, and dysesthesia (sensory alteration) most prominent distally, particularly in the feet. Truncal neuropathy involves thoracic dermatomes, and symptoms can be misattributed to internal organs. Truncal pain can be severe, with sleep disruption often noted, and patchy sensory deficits can be observed on examination. The onset of symptoms in truncal neuropathy often coincides with extremes of blood sugar levels or with weight loss or gain (Waldman 2002).

Treatment of diabetic neuropathy consists first of improved control of blood sugar, with insulin often providing better symptom improvement and ultimate pain prevention than oral hypoglycemic agents (Waldman 2002). As with other neuropathic pain syndromes, pharmacologic options include anticonvulsants and dual-acting antidepressants (i.e., with serotonergic and noradrenergic effects). Tricyclic antidepressant use is limited by adverse effects in elderly patients, as discussed in Chapter 4 of this volume, "Antidepressants."

Specific agents and recommended doses are as follows (lidocaine 5% patches, providing topical analgesia to epidermal and dermal layers of skin, can be used in tandem with these agents [White et al. 2003]):

- Gabapentin started at 100–300 mg three times a day, titrated slowly to 3,600 mg or the highest tolerated dose (Backonja et al. 1998). There is some evidence that doses above 1,600 mg/day are required (Mendell and Sahenk 2003).
- Pregabalin started at 150 mg/day (divided two or three times a day) and titrated over 1 week to 150 mg two times a day (McEvoy et al. 2006). Some patients require doses up to 300 mg two times a day (Freynhagen et al. 2005).
- Venlafaxine XR at a target dosage of 150–225 mg/day (Rowbotham et al. 2004).
- Duloxetine at a target dosage of 60 or 120 mg/day (Goldstein et al. 2005).

Fractured Ribs

In elderly patients, rib fracture may be a consequence of a fall or even minor trauma (e.g., coughing) in those with osteoporosis. The severity of pain and functional disability depends on whether the fracture is partial or complete, whether bone fragments are free-floating, the number of ribs involved, and the degree of injury to surrounding nerves and pleura (Waldman 2002). Pneumothorax or hemopneumothorax that may be associated will require treatment, and pulmonary function may be compromised, placing the patient at risk for pneumonia. Plain radiographs of the ribs and chest wall (not chest X rays) are needed for diagnosis. Treatment involves application of heat/cold packs and use of an elastic rib belt, as well as analgesic therapy using the WHO ladder. When opioids are used, careful attention has to be paid to pulmonary status to avoid complicating pneumonia, because these agents suppress the cough reflex. For patients whose pain is refractory to these treatments, local injection of an anesthetic may provide relief (Waldman 2002).

Gout

Gout is an intermittent, exquisitely painful inflammatory monoarthritis usually involving the joints of the distal lower extremity but also including the hand, wrist, or elbow. Urate crystal deposits (*tophi*) may be palpated in the hands, feet, elbows, or ears. Acute gout is distinguished from septic arthritis by joint aspiration and examination of synovial fluid (Gershwin and Hamilton 1998). Gout is a chronic disease that requires adherence to a low-purine diet and treatment with allopurinol to lower serum urate levels. When acute flares occur, colchicine, high-dose NSAIDs, and/or intra-articular steroids should be used.

Herpes Zoster (Acute) and Postherpetic Neuralgia

Reactivation of the varicella zoster virus causes the syndrome of acute herpes zoster (*shingles*). Most commonly, the ensuing skin eruption involves the distribution of thoracic nerves or the first division of the trigeminal nerve. The syndrome is more common in elderly patients and in those with deficient immunity. Early and aggressive treatment is indicated to prevent the development of postherpetic neuralgia. Sympathetic nerve blocks can be used in tandem with opioid medications. Gabapentin may be a useful adjunct, and antiviral agents may be indicated. Cold packs, topical aluminum sulfate as a tepid soak (for crusting/weeping lesions), and zinc oxide (as a protectant during healing when temperature sensitivity occurs) may be helpful (Waldman 2002).

Postherpetic neuralgia is characterized by pain in the area affected by acute herpes zoster that persists more than 1 month beyond lesion healing (Gershwin and Hamilton 1998). Incidence is highest among elderly patients. The pain is constant and burning, often accompanied by lancinating neuritic pain. Pain may be made worse by movement or sensory stimulation of the affected skin (Waldman 2002). The syndrome is best prevented by early and aggressive treatment of acute herpes zoster, as discussed above.

When postherpetic neuralgia does develop, gabapentin and pregabalin are drugs of choice, both with U.S. Food and Drug Administration–approved labeling for this indication (Backonja et al. 1998; Frampton and Foster 2005). Gabapentin should be initiated at a dosage of 300 mg three times a day (if tolerated) and titrated to clinical effect, with dosages up to 3 g/day required in some cases. Gabapentin can be used in tandem with local analgesia in the form of lidocaine patches over the affected area, applied every 24 hours (White et al. 2003).

Pregabalin has been shown in several controlled trials to be effective in relieving pain and pain-related insomnia at dosages ranging from 150 to 600 mg/day (divided two or three times a day), although dosages above 300 mg/day apparently confer no additional benefit (Frampton and Foster 2005; Sabatowski et al. 2004). Pregabalin should be initiated at a dosage of 150 mg/day (divided two or three times a day) and increased as tolerated to 300 mg/day (divided two or three times a day) within 1 week based on efficacy and tolerability (McEvoy et al. 2006). Dose must be reduced for renal impairment according to details contained in the package insert. Because the drug is hemodialyzed, a supplement should be given after each dialysis session.

Osteoarthritis

Osteoarthritis is a highly prevalent, painful condition among elderly patients caused by wear and tear and inflammation of joints, including the spine, shoulder, hip, and all extremity joints. The condition may show exacerbations and remissions with relative subsidence of pain. The pain is generally worsened by activity and improved with rest and heat. As the patient ages, mobility may be lost along with functional ability, and muscle wasting may occur; ambulation aids may be needed. Regular graded exercise can mitigate these developments. Treatment should be initiated with acetaminophen at 3–4 g/day in divided doses. If this is not effective, the next step of treatment should be with an NSAID. If this fails or if the patient has a contraindication to NSAIDs, tramadol should be tried (Sarzi-Puttini et al. 2005). If the patient has severe pain and these pharmacologic treatments have failed or been poorly tolerated, opioids should be considered. Other options include topical analgesics such as capsaicin cream, intra-articular steroid injections, and intra-articular hyaluronic acid injections to restore viscoelasticity of the synovial fluid (Sarzi-Puttini et al. 2005).

Phantom Limb Pain

Patients who have undergone amputation of a limb or part of a limb may have the postoperative experience of pain or other sensations that seem to arise from the absent limb. This is a highly distressing experience, termed *phantom limb pain,* often requiring reassurance that this is a normal postamputation phenomenon that has a physiological basis in deafferentation. For many patients, phantom limb sensations subside with time. Those who go on to have persistent phantom limb pain may also report abnormal phantom limb positions and movements. It is widely believed that long-term changes in central pain pathways from persistent painful input occurring before the amputation may be responsible for this phenomenon and that once these changes have occurred, the syndrome can be difficult to treat. It is best prevented by early surgical intervention (if amputation is inevitable) and possibly by early use of NMDA antagonists such as memantine and drugs such as gabapentin or pregabalin. These drugs have been shown in animal studies to prevent cortical reorganization. In at least one randomized controlled study in humans memantine has been shown to prevent phantom limb pain (Flor 2002). Once the phantom limb pain syndrome has developed, it should be treated aggressively with a combination of modalities:

- Gabapentin up to 3,600 mg/day in divided doses
- Alternative anticonvulsants such as carbamazepine or phenytoin
- Antidepressants such as duloxetine or venlafaxine
- Sympathetic nerve blocks with anesthetic and steroid
- TENS, sensory discrimination training (Flor 2002)

Among elderly patients, opioids have a more limited role in treatment, but potent, long-acting agents such as methadone, morphine, or oxycodone may be helpful (Waldman 2002).

Polymyalgia Rheumatica

Polymyalgia rheumatica is a large-joint synovitis seen primarily in geriatric patients that presents with the acute or subacute onset of proximal aching and stiffness in the neck, shoulder girdle, and pelvic girdle; it is most commonly seen in Scandinavians. Up to 20% of patients have an associated temporal arteritis (Gershwin and Hamilton 1998). The diagnosis is made on clinical grounds: the erythrocyte sedimentation rate (ESR) is elevated, there may be a normochromic, normocytic anemia, and alkaline phosphatase may be moderately elevated. Bone scans have shown uptake in affected joints (shoulder and hip). Rapid resolution of symptoms may be seen with 10–20 mg/day of prednisone, which should be tapered slowly over 6 months to 5 mg/day, then stopped after 12–18 months. If the patient also shows evidence of temporal arteritis (diplopia, temporal pain), immediate initiation of higher-dose steroid (e.g., oral prednisone at 60 mg/day) is indicated, along with temporal artery biopsy (Gershwin and Hamilton 1998). These patients should be referred for urgent consultation by a specialist to avoid the serious complication of blindness.

Postoperative Pain

For the time-limited indication of postoperative pain, most patients receive opioids as monotherapy. Epidural analgesia or patient-controlled analgesia is often used for the first 48 hours postoperatively, and then oral or intravenous analgesics are prescribed on an as-needed basis. For those still in significant pain after 48 hours, scheduled doses of opioids should be considered. Elderly patients may prefer oral to parenteral analgesics, and morphine to other opioids (Sauaia et al. 2005).

A subset of patients who have undergone thoracic surgery may have persistent pain that appears to have both nociceptive and neuropathic components, a condition known as *postthoracotomy syndrome*. This is a consequence of factors such as compression and stretch injuries to nerves, cutaneous neuroma formation, and rib fractures (Waldman 2002). A workup is necessary to rule out other thoracic or abdominal pathologies leading to pain. The condition can be treated with the application of heat/cold packs, use of an elastic rib belt, and administration of analgesics or adjuvants, including acetaminophen, NSAIDs, opioids, gabapentin, and dual-acting antidepressants, such as venlafaxine or duloxetine. Those with pain refractory to these measures may benefit greatly from intercostal nerve block (Waldman 2002).

Rheumatoid Arthritis

Rheumatoid arthritis is an inflammatory and erosive joint disease with onset most frequently in middle or old age. Compared with diseases with onset before 60 years of age, elderly-onset disease more often has an acute onset with constitutional symptoms (e.g., weight loss, fatigue) (Olivieri et al. 2005). Radiographic study of hands and feet as well as other affected areas may initially show only soft tissue involvement and later show joint space narrowing and joint erosion. High titers of serum rheumatoid factor ($\geq$1:320) are specific for rheumatoid arthritis. Symptomatic treatment consists of physical and occupational therapy, exercise, use of assistive devices, and heat/cold packs. NSAIDs can be used on a scheduled basis to control pain and swelling. Judicious use of low-dose prednisone is sometimes indicated. Disease-modifying antirheumatic drugs are the most important component of treatment and should be initiated as early as possible in the disease course. These drugs prevent joint destruction, improve function, and reduce mortality in elderly patients just as in younger patients. These agents include methotrexate, hydroxy-chloroquine, sulfasalazine, and the anticytokines etanercept, infliximab, adalimumab, and anakinra. These agents should be managed by specialists in rheumatology and are not discussed further in this chapter.

Temporal Arteritis

New-onset, persistent headache that may be associated with tender, palpable vessels underlying the lateral face and scalp characterizes *temporal arteri-*

tis, a disease primarily affecting those over 60 years of age. Diplopia is commonly associated with this disease. Systemic symptoms may be present, suggesting an additional diagnosis of polymyalgia rheumatica (discussed above). Jaw claudication is highly suggestive of temporal arteritis, but this symptom is not always present. Elevated ESR (>45 mm/hour) is characteristic, but nonspecific; temporal artery biopsy is required for definitive diagnosis. Immediate initiation of higher-dose prednisone (60 mg/day) is indicated to avoid loss of vision (Gershwin and Hamilton 1998). Biopsy should follow steroid dosing to avoid delay. As noted above, patients with characteristic symptoms should be referred for urgent consultation by a specialist.

Trigeminal Neuralgia

Most common in 50- to 70-year olds, the *trigeminal neuralgia*—also known as *tic douloureux*—is characterized by excruciating paroxysmal pain that results from compression of the trigeminal nerve (cranial nerve V) as it leaves the brain stem (Gershwin and Hamilton 1998). Causes include tortuous blood vessels, neuromas, bony abnormalities, and aneurysms. In most patients, no anatomic abnormality can be identified. Acute attacks can be triggered by stimulation of the nerve along its peripheral course by activities such as brushing teeth or chewing, or by cold wind on the face. Patients are prone to anticipatory anxiety and persistent depression, which is associated with suicidality in some cases. In the minority of cases, a surgical intervention is indicated. In all others, symptoms should be controlled with medications. Once the pain syndrome has been diagnosed, the patient should be referred for magnetic resonance angiography/MRI to rule out posterior fossa or brain stem lesions and demyelinating disease (Waldman 2002). In addition, if the first division of CNV is affected, referral to an ophthalmologist is indicated. Drugs that have been found effective in the treatment of trigeminal neuralgia include carbamazepine, oxcarbazepine, gabapentin, valproate, lamotrigine, phenytoin, clonazepam, lidocaine, and baclofen. The most evidence exists at present for the efficacy of carbamazepine, and this drug is considered the mainstay of therapy. Carbamazepine should be started at a low dose and titrated slowly to symptom control or to a target dosage of 1,200 mg/day (Waldman 2002).

Nonpharmacologic Therapies

Elderly patients prefer pain treatments that they consider low risk, such as massage, topical analgesics, hot/cold packs, and activities that serve to distract from pain, such as music, prayer, humor, and social visits (Davis and Srivastava 2003). However, pain clinicians are more likely to prescribe medications, physical therapy, and exercise. Some elders, particularly the oldest old (>80 years of age), avoid exercise because of the risk of falling. Many other treatments for pain exist, including TENS, ultrasound, acupuncture, and spinal cord stimulation. Specific psychotherapeutic approaches include relaxation training, hypnosis, cognitive-behavioral therapy, and biofeedback. Cognitive-behavioral therapy was found in a randomized trial of group versus individual treatment to be effective in ameliorating interference of pain in daily activities and depression in a cohort of patients with chronic pain (Turner-Stokes et al. 2003).

Chapter Summary

- The goal of chronic pain management in the elderly patient is improvement to the point that the patient's function is satisfactory; it is not necessarily the elimination of pain or use of the lowest possible dose of analgesic medication.
- There is no evidence that elderly patients have different physiological responses to pain compared with younger individuals.
- Since pain by nature waxes and wanes in intensity, it is not uncommon to see patients appear more mobile and less distressed at times, which should not be taken as evidence that the patient's report of pain is exaggerated.
- When analgesic medications are used for intermittent pain such as headache, they can be used on an as-needed basis, but when they are used for ongoing pain, they should be prescribed on a scheduled basis.
- Two types of pain are recognized: nociceptive, resulting from tissue injury, and neuropathic, resulting from malfunctioning nerves. Treatment of the two types differs.
- Nociceptive pain may respond to opioids, nonsteroidal anti-inflammatory drugs, salicylates, and acetaminophen as well as surgical interventions, whereas neuropathic pain may respond less well to opioids and have a variable but better response to antidepressants, anticonvulsants, and sympatholytics.
- Opioid medications of choice in elderly patients include codeine, hydrocodone, hydromorphone, morphine, oxycodone, oxymorphone, and tramadol.
- Nonopioid medications of choice include acetaminophen, salicylates, ibuprofen, and (for short-term use) naproxen.
- Of the numerous medications studied for treatment of neuropathic pain, the most effective appear to be gabapentin, pregabalin, carbamazepine, venlafaxine, and possibly duloxetine.
- Various psychotropic adjuvants can be used to improve pain control or to mitigate adverse effects of opioids.
- When opioids are to be discontinued, the recommended rate of taper is slow: 10% every 24–72 hours.

References

Amanzio M, Pollo A, Maggi G, et al: Response variability to analgesics: a role for non-specific activation of endogenous opioids. Pain 90:205–215, 2001

Armstrong SC, Cozza KL: Pharmacokinetic drug interactions of morphine, codeine, and their derivatives: theory and clinical reality, part I. Psychosomatics 44:167–171, 2003

Backonja M, Beydoun A, Edwards KR, et al: Gabapentin for the symptomatic treatment of painful neuropathy in patients with diabetes mellitus. JAMA 280:1831–1836, 1998

Benson GD, Koff RS, Rolman KG: The therapeutic use of acetaminophen in patients with liver disease. Am J Ther 12:133–141, 2005

Bernabei R, Gambassi G, Lapane K, et al: Management of pain in elderly patients with cancer. SAGE Study Group. Systematic Assessment of Geriatric Drug Use via Epidemiology. JAMA 279:1877–1882, 1998

Borer JS, Simon LS: Cardiovascular and gastrointestinal effects of COX-2 inhibitors and NSAIDs: achieving a balance. Arthritis Res Ther 7 (suppl 4):S14–S22, 2005

Bruera E, Strasser F, Shen L, et al: The effect of donepezil on sedation and other symptoms in patients receiving opioids for cancer pain: a pilot study. J Pain Symptom Manage 26:1049–1054, 2003

Cheville A, Caraceni A, Portenoy RK: Pain: definition and assessment, in Pain: What Psychiatrists Need to Know. Edited by Massie MJ. Washington, DC, American Psychiatric Press, 2000, pp 1–22

Chodosh J, Solomon DH, Roth CP, et al: The quality of medical care provided to vulnerable older patients with chronic pain. J Am Geriatr Soc 52:756–761, 2004

Cozza KL, Armstrong SC, Oesterheld JR: Concise Guide to Drug Interaction Principles for Medical Practice, 2nd Edition. Washington, DC, American Psychiatric Publishing, 2003

Davis MP, Srivastava M: Demographics, assessment, and management of pain in the elderly. Drugs Aging 20:23–57, 2003

Desbiens NA, Mueller-Rizner N, Connors AF Jr, et al: Pain in the oldest-old during hospitalization and up to one year later. HELP Investigators. Hospitalized Elderly Longitudinal Project. J Am Geriatr Soc 45:1167–1172, 1997

Fick DM, Cooper JW, Wade WE, et al: Updating the Beers criteria for potentially inappropriate medication use in older adults. Arch Intern Med 163:2716–2724, 2003

Fine PG, Busch MA: Characterization of breakthrough pain by hospice patients and their caregivers. J Pain Symptom Manage 16:179–183, 1998

Flor H: Phantom-limb pain: characteristics, causes, and treatment. Lancet Neurol 1:182–189, 2002

Frampton JE, Foster RH: Pregabalin in the treatment of postherpetic neuralgia. Drugs 65:111–118, 2005

Freynhagen R, Strojek K, Griesing T, et al: Efficacy of pregabalin in neuropathic pain evaluated in a 12-week, randomised, double-blind, multicentre, placebo-controlled trial of flexible- and fixed-dose regimens. Pain 115:254–263, 2005

Fuller MA, Sajatovic M: Drug Information Handbook for Psychiatry, 5th Edition. Hudson, OH, Lexi-Comp, 2005

Gershwin ME, Hamilton ME: The Pain Management Handbook: A Concise Guide to Diagnosis and Treatment. Totowa, NJ, Humana Press, 1998

Goldstein DJ, Lu Y, Detke MJ, et al: Duloxetine vs. placebo in patients with painful diabetic neuropathy. Pain 116:109–118, 2005

Likar R, Sittl R: Transdermal buprenorphine for treating nociceptive and neuropathic pain: four case studies. Anesth Analg 100:781–785, 2005

Lotsch J, Zimmermann M, Darimont J, et al: Does the A118G polymorphism at the mu-opioid receptor gene protect against morphine-6-glucuronide toxicity? Anesthesiology 97:814–819, 2002

Massie MJ (ed): Pain: What Psychiatrists Need to Know. Washington, DC, American Psychiatric Press, 2000

McCormack K: Signal transduction in neuropathic pain, with special emphasis on the analgesic role of opioids—part II: moving basic science towards a new pharmacotherapy. Pain Reviews 6:99–131, 1999

McEvoy GK, Snow EK, Kester L, et al: AHFS Drug Information. Bethesda, MD, American Society of Health-System Pharmacists, 2006

Mendell JR, Sahenk Z: Painful sensory neuropathy. N Engl J Med 348:1243–1255, 2003

Olivieri I, Palazzi C, Peruz G, et al: Management issues with elderly onset rheumatoid arthritis: an update. Drugs Aging 22:809–822, 2005

Pilotto A, Franceschi M, Leandro G, et al: NSAID and aspirin use by the elderly in general practice. Drugs Aging 20:701–710, 2003

Poulsen L, Arendt-Nielsen L, Brosen K, et al: The hypoalgesic effect of tramadol in relation to CYP2D6. Clin Pharmacol Ther 60:636–644, 1996

Poulsen L, Riishede L, Brosen K, et al: Codeine in postoperative pain. Study of the influence of sparteine phenotype and serum concentrations of morphine and morphine-6-glucuronide. Eur J Clin Pharmacol 54:451–454, 1998

Rowbotham MC, Twilling L, Davies PS, et al: Oral opioid therapy for chronic peripheral and central neuropathic pain. N Engl J Med 348:1223–1232, 2003

Rowbotham MC, Goli V, Kunz NR, et al: Venlafaxine extended release in the treatment of painful diabetic neuropathy: a double-blind, placebo-controlled study. Pain 110:697–706, 2004

Sabatowski R, Galvez R, Cherry DA, et al: Pregabalin reduces pain and improves sleep and mood disturbances in patients with post-herpetic neuralgia: results of a randomised, placebo-controlled trial. Pain 109:26–35, 2004

Sarzi-Puttini P, Cimmino MA, Scarpa R, et al: Osteoarthritis: an overview of the disease and its treatment strategies. Semin Arthritis Rheum 35 (suppl 1):1–10, 2005

Sauaia A, Min S-J, Leber C, et al: Postoperative pain management in elderly patients: correlation between adherence to treatment guidelines and patient satisfaction. J Am Geriatr Soc 53:274–282, 2005

Semla TP, Beizer JL, Higbee MD: Geriatric Dosage Handbook, 11th Edition. Hudson, OH, Lexi-Comp, 2006

Slatkin N, Rhiner M: Treatment of opioid-induced delirium with acetylcholinesterase inhibitors: a case report. J Pain Symptom Manage 27:268–273, 2004

Slatkin NE, Rhiner M, Bolton TM: Donepezil in the treatment of opioid-induced sedation: report of six cases. J Pain Symptom Manage 21:425–438, 2001

Turner-Stokes L, Erkeller-Yuksel FE, Miles A, et al: Outpatient cognitive behavioral pain management programs: a randomized comparison of a group-based multidisciplinary versus an individual therapy model. Arch Phys Med Rehabil 84:781–788, 2003

Waldman SD: Atlas of Common Pain Syndromes. Philadelphia, PA, WB Saunders, 2002

Webster L, Andrews M, Stoddard G: Modafinil treatment of opioid-induced sedation. Pain Med 4:135–140, 2003

White WT, Patel N, Drass M, et al: Lidocaine patch 5% with systemic analgesics such as gabapentin: a rational polypharmacy approach for the treatment of chronic pain. Pain Med 4:321–330, 2003

Wiffen P, Collins S, McQuay H, et al: Anticonvulsant drugs for acute and chronic pain (review). The Cochrane Database of Systematic Reviews, Issue 2, Article No: CD001133. DOI: 001110.001002/14651858.CD14001133.pub14651852, 2005

Generic name	acetaminophen
Trade name	Tylenol and others
Class	Antipyretic/Analgesic
Half-life	1–3 hours (may be longer in elderly)
Mechanism of action	Inhibits synthesis of prostaglandins centrally, blocks pain impulse generation peripherally, inhibits hypothalamic heat-regulating center
Available preparations	See Table 10–3
Starting dose	325 mg every 6 hours
Titration	As needed and tolerated to maximum daily dose of 4 g
Typical daily dose	650 mg every 6 hours
Dose range	325–1,000 mg every 6 hours
Therapeutic serum level	Not established

Comments: First-line analgesic in the elderly. Absorption is incomplete and varies by dosage form. Absorption delayed by food. Onset of action in < 1 hour. Time to peak levels is 10–60 minutes. Duration of action is 4–6 hours. Metabolized in the liver to sulfide and glucuronide metabolites; small amount metabolized by microsomal oxidases to the highly reactive intermediate *N*-acetyl-imidoquinone, which is conjugated and inactivated by glutathione. At acetaminophen doses > 4 g/day, glutathione is depleted and the toxic intermediate accumulates; this is thought to cause hepatic cell necrosis. Glutathione may be depleted at doses < 4 g/day in alcoholic and fasting patients. Eliminated in urine, mostly as metabolites. *Drug interactions:* See Table 10–6. *Adverse effects:* Rash, laboratory abnormalities (increased chloride, uric acid, glucose, bilirubin, alkaline phosphatase, and ammonia; decreased sodium, bicarbonate, and calcium), blood dyscrasias, nephropathy, nephrotoxicity with chronic overdose, and hepatotoxicity.

Generic name	aspirin (acetylsalicylic acid)
Trade name	(various)
Class	Salicylate
Half-life	6–12 hours (dose-dependent)
Mechanism of action	Inhibits prostaglandin synthesis, acts on hypothalamic heat-regulating center, blocks prostaglandin synthetase to prevent formation of thromboxane A_2 (platelet aggregating substance)
Available preparations	See Table 10–3
Starting dose	325 mg every 6 hours
Titration	As needed and tolerated
Typical daily dose	650 mg every 6 hours for analgesia
Dose range	325–1,000 mg every 6 hours
Therapeutic serum level	About 100 µg/mL for analgesia, antipyresis, antiplatelet effects; 150–300 µg/mL for anti-inflammatory effect

Comments: Used for a variety of indications beyond analgesia in the geriatric population. Absorbed from the stomach and small intestine. Taken with food or milk to minimize GI distress. Distributed readily into most body fluids and tissues. Time to peak plasma concentration 1–2 hours. More than 90% protein bound at therapeutic concentrations. Metabolized by hepatic microsomal enzymes. Discontinue if tinnitus, dizziness, or impaired hearing develop. High incidence of GI adverse effects. Can compromise renal function, especially at low baseline creatinine clearance (<30 mL/min). Use with caution in patients with platelet or bleeding disorders, renal dysfunction, hepatic disease, peptic ulcer disease, dehydration, vitamin K deficiency, and asthma and other certain conditions. *Drug interactions:* See Table 10–6. *Adverse effects:* Bleeding, acidosis, hypernatremia with buffered forms, GI ulceration, tinnitus, hearing loss, rhabdomyolysis, renal failure, hepatotoxicity, and others. In general, adverse effects other than GI bleeding are uncommon with low doses and serum levels. Misoprostol and proton pump inhibitors may help prevent drug-induced ulceration.

Generic name	celecoxib
Trade name	Celebrex
Class	COX-2-selective NSAID
Half-life	11 hours
Mechanism of action	Inhibits cyclooxygenase-2, resulting in decreased formation of prostaglandin precursors
Available preparations	See Table 10–3
Starting dose	100 mg bid
Titration	Not needed except for certain indications, such as rheumatoid arthritis
Typical daily dose	100 mg bid
Dose range	100–200 mg bid
Therapeutic serum level	Not established

Comments: Other COX-2-selective drugs have been withdrawn from the market because of concern regarding increased cardiovascular risks. Time to peak is 3 hours. Delayed peak levels and increased concentration when taken with high-fat foods. 97% protein bound. Metabolized in the liver to inactive metabolites, which are eliminated in urine. *Drug interactions:* See Table 10–6. *Adverse effects:* Headache, peripheral edema, insomnia, dizziness, rash, dyspepsia, diarrhea, abdominal pain, nausea, flatulence, back pain, upper respiratory tract infection, and sinusitis. Numerous serious but uncommon adverse effects.

Generic name	codeine
Trade name	(generic)
Class	Opioid analgesic (weak)
Half-life	3–4 hours
Mechanism of action	Binds to opioid receptors in the central nervous system
Available preparations	See Table 10–2
Equianalgesic dose	200 mg oral codeine = 10 mg iv morphine
Starting dose	15 mg every 4–6 hours
Titration	As needed and tolerated
Typical daily dose	30 mg every 6 hours
Dose range	15–120 mg every 4–6 hours
Therapeutic serum level	Not established

Comments: A first-line opioid for analgesia in elderly patients. Adequately absorbed orally. Onset of action in 30–60 minutes; peak action in 60–90 minutes. Duration 4–6 hours (may be more in elderly). 7% protein bound. Given as a prodrug; metabolized in the liver via CYP2D6 to morphine (the active drug). Excreted in urine. Drug interactions: See Table 10–6. Adverse effects: Drowsiness, constipation, tachycardia, bradycardia, hypotension, dizziness, light-headedness, confusion, delirium, dry mouth, nausea, vomiting, increased transaminases, decreased urination, weakness, blurred vision, dyspnea, dependence, and seizures.

Generic name	fentanyl
Trade name	Actiq, Duragesic, Sublimaze
Class	Opioid analgesic (potent)
Half-life	Transmucosal: 6.6 hours (range 5–15 hours) Transdermal: 17 hours Injection: 2–4 hours
Mechanism of action	Binds many CNS receptors to increase pain threshold, alter pain reception, and inhibit ascending pain pathways
Available preparations	See Table 10–2
Equianalgesic dose	0.1 mg iv fentanyl = 10 mg iv morphine
Starting dose	Transmucosal: 200-µg lozenge iv: 50 µg
Titration	N/A (used prn)
Typical daily dose	Transmucosal: 200-µg lozenge prn (not earlier than 15 minutes after last lozenge dose completed; not to exceed four doses within 24 hours) iv: 50–100 µg every 2 hours prn
Dose range	N/A
Therapeutic serum level	Not established

Comments: May be a drug of choice for elderly patients when used only inter-mittently for breakthrough pain; when used continuously (e.g., transdermal patch), drug accumulation limits use. Rapidly absorbed from buccal mucosa (25%) and in GI tract when swallowed with saliva (75%). Highly lipophilic drug, with extensive distribution to fat stores and brain, and drug accumula-tion with repeated dosing. Metabolized in the liver, primarily via CYP3A4. Eliminated in urine, mostly as metabolites. Pharmacokinetics of transdermal system not known for elderly patients. Lozenges should only be used in patients already tolerant to opioids. Care should be taken to avoid overdose when lozenges are used in combination with other opioids. *Drug interactions:* See Table 10–6. *Common adverse effects (>10%):* Hypotension, bradycardia, res-piratory depression, CNS depression, confusion, drowsiness, sedation, nausea, vomiting, constipation, dry mouth, weakness, and diaphoresis. Many other less common adverse effects, some serious.

Generic name	gabapentin
Trade name	Neurontin (generic available)
Class	Anticonvulsant structurally related to γ-aminobutyric acid (GABA)
Half-life	5–7 hours
Mechanism of action	Unknown; no direct GABA-mimetic action
Available preparations	Tablets: 100, 300, 400, 600, 800 mg Capsules: 100, 300, 400 mg Oral solution: 250 mg/5 mL
Starting dose	100 mg tid
Titration	Increase by 100 mg tid as often as every 24 hours (as tolerated)
Typical daily dose	2,400 mg (divided tid)
Dose range	1,600–3,600 mg/day (divided tid to qid)
Therapeutic serum level	Not established

Comments: A first-line drug for treatment of neuropathic pain in elderly patients. 50%–60% absorbed from proximal small bowel via L-amino transport system. Reduced bioavailability at higher doses because of saturable absorption. Less than 3% protein bound. Not metabolized; excreted in urine as unchanged drug. Clearance declines with age. Dosage adjustment required for renal failure; administered after hemodialysis. Avoid abrupt withdrawal upon discontinuation (seizure risk). *Drug interactions:* Additive effects with other CNS depressants. *Relatively common adverse effects:* Somnolence, dizziness, ataxia, fatigue, peripheral edema, diarrhea, tremor, weakness, nystagmus, and diplopia. Induction of rapid cycling reported in some patients with bipolar disorder. At high doses, asterixis and encephalopathy reported. *Uncommon but serious adverse effect:* Acute renal failure.

Generic name	hydrocodone/acetaminophen
Trade name	Vicodin, Lortab, others (generic available)
Class	Opioid-nonopioid analgesic combination
Half-life	3.8 hours
Mechanism of action	Binds to μ and κ opioid receptors to block pain perception
Available preparations	See Table 10–2
Starting dose	2.5 mg hydrocodone every 6 hours
Titration	As needed and tolerated
Typical daily dose	5 mg hydrocodone every 6 hours
Dose range	2.5–5 mg hydrocodone every 4–8 hours (not to exceed 4 g/day acetaminophen)
Therapeutic serum level	Not established

Comments: A first-line drug for analgesia in elderly patients. Onset of analgesia in 10–20 minutes, duration 3–6 hours. Administered as a prodrug; metabolized in the liver via CYP2D6 and 3A4 and eliminated in urine. Carries same warnings regarding hepatotoxicity as acetaminophen. *Drug interactions:* See Table 10–6. *Adverse effects:* Bradycardia, hypotension, respiratory depression, cardiac arrest, circulatory collapse, dizziness, drowsiness, mood changes, light-headedness, cognitive impairment, hypoglycemia, constipation, nausea, vomiting, urinary retention, blood dyscrasias, hepatitis, hepatic necrosis, and nephrotoxicity.

Generic name	hydromorphone
Trade name	Dilaudid (generic available)
Class	High-potency opioid analgesic
Half-life	2–4 hours
Mechanism of action	Binds to opioid receptors in CNS, inhibiting ascending pain pathways and altering perception and response to pain
Available preparations	See Table 10–2
Equianalgesic dose	1.5 mg iv hydromorphone = 7.5 mg oral hydromorphone = 10 mg iv morphine
Starting dose	Oral: 1 mg every 6 hours iv: 0.5 mg every 6 hours
Titration	As needed and tolerated
Typical daily dose	Oral: 1 mg every 6 hours iv: 0.5 mg every 6 hours
Dose range	Oral: 0.5–2 mg every 4–6 hours iv: 0.25–1 mg every 4–6 hours
Therapeutic serum level	Not established

Comments: A first-line opioid for analgesia in elderly patients. Onset of analgesia with iv use < 5 minutes; oral, 15–30 minutes. Peak effect with oral use, 30–60 minutes. Bioavailability 62%. Duration of analgesia 4–6 hours. About 20% protein bound. Metabolized in the liver via glucuronidation to inactive metabolites, which are renally excreted. *Drug interactions:* See Table 10–6. *Adverse effects:* Hypotension, peripheral vasodilation, tachycardia, bradycardia, respiratory depression, dizziness, light-headedness, restlessness, hallucinations, seizures, urticaria, antidiuretic hormone release, nausea, vomiting, constipation, dry mouth, biliary tract and ureteral spasm, increased transaminases, trembling, weakness, myoclonus, and others.

Generic name	ibuprofen
Trade name	Motrin, Advil, others
Class	Nonsteroidal anti-inflammatory drug
Half-life	2–4 hours
Mechanism of action	Inhibits prostaglandin synthesis by decreasing activity of cyclooxygenase
Available preparations	See Table 10–3
Starting dose	Analgesia: 200 mg every 4–6 hours prn Inflammatory disease (e.g., osteoarthritis): 400 mg tid
Titration	As needed and tolerated
Typical daily dose	Analgesia: 200 mg every 4 hours prn Inflammatory disease: 400 mg tid
Dose range	Analgesia: up to 400 mg every 4–6 hours prn (not to exceed 1.2 g/day) Inflammatory disease: up to 800 mg tid
Therapeutic serum level	Not established

Comments: A first-line analgesic for elderly patients. Onset of analgesia in 30–60 minutes; duration, 4–6 hours. Anti-inflammatory effects take up to 1 week and peak at 1–2 weeks. Rapidly absorbed orally. 90%–99% protein bound. Metabolized in the liver via oxidation to two inactive metabolites. Excreted in urine and feces. *Drug interactions:* See Table 10–6. Relatively common adverse effects include dizziness, rash, heartburn, nausea, epigastric pain, and tinnitus. *Uncommon but serious adverse effects (<1%):* Acute renal failure, GI ulceration, GI bleeding, bone marrow suppression, and blood dyscrasias.

Generic name	lidocaine patch
Trade name	Lidoderm
Class	Local anesthetic
Half-life	Unknown
Mechanism of action	Inhibits ionic fluxes required for nerve conduction; acts to stabilize neuronal membranes
Available preparations	10 x 14-cm patch
Starting dose	1–3 patches over affected area of intact skin
Titration	N/A
Typical daily dose	1–3 patches over affected area of intact skin for 12 hours out of any 24-hour period
Dose range	As above
Therapeutic serum level	N/A

Comments: May be useful for neuropathic pain syndromes such as postherpetic neuralgia as an adjunct to usual therapy (see text). Patch is applied over an affected area of intact skin and maintained in place for 12 hours in any 24-hour period. Up to three patches may be applied in tandem to cover a larger area. Absorption of lidocaine dose is 1%–5%. Serum levels achieved are one-tenth those required for treatment of cardiac arrhythmias. It is not known if lidocaine is metabolized in the skin. *Drug interactions:* Not expected, but caution is urged if used in combination with other Class I antiarrhythmic drugs. *Adverse effects:* Eye irritation with eye exposure, increased absorption if applied over nonintact skin.

Generic name	morphine
Trade name	Avinza, Kadian, Roxanol, and others (generics available)
Class	High-potency opioid analgesic
Half-life	2–4 hours (immediate-release [IR] forms)
Mechanism of action	Binds to opioid receptors in CNS, inhibiting ascending pain pathways and altering perception of and response to pain
Available preparations	See Table 10–2
Starting dose	Oral: 5–10 mg every 4–6 hours (plus prn every 2 hours for breakthrough pain) iv: 1–2 mg every 4 hours (plus prn every 2 hours)
Titration	As needed and tolerated
Typical daily dose	Oral: 5–10 mg every 4–6 hours (plus prn every 2 hours) iv: 2–5 mg every 4 hours (plus prn every 2 hours)
Dose range	No ceiling dose
Therapeutic serum level	Not established

Comments: A first-line opioid for analgesia in elderly patients. Variable oral absorption; increased with food (especially a high-fat meal). Hydrophilic, so volume of distributed drug is relatively decreased in elderly patients. Metabolized in the liver via glucuronidation to form the active metabolite M6G, which is 50 times more potent than parent compound. 6%–10% excreted unchanged in urine. *Drug interactions:* See Table 10–6. *Common adverse effects (>10%):* Hypotension, bradycardia, drowsiness, dizziness, confusion, pruritus, nausea, vomiting, constipation, dry mouth, urinary retention, and weakness. *Less common but serious adverse effects:* Respiratory depression, hallucinations, and muscle rigidity.

Generic name	naproxen
Trade name	Aleve, Naprosyn, others (generic available)
Class	Nonsteroidal anti-inflammatory drug
Half-life	12–17 hours
Mechanism of action	Inhibits prostaglandin synthesis by decreasing activity of cyclooxygenase
Available preparations	See Table 10–3
Starting dose	200 mg every 12 hours
Titration	Slowly, as needed and tolerated
Typical daily dose	200 mg every 12 hours
Dose range	Up to 600 mg in 24 hours
Therapeutic serum level	Not established

Comments: A first-line analgesic only for short-term use in elderly patients. Onset of analgesia in 1 hour; duration 7 hours. Onset of anti-inflammatory effects takes up to 2 weeks, with peak effects in 2–4 weeks. Completely absorbed orally. More than 99% protein bound. Metabolized in the liver. *Drug interactions:* See Table 10–6. *Adverse effects:* Edema, dizziness, drowsiness, headache, pruritis, rash, constipation, nausea, abnormal renal function, hemolysis, ecchymosis, increased bleeding time, increased liver function test values, tinnitus, and dyspnea. As with other NSAIDs, uncommon but serious adverse effects include renal failure, blood dyscrasias, and blood pressure changes.

Generic name	oxycodone
Trade name	OxyContin, OxyIR, others (generic available)
Class	Opioid analgesic
Half-life	IR: 3.2 hours Controlled-release (CR): 4.5 hours (may be longer in elderly)
Mechanism of action	Binds to opioid receptors in CNS, inhibiting ascending pain pathways and altering perception of and response to pain
Available preparations	See Table 10–2
Starting dose	IR: 2.5–5 mg every 6 hours CR: 10 mg every 12 hours
Titration	As needed and tolerated
Typical daily dose	20 mg of CR every 12 hours and 5 mg of IR every 4 hours; prn for breakthrough pain
Dose range	No ceiling dose
Therapeutic serum level	Not established

Comments: A first-line opioid for analgesia in elderly patients. Analgesia reached within 10–15 minutes; peak at 30–60 minutes; duration 4–5 hours (IR) and 12 hours (CR). Metabolized in the liver; substrate of CYP2D6. Eliminated in urine. *Drug interactions:* See Table 10–6. *Common adverse effects (>10%):* Fatigue, drowsiness, dizziness, somnolence, pruritus, vomiting, constipation, and weakness. *Less common adverse effects (1%–10%):* Orthostasis, restlessness, malaise, confusion, anorexia, stomach cramps, gastritis, dry mouth, biliary spasm, decreased urination, dyspnea, hiccups, and diaphoresis. *Uncommon but serious adverse effects:* syndrome of inappropriate antidiuretic hormone, urinary retention, and death due to overdose from crushing CR tablets.

Generic name	oxymorphone
Trade name	Numorphan
Class	Opioid
Half-life	2 hours
Mechanism of action	Binds to opioid receptors in CNS, inhibiting ascending pain pathways and altering perception and response to pain
Available preparations	See Table 10–2
Starting dose	iv: 0.5 mg every 4–6 hours (plus prn every 2 hours) pr: 5 mg every 4–6 hours
Titration	As needed and tolerated
Typical daily dose	iv: 1 mg every 4–6 hours (plus prn every 2 hours) pr: 5 mg every 4–6 hours
Dose range	No ceiling dose
Therapeutic serum level	Not established

Comments: A first-line opioid for analgesia in elderly patients. Onset of analgesia with intravenous use within 5 minutes; onset within 15–30 minutes with rectal administration. Duration of analgesia is 3–4 hours (may be longer in elderly). Metabolized by conjugation in the liver; excreted in urine. *Drug interactions:* See Table 10–6. *Common adverse effects:* Hypotension, fatigue, drowsiness, dizziness, nausea, vomiting, constipation, weakness, and histamine release. *Less common adverse effects:* Dyspnea, dry mouth, and biliary and ureteral spasm.

Generic name	pregabalin
Trade name	Lyrica
Class	Anticonvulsant
Half-life	4.6–6.8 hours
Mechanism of action	Binds to the α_2-δ protein subunit of voltage-gated calcium channels and reduces excitatory neurotransmitter release
Available preparations	Capsules: 25, 50, 75, 100, 150, 200, 225, 300 mg
Starting dose	150 mg/day (divided bid or tid)
Titration	As tolerated over 1 week to 300 mg/day (divided bid or tid)
Typical daily dose	150 mg bid
Dose range	150–300 mg/day (divided bid or tid)
Therapeutic serum level	Not established for pain

Comments: A first-line drug for treatment of postherpetic neuralgia and diabetic neuropathic pain. Rapidly absorbed orally; 1.3 hours to peak concentration. Bioavailability 90%. Not substantially metabolized. Renally excreted 98% as unchanged drug. Clearance directly proportional to creatinine clearance, so dose adjustment needed in renal impairment. Hemodialyzed; supplement should be administered after each dialysis session. *Common adverse effects:* Dizziness, somnolence, peripheral edema, headache, dry mouth, and diarrhea.

Generic name	tramadol, tramadol ER, tramadol/acetaminophen
Trade name	Ultram (generic available), Ultram ER, Ultracet
Class	Opioid
Half-life	6 hours (metabolite, 7 hours); longer in elderly
Mechanism of action	Binds to μ opioid receptors in CNS, causing inhibition of ascending pain pathways, altering perception of and response to pain. Also inhibits reuptake of serotonin and norepinephrine.
Available preparations	See Table 10–2
Dose	Tramadol: 50 mg tid Tramadol/acetaminophen: 2 tablets every 4–6 hours
Titration	Tramadol: increase by 50 mg every week to target dose
Ceiling dose parameters	Tramadol not to exceed 400 mg/day (300 mg for patients >75 years of age) Tramadol/acetaminophen not to exceed 8 tablets/24 hours (use not to exceed 5 days)
Therapeutic serum level	Not established

Comments: A first-line opioid for analgesia in elderly patients. Rapidly and completely absorbed. Bioavailability 75%. 20% protein bound. Given as prodrug and metabolized extensively in the liver, in part via CYP2D6 to active drug. Eliminated in urine. *Drug interactions:* See Table 10–6. *Common adverse effects (>10%):* Dizziness, headache, somnolence, vertigo, constipation, and nausea. *Less common adverse effects (1%–10%):* Vasodilation, agitation, confusion, impaired coordination, hallucinations, tremor, rash, anorexia, diarrhea, dry mouth, urinary retention, hypertonia, and visual disturbance. *Uncommon but serious adverse effects:* Serotonin syndrome with other serotonergic medications, dyspnea, renal insufficiency, and GI bleeding. See also acetaminophen adverse effects.

Index

*Page numbers printed in **boldface** type refer to tables or figures.*

serum levels of, 132
summary of, 132
Fluphenazine decanoate, 71, 76
dosage of, 76
switching from oral drug to, 82
Flurazepam, 53
Beers criteria for potentially
inappropriate use of, 13
contraindicated for geriatric
patients, 333, 345
half-life of, 336
metabolic pathways for, 333
pharmacokinetics of, 336
Flurbiprofen, 621
Flushing
in neuroleptic malignant syndrome,
500
pain and, 609
Flutamide, 48
Fluvastatin, 37, 41, 44
Fluvoxamine
Beers criteria for potentially
inappropriate use of, 21
drug interactions with, 154
benzodiazepines, 340, 341
clozapine, 67
cytochrome P450 metabolism
and, 36, 37, 38, 41, 45,
145, 148, 154
lithium, 270
methadone, 159, 471
olanzapine, 68, 158
ramelteon, 342, 398
warfarin, 156, 193
mechanism of action of, 151
receptor binding profile of, 152

serotonin syndrome and, 199, 200
withdrawal syndrome with, 181
Folate, 6
during alcohol withdrawal, 425
to lower homocysteine levels, 411
for periodic limb movements of
sleep, 376
Folliculitis, lithium exacerbation of, 295
Food interactions
with clozapine, 68
cytochrome P450 metabolism and, 42
with ethanol, 407
with levodopa/carbidopa, 493, 535
with lithium, 268
with monoamine oxidase inhibitors,
155, 162, 186, 202
with olanzapine, 68
with selegiline, 606
Formamide, 37
"Foxy methoxy" (5-methoxy-N,N-
diisopropyltryptamine), 200
Fractures
rib, 649
vertebral compression, 646
Frontotemporal dementia (FTD), 486,
543, 570
age at onset of, 570
diagnostic criteria for, 571
treatment of, 570
FTA-ABS (fluorescent treponemal
antibody absorption) test, 549
FTD. See Frontotemporal dementia
Furafylline, 41
Furosemide
interaction with celecoxib, 623
UGT metabolism and, 48

consultation for, 1
factors affecting drug choice, 4
genetic heterogeneity and, 27
improving treatment adherence, 8–12
maximizing therapeutic effects,
2–8
accurate diagnosis, 2
adequate drug trial, 4
drug level monitoring, 4
proven treatments, 2–4, **5–7**
minimizing adverse effects and drug
interactions, 12–24
Beers criteria for potentially
inappropriate medication
use, **13–22**
between-dose fluctuation of
drug levels, 12
dosage adjustments, 12
early detection of adverse effects,
23–24
polypharmacy, 1, 2, 12, 23
nonpharmacologic therapies and, 2
pharmacodynamics and aging, 53
pharmacokinetics and aging, 27,
28–53 (*See also*
Pharmacokinetics)
prn medications, 8
screening procedures for, 2, **3**
summary guidelines for, **23**
treatment plan for, 8, 10
Gestodene, **41**
GFR (glomerular filtration rate), 51, 145
GGT (γ-glutamyltransferase), alcohol
use and, 410–411
GHB (γ-hydroxybutyrate), laboratory
screening for, 406

Ginkgo biloba
for Alzheimer's disease, 558–560, 565
interaction with selective serotonin
reuptake inhibitors, **158**
in mild cognitive impairment, 574
Glasgow Coma Scale, 353
Glaucoma, psychotropic drug use in
patients with
anticholinergic drugs, 188
antidepressants, **166**, 188
antipsychotics, **75**, 88
biperiden, 524
desipramine, 240
dextroamphetamine, 241
diphenhydramine, 531
levodopa/carbidopa, 535
procyclidine, 538
trihexyphenidyl, 541
Glimepiride, **37**
Glipizide, **37**, 44
Glitazones, **41**
Glomerular filtration rate (GFR), 51,
145
Glucose-6-phosphate dehydrogenase
(G6PD) deficiency, use of aspirin
in, 636
Glucose dysregulation, drug-induced
antipsychotics, 74, 85, 96, **97**,
101–102
clozapine, 131
lithium, 291, 296
monitoring for, **100**
nortriptyline, 250
olanzapine, 135
quetiapine, 137
risperidone, 139

The following contributor to this book has indicated a financial interest in or other affiliation with a commercial supporter, a manufacturer of a commercial product, a provider of a commercial service, a nongovernmental organization, and/or a government agency, as listed below:

Ronald W. Pies, M.D.   Stipends for occasional lectures, writing, or conference participation from Alkermes, Cephalon, Glaxo-Smith-Kline, and other pharmaceutical companies. *Grant Support:* May 2001–June 2006—Part-time consulting work for Fusion Medical Education. Occasional unrestricted grant support for writing projects from several pharmaceutical companies, including Alkermes, Cephalon, and Glaxo-Smith-Kline. Dr. Pies currently remains an unpaid psychiatric consultant to Fusion Medical Education and has no formal ties to named client companies. He does not otherwise receive direct funding from any pharmaceutical or related corporate entity on a regular basis.